HANDBOOK OF
Clinical
Hypnosis

SECOND EDITION

HANDBOOK OF
Clinical
Hypnosis

SECOND EDITION

EDITED BY

Steven Jay Lynn
Judith W. Rhue
Irving Kirsch

AMERICAN PSYCHOLOGICAL ASSOCIATION
WASHINGTON, DC

Second Printing: April 2014

Published by
American Psychological Association
750 First Street, NE
Washington, DC 20002
www.apa.org

To order
APA Order Department
P.O. Box 92984
Washington, DC 20090-2984
Tel: (800) 374-2721; Direct: (202) 336-5510
Fax: (202) 336-5502; TDD/TTY: (202) 336-6123
Online: www.apa.org/books/
E-mail: order@apa.org

In the U.K., Europe, Africa, and the Middle East, copies may be ordered from
American Psychological Association
3 Henrietta Street
Covent Garden, London
WC2E 8LU England

Typeset in Goudy by Circle Graphics, Columbia, MD.

Printer: Edwards Brothers, Inc., Ann Arbor, MI
Cover Designer: Berg Design, Albany, NY

The opinions and statements published are the responsibility of the authors, and such opinions and statements do not necessarily represent the policies of the American Psychological Association.

Library of Congress Cataloging-in-Publication Data

Handbook of clinical hypnosis / edited by Steven Jay Lynn, Judith W. Rhue, and Irving Kirsch. — 2nd ed.
      p. cm.
  Includes bibliographical references and index.
  ISBN-13: 978-1-4338-0568-4 (alk. paper)
  ISBN-10: 1-4338-0568-5 (alk. paper)
1. Hypnotism—Therapeutic use. I. Lynn, Steven J. II. Rhue, Judith W. III. Kirsch, Irving, 1943-

  RC495.H356 2010
  615.8'512—dc22

                                    2009029008

British Library Cataloguing-in-Publication Data

A CIP record is available from the British Library.

Printed in the United States of America
Second Edition

To my beloved grandchildren, Kelly and Tyler, the future
—*Steven Jay Lynn*

To the beautiful Alexandra, the handsome Grant,
and the ever swift Steven
—*Judith W. Rhue*

In memory of my brother Sol
—*Irving Kirsch*

CONTENTS

CONTRIBUTORS

Elgan L. Baker, Meridian Psychological Associations, Indianapolis, IN

Sean M. Barnes, Binghamton University, Binghamton, NY

Amanda J. Barnier, Macquarie University, Sydney, Australia

Peter B. Bloom, University of Pennsylvania School of Medicine, Philadelphia

Antonio Capafons, University of Valencia, Valencia, Spain

Etzel Cardeña, Lund University, Lund, Sweden

John F. Chaves, State University of New York at Stoneybrook

Alison S. Cole, Binghamton University, Binghamton, NY

Gep Colletti, Binghamton University, Binghamton, NY

James R. Council, North Dakota State University, Fargo

Nicholas A. Covino, Massachusetts School of Professional Psychology, Boston

Daniel David, Babes-Bolyai University, Cluj-Napoca, Romania

Amanda Deming, Binghamton University, Binghamton, NY

Marlene R. Eisen, private practice, Evanston, IL

Salomao Faintuch, Beth Israel Deaconess Medical Center, Boston, MA

Jeffrey D. Gfeller, Saint Louis University, Saint Louis, MO

Don E. Gibbons, independent practice, Ship Bottom, NJ

Donald R. Gorassini, Kings University College, London, Ontario, Canada

Joseph P. Green, The Ohio State University, Lima

Peter W. Halligan, Cardiff University, Cardiff, United Kingdom

Michael N. Hallquist, Western Psychiatric Institute, Pittsburgh, PA

Michael Heap, The University of Sheffield, Sheffield, United Kingdom

Mark P. Jensen, University of Washington, Seattle

Stephen Kahn, private practice, Chicago, IL

Irving Kirsch, University of Hull, Hull, United Kingdom

Stanley Krippner, Saybrook Graduate School, San Francisco, CA

Elvira Lang, Beth Israel Deaconess Medical Center, Boston, MA

Stephen R. Lankton, Editor-in-Chief, *American Journal of Clinical Hypnosis;*
    private practice, Phoenix, AZ

Eleanor Laser, Beth Israel Deaconess Medical Center, Boston, MA

Jean-Roch Laurence, Concordia University, Montreal, Quebec, Canada

Arnold A. Lazarus, The Lazarus Institute, Skillman, NJ

Steven Jay Lynn, Binghamton University, Binghamton, NY

Abigail Matthews, Binghamton University, Binghamton, NY

William J. Matthews, University of Massachusetts, Amherst

Giuliana Mazzoni, University of Hull, Hull, England

David I. Mellinger, Kaiser Permanente Behavioral Health Care,
    Los Angeles, CA

M. Elena Mendoza, University of Valencia, Valencia, Spain

Guy H. Montgomery, Mount Sinai School of Medicine, New York, NY

William P. Morgan, University of Wisconsin, Madison

Michael R. Nash, University of Tennessee, Knoxville

David A. Oakley, University College London, London, United Kingdom

David R. Patterson, University of Washington, Seattle

Cornelia M. Pinnell, Argosy University, Phoenix, AZ

Judith Pintar, University of Illinois at Urbana–Champaign

Judith W. Rhue, Ohio University, Athens

Pamela Sadler, Wilfrid Laurier University, Waterloo, Ontario, Canada

Gloria Maria Martinez Salazar, Beth Israel Deaconess Medical Center,
    Boston, MA

Alan Scoboria, University of Windsor, Windsor, Ontario, Canada

David Spiegel, Stanford University, Stanford, CA

Aaron J. Stegner, University of Wisconsin, Madison

Graham F. Wagstaff, University of Liverpool, Liverpool, United Kingdom

David M. Wark, University of Minnesota, Minneapolis

John C. Williams, Binghamton University, Binghamton, NY

Erik Woody, University of Waterloo, Waterloo, Ontario, Canada

Michael D. Yapko, independent practice, Fallbrook, CA

PREFACE

Fifteen years have passed since the first edition of this handbook was published. During that time, the evidential base supporting the efficacy of hypnosis in the treatment of many conditions has increased substantially (Alladin, Sabatini, & Amundson, 2007; Lynn, Kirsch, Barabasz, Cardeña, & Patterson, 2000). It is not surprising that the most extensive and compelling evidence is for the use of hypnosis to reduce pain. Reviews indicate that 75% of the population can benefit from hypnotic suggestions for pain relief (Montgomery, DuHamel, & Redd, 2000) and that its effectiveness extends to a wide variety of clinical conditions and types of pain (Paterson & Jensen, 2003; see also chap. 21, this volume). Indeed, a recent Cochrane review concluded that hypnosis was the most promising of several psychological procedures assessed for acute pain management in adolescents and children, outperforming distraction and various cognitive–behavioral interventions (Uman, Chambers, McGrath, & Kisely, 2006). Although best established for managing pain, data support the use of hypnosis as an adjunctive procedure in the treatment of a wide variety of conditions, including anxiety disorders, depression, obesity, nausea, and irritable bowel syndrome. Thus, the time seemed right for a new edition, in which more recent research and treatment innovations could be presented, as a sequel to our highly acclaimed first handbook.

As in the first edition, we have endeavored to bring eminent scholars and clinicians together to create a thoroughly up-to-date, authoritative, and comprehensive textbook of clinical hypnosis that represents the gamut of theoretical orientations and clinical applications. As before, our goal is to advance a scientifically rigorous yet compassionate approach to hypnotherapy, with chapters written by those individuals from whom we would like to learn. To reflect recent developments in psychological hypnosis, our virtually encyclopedic treatment of the topic covers new approaches to understanding the cognitive neuroscience of hypnosis, acceptance and mindfulness-based clinical interventions, advances in medical and surgical applications of hypnosis and sport psychology, hypnosis in the popular media, and new developments in treating an array of disorders that touch virtually all aspects of the human experience.

The majority of contributions are organized in a uniform way so as to facilitate comparisons across theories and treatment modalities and to maximize the accessibility of each approach for the reader. With few exceptions, each chapter introduces a particular theory or technique, then discusses clinical applications and clinical material (often case studies), and concludes with an appraisal of relevant research and final comments by the authors.

The handbook is divided into parts that cover general considerations and background knowledge, hypnosis theoretical models, hypnotic methods, specific applications, and contemporary issues. Part I includes chapters relevant to understanding the foundations of clinical hypnosis. Represented here are chapters on the definition of and rationale for using hypnosis; the fascinating history of hypnosis; the what, why, and how of measurement of hypnotizability; and the neurological underpinnings of responding during hypnosis. Part II presents the major modes and models of hypnotherapy, which include psychoanalytic and psychodynamic, dissociation, cognitive–behavioral, Ericksonian, and multimodal approaches. Parts III, IV, and V of the book describe, respectively, a variety of useful hypnotic techniques and strategies for maximizing hypnotic responsiveness, specific interventions that are used in treating a wide variety of psychological disorders ranging from anxiety disorders to dissociative identity disorders, and the application of hypnotic techniques to health and sport psychology. In Part VI, issues germane to popular images of hypnosis in our culture, training, forensic hypnosis, and understanding hypnosis from a cross-cultural perspective are discussed.

Like the first edition, this book is intended for anyone who wishes to learn about clinical hypnosis. It introduces the novice hypnotherapist to the basics of hypnotherapy and the many potential uses of hypnosis. It is thus ideally suited for use as a textbook for graduate and postgraduate courses and workshops. For the trained hypnotherapist, and even the seasoned clinician, this handbook can be used as a reference volume that contains many suggestions for applying techniques and strategies relevant to the nitty-gritty work of the practitioner. Finally, hypnosis researchers and theoreticians will find much of value in this book. We hope that the research summaries and suggestions for future studies contained herein will spur creative investigations at the interface of research and practice for years to come and infuse the artistry of clinical work with insights derived from psychological science.

REFERENCES

Alladin, A., Sabatini, L., & Amundson, J. K. (2007). What should we mean by empirical validation in hypnotherapy: Evidence-based practice in clinical hypnosis. *International Journal of Clinical and Experimental Hypnosis, 55*, 115–131.

Lynn, S. J., Kirsch, I., Barabasz, A., Cardena, E., & Patterson, D. (2000). Hypnosis as an empirically supported adjunctive technique: The state of the evidence. *International Journal of Clinical and Experimental Hypnosis, 48*, 342–361.

Montgomery, G. H., DuHamel, K. N., & Redd, W. H. (2000). A meta-analysis on hypnotically induced analgesia: How effective is hypnosis? *International Journal of Clinical and Experimental Hypnosis, 48*, 138–153.

Patterson, D., & Jensen, M. (2003). Hypnosis and clinical pain. *Psychological Bulletin, 129*, 495–521.

Uman, L. S., Chambers, C. T., McGrath, P. J., & Kisley, S. (2006). Psychological interventions for needle-related procedural pain and distress in children and adolescents. *The Cochrane Database for Systematic Reviews, 4*. doi: 10.1002/14651858.CD005179.pub2

I

FOUNDATIONS AND GENERAL CONSIDERATIONS

1

FOUNDATIONS AND
GENERAL CONSIDERATIONS

1

AN INTRODUCTION TO CLINICAL HYPNOSIS

STEVEN JAY LYNN, IRVING KIRSCH, AND JUDITH W. RHUE

Hypnosis is a word that conjures many associations. There is a certain magic in the ability of mere words to produce profound changes in a person's mood, thoughts, and behaviors. There is a compelling quality to participants' reports of involuntary experiences that often accompany hypnotic behaviors. And there is an almost eerie feeling of surprise and amazement when people who experience hypnosis demonstrate classical hypnotic phenomena such as positive and negative hallucinations, alterations in pain sensitivity, and amnesia on command.

No wonder then, that hypnosis has long been associated with terms such as *mystery*, *mysticism*, and the *supernatural*. Yet, at the same time that the media and stage hypnotists have exploited and advanced these misconceptions of hypnosis (see chap. 27), scientists have placed hypnosis on a firm empirical footing, and clinicians have devised ever more creative ways of serving their clientele with hypnotic stratagems and techniques.

No student of contemporary psychology can ignore the surge of interest in hypnosis in the past few decades. Hypnosis has always captured the attention of some of the most creative thinkers in the field of psychology, including Sigmund Freud, William James, Wilhelm Wundt, Clark Hull, T. X. Barber, and Ernest Hilgard, among others. Today, hypnosis and hypnotic phenomena are studied with state-of-the-science neuroimaging techniques (see chap. 4, this volume), hypnosis research is routinely published in premiere psychology journals, and hypnosis has informed cognitive science (and vice versa) in meaningful ways (Barnier, Dienes, & Mitchell, 2008; Raz et al., 2006; see also chap. 6, this volume). Accordingly, it seems fair to claim that the scientific community has increasingly recognized that hypnosis is a fruitful and legitimate area of scientific inquiry and that hypnosis has moved firmly into the orbit of mainstream psychology.

Clinicians have good reason to familiarize themselves with hypnosis and hypnotic methods. Reviews and meta-analytic studies consistently document the effectiveness or promise of hypnosis in treating a wide variety of psychological and medical conditions, ranging from acute and chronic pain to obesity (e.g., Brown, 2007; Brown & Hammond, 2007; Elkins, Jensen, & Patterson, 2007; Flammer & Alladin, 2007; Flammer & Bongartz, 2003; Flory, Martinez Salazar, & Lang, 2007; Lynn, Kirsch, Barabasz, Cardeña, & Patterson, 2000; Neron & Stephenson, 2007). Furthermore, meta-analyses have shown that hypnosis enhances the effectiveness of both psychodynamic and cognitive–behavioral psychotherapies (Kirsch, 1990; Kirsch, Montgomery, & Sapirstein, 1995).

Although hypnosis is a useful adjunct to many psychotherapeutic approaches, the media and some practitioners often treat hypnotherapy as if it were a particular approach to psychotherapy, on a par with psychoanalysis, client-centered therapy, behavior therapy, and other therapeutic modalities (e.g., Smith, Glass, & Miller, 1980). In the 19th century, hypnotherapy was actually a distinct mode of treatment. Auguste Liebault (1823–1904), for example, offered his patients a choice between traditional medical treatment, for which a standard fee would be charged, and hypnotherapy, which he would administer without charge (Gravitz, 1991). In those days, hypnotherapy consisted of administering a hypnotic induction and suggesting the alleviation of the symptom for which the patient sought relief.

A careful reading of the chapters in this handbook makes it evident that this is no longer the case. Although direct suggestion of symptom relief is still used for some purposes, such as for the treatment of warts (see chap. 22) and pain (see chap, 21), it is the exception rather than the rule. More frequently, the use of hypnosis in contemporary hypnotherapy is embedded within some broader therapeutic approach. Thus, one can speak of psychodynamic hypnotherapy, cognitive–behavioral hypnotherapy, or Ericksonian hypnotherapy, as discussed in the chapters in Part II of this volume.

Just as most psychotherapists identify their orientation as eclectic, hypnotherapy often involves a blending of ideas and techniques from different theoretical perspectives. Many of the chapters in this volume devoted to the treatment of specific presenting problems include elements of psychodynamic and cognitive–behavior theory. Thus, most clinical applications of hypnosis can be referred to as *eclectic hypnotherapy*. As it is practiced today, *hypnotherapy* can be defined as the addition of hypnosis to accepted psychological or medical treatment. As such, it should be practiced only by professionals who have the appropriate training and credentials to provide the treatment that is being augmented by hypnosis.

DEFINING HYPNOSIS

Our definition of hypnotherapy assumes that one knows what is meant by the term *hypnosis*. But what is hypnosis? For more than a century, hypnosis was defined as a special state that is different from normal waking consciousness (American Psychological Association Division of Psychological Hypnosis, 1985; James, 1890). The media continues to popularize this view in movies, television programs, and on the Internet, depicting the hypnotized subject as deeply entranced and highly responsive to all manner of suggestions.

However, the question of whether hypnosis is an altered state of consciousness is today the subject of intense controversy among scientists (Kallio & Revonsuo, 2003). As early as the 1950s, Theodore Sarbin (1950) and, later, T. X. Barber (1969) rejected the idea that hypnotic phenomena were due to an altered state of consciousness unique to hypnosis and instead asserted that these phenomena were the direct byproduct of motivated responses to imaginative suggestions. During the 1960s and 1970s, the altered state issue was the most contentious issue in the field (Sheehan & Perry, 1976). Despite various pronouncements of convergence (e.g., most researchers only use the term *hypnotic state* in a descriptive sense to denote subjective changes that hypnotized persons report experiencing) in the altered state debate (Kirsch & Lynn, 1995; Spanos & Barber, 1974), the controversy has continued (for a review, see Lynn, Kirsch, & Hallquist, 2008). Indeed, contributors to this volume differ in their views of hypnosis as an altered or mundane state of consciousness, as revealed by the fact that some use the term *trance* descriptively to describe what transpires during hypnosis, whereas other contributors studiously avoid this term. Clearly, defining hypnosis as an altered state begs the question. The field needs a theoretically neutral definition that is not inconsistent with any prominent theories.

Fortunately, there is general agreement about the kinds of phenomena that are observed in what has been termed *the domain of hypnosis* (Hilgard, 1973; Kihlstrom, 2008). Many of these fascinating phenomena, such as selective amnesia and diminished perception of pain, are the direct byproducts of suggestions. In keeping with this observation, some years ago, the American

Psychological Association (APA) Division of Psychological Hypnosis (1985) officially adopted the following definition:

> Hypnosis is a procedure during which a health professional or researcher suggests that a client, patient, or subject experience changes in sensations, perceptions, thoughts, or behavior. The hypnotic context is generally established by an induction procedure. Although there are many different hypnotic inductions, most include suggestions for relaxation, calmness, and well-being. Instructions to imagine or think about pleasant experiences are also commonly included in hypnotic inductions.

In actuality, practitioners use a wide variety of inductions that are described in subsequent chapters of this handbook. The reader will encounter inductions that foster a more alert or "waking" experience of hypnosis, in addition to more traditional inductions that emphasize relaxation and altered states of awareness.

Almost two decades after the first definition was crafted, the Executive Committee of the APA Division of Psychological Hypnosis (2004) revised the definition to encompass the widely used clinical technique of self-hypnosis, described as "the act of administering hypnotic procedures on one's own" (p. 13). The reformulated definition also acknowledged that "many believe that hypnotic responses and experiences are characteristic of a hypnotic state. While some think that it is not necessary to use the word 'hypnosis' as part of the hypnotic induction, others view it as essential" (p. 13). The new definition also noted that responsiveness to suggestion can be assessed by standardized scales in clinical and research settings; that scores can be grouped into low, medium, and high categories; and that "the salience of evidence for having achieved hypnosis increases with the individual's score" (p. 13). The definition of hypnosis has proven to be a controversial issue in general (e.g., Fellows, 1995; Hasegawa & Jamieson, 2002; Kallio & Revonsuo, 2003; Spiegel, 1998; Wagstaff, 1998). However, the definitions of hypnosis generated by the APA constitute a mostly theoretically neutral and useful platform for understanding hypnosis and hypnotic phenomena (Lynn & Kirsch, 2006).

Although controversy about whether hypnosis is an altered state of consciousness persists, there is broad agreement among workers in the field that many popular beliefs about hypnosis, no doubt perpetuated by the media, are not in agreement with scientific evidence. In a recent survey of popular beliefs about hypnosis, Green, Page, Rasekhy, Johnson, and Bernhardt (2006) determined that at least 40% of students in the United States endorsed the beliefs that during hypnosis people (a) "give up their free will to the hypnotist" and can be made to do things against their will, (b) are "only aware of what the hypnotist is suggesting and not aware of anything else," (c) can be made to do things they normally would not do, (d) "can be made to tell the truth about things they would normally lie about," and (e) respond based on the skill of the hypnotist. It is of interest to note that students sampled in Australia, Germany, and Iran hold similarly inaccurate beliefs about hypnosis.

Despite pervasive and far-reaching misconceptions about hypnosis, research has played an influential role in demystifying hypnosis. With increasing confidence, clinicians can practice with the assurance that there is an empirical basis to many of their clinical intuitions and the information they share with clients. Research-based information can be incorporated into clinical hypnosis with many clients who, before hypnotic work can begin in earnest, require education that disabuses them of misconceptions about hypnosis that can interfere with a complete response to hypnotic suggestions (Lynn, Kirsch, Neufeld, & Rhue, 1996; Nash, 2001).

Clinicians can now rely on the following empirically derived information to educate their clients and inform their practice:

- The ability to experience hypnotic phenomena does not indicate gullibility or weakness (Barber, 1969).
- Hypnosis is not a sleeplike state (Banyai, 1991).
- Hypnosis depends more on the efforts and abilities of the subject than on the skill of the hypnotist (Barber, 1985; Hilgard, 1965).
- Subjects retain the ability to control their behavior during hypnosis, to refuse to respond to suggestions, and to even oppose suggestions (see Lynn et al., 2008; Lynn, Rhue, & Weekes, 1991).
- Spontaneous amnesia is relatively rare (Simon & Salzberg, 1985); informing clients that they will be able to remember everything that they are comfortable remembering about the session can prevent its unwanted occurrence.
- Suggestions can be responded to with or without hypnosis; the function of a formal induction is primarily to increase suggestibility to a minor degree (see Barber, 1969; Braffman & Kirsch, 1999; Hilgard, 1965).
- Hypnosis is not a dangerous procedure when practiced by qualified clinicians and researchers (see Lynn, Martin, & Frauman, 1996).
- Most hypnotized subjects are neither faking nor merely complying with suggestions (Kirsch, Silva, Carone, Johnston, & Simon, 1989).
- Hypnosis does not increase the accuracy of memory or foster a literal reexperiencing of childhood events (Nash, 1987; see also chap. 29, this volume).

- Direct, traditionally worded hypnotic techniques generally appear to be just as effective as permissive, open-ended, indirect suggestions (Lynn, Neufeld, & Mare, 1993; Robin, Kumar, & Pekala, 2005).
- A wide variety of hypnotic inductions can be effective (e.g., inductions that emphasize alertness can be just as effective as inductions that promote physical relaxation; Banyai, 1991; see also chaps. 10 and 11, this volume).
- Most hypnotized subjects do not describe their experience as "trance" but as focused attention on suggested events (McConkey, 1986).
- Hypnosis is not a reliable means of recovering repressed memories, but it might increase the danger of creating false memories (Lynn, Barnes, & Matthews, 2008; see also chap. 29, this volume).

It is of interest to note that when participants experience hypnosis, it can counter many of their prior, media-derived beliefs about hypnosis. More specifically, Green (2003) discovered that after participants are hypnotized, they are less likely to believe that (a) hypnosis is an altered state of consciousness, (b) the experience of hypnosis depends on the ability of the hypnotist, (c) suggestions are so powerful that they cannot be resisted, (d) hypnotized individuals are not conscious of their surroundings, and (e) hypnosis can make subjects tell the truth about things they normally would lie about.

HYPNOTIC SUGGESTIBILITY

The majority of people can be hypnotized to a moderate degree. In fact, only about 10% to 15% of the population will respond to only a few suggestions, whereas an equal percentage of individuals will respond to the great majority of suggestions they are given. There is a remarkable degree of consistency in suggestibility scores across cultures, as indexed by widely used scales of hypnotic suggestibility. For example, Jacquith, Rhue, Lynn, and Seevaratnam (1996) found that college students tested in Malaysia, Malaysian students who had resided in the United States for an average of 2.5 years, and native-born U.S. college students scored comparably in terms of suggestibility. Zachariae, Jorgensen, and Christensen (2000) determined that Danish students' mean scores were comparable with scores obtained in samples in the United States (Coe, 1964; Shor & Orne, 1963), whereas Lamas, del Valle-Inclan, Blanco, and Diaz (1989) reported that Spanish participants responded comparably with other normative samples, including those obtained in Germany (Bongartz,

1985). Moreover, data collected from three samples of Romanian participants revealed that normative data were consistent with earlier normative data (e.g., score distribution, item difficulty levels, reliability) collected from samples in Australia (Sheehan & McConkey, 1979), Canada, Denmark, Finland, German, Italy, Spain, and the United States (David, Montgomery, & Holdevici, 2003). Similarly, Carvalho, Kirsch, Mazzoni, and Leal (2008) reported normative data for Portuguese students that were congruent with American and Canadian reference samples. Indeed, mean scores on the Harvard Group Scale of Hypnotic Susceptibility range from 6.5 to 7.39 suggestions passed (total suggestions = 12) across Finnish, Spanish, German, and American samples. Mean scores on the Waterloo-Stanford Group C Scale of Hypnotic Susceptibility range from 5.47 to 5.81 across Portuguese, American, and Canadian samples.

Clinically speaking, in many instances, hypnotic suggestibility is not measured prior to treatment (e.g., on the operating table; see chap. 23), and some clinicians clearly view assessment as more integral to hypnotic treatment than others. However, in instances in which high suggestibility is a prerequisite (e.g., a surgical procedure in which hypnosis is used as a sole anesthetic in a person allergic to standard anesthetics), the assessment of hypnotic suggestibility is imperative. High suggestibility is not necessary to respond to many therapeutic suggestions (e.g., relaxation, imagery) at the core of hypnotic treatments. Indeed, there is not a particularly close relation between hypnotic suggestibility and treatment gains. Nevertheless, suggestibility is not completely irrelevant to outcome. In no study reported to date is high hypnotic suggestibility associated with a negative treatment outcome (Lynn & Kirsch, 2006). Moreover, the findings regarding suggestibility and treatment outcome, although not entirely consistent, are at least somewhat promising in the following conditions or disorders: smoking cessation, obesity, warts, anxiety, somatization, conversion disorders, and asthma (Lynn, Shindler, & Meyer, 2004). In chapter 3 of this volume, Barnier and Council examine the issue of the assessment of suggestibility and provide readers with a variety of practical options for evaluating suggestibility in clinical and research contexts.

INDICATIONS AND CONTRAINDICATIONS
FOR THE USE OF HYPNOSIS IN THERAPY

The chapters of this volume demonstrate the wide range of clinical problems to which hypnosis can be applied. These include anxiety disorders, depression, posttraumatic stress, dissociative identity disorder, psychosomatic disorders, pain conditions, eating disorders, and smoking. Indeed, hypnosis can be used in treating virtually any condition for which a psychological intervention is indicated. Notably, each of these clinical problems was ranked highly in terms of the extent to which research on the topic will contribute to knowledge regarding clinical practice by a panel of experts in a survey commissioned by the APA Division of Psychological Hypnosis (Lynn, Matthews, & Stafford, 2008).

There are many reasons for adding hypnotic procedures to treatment plans. The hypnotic situation provides a context that facilitates active and experiential learning (Barber, 1985; see also chap. 15, this volume). Clients can detach from their everyday concerns and focus on therapeutic thoughts, images, and suggestions. Therapists can talk to clients in a deeply personal and meaningful way and can say virtually anything they believe will be beneficial (Barber, 1985, p. 349) while urging clients to transcend entrenched and self-limiting beliefs and long-standing patterns of avoidance. The goal-directed, positive nature of the encounter with the hypnotist may increase clients' rapport with the therapist and enhance the treatment alliance (see chap. 5). For clients with positive attitudes toward hypnosis, the hypnotic context may enhance their confidence in the effectiveness of therapy and thereby produce a placebo effect, without the deception that is generally associated with placebos (Kirsch, 1990; see also chap. 7, this volume).

Moreover, hypnosis is a useful self-control technique in its own right that can promote self-soothing and build personal resources (see chap. 8). Clients can be taught *cue-controlled relaxation* or *anchoring,* as it is sometimes called, whereby they pair an image or verbal cue with a well-practiced or conditioned response to relaxation or other suggested experiences. In many of the chapters in this volume, therapists use soothing images of a safe place, or posthypnotic suggestions and self-hypnosis, to facilitate coping in everyday life, thereby generalizing treatment gains. In a related manner, hypnosis can be used to augment desensitization to fears and provide an optimum level of exposure to anxiety-eliciting stimuli in a gradual, safe, and controlled manner (Lynn, Kirsch, Neufeld, & Rhue, 1996; Schoenberger et al., 1996).

Hypnotic suggestions can also produce changes in perception among hypnotizable clients. An example of the use of this phenomenon is in the administration of suggestions to decrease the intensity of withdrawal symptoms and to increase the aversiveness of tobacco smoke in smoking cessation treatments (see chap. 24). Yet hypnosis is not a panacea. It is simply not effective with all clients, and it should be used only after careful deliberation on the part of the therapist. The use of hypnosis, or any other therapeutic intervention for that matter, should be preceded by an evaluation of the client. At a minimum, this assessment should include information pertinent to the client's mental status, life history, and current psychological problems and dynamics. Important areas of inquiry include the client's treatment motivation, needs, character structure, life situation, beliefs about hypnosis, and perceived strengths and weaknesses.

Delving into the archive of life experiences can be a source of useful suggestions that tap into the client's resources; acquiring knowledge of hypnosis-specific attitudes and expectations can prove invaluable in preparing the client for hypnosis, as described in the next section.

It is essential that the decision to use hypnosis be justified by what is learned in the initial assessment, by the therapist's general theoretical orientation, and by the specific goals and objectives of psychotherapy. Before hypnosis is undertaken, it is imperative that therapists establish a strong therapeutic alliance, know what they wish to accomplish, and have a clear idea about how hypnotic communications can facilitate treatment. In addition, careful planning and preparation of therapeutic communications and suggestions is essential before hypnosis is induced. Ultimately, the pros and cons of hypnosis must be carefully weighed against those of nonhypnotic treatment.

Therapists would do well to examine their motives for using hypnosis (or any other psychotherapy technique) and to monitor their actions and reactions and those of the client. Given these considerations, in our own clinical practice, we do not make the decision to use hypnosis on a casual or cursory basis. Before we induce hypnosis, we routinely ask ourselves a number of questions, the first and foremost of which are: Why use hypnosis at this particular juncture in therapy? What is to be gained? Can hypnosis accelerate treatment? Can it promote generalization of treatment effects? What are the client's motives for requesting hypnotherapy? Is the client's request a test of whether we truly care and will yield to the client's wishes or whims? In contrast, what are our motives? Do we wish to use hypnosis because we feel guilty that we are not doing more for the client? Are we bored or angry with the client and hungering for "a quick fix" in therapy that only hypnosis can provide?

Affirmative answers to the last two questions should lead a therapist to reevaluate the use of hypnosis or to postpone hypnotherapy until these issues are adequately addressed or resolved. For example, clients sometimes request hypnotherapy thinking that hypnosis will do the work for them. Unrealistic expectations of this sort set up both the therapist and client for failure. The client may feel like a failure when yet one more intervention fails to make a difference, and the therapist can be discredited or diminished when a highly touted intervention meets with little success. The client's experience may lead to the despondent conclusion "I tried hypnosis, and even that didn't work!"

We would be equally leery of using hypnosis to bypass the cautions that normally would be considered before abreactive or uncovering work was undertaken. Clients can have intense abreactive reactions during hypnosis, as they can in nonhypnotic contexts. It has been our observation that the hypnotic context may give some clients license to express thoughts and feelings that they ordinarily would not express in psychotherapy. This can be one of the advantages of using hypnosis. But if therapists are not trained or prepared to work with clients who experience abreactions, then they ought to avoid techniques, hypnotic or otherwise, that promote regressive experiences.

It would also be wise for therapists to postpone hypnotherapy or not use hypnosis with borderline or dissociative clients who are not yet stabilized in treatment. Regressive or altered bodily experiences that often accompany hypnosis could well disrupt these clients' psychological equilibrium. As in non-hypnotic treatment, the following questions need to be considered: Is the client's condition sufficiently stabilized to justify treatment that focuses on abreaction or uncovering? Are there conscious or subconscious motivations to resist responsibility for current actions and to affix blame on events or persons from the past? Does the client wish to arrive at a facile understanding of his or her problems by way of viewing his or her present through the lens of a past rife with abuse?

Besides these general concerns, there are questions that relate directly to the establishment of a hypnotic context for doing uncovering work: Does the client view hypnosis as a magic cure, as a royal road to the unconscious, or as a window to the past? Does the client's request for hypnosis to recall past events represent an attempt to control the therapy hour to avoid dealing with issues that trouble him or her in the present? In chapter 10, Gibbons and Lynn present the "nuts and bolts" of administering hypnotic inductions that are meant to introduce the reader to the use of hypnotic techniques. Many issues pertinent to the indications and counterindications of hypnosis and the management of client reactions are discussed in the chapter on the prevention and management of negative effects in hypnotherapy (see chap. 10).

If the clinician decides to proceed with hypnosis, some clients will nevertheless be ambivalent, resistant, or unable to experience hypnotic effects at all. It is, of course, impossible to know precisely how a client will respond to a hypnotic intervention prior to inducing hypnosis itself. Yet, even when hypnosis is not entirely successful, much can be learned about the client. For example, it is possible to better understand clients' resistance or ambivalence to treatment; their creative abilities and comfort with relaxation, imagination, and fantasy; their feelings about the therapist and the therapeutic alliance; and the needs, wishes, and fears that they are projecting onto the therapist and the hypnotic relationship. Whether and how this knowledge can be exploited depend, in part, on the therapist's acumen and the degree to which insight derived from clients' reaction to hypnosis is relevant to the therapist's particular brand of psychotherapy.

Because hypnosis is not a form of psychotherapy, the best guarantee of competent practice is adequate training in the psychotherapy that is used. The limited information we provide is not intended to be a substitute supervised training in the use of hypnotic inductions and the administration of therapeutic suggestions.

SOME WORDS OF CAUTION

Inducing hypnosis is notoriously easy to learn. This has led to a pro-liferation of self-described hypnotherapists who have learned how to induce hypnosis but have not been adequately trained in psychotherapy. In fact, we were somewhat hesitant about providing detailed instructions here. However, this volume is intended for professionals and graduate students and not for a lay audience. Therapists who wish to add hypnosis to their clinical repertoire should learn the standard procedures of hypnotic induction, as described by Gibbons and Lynn in this volume (see chap. 10); a handbook of this sort would be incomplete without this information. In any case, hypnotic induc-tions have also been printed in other professional volumes. Nevertheless, we caution readers against sharing this information with nonprofessionals. Only persons with appropriate training and credentials should practice hypnotherapy.

The chapters in this volume illustrate a wide variety of hypnotic tech-niques. These techniques include, but are not limited to, suggested hypnotic dreams, analgesia, metaphors, and communications couched in indirect language. One technique that is widely used by therapists of diverse persua-sions is age regression. Events that are remembered during hypnosis may seem particularly compelling to both the therapist and client when they are associated with intense affect, reminiscent of childhood displays of emotion. However, memory studies (e.g., Lynn & McConkey, 1998) have challenged the idea that all events are stored with perfect accuracy in memory. A traumatic history, for example, consists not only of past childhood events but also of the person's interpretations, embellishments, and distortions of those events from the perspective of present events, accomplishments, behaviors, and relationships that constitute life in the present. Indeed, the memory literature indicates that ordinary memory is fallible and that certain sub-jects place an inordinate degree of confidence in their remembrances, even to the point of being convinced that events that did not take place actually did occur (Lynn & McConkey, 1998).

Practitioners of hypnosis need to be cognizant that hypnosis does not foster a literal reexperiencing of childhood events, much less of recent events (see chap. 29). Hypnosis is not a key to unlocking the vault of memory. In his exhaustive review of over 100 years of hypnosis research on temporal regression, Nash (1987) failed to find any special correspondence between the behavior and experience of hypnotized adults and that of children. The conclusion he arrived at is that whereas the products of hypnotic age regres-sion are often clinically useful, the client's response cannot be accepted at face value.

The point is that hypnosis in no way obviates the hazards of memory distortion associated with ordinary psychotherapy. In fact, hypnosis may exacerbate memory problems. That is, hypnosis can increase confidence of recalled events with little or no change in the level of accuracy (Lynn, Barnes, & Matthews, 2008; see also chap. 30, this volume). Moreover, high and medium hypnotizable subjects are at particular risk of suggestion-related memory distortions both within and apart from the hypnotic context (Lynn et al., in press). Although there is disagreement in the field and among the authors of this volume about the risk and the role of hypnosis in producing false recollections and eliciting traumatic memories, it is safe to say that there is virtually universal agreement that therapists need to exercise vigilance to avoid inadvertently administering suggestions that produce or legitimize pseudomemories across hypnotic and nonhypnotic contexts. In addition, it seems prudent to evaluate the credibility of purportedly repressed memories uncovered during therapy in light of the client's hypnotic suggestibility and the nature of the procedures used to uncover the remembrances.

It should be obvious by this point that hypnosis is a broad and complex subject, and, that to describe the topic fully in this volume, we have included chapters written by an elite but diverse group of researchers and practitioners who, as we have indicated, do not always agree with one another on vital aspects of clinical hypnosis, such as the need to assess hypnotic suggestibility, what kind of induction techniques are preferable, whether to use traditional or alert–awake suggestions (or both), and the advisability of using hypnosis to recall traumatic events. In addition, researchers and clinicians have disagreed for many years on the question of whether hypnosis produces a unique altered state of consciousness; this dispute is also discussed in this volume. This diversity of opinion reflects the subjective nature of the hypnotic experience for client and clinician alike, as well as the unsettled, continuously evolving field of clinical hypnosis itself. As such, the chapters that follow should be taken to represent their authors' views on these aspects of hypnosis. There is no single "proper" way to practice clinical hypnosis; rather, this handbook will present a comprehensive treatment of the topic, allowing practitioners to make their own decisions about what kinds of hypnotic procedures will work best for their clients.

REFERENCES

American Psychological Association, Division 30. (2004, Winter/Spring). Hypnosis: A definition. *Psychological hypnosis: A bulletin of Division 30*, 13.

American Psychological Association Division of Psychological Hypnosis (1985, August). *A general definition of hypnosis and a statement concerning its application and efficacy* (Report submitted to the Council of Representatives of the American Psychological Association). Washington, DC: Author.

Banyai, E. (1991). Toward a social–psychobiological model of hypnosis. In S. J. Lynn & J. W. Rhue (Eds.), *Theories of hypnosis: Current models and perspectives* (pp. 564–598). New York: Guilford Press.

Barber, T. X. (1969). *Hypnosis: A scientific approach.* New York: Van Nostrand Reinhold.

Barber, T. X. (1985). Hypnosuggestive procedures as catalysts for psychotherapies. In S. J. Lynn & J. P. Garske (Eds.), *Contemporary psychotherapies: Models and methods* (pp. 333–376). Columbus, OH: Merrill.

Barnier, A. J., Dienes, Z., & Mitchell, C. J. (2008). How hypnosis happens: New cognitive theories of hypnotic responding. In M. Nash & A. Barnier (Eds.), *The Oxford handbook of hypnosis: Theory, research, and practice* (pp. 141–178). New York: Oxford University Press.

Bongartz, W. (1985). German norms for the Harvard Group Scale of Hypnotic Susceptibility, Form A. *International Journal of Clinical and Experimental Hypnosis, 33,* 131–140.

Braffman, W., & Kirsch, I. (1999). Imaginative suggestibility and hypnotizability: An empirical analysis. *Journal of Personality and Social Psychology, 77,* 578–587.

Brown, D. (2007). Evidence-based hypnotherapy for asthma: A critical review. *International Journal of Clinical and Experimental Hypnosis, 55,* 220–247.

Brown, D., & Hammond, D. C. (2007). Evidence-based clinical hypnosis for obstetrics, labor and delivery, and preterm labor. *International Journal of Clinical and Experimental Hypnosis, 55,* 355–371.

Carvalho, C., Kirsch, I., Mazzoni, G., & Leal, I. (2008). Portuguese norms for the Waterloo-Stanford Group C (WSGC) Scale of Hypnotic Susceptibility. *International Journal of Clinical and Experimental Hypnosis, 56,* 295–305.

Coe, W. C. (1964). Further norms for the Harvard Group Scale of Hypnotic Susceptibility, Form A. *International Journal of Clinical and Experimental Hypnosis, 12,* 184–190.

Elkins, G., Jensen, M. P., & Patterson, D. R. (2007). Hypnotherapy for the management of chronic pain. *International Journal of Clinical and Experimental Hypnosis, 55,* 275–287.

Fellows, B. J. (1995). Critical issues arising from the APA definition and description of hypnosis. *Contemporary Hypnosis, 12,* 74–81.

Flammer, E., & Alladin, A. (2007). The efficacy of hypnotherapy in the treatment of psychosomatic disorders: Meta-analytical evidence. *International Journal of Clinical and Experimental Hypnosis, 55,* 251–274.

Flammer, E., & Bongartz, W. (2003). On the efficacy of hypnosis: A meta-analytic study. *Contemporary Hypnosis, 20,* 179–197.

Flory, N., Martinez Salazar, G. M., & Lang, E. V. (2007). Hypnosis for acute distress management during medical procedures. *International Journal of Clinical and Experimental Hypnosis, 55,* 303–371.

Gravitz, M. A. (1991). Early theories of hypnosis: A clinical perspective. In S. J. Lynn & J. W. Rhue (Eds.), *Theories of hypnosis: Current models and perspectives* (pp. 19–42). New York: Guilford Press.

Green, J. P. (2003). Beliefs about hypnosis: Popular beliefs, misconceptions, and the importance of experience. *International Journal of Clinical & Experimental Hypnosis, 51*, 369–381.

Green, J. P., Page, R. A., Rasekhy, R., Johnson, L. K., & Bernhardt, S. E. (2006). Cultural views and attitudes about hypnosis: A survey of college students across four countries. *International Journal of Clinical and Experimental Hypnosis, 54*, 263–280.

Hasegawa, H., & Jamieson, G. A. (2002). Conceptual issues in hypnosis research: Explanations, definitions and the state/non-state debate. *Contemporary Hypnosis, 19*, 103–117.

Hilgard, E. R. (1965). *Hypnotic susceptibility*. New York: Harcourt, Brace & World.

Hilgard, E. R. (1973). The domain of hypnosis: With some comments on alternate paradigms. *American Psychologist, 28*, 72–982.

Jacquith, L., Rhue, J., Lynn, S. J., & Seevaratnam, J. (1996). Cross-cultural aspects of hypnotizability and imagination. *Contemporary Hypnosis, 13*, 74–79.

James, W. (1890). *Principles of psychology* (Vols. 1–2). New York: Holt.

Kallio, S., & Revonsuo, A. (2003). Hypnotic phenomena and altered states of consciousness: A multilevel framework of description and explanation. *Contemporary Hypnosis, 20*, 111–164.

Kihlstrom, J. F. (2008). The domain of hypnosis revisited. In M. R. Nash & A. J. Barnier (Eds.), *The Oxford handbook of hypnosis: Theory, research, practice* (pp. 21–52). New York: Oxford University Press.

Kirsch, I. (1990). *Changing expectations: A key to effective psychotherapy*. Pacific Grove, CA: Brooks/Cole.

Kirsch, I., & Lynn, S. J. (1995). The altered state of hypnosis: Changes in the theoretical landscape. *American Psychologist, 50*, 846–858.

Kirsch, I., Montgomery, G., & Sapirstein, G. (1995). Hypnosis as an adjunct to cognitive behavioral psychotherapy: A meta-analysis. *Journal of Consulting and Clinical Psychology, 63*, 214–220.

Kirsch, I., Silva, C. E., Carone, J. E., Johnston, J. D., & Simon, B. (1989). The surreptitious observation design: An experimental paradigm for distinguishing artifact from essence in hypnosis. *Journal of Abnormal Psychology, 98*, 132–136.

Lamas, J. R., del Valle-Inclan, F., Blanco, M. J., & Diaz, A. A. (1989). Spanish norms for the Harvard Group Scale, Form A. *International Journal of Clinical and Experimental Hypnosis, 37*, 264–273.

Lynn, S. J., Barnes, S., & Matthews, A. (2008). Hypnosis and memory: From Bernheim to the present. In K. Markman, W. Klein, & J. Suhr (Eds.), *Handbook of imagination and mental simulation* (pp. 103–119). New York: Psychology Press.

Lynn, S. J., & Kirsch, I. (2006). *Essentials of clinical hypnosis.* Washington, DC: American Psychological Association.

Lynn, S. J., Kirsch, I., Barabasz, A., Cardeña, E., & Patterson, D. (2000). Hypnosis as an empirically supported adjunctive technique: The state of the evidence. *International Journal of Clinical and Experimental Hypnosis, 48,* 343–361.

Lynn, S. J., Kirsch, I., & Hallquist, M. (2008). Social–cognitive theories of hypnosis. In M. R. Nash & A. Barnier (Eds.), *The Oxford handbook of hypnosis* (pp. 111–140). New York: Oxford University Press.

Lynn, S. J., Kirsch, I., Neufeld, V., & Rhue, J. (1996). Clinical hypnosis: Assessment, applications, and treatment considerations. In S. J. Lynn, I. Kirsch, & J. W. Rhue (Eds.), *Casebook of clinical hypnosis* (pp. 3–30). Washington, DC: American Psychological Association.

Lynn, S. J., Martin, D., & Frauman, D. C. (1996). Does hypnosis pose special risks for negative effects? *International Journal of Clinical and Experimental Hypnosis, 44,* 7–19.

Lynn, S. J., Matthews, A., & Stafford, J. (2008). *A survey of expert opinion of the future of hypnosis.* Unpublished manuscript.

Lynn, S. J., & McConkey, K. M. (1998). *Truth in memory.* New York: Guilford Press.

Lynn, S. J., Neufeld, V. R., & Mare, C. (1993). Direct versus indirect suggestions: A conceptual and methodological review. *International Journal of Clinical and Experimental Hypnosis, 41,* 124–152.

Lynn, S. J., Rhue, J. W., & Weekes, J. R. (1990). Hypnotic involuntariness: A social–cognitive analysis. *Psychological Review, 97,* 169–184.

Lynn, S. J., Shindler, K., & Meyer, E. (2004). Clinical correlates of high hypnotizability. In M. Heap, R. J. Brown, & D. Oakley (Eds.), *The highly hypnotizable person: Theoretical, experimental, and clinical issues* (pp. 187–212). New York: Brunner-Routledge.

McConkey, K. M. (1986). Opinions about hypnosis and self-hypnosis before and after hypnotic testing. *International Journal of Clinical and Experimental Hypnosis, 34,* 311–319.

Nash, M. R. (1987). What, if anything, is regressed about hypnotic age regression? A review of the empirical literature. *Psychological Bulletin, 102,* 42–52.

Nash, M. R. (2001). The truth and hype of hypnosis. *Scientific American, 285,* 46–55.

Neron, S., & Stephenson, R. (2007). Effectiveness of hypnotherapy with cancer patients' trajectory: Emesis, acute pain, and analgesia and anxiolysis in procedures. *International Journal of Clinical and Experimental Hypnosis, 55,* 336–354.

Robin, B. R., Kumar, V. K., & Pekala, R. J. (2005). Direct and indirect scales of hypnotic susceptibility: Resistance to therapy and psychometric comparability. *International Journal of Clinical and Experimental Hypnosis, 52,* 135–147.

Sarbin, T. R. (1950). Contributions to role-taking theory: 1. Hypnotic behavior. *Psychological Review, 57,* 225–270.

Schoenberger, N. E. (1996). Cognitive–behavioral hypnotherapy for phobic anxiety. In S. J. Lynn, I. Kirsch, & J. W. Rhue (Eds.), *Casebook of clinical hypnosis* (pp. 33–49). Washington, DC: American Psychological Association.

Sheehan, P. W., & McConkey, K. M. (1979). Australian norms for the Harvard Group Scale of Hypnotic Susceptibility, Form A. *International Journal of Clinical and Experimental Hypnosis, 27*, 294–304.

Sheehan, P. W., & Perry, C. W. (1976). *Methodologies of hypnosis.* Hillsdale, NJ: Erlbaum.

Shor, R. E., & Orne, E. C. (1963). Norms on the Harvard Group Scale of Hypnotic Susceptibility, Form A. *International Journal of Clinical and Experimental Hypnosis, 11*, 39–47.

Simon, M. J., & Salzberg, H. C. (1985). The effect of manipulated expectancies on posthypnotic amnesia. *International Journal of Clinical and Experimental Hypnosis, 33*, 40–51.

Smith, M. L., Glass, G. V., & Miller, T. I. (1980). *The benefits of psychotherapy.* Baltimore, MD: Johns Hopkins University Press.

Spanos, N. P., & Barber, T. X. (1974). Toward a convergence in hypnosis research. *American Psychologist, 29*, 500–511.

Spiegel, D. (1998). Using our heads: Effects of mental state and social influence on hypnosis. *Contemporary Hypnosis, 15*, 175–177.

Wagstaff, G. (1998). The semantics and physiology of hypnosis as an altered state: Towards a definition of hypnosis. *Contemporary Hypnosis, 15*, 149–165.

Zachariae, R., Jorgensen, M. M., & Christensen, S. (2000). Hypnotizability and absorption in a Danish sample: Testing the influence of context. *International Journal of Clinical and Experimental Hypnosis, 48*, 306–314.

2

IL N'Y A PAS D'HYPNOTISME: A HISTORY OF HYPNOSIS IN THEORY AND PRACTICE

JUDITH PINTAR

When Scottish surgeon James Braid popularized the word *hypnosis* in 1843, he was applying the term to a constellation of existing techniques that had long been in and out of practice. The associated hypnotically induced phenomena he described had been variously understood to be medical, psychological, spiritual, and even occult in their essential character.

The tangled histories of mesmerism and hypnosis challenge commonsense notions about the progress of scientific discovery. Competing medical and popular theories about the nature of hypnosis, varying techniques for its clinical and nonclinical use, and contradictory claims about its efficacy have coexisted for more than 2 centuries and, to a surprising extent, still do. For this reason, it is problematic to present discredited theories and practices as scientific stepping-stones that led to the discovery of hypnosis in its "true" modern form. This chapter suggests that the multiplicity of historic techniques and behavioral manifestations produced by hypnotic participants through time are empirically significant in themselves.

Hypnotic practitioners, subjects, researchers, observers, and skeptics have episodically constructed, deconstructed, and reconstructed hypnosis across decades and centuries and countless intellectual generations. This lively collaborative process has occurred in conjunction with, and often at odds with, the contributions of spiritual seekers and has also had to contend with the fantastical imaginings of novelists, playwrights, filmmakers, and their audiences. Contemporary researchers have tried to lay to rest popular myths that interfere with effective clinical applications of hypnosis; for example, the assumption that hypnotic subjects who score high on measures of suggestibility are gullible or weak willed or that a real hypnotic induction requires subjects to attain a state of consciousness physiologically related to sleep (Kirsch & Lynn, 1995). Yet these beliefs continue to be enshrined in popular stories and films that make hypnosis central in their plots (see chap. 27, this volume).

Reviewing the historical and cultural conditions within which hypnotic practitioners and their subjects emerged contributes to the onion-peeling task of determining which phenomena that may occur as part of a hypnotic induction are essential and which are cultural artifacts or epiphenomenal products of suggestion. Making these distinctions can be as challenging for modern hypnotists as it was for 18th century theorists and practitioners of the antecedents of hypnosis.[1]

EXORCISM AND MESMERISM

It is as inaccurate to say that exorcism was "actually" mesmerism as it would be to say that mesmerism was "actually" hypnosis. Yet the striking continuities between these culturally specific practices has typically lead historians to begin the story of hypnosis with Franz Anton Mesmer (1734–1815), who appeared on the medical stage in Germany and Austria at the same time that Father Johann Joseph Gassner (1727–1779), the celebrated exorcist, was leaving it.[2] The ritual of healing practiced by Gassner was straightforward. He would command in Latin that, in the name of Jesus, any unnatural aspect of a patient's disease should manifest immediately. If the symptoms did not immediately appear, Gassner concluded that the illness was purely physical and sent the patient to a medical doctor. If the exorcism produced symptoms, typically convulsions, Gassner would cast out the demon through words and touch and declare the patient healed (Ellenberger, 1970).

In 1775, a young German doctor, Franz Mesmer, was invited by Prince-Elector Max Joseph of Bavaria to help a commission to investigate Gassner's work. Mesmer had completed his doctoral dissertation at the University of

---

[1]For a more comprehensive narrative of the history of hypnosis presented along these lines, see *Hypnosis: A Brief History* (Pintar & Lynn, 2008).

[2]In addition to Mesmer's own writing, the most helpful secondary sources illuminating the life of Franz Mesmer are *The Discovery of the Unconscious* (Ellenberger, 1970), *A History of Hypnotism* (Gauld, 1992), and *Mesmer and Animal Magnetism* (Pattie, 1994).

Vienna almost 10 years earlier. His thesis, which was firmly based in Newtonian physics, was an analysis of the gravitational effects of heavenly bodies upon the human body, and, correspondingly, upon illness. He proposed the existence of a universal force, termed *animal gravity* that exerts a "tidal" influence upon us (Mesmer, 1980, p. 14). Despite the fact that this dissertation plagiarized an existing work by Richard Mead, a student of Isaac Newton (Pattie, 1956, pp. 275–287), at the age of 33, Mesmer became a doctor of medicine. Following a conventional route, he set up a medical practice in Vienna in 1767, using the common healing techniques of the time. Mesmer was unhappy with having to bleed and blister his patients. Rather than terrorizing his patients with painful procedures, Mesmer began instead to use touch to establish rapport. He discovered that this simple technique could produce dramatic effects.

In 1774, Mesmer began to treat a 27-year-old woman who presented complicated symptoms that included toothaches, convulsions, and vomiting. Franzl Oesterline required such constant attention that she was moved into his house. At these close quarters, Mesmer was able to observe an astronomical influence on the periodicity of her symptoms, just as his dissertation had predicted he would. Ordinary medical techniques provided the girl with no relief, so he decided to try to influence the gravitational effects himself. Mesmer attached magnets to Oesterline's body after having her swallow a lead solution. He discovered that he was able to evoke her disabling symptoms on command. After a series of productive sessions, Oesterline's illness was flushed from her body. She experienced the magnetic fluid rushing downward and through her, carrying it away (Mesmer, 1980, p. 48).

Mesmer distinguished the medium of healing, the magnet, from the source of the healing, the invisible fluid, which he believed could be transferred between a magnetist and a patient. His investigations into the movement of the fluid, which he termed *animal magnetism*, convinced him that illness and healing were both connected to the presence and quality of this magnetic fluid. With proper training in Mesmer's techniques, which included passing hands, magnets, and other magnetized objects across the body of a patient, Mesmer believed that any healthy person could heal another by channeling magnetic fluid into them. At the critical point of healing, it was expected that the patient would experience a dramatic and even violent relapse of symptoms. The appearance of this *crisis* indicated that the illness was being driven out.

Mesmer's unconventional medical practice, which used magnets and touch to treat both physiological and what would now be considered psychological conditions, brought him to the attention of the medical community and the public in Vienna and beyond. It was in 1775, the same year that Mesmer produced his first pamphlet on animal magnetism, that he demonstrated his techniques to the Academy of Science in Munich in coordination with an investigation into the practices of the exorcist, Gassner. There was substantial similarity between Mesmer's cures and Gassner's. They both made use of words and touch to produce symptoms and to resolve them following a violent crisis. In both cases, their patients believed that they had been healed. It is not the case, however, that mesmerism replaced exorcism. Their practices overlapped in both time and geography and were not mutually exclusive. Intellectual conditions were more conducive to supporting Mesmer's healing rituals than Gassner's because of the explanations that each offered about why they worked. The supernatural narrative essential to Gassner's cure was out of step with the new rational approach of the enlightenment (Ellenberger 1970, p. 56).

Mesmer accomplished a symbolic coup by rhetorically assimilating Gassner's healings into his new scientific paradigm. He claimed that although Gassner was undoubtedly a powerful healer, his power was not supernatural but simply reflected the exceptional portion of animal magnetism he possessed and shared with others. Due in some part to Mesmer's testimony, Gassner was exiled to a provincial Catholic community where his exorcisms were controlled by the church until his death in 1779 (see Midelfort, 2005).

Mesmer enjoyed widespread popularity as a traveling healer across central Europe during this period, much as Gassner had done. Unfortunately, back in Vienna the mainstream scientific and medical community, including Mesmer's colleagues and old teachers, continued to reject his ideas and to withhold their professional respect. Demoralized but not beaten, he decided eventually to try his luck in Paris, where he began magnetizing patients in 1778, starting off on a path to healing that he would vigorously promote and defend for the next 2 decades.

In 1779, Mesmer published his theory of animal magnetism, which declared that an invisible universal fluid, physical and tangible in its effects like electricity or magnetism, existed between everyone and everything. Because disease results from poor distribution of magnetic fluid, according to Mesmer, health could be restored by reestablishing magnetic equilibrium. All other medical approaches that produced healing could be explained by this theory of disease, which he viewed as universal. "There is only one illness and one healing," Mesmer confidently declared (cited by Ellenberger, 1950, p. 63). For Mesmer, all effective methods of healing involved the channeling of animal magnetism from the doctor to the patient, regardless of whether the doctor was aware that this was happening.

CRISIS AND SLEEP

By 1780, Mesmer was treating upward of 200 people a day. He devised an unusual way to treat greater numbers of people simultaneously. He filled a large tub with magnetized water. While people were standing around this *baquet*, placing their bodies directly against iron rods and holding on to a rope, Mesmer, wearing a velvet cape, played to them on his glass harmonica, an instrument invented by Benjamin Franklin that produced ethereal tones. Ideally, Mesmer's patients would achieve a crisis of convulsions or other dramatic symptoms. There was a special room set aside for this purpose, where they would be safe during that stage of their healing.

Despite his experience in Vienna, Mesmer expected that his success in Paris would lead to acknowledgment and respect from the French Academy of Science. He was therefore disappointed and bewildered that once again mainstream professional respect would be denied him. Charles D'Eslon (1739–1786), Mesmer's most important student, also felt the disdain of the Academy. Before his association with Mesmer, D'Eslon had been a respected doctor. His practice of animal magnetism led to his expulsion from the Academy. Despite his professional sacrifices on behalf of Mesmer's techniques, their relationship was a rocky one. Mesmer accused D'Eslon of stealing his patients after D'Eslon's clinic opened in 1782 and began offering magnetic treatments at a lower cost than did Mesmer's (Crabtree, 1993, p. 23).

Mesmer took steps to protect his financial and intellectual interests in the techniques of magnetism. One of the most successful was the creation of a secret society, the Society of Harmony, which was established in 1783 with the help of lawyer Nicholas Bergasse (1750–1832). Incorporating aspects of the Masonic tradition (see Gravitz, 1997, pp. 266–270), students could learn the techniques of magnetism if they paid the subscription fee and signed a confidentiality agreement. Branches of the society soon appeared across France. Even though the popularity of magnetism was growing and Mesmer personally prospered, he continued to struggle over issues of control. Mesmer's relationship with Bergasse suffered because they disagreed about who had the right to teach magnetism and to write about it. Eventually, Mesmer would expel Bergasse from the society he helped to form.

The year after the Society of Harmony was inaugurated, the French Academy of Science and the Paris Faculty of Medicine initiated an investigation into the practice of animal magnetism.[3] Benjamin Franklin, then the American ambassador to France, was included in the commission, although his direct involvement was limited. The commission was specifically interested in claims about the existence of the universal fluid. Its members were ambivalent at best on the question of whether animal magnetism actually produced any cures. Although Mesmer was incensed that the commission studied D'Eslon's clinic, rather than his own, this saved him from direct censure. After observation and

---

[3]A full exploration of the work of the Franklin Commission and its findings was provided in the 50th anniversary special issue of the *International Journal of Clinical and Experimental Hypnosis*, "Mesmer, Franklin, and the Royal Commission" (Nash, 2002).

experimentation, the commission rejected the reality of magnetic fluid and condemned D'Eslon's practice. Their report suggested insofar as the techniques of animal magnetism cured anyone, the positive effects were the result of the patient's imagination and expectancies (Bailly, 1784, cited by Crabtree, 1993).

Mesmer argued successfully that because the commission had investigated the practice of D'Eslon, rather than his own, their conclusions should not extend to him. However, he could not evade the public ridicule that followed the report. Mesmer was vilified and lampooned in popular songs and on stage. Animal magnetism was the object of scathing academic scrutiny. Even Mesmer's supporters and students continued to take his work in directions of which he did not approve. Bergasse politicized mesmerism to support the philosophical justifications for the French Revolution, for example (see Darnton, 1968), whereas a growing number of his followers saw mesmerism as a supernatural path to acquiring occult knowledge. This interpretation made the physical reality of magnetic fluid, on which Mesmer had staked his life and reputation, irrelevant.

It may be that Mesmer was simply tired of fighting for acceptance of his theories and techniques. Leaving the battle in the hands of others, at the end of the 18th century, he left Paris, wandered across Europe, and finally settled on the shores of Lake Constance, the region where he had been born, and he continued a local private practice. Mesmer died in 1815. Mesmerism did not, however, die with its namesake. It was to experience a profound transformation in the hands another of his students, Armand-Marie-Jacques de Chastenet, the Marquis de Puységur (1751–1825).

The eldest of three brothers who all had an interest in animal magnetism, the Marquis de Puységur inherited the family's title and ancestral lands. He had trained with Mesmer during the 1780s, but he left Paris to practice the techniques on behalf of the men and women who lived on his own estate. The healing of Oesterline provided Mesmer a breakthrough moment in his theory of animal magnetism. Something similar happened to Puységur when he healed a 23-year-old peasant on his estate, Victor Race. In 1784, Puységur mesmerized the young man, who had congestion and fever, and effected a successful healing. What was strange about the event was that Race did not go through the crisis that Mesmer believed was a necessary stage in the healing, a stage so crucial that Mesmer judged a patient to have been genuinely mesmerized only if he or she achieved a crisis.

When Puységur mesmerized Victor Race, he appeared to fall asleep, although he was still able to speak. Puységur coined the terms *magnetic somnambulism* and *magnetic sleep* to refer to the strange state of consciousness that Race had achieved.[4] Puységur soon found that few of his subjects went through

---

[4]For an insightful account of the practice of Puységur and his place within the larger history of psychology, see *From Mesmer to Freud: Magnetic Sleep and the Roots of Psychological Healing* (Crabtree, 1993).

crises while mesmerized but instead would enter into this state of consciousness in which they were neither asleep nor awake. Because this phenomenon was so dramatically different from what Mesmer had taught his followers to expect, it brought about a definitive schism in the already fractured community. Many mesmerists remained loyal to Mesmer, practicing Mesmerism as the master had taught them and invoking violent crises in their patients. Increasingly, magnetists began to prefer Puységur's approach, which, though similar in technique to Mesmer's, looked to magnetic sleep rather than to the crisis as the key indication that a patient was mesmerized and that healing was taking place.

Puységur's approach to animal magnetism differed from Mesmer's in another significant way. Mesmer's view rested on the objective reality of magnetic fluid and its role in illness and healing. He rejected all judgments of his healings as products of imagination. Puységur, however, was ambivalent on the subject of the tangibility of magnetic fluid. The issue had no direct bearing on his practice and so the charge of "imagination" was not a threatening one. What mattered for Puységur was that healing clearly was occurring as a result of a rapport he established between himself and his subjects. He did not care whether the healing occurred as a result of a psychological connection rather than a transfer of a universal fluid.

Puységur's work transformed prevailing definitions of what it meant to be mesmerized. The dramatic crises produced by Mesmer were increasingly seen to be products of suggestion rather than being essential to the experience. This is not so different from the critical effect that Mesmer's techniques had on Gassner's exorcisms. By arguing that verbal confrontations with demons were superfluous, Mesmer was able to reframe exorcism as a form of animal magnetism. Comparing the healing work of Gassner, Mesmer, and Puységur, it is clear that the methods used by each presupposed a particular cause of illness that necessitated a particular cure. Because Gassner believed the presence of a demon could cause bodily illness, the offending spirit had to be cast out. Mesmer needed to produce equilibrium in the magnetic fluid flowing through his patients because he believed that their illnesses were caused by its disruption or its inadequacy. Because Puységur came to understand that healing would follow the induction of a somnambulistic state, he correspondingly theorized that the illness resulted from a condition he referred to as *disordered somnambulism* (Puységur, 1784, cited by Crabtree, 1993, p. 48).

The astonishing effects of mesmerism experienced by Victor Race came to be seen as normative, or at least expectable, even when they were not understood to be essential. These phenomena included posttrance amnesia as well as dissociation of identity. While magnetized, Race often spoke with a different vocabulary and accent, as though he were of a higher social status than his own (Gauld, 1992, p. 60). More significantly for Puységur, Race seemingly developed paranormal abilities. He was able to diagnose his own illnesses as well as those suffered by people who were not in the room and whom he did not personally know. Race was not the only subject who purportedly proved capable of telepathic and clairvoyant wonders while mesmerized though completely incapable of performing them in a normal, waking state. In fact, the association of the mesmeric trance with extraordinary cognitive functioning occurred so frequently that Puységur's theory of mesmerism had to be altered to account for it.

Despite significant differences between Mesmer's theory and practice of animal magnetism and Puységur's approach, what Puységur was doing was still considered to be mesmerism. Mesmer's name persisted for another half century or more to describe the practice of the next generation of magnetists. Still, it was the influence of Puységur on the techniques and practice introduced by Mesmer that made them attractive on so many cultural levels in the middle and end of the 19th century in both Europe and the United States. Puységur died in 1825, only 10 years after Mesmer's death. His work was soon overshadowed by the theoretical innovations, performances, and research of his colorful contemporaries and the mesmerists who were to appear next on the scene, but his influence is easily detectable in everything they did.

BODY AND SOUL

The conflict between *fluidists*, who still professed a belief in the tangibility of animal magnetism, and *animists*, whose explanation for mesmeric phenomena was more purely psychological, occupied mesmerists for the first few decades of the 19th century. There was also an intermediate position characterized by a distinct ambivalence on the subject. For this group, the fact that mesmeric techniques demonstrably worked was more important than the unresolved question of why they worked. Still, the animists clearly were gaining ground.

One of the first of this number was an ordained Catholic priest named Jose-Custodio de Faria (1756–1819). Beginning as early as 1815, Abbe Faria attracted enormous crowds to his demonstrations of animal magnetism on the stage. He had an exotic presence, which he cultivated. His method of invoking the somnambulistic state in his subjects was idiosyncratic. He commanded them in a loud voice to "Sleep!" If that did not work, he would repeat the imperious command, only louder (Bertrand, 1826, p. 247, cited by Gauld, 1992). Sometimes he would mesmerize his entire audience into a somnambulistic state. Faria was so successful in these demonstrations that critics accused him of sorcery, but he vehemently denied this charge.

Faria rejected the idea that he possessed any secret power. He was an animist, so he also did not believe in the physical existence of any type of magnetic fluid. His explanation for what was going on was wholly psychological: To the extent that there was any power at work, its source was the will and the belief of the participants. He believed that his techniques would only work if his subjects accepted the possibility of magnetism, if they expected him to have power over them, and if they believed that a particular object had indeed been magnetized. If any of these conditions were lacking, animal magnetism would not work, because it had no power that was not conferred by the participants (Crabtree, 1993, pp. 122–123). In his attachment to this view, Faria's approach to animal magnetism comes across as distinctly modern. He also recognized the role of suggestion, believing that suggestions given by mesmerists to their subjects had an effect both while subjects were entranced and when they were not.

Faria's writings were not particularly influential during his lifetime but achieved salience later in the century. Most of the terms he coined did not catch on, though the ideas themselves were perceptive. Faria observed, for example, that not everyone could achieve the state of lucid sleep with the same ease or ability. Those who seemed to have an aptitude for this he referred to as *natural epoptes* (Faria, 1906, p. 27, cited by Gauld, 1992, p. 274). Better known than Faria's writing was the work of two men he influenced: the fluidist General François Joseph Noizet (1792–1885), and Alexandre Bertrand (1795–1831), an animist whose views were to be a significant source in the development of a more psychological view of mesmerism.

Through systematic, empirical research, Bertrand was able to test Faria's theoretical belief in the power of the subject's belief and expectation. Most significantly, by systematically manipulating the expectancy of the subjects, he found that their beliefs could be altered through suggestion. This discovery was devastating to the position of the fluidists. If the subjects of fluidists experienced the physical reality of magnetic fluid whereas the subjects of animists did not, it indicated that the tangibility of the fluid was a product of expectation and suggestion, rather than being essential to the process (Bertrand, 1826, cited by Gauld 1992, p. 132). Bertrand's conclusions about mesmerism following his experiments differed greatly from those of the Franklin Commission, which had conducted similar experiments. Although the commission considered the entire endeavor to be wholly discredited, Bertrand believed he had only disproved the existence of the magnetic fluid. Following Puységur, Bertrand maintained that the defining characteristic of mesmerism was the altered state.

Chief among the spokesmen for mesmerism in the first half of the 19th century was Joseph Deleuze (1753–1835), a student of Puységur. His two-volume treatise, published in 1813, *Histoire Critique de Magnétisme Animal*, was widely read, and in translation became the most influential work on mesmerism in the English language. Deleuze encouraged open practice of the techniques and a free sharing of common knowledge. Many of his observations of mesmerism seem to anticipate modern understandings of hypnosis. For example, he tempered the emphasis on magnetic sleep that had begun with Puységur, noting that only about a tenth of mesmerized subjects entered into a somnambulistic trance state. He also recorded the effective use of mesmerism in relief of pain, both during surgical operations and childbirth (Gauld, 1992, p. 118).

The work of Deleuze was translated into English by Thomas Hartshorn and introduced into the United States during the 1830s. Although there had been lectures on magnetism given in the United States during the first decades of the 1800s, it was Charles Poyen St. Sauveur (d. 1844) who was responsible for the first real wave of interest in mesmerism in the United States (Poyen, 1837). As a medical student in Paris he had first been exposed to the techniques, but his interest became serious after a visit to the French West Indies. Poyen presented himself as a professional practitioner when he arrived in Massachusetts in 1836. His lectures and training sessions swiftly became a popular sensation. Providence, Rhode Island, where he established his practice, was considered to be "the Mecca of American magnetism" (Gauld, 1992, p. 181). When Poyen arrived in the United States, he found a population that was actively exploring spiritual movements and experimenting with progressive reforms. Particularly on the east coast, abolitionists, suffragists, vegetarians, homeopaths, phrenologists, and followers of the Swedish mystic Emanuel Swedenborg were everywhere. Poyen found an audience, it can safely be said, that was receptive to his message.[5]

Mesmerism was connected to several religious movements in the United States, influencing the development of spiritualism, Christian Science, and New Thought. Andrew Jackson Davis (1826–1910), later known as the "Seer of Poughkeepsie," attended a lecture on mesmerism in 1843. Though he failed that evening to be mesmerized when he was brought on stage, Davis eventually found a mesmerist more to his liking. Believing himself to be gifted with clairvoyance and the power to diagnose and treat disease, Davis soon began to lecture on magnetism and spiritual philosophy (see Davis, 1859). Eventually he claimed to be a psychic channel for Swedenborg himself (Bush, 1847, p. 17).

Christian Science also has a genealogy that can be, controversially, traced back to mesmerism. Phineas Parkhurst Quimby (1802–1846) was inspired by

---

[5]See *Mesmerism and the American Care of Souls* (Fuller, 1982) for a detailed discussion of the history of mesmerism and related techniques in relationship to religious movements in 19th century United States.

one of Poyen's demonstrations. His particular interest in mesmerism, however, was not trance channeling but healing. In 1862, Quimby treated Mary Patterson, better known by her married name, Mary Baker Eddy. She would become the founder of Christian Science, a religion that is closely identified with its approach to healing based on faith rather than on medical intervention. The exact nature of Eddy's intellectual debt to Quimby became a flash point for controversy between Quimby's followers and Eddy's. The rancor between defenders and detractors of Christian Science because of it has persisted into the present day. There is also academic disagreement over the lineage between Quimby and Eddy and the philosophical and religious movement known as *New Thought*, which encouraged individuals to seek direct personal experience of spirituality and the divine (see Caplan, 1998, pp. 65–88; Taves, 1999, pp. 213–225).

MAGNETISM AND HYPNOTISM

In the idiosyncratically religious United States, mesmerism traveled in spiritual directions. In Europe, where mesmerists had also inspired mystics and romanticists, its movement in a spiritual direction was curtailed by the correcting influence of scientific positivism (Ellenberger, 1970, p. 86, 91). One of the more odd theories to arise at the intersection of mysticism and rationalism was phrenology, a system that associated emotional and cognitive phenomena with particular areas of the skull. Beginning in the 1840s, mesmerism and phrenology in the United States and the United Kingdom became entwined in the practice known as phrenomagnetism. Its proponents believed that if magnetic fluid were directed at a particular spot on the skull, symptoms associated with a phrenological "organ" could be invoked (Fuller, 1982, pp. 53–54).

Mesmerism was popularized in Britain in the 1830s by the writings of J. C. Colquhoun (1785–1854), an Edinburgh lawyer who had studied magnetism in both French and German. It was also made popular by the demonstrations of "Baron" Dupotet de Sennevoy (1796–1881), another larger-than-life character who arrived in England in 1837. In private rooms and hospitals, Dupotet provided dramatic demonstrations of mesmeric phenomena, including subjects' apparent insensibility to pain. His work drew the attention of John Elliotson (1791–1868), a doctor at London University and a devoted phrenologist, who invited him into the University hospital and allowed him to work with some of the patients there. Elliotson soon began his own experiments and demonstrations with both mesmerism and phrenomagnetism. He gained notoriety through a dramatic public conflict with Thomas Wakely (1795–1862), the founder and editor of the reformist medical journal, *The*

Lancet.[6] Wakely became a brutal skeptic of mesmerism and eventually brought about the episode that led to Elliotson resigning from his positions at London Hospital and University. Elliotson's star somnambulists, two young Irish girls who had produced mesmeric crises before large crowds at London University hospital, were publicly debunked by Wakely, who caused them to have seizures when they were not actually mesmerized. Wakely, like the Franklin commission before him, believed that his expectancy-manipulating experiments discrediting the existence of magnetic fluid should have ended the debate over magnetism (Gauld, 1992, pp. 202–203). Elliotson, like generations of supporters of mesmerism before him, was nonplussed by the experiment's results.

Elliotson was both a fluidist and a phrenomagnetist; thus, he believed in the tangible physical reality of some sort of force that could exert an effect on mesmerized subjects. He was not particularly interested in proving its existence, and he did not feel it necessary to explain exactly how it worked. Despite bad press, Elliotson continued to practice mesmerism privately. He was not a sophisticated theorist but took a pragmatic approach to mesmerism. Elliotson's own publication, *The Zoist: A Journal of Cerebral Psychology and Mesmerism and Their Applications to Human Welfare*, which was published from 1843 to 1856, emphasized the practical and applied aspects of mesmerism and did not delve deeply into the larger theoretical questions. Elliotson wanted to reduce human suffering and intended to explore whatever techniques seemed promising in this regard. He was particularly enthusiastic about reports that mesmerism could control the experience of painful medical procedures.

One of the contributors to *The Zoist* was James Esdaile (1805–1855), a Scottish surgeon who had lived and worked in India near Calcutta. It was through his writings that mesmeric analgesia began to attract significant professional attention in Britain (Winter, 1998). Esdaile claimed that mesmerism was much less dangerous to his patients than ether or chloroform, which had recently come into use (Esdaile, 1846). His dramatic writings, which appeared in *The Zoist*, documented painless operations and were persuasive even to skeptics. The excitement engendered by the work of Esdaile reflected the interests and priorities of the surgeons of that era, who had significant interest in reducing the pain of their procedures.

A Scottish surgeon, James Braid (1795–1860), was to have a significant role in the evolution of mesmerism. Braid's interest in the subject began at a performance in 1841 given by Charles Lafontaine (1803–1892), a stage hypnotist from Switzerland. Initially skeptical, but still curious, Braid immediately

---

[6]*Mesmerized: Powers of Mind in Victorian Britain* (Winter, 1998) provides an incisive social and cultural analysis of mesmerism in this era.

began experimenting on a friend, his wife, and then on a manservant. Braid consistently induced in his subjects what he considered to be a special state of consciousness related to, but different from, ordinary sleep. He believed it was triggered by relaxation, controlled breathing, and a fixed stare, which led to a "derangement" of the circulatory, and respiratory, and muscular systems (Braid, 1843).

Braid rejected completely the existence of magnetic fluid; he was a doctor, not a mystic. By highlighting the physiological conditions that occurred during a hypnotic induction, most famously eye fixation, Braid was asserting that "nervous sleep" was a physical process, not an imaginary one, and that it was capable of ameliorating symptoms of physical ailments, as long as a proper state were achieved. Braid identified in his hypnotic subjects several discrete stages of hypnosis that he referred to as *torpor, catalepsy*, and *anesthenia*. Although the French mesmerist Hénin de Cuvillers (1755–1841) had begun using words adapted from *hypnos*, the Greek word for "sleep," to describe animal magnetism 2 decades before, Braid's 1843 article, *Neurypnology, or the Rationale of Nervous Sleep*, is generally credited with introducing the terms *hypnotism* and *hypnotize*, into common usage.

In formalizing his views, Braid tried to divorce mesmeric phenomena from its prior association with magnets and invisible fluids, and wed it instead to the phenomena of magnetic sleep. When Braid died in 1860, his innovations in technique had not inspired any particular revolution in Britain or in France. Eugene Azam (1822–1899), a professor of medicine at Bordeaux, was apparently influenced by Braid's terminology and his emphasis on clear stages of nervous sleep. Still, historians contest the claim that Braid had a direct influence on later hypnotic theory (Gauld, 1992, p. 287). Whether or not Braid himself was responsible for changes that followed him, his transformation of the available vocabulary corresponded with a significant shift in theoretical understanding and clinical practice.

The dramatic popularity of techniques associated with both mesmerism and hypnosis in France during the last decades of the 19th century can be more confidently credited to the work of Charles Richet (1850–1935), a professor of physiology who would be awarded the Nobel Prize in 1913 in recognition of his research on anaphylaxis. Making use of the mesmerizing hand passes developed by Mesmer a century before, Richet experimented with hypnosis in a mainstream medical setting. Richet's subjects reportedly experienced hallucinations, demonstrated hyperideation (i.e., ideation characterized by unusually energetic speech and action), automation (i.e., obeying orders like automatons), and posthypnotic amnesia.

Elsewhere in Europe during this period, Carl Hansen (1833–1897), a magnetic demonstrator from Denmark, was putting his subjects into cataleptic states and evoking dramatic muscular rigidity. During the period of Hansen's popularity, most demonstrations seem to have been staged for their entertainment value, whereas German scientists pursued theoretical issues related to mesmerism rather than to clinical or therapeutic ones (Gauld, 1992, p. 305). In France, however, the most exciting events were happening in the clinical setting.

SALPÊTRIÈRE AND NANCY

Jean-Martin Charcot (1825–1893) spent 30 years at the Salpêtrière women's asylum, first as a medical student and then becoming chief of medicine there in 1862 (see Micale, 1985). As a well-regarded neurologist, Charcot developed protocols for diagnosis prior to engaging in his exploration of hypnosis, which he began in 1878. His early experiences in neurology influenced his particular approach to psychiatric diagnosis as well. When faced with a ward of women who suffered from convulsions, some of whom appeared to be afflicted with epileptic conditions, and others whose convulsions arose from hysteria, he was fascinated to discover that the women with hysterics had learned through observation how to have "epileptoid attacks" (Ellenberger, 1970, p. 90).

For a period of about 4 years, from 1878 to 1882, Charcot analyzed his patients with hysteria with the aid of hypnotic techniques. Following the approach taken by both Braid and Richet, Charcot identified discrete stages of hypnosis that were both descriptive and predictive of a "real" hypnotic experience. He found that he could observe the same stages reoccurring in all of his patients. When they were experiencing the stage of *catalepsy*, they behaved like automatons, responding to his physical suggestions. Entering the stage he termed *lethargy*, they were nonresponsive to suggestion and became effectively insensible. If they achieved *somnambulism*, the final stage, they regained their capacity for conversation and responded enthusiastically to his suggestions.

Charcot examined his patients in front of doctors, students, and the press every Tuesday morning at the Salpêtrière. Sometimes the general public was allowed to observe as well. What they saw dependably every week was Charcot's ability to draw his female patients through the stages of hypnosis, a ritual he referred to as *grande hypnotisme*. His most famous subject, Blanche Wittman, was noted for putting on a particularly good show (Ellenberger, 1970, p. 99). Charcot also offered Friday morning lectures, disseminating what he believed to be the theoretical implications of the demonstrations.

Charcot had observed that the behaviors associated with *grande hypnotisme* closely resembled the symptoms of hysteria, an illness that was believed to arise from a combination of physical or psychic trauma and an inherited predisposition to the disease (see Micale, 1995). Epileptic-like seizures were typically followed by periods of delirium and sensibility, as well as a susceptibility to suggestion. It soon became necessary to account for the fact that the most prominent characteristics of the hypnotic state, which could be witnessed every Tuesday at the Salpêtrière, and the accepted diagnostic symptoms of hysteria, were nearly identical. Charcot provided an explanation for this overlap: The capacity to be hypnotized, he declared, was a manifestation of hysteria.

Charcot was inducted as a member of the *Académie des Sciences* in 1883, by which time he had fully developed his theory of *grand hypnotisme*. This honor, which had been denied to Franz Mesmer a century before, reflects not only the professional regard in which Charcot was held but also the extent to which his techniques had achieved mainstream status. All of this began to change when researchers and practitioners of the "Nancy School" of hypnosis challenged Charcot and his followers at the Salpêtrière.

The father figure, though not the driving force of the Nancy School, was Ambroise-Auguste Liébault (1823–1904). Born in the French village near Nancy, he began his professional career in 1850 as a conventional doctor in Strasbourg. After reading an old volume on animal magnetism, he began to use animal magnetism to treat his patients, regardless of whether they suffered from arthritis or tuberculosis. Liébault's method was both old and new. He used the gentle physical touch promoted by the earliest magnetists, but he also suggested to his patients that they should sleep. Liébault was a fluidist for the first 3 decades of his practice and was only persuaded away from his belief in the presence of a tangible force by the experiments of Hippolyte Bernheim (1840–1919). Using placebo-controlled experiments, Bernheim was able to demonstrate to Liébault that unmagnetized objects had the same power as magnetized ones, as long as the subject believed them to be magnetized (Gauld, 1992, p. 324).

Bernheim, who was a professor of medicine at Nancy, began his study of hypnosis after meeting Liébault in 1882. Four years later, he published his first critique of Charcot's work at the Salpêtrière. The Nancy School of hypnosis came into existence to challenge Charcot's mainstream and institutionalized theory of *grande hypnotisme*. A pamphlet war ensued. The Salpêtrière position was straightforward: Hypnosis was an abnormal phenomenon related to hysteria and characterized by three clearly defined stages. The Nancy School rejected the connection between hysteria and hypnosis. They also denied the pathology of suggestibility. Everyone, not only hysterics, they believed, was capable of hypnotic responsiveness. Finally, and most damningly, they claimed that the three stages of *grand hypnotisme* were themselves only products of suggestion (Gauld, 1992). Defenders of Charcot countered that if the stages of hypnosis were simply products of suggestion, then all phenomena produced in a hypnotic context must be products of suggestion, and if that were so, how would it ever be possible to say whether someone was hypnotized or not (Gauld 1992, p. 331)?

When details of the life of the patients with hysteria in the Salpêtrière were more closely examined, it was impossible for Charcot's supporters to deny the role of suggestion in their clinic. Some commentators charged that Charcot's subjects were "faking" their performances in his weekly demonstrations or, more kindly, that they were simply fulfilling powerful expectations. Certainly, everyone inside the Salpêtrière, and many people outside of it, knew exactly what to expect from each of the three stages. In addition, the details of animal magnetism had been in mainstream popular consciousness already for a century.

An account by Pierre Janet (1859–1947) of what had occurred is critical but sympathetic. He believed that the three stages of the *grand hypnotisme* were produced in subjects as a result of deliberate training by student magnetizers and without the knowledge or approval of Charcot. According to Janet, Charcot's real error arose as a result of his attempt to classify hysterical diseases as he had done for neurological ones. He simply oversimplified the conditions he was describing, and this error was compounded by Charcot's lack of interest in the details of his subjects' lives (see Janet, 1925, pp. 186–192). When Charcot died in 1893, although he had never publicly revised his views, *grand hypnotisme* was no more. Charcot's approach was displaced entirely by the Nancy position, which conceived of hypnosis as a treatment for both physiological and psychological illness through psychological means.

The collective transformation in understanding hypnosis is illustrated well in Janet's intellectual career. Janet became a doctor in 1893 and also worked with psychiatric patients at Salpêtrière. Janet agreed with Charcot that hypnosis could be accurately characterized as hysterical somnambulism. He observed in his hypnotic subjects at the Salpêtrière many of the same symptoms associated with hysteria: not only somnambulism but also hysterical paralysis and automatic writing as well. He at first rejected the view that these phenomena were only products of his suggestion. He wanted to know why such suggestions, if that was what they were, only seemed to have power over certain people. Janet's theory was that patients with hysteria lacked critical cognitive functions that resulted in a diminished consciousness. The problem with this idea was that it implied that only patients with hysteria were hypnotizable, which clearly was not the case. Faced with this contradiction, Janet eventually moved in the direction of the Nancy position and acknowledged that normal, psychologically healthy people could also be hypnotized, and could exhibit all the symptoms of pathological hysteria.

HYPNOTHERAPY AND PSYCHOTHERAPY

Despite the fact that the Nancy School approach to hypnosis spread across Europe and the United States, the Nancy School itself lost its raison d'etre once the battle against the Salpêtrière had been won. There is substantial disagreement over why the use of hypnosis by mainstream medical practitioners declined following the victory of the Nancy School approach. Some point to Bernheim, who did not tone down his rhetoric. Though he was at first willing to allow the possibility that hypnosis created a "state" of heightened suggestibility, he eventually rejected this concept as well. He was convinced by the results of his experimental research that ordinary people are as suggestible in their everyday waking states as they are when they have been through a hypnotic induction. Declaring that every behavioral marker produced by hypnosis is a product of suggestion and that techniques of hypnosis were therapeutic to subjects only because it was suggested to them that they would be so, Bernheim publicly concluded at a conference in 1897, "*Il n'y a pas d'hypnotisme* [There is no (such thing as) hypnotism]." Peeling the onion of hypnosis as far as he could, Bernheim decided that it was made of peels all the way down. This was the conclusion that the defenders of the Salpêtrière had earlier feared: How can hypnosis be measured, if everything produced by hypnosis is a product of suggestion?

By claiming that hypnosis did not actually exist, Bernheim appeared to be taking the position held by those in past generations who had been most dismissive of mesmerism and hypnosis. From the Franklin Commission to Wakely, critics discredited some phenomenon as being a product of suggestion and believed they had therefore disproved mesmerism as a whole. Bernheim's recognition of the intrinsic role of suggestion in hypnosis, however, reflected an entirely different train of thought that can be traced back to the 18th century. After the release of the Franklin Commission report dismissing the physical existence of animal magnetism, Charles D'Eslon responded, "If the medicine of the imagination is the most efficient, why do we not make use of it?" (Binet & Féré, 1888, p. 17). A few decades later, Alexandre Bertrand titled the preface to his book, *Traité du Somnambulisme* (1823), "How the Author Came to Realize That Animal Magnetism Does Not Exist." Influenced by the work of Bertrand, Joseph Delboeuf (1831–1896), a rationalist-philosopher-turned-experimental-psychologist, conducted his own empirical research, which convinced him that the suggestion operated without the need for a trance state, and penned an article entitled, "So It Turns Out There's No Such Thing As Hypnosis" (Delboeuf, 1891). These men were not debunking hypnosis but rather arguing that the power of suggestion, as opposed to magnetic fluid or hysteria, was the real cause of its attendant phenomena.

Other than Bernheim, the man most frequently held responsible for the disappearance of hypnosis from the mainstream is Sigmund Freud, who studied with both Charcot and Bernheim. Hypnotherapy and psychotherapy at that historical moment were virtually synonymous, and hypnosis was a central feature in Freud's clinical technique. Eventually, Freud replaced hypnosis with his own therapeutic innovations, which resulted in the exile of hypnosis from the psychoanalytic mainstream for decades. This narrative, although factually accurate, requires a caveat. It was not Bernheim's peeled-onion style of hypnosis that Freud abandoned. He did not view the somnambulistic trance state to be a product of suggestion but rather as an essential feature of hypnosis. It was only the deliberate induction of somnambulism that Freud rejected. He still incorporated other hypnotic and arguably mesmeric techniques into his practice. Freud's use of touch and rapport, suggestion and catharsis, would all have been intimately familiar to Mesmer, though, of course, Freud's explanation for what he was doing would have been a surprise.

If mainstream medical establishments hastened to distance themselves once again from the chimerical hypnotic tradition (though not necessarily its techniques by other names), there was no corresponding decline of interest in hypnosis occurring in popular culture. Stage hypnotists continued their successful performances across Europe and the United States, and a plethora of novels and plays on the topic appeared during this period. The explosion of popular interest continued through the turn of the century and into the 20th century, incorporating versions of mesmerism and hypnosis into literature and into film (see chap. 27).

At the same time, there continued to be an enthusiastic international and multidisciplinary community of scholars whose interests originated in issues raised by the practice of hypnosis. In addition to Pierre Janet, a group of men that included Frederic W. H. Myers (1843–1901), Edmund Gurney (1847–1888), Frank Podmore (1856–1910), Alfred Binet (1857–1911), Max Dessoir (1867–1947), Théodore Flournoy (1854–1921), Morton Prince (1862–1939), and, most famously, William James (1842–1910) were all engaged in a quest to understand human consciousness and the nature of the self, in a train of intellectual thought that continued outside the psychoanalytic mainstream.

HYPNOSIS IN THE 20TH CENTURY

Histories of hypnosis frequently leave a gap of almost half a century between the colorful 19th-century adventures in hypnosis and the golden age that purportedly began in the 1960s. When understood as a kind of historical rounding error, the gap disappears. The hypnosis researchers who represent the final generation of the 19th century, including Pierre Janet, Morton Prince, and Joseph Jastrow (1863–1944) survived for decades into the 20th century, researching and writing. Their students trained other students during the first half of the 20th century; the mature professional work of this latter group of students came of age beginning in the 1950s and 1960s.

The investigations of Milton Erickson (1902–1980) in the first half of the 20th century, for example, were particularly influential on the second half. Erickson's clinical innovations in the practice of hypnosis are credited with inspiring its renaissance, arousing an entire new generation of practitioners. At once creative and controversial, Erickson established an approach to the use of hypnosis in a clinical setting that influenced practitioners both marginal and mainstream (Erickson, Rossi, & Rossi, 1976). As a student at the University of Wisconsin in Madison during the 1920s, Erickson was encouraged by Jastrow, the head of the psychology department. A friend and colleague of William James, Jastrow was fascinated by everyday dissociations. Erickson had a more problematic relationship with another professor in the department, Clark Hull (1884–1952), who disapproved of Erickson's inclination to blur the boundary between lab and clinic.

Clark Hull conducted some of the most significant experimental work on hypnosis that occurred during the first half of the 20th century. He established a rigorous empirical approach to the study of hypnosis that would become the standard in contemporary research. Among other instruments, he developed the first scales for measuring suggestibility. Although he was able to establish through research the validity of some phenomena associated with hypnosis, including hypnotic anesthesia, other traditions he persuasively debunked. For example, Hull (1933) demonstrated that hypnotic trance states were unrelated to sleep and that they did not produce extraordinary cognitive abilities.

Frank A. Pattie (1901–1999) was also researching hypnotically induced tactile anesthesia during the 1930s (Pattie, 1937). The decade before, Pattie had been one of a group of hypnosis and personality researchers who studied with Morton Prince at Harvard. Pattie's best-known work, *Mesmer and Animal Magnetism: A Chapter in the History of Medicine* (1994), was not published until the end of his long life, the culmination of half a century of research. In addition to Pattie, the group at Harvard included William Taylor (1894–1976), Paul Young (1892–1991), and Henry Murray (1893–1988), who authored a biography of Prince. Murray earned his real significance within the history of hypnosis because of the encouragement he offered to Robert Winthrop White (1893–1988).

After the death of Morton Prince, Murray turned the attention of the Harvard Psychological Clinic to the study of personality (Murray, 1938). White's contribution to the massive study was a study on hypnotic receptivity.

Although White's research on hypnosis only continued for a few more years, it was particularly significant for the future of hypnosis because it reframed the crucial question that had been left unresolved since the turn of the century: Which aspects of hypnosis are essential and which are epiphenomenal products of suggestion? This question was taken up as a crucial research task by White and would provide the starting point for decades of research that would follow.

Although White believed that hypnotic behavior occurred within an objective and measurable altered state of consciousness, he also maintained that hypnotic subjects were susceptible to the spoken and unspoken wishes of the hypnotist, famously stating, "Hypnotic behavior is meaningful, goal-directed striving, its most general goal by the subject being to behave like a hypnotized person as this is continuously defined by the operator and understood" (1941, p. 483). After White left the field, the debate that followed him sought a balance between his two convictions: On one hand was the belief in the reality of an altered state of consciousness, and on the other was an acknowledgement of social psychological processes at work between hypnotist and subject. Beginning in the 1950s and continuing for the next 2 decades, a polarization occurred between researchers, theorists, and practitioners of hypnosis whose opposing positions were characterized as *altered state* or *nonstate* theories of hypnosis.

Most altered state theorists set out to explain hypnosis by describing cognitive processes of dissociation. Ernest R. Hilgard (1904–2001), considered to be the most influential of the early state theorists, introduced *neodissociation theory*, based on a view of the human mind as a set of hierarchical cognitive systems controlled by an *executive ego* (1977). Hilgard suggested that when a person is hypnotized, his executive ego becomes divided into two parts, separated by a barrier of amnesia. If the individual receives a suggestion to lift his arm, the executive ego must give the command, but the amnesiac barrier prevents it from being aware that it has done so. This results in the illusory sensation frequently reported by hypnotic subjects that their actions while under hypnosis are nonvolitional.

In Hilgard's view, this type of dissociation occurs in ordinary, non-hypnotic circumstances as well; for example, when one finds oneself driving home instead of going to the store as one had intended. Because of this descriptive overlap between hypnotic and ordinary circumstances, Hilgard's work is no longer described purely as an altered state theory. Kenneth S. Bowers (1937–1996), a colleague of Hilgard's, believed that the concept of an amnesiac barrier weakened the neodissociation approach. Bowers's theory of *dissociated control,* in which hypnotic responses are believed to be directly and automatically activated by suggestions, bypassing executive control, emerged as a significant alternative to Hilgard's model (Bowers, 1992). Bowers's theory was further refined and expanded by his colleague Erik Woody (Woody

& Bowers, 1994; Woody & Farvolden, 1998), who proposed ways of integrating variants of dissociation theory under the umbrella of a more encompassing scheme (see chap. 6, this volume).

Through his own explorations of the dissociations that occur between experience and memory, and between pain and the experience of pain, John F. Kihlstrom also extended neodissociation theory in significant ways (Kihlstrom, 1992). Most significantly, he is recognized for incorporating new models of cognitive psychology into hypnosis theory and research (Kihlstrom, 1998) and for cultivating the center ground in the state debate (Kihlstrom, 2003). Kihlstrom collaborated with Martin T. Orne (1927–2000), a student of Robert White. Orne's Unit for Experimental Psychiatry at the University of Pennsylvania became one of the most influential hypnosis laboratories in the United States. It was there that Orne developed what has been called a *phenomenological model* of hypnosis (Spanos & Chaves, 1991), which incorporated aspects of both the state and nonstate approaches to focus on the distinctions between hypnotic and waking cognition (Orne, 1959, 1979). Peter W. Sheehan (see Sheehan, 1991) and Kevin M. McConkey (see McConkey, 1991) are two important theorists who continue to work along these lines.

Finally, the psychodynamic tradition has also contributed to the altered state approach to hypnosis. Erika Fromm, Michael Nash, and Elgan Baker have all made use of psychodynamic terminology and theory to describe hypnosis and its attendant phenomena. They emphasize the effect of hypnosis on primary process thinking, including most particularly its enhancement of imagination (see, e.g., Fromm & Nash, 1997).

In contrast to theorists and clinicians who take an altered state perspective, those who prefer the nonstate position reject dissociation as an explanatory phenomenon though they may accept it as a descriptive one. If the subjective experience of dissociation occurs, it is considered to be a product of suggestion rather than its causal agent. In other words, they feel that the expectations and beliefs held by hypnotic participants about what will happen to them when they are hypnotized are sufficient to explain all hypnotic responses.

Theodore R. Sarbin (1911–2005) was among the earliest of the nonstate theorists. Sarbin, whose *role theory* was influential across the field of psychology, found that when it was applied to the study of hypnosis, he was able to gain insight into the relationship between the hypnotist and the subject and the "scripts" that each would follow, whether or not they were conscious of these. Along with his colleague William C. Coe (1930–2004), Sarbin identified multiple variables that affected hypnotic responsiveness. Many of these were associated with expectations and imagination (Coe & Sarbin, 1991). Sarbin believed that in both the hypnotic context and in ordinary life, "believed-in-imaginings" have the power to distort perceptions of reality (Sarbin, 1972).

Another influential nonstate theorist, Theodore X. Barber (1927–2005), criticized "the altered state" model for using hypnotic responsiveness both to explain the hypnotic state as well as to indicate its presence (Barber, 1969). Based on research conducted through the 1960s and into the early 1970s, Barber found that hypnotic responsiveness could result from a wide number of factors. Like Sarbin, he was interested in expectancies, but he also focused on the particular wording and vocal tone of suggestions, the way that subjects' responsiveness was assessed, and the physical behavior of the experimenter in all stages (see, e.g., Barber & Calverley, 1964; Barber, Spanos, & Chaves, 1974). He was particularly intrigued by individual differences in imaginative capacity, but he still maintained that hypnosis could have positive therapeutic effects on people regardless of their innate abilities (Barber, 1969, p. 282; see also chap. 7, this volume).

Arguably the most influential nonstate theorist of the late 20th century was Nicholas P. Spanos (1942–1994), who combined Sarbin's role theory with Barber's cognitive–behavioral work and extended them in unexpected ways. Spanos and his colleagues, including John Chaves (1941–2008), who was instrumental in establishing the credibility of hypnosis in the dental profession, focused on social psychological processes. They were interested in how hypnotic participants come to understand their role and the communicative dynamics that might influence their interpretation of hypnotic suggestions (Spanos, 1991; Spanos & Chaves, 1989). Graham Wagstaff, of the University of Liverpool, is another important social-cognitive theorist who was strongly influenced by Barber, Sarbin, and Orne (Wagstaff, 2001).

Also working within the nonstate tradition, Irving Kirsch developed his *response expectancy theory* to describe the relationship between a subject's expectancy and the subjective sense of nonvolition during a hypnotic induction. Kirsch has argued that the role of expectancy in hypnotic response is related to the same internal processes that allow a placebo to produce significant alterations in subjective mental and emotional states, including anxiety and depression as well as objective physiological conditions, such as pain (Kirsch, 1994). Steven Jay Lynn's *integrative model* looks at hypnotic subjects as creative problem solvers, who integrate situational, personal, and interpersonal variables in creative ways during a hypnotic session (Lynn & Sivec, 1992). *Response set theory*, a collaboration between Kirsch and Lynn, incorporates aspects of both response expectancy theory and the integrative model to examine the automaticity of ordinary life as well as the subjective sense of nonvolition in the hypnotic context (Kirsch & Lynn, 1997). Response set theory proposes that most actions are initiated automatically, rather than being the result of a fully conscious intention. In other words, it is one's experience of volition in everyday life that is an illusion. The involuntary or automatic actions that seem wondrous in the hypnotic context are actually ubiquitous and quite ordinary occurrences in people's waking lives (Kirsch & Lynn, 1999; Lynn, 1997).

CONTROVERSY AND DEBATE

The terms *state* and *nonstate* began to fall out of use during the 1980s and were replaced by the more descriptively useful terms *special process* and *social-cognitive*. Despite some degree of convergence between the two sides, there remains a difference between theorists and researchers who perceive hypnotic behavior to be essentially different from nonhypnotic behavior because it is produced by a trance state or through a related process of dissociation (Spanos, 1982) and those who believe that hypnotic behavior can be explained completely using the same variables that account for nonhypnotic behavior.

The controversy is, arguably, irresolvable because neurological research begins with different premises and considers different types of evidence from research that focuses on social–psychological processes. Still, in recent years the war between the state and nonstate theorists has become decidedly less raucous. This may be due, in part, to the fact that the turn of the millennium was marked by a dramatic and deeply emotional conflict over the relationship of hypnosis to memory that redrew long-standing battle lines into new configurations.

The controversy began with high profile child abuse investigations during the 1980s and into the 1990s. The use of hypnosis to "recover" traumatic memories was increasingly questioned as it became implicated in the creation of *false memories* (see Lynn & McConkey, 1998). At the same time, sensationalized accounts of hypnotists iatrogenically creating multiple personalities in their vulnerable, dissociative clients began to emerge in the press and eventually in the courts. Researchers and clinicians frequently found themselves at odds with one another in often-rancorous debates. Slowly, a consensus position emerged: Hypnotically induced memories are not necessarily any more accurate than nonhypnotic memories, and hypnosis improperly used can in fact lead to dramatically inaccurate recall (see Garry & Polaschek, 2000).

The professional integrity of hypnosis and its practitioners was ensured by the professional acknowledgment of the potential misuse of hypnosis (American Psychological Association [APA], 1995) as well as by clear and consistent messages about its safety and benefits. There is now an impressive mountain of empirical evidence attesting to the positive effects of hypnosis on a wide range of physical and psychological ailments, from control of anxiety to pain management (reviewed by Pinnell & Covino, 2000). The mainstream position that hypnosis now enjoys in the medical and psychotherapeutic world is also due to the organization of influential hypnosis societies and interest groups that have provided training to individuals across professions, from social work to dentistry.

In 2004 the Executive Committee of the APA Division of Psychological Hypnosis (APA, Division 30, 2005) revised the definition of hypnosis to include clinical techniques of self-hypnosis and to acknowledge the continuing coexistence of competing models, as follows: "Many believe that hypnotic responses and experiences are characteristic of a hypnotic state. While some think that it is not necessary to use the word 'hypnosis' as part of the hypnotic induction, others view it as essential" (para. 1). What is remarkable about this definition is its pragmatism, a sensibility that has been the strong suit of hypnosis through the centuries.

When Bernheim declared, "*Il n'y a pas d'hypnotisme!*" he was making the wry observation that hypnosis apparently works even if it does not "exist" in the way that most hypnotists of his day believed that it did. The dizzying historical array of colorful, contradictory, and discredited epiphenomena associated with hypnosis has proved to be empirically significant in itself, shedding light on the biological, social, and cultural dynamics of suggestibility that lie at the heart of hypnosis, whether or not one believes that suggestions require, or are enhanced by, a trance state.

History has also amply demonstrated that hypnosis can produce positive effects even when key epistemological questions remain unresolved. Modern hypnosis did not evolve in a neat linear fashion, truth replacing misconception in landmark breakthroughs leading to broad consensus. Instead, disagreement, ambiguity, and incongruity over and over again provided the engine for significant innovations in research, theory, and practice. As prevailing understandings of hypnosis are challenged by breakthroughs in neurobiology, are extended by investigations of non-Western perspectives (see chap. 29), and are informed by the development of new clinical uses, perplexing contradictions are likely to continue to provide inspiration into the foreseeable future and beyond.

REFERENCES

American Psychological Association, Division 17, Committee on Women & Division 42, Trauma and Gender Issues Committee (1995, July). *Psychotherapy guidelines for working with clients who may have an abuse or trauma history*. Washington, DC: Author.

American Psychological Association, Division 30, Society of Psychological Hypnosis. (2005). New Definition: Hypnosis. Retrieved from http://www.apa.org/divisions/div30/define_hypnosis.html

Barber, T. X. (1969). *Hypnosis: A scientific approach*. New York: Van Nostrand Reinhold.

Barber, T. X., & Calverley, D. S. (1964). Toward a theory of hypnotic behavior: Effects on suggestibility of defining the situation as hypnosis and defining responses to suggestions as easy. *Journal of Abnormal and Social Psychology, 68,* 585–592.

Barber, T. X., Spanos, N. P., & Chaves, J. F. (1974). *Hypnosis, imagination, and human potentialities.* New York: Pergamon Press.

Bernheim, H. (1897). *L'hypnotisme et la suggestion* [Hypnotism and suggestion]. Paris: O. Doin.

Bertrand, A. J. F. (1823). *Traité du somnabulisme et des différentes modifications qu'il présente.* Paris: Dentu.

Binet, A., & Fere, C. (1888). *Animal magnetism.* New York: Appleton-Century-Crofts.

Bowers, K. S. (1992). Imagination and dissociation in hypnotic responding. *International Journal of Clinical and Experimental Hypnosis, 40,* 253–275.

Braid, J. (1899). *Neurypnology, or the rationale of nervous sleep considered in relation to animal magnetism or mesmerism.* London: George Redway. (Original work published 1843)

Bush, G. (1847). *Mesmer and Swedensborg; Or, the relation to the development of Mesmerism to the doctrines and disclosures of Swedenborg.* New York: John Allen.

Caplan, E. (1998). *Mind games: American culture and the birth of psychotherapy.* Berkley: University of California Press.

Coe, W. C., & Sarbin, T. R. (1991). Role theory: Hypnosis from a dramaturgical and narrational perspective. In S. J. Lynn & J. W. Rhue (Eds.), *Theories of hypnosis: Current models and perspectives* (pp. 303–323). New York: Guilford Press.

Crabtree, A. (1993). *From Mesmer to Freud: Magnetic sleep and the roots of psychological healing.* New Haven, CT: Yale University Press.

Darnton, R. (1968). *Mesmerism and the end of the Enlightenment in France.* Cambridge, MA: Harvard University Press.

Davis, A. J. (1859). *The magic staff: An autobiography of Andrew Jackson Davis.* New York: J. S. Brown & Co.

Ellenberger, H. F. (1970). *The discovery of the unconscious: The history and evolution of dynamic psychiatry.* New York: Basic Books.

Erickson, M. H., Rossi, E. L., & Rossi, S. I. (1976). *Hypnotic realities: The induction of clinical hypnosis and forms of indirect suggestion.* New York: Irvington Publishers.

Esdaile, J. (1846). *Mesmerism in India and its practical applications in surgery and medicine.* London: Longman, Brown, Green, and Longmans.

Franklin Commission. (2002). Mesmer, Franklin, and the Royal Commission [50th Anniversary Special Issue]. *International Journal of Clinical and Experimental Hypnosis, 50*(4).

Fromm, E., & Nash, M. R. (1997). *Psychoanalysis and hypnosis.* Madison, CT: International Universities Press, Inc.

Fuller, R. C. (1982). *Mesmerism and the American cure of souls.* Philadelphia: University of Pennsylvania Press.

Garry, M., & Polaschek, D. (2000). Imagination and memory. *Current Directions in Psychological Science, 9*, 6–10.

Gauld, A. (1992). *A history of hypnotism*. Cambridge, England: Cambridge University Press.

Gravitz, M. A. (1997). Early historical interactions between Mesmerism and Masonry. *American Journal of Clinical Hypnosis, 39*, 266–270.

Hilgard, E. R. (1977). *Divided consciousness: Multiple controls in human thought and action*. New York: Wiley.

Hull, C. L. (1933). *Hypnosis and suggestibility: An experimental approach*. New York: Appleton-Century-Crofts.

Janet, P. (1925). *Psychological healing: A historical and clinical study*. New York: Macmillan.

Kihlstrom, J. F. (1992). Hypnosis: A sesquicentennial essay. *International Journal of Clinical and Experimental Hypnosis, 40*, 301–314.

Kihlstrom, J. F. (1998). Dissociations and dissociation theory in hypnosis: Comment on Kirsch and Lynn. *Psychological Bulletin, 132*, 186–191.

Kihlstrom, J. F. (2003). The fox, the hedgehog, and hypnosis. *International Journal of Clinical & Experimental Hypnosis, 51*, 166–189.

Kirsch, I. (1994). Clinical hypnosis as a nondeceptive placebo: Empirically derived techniques. *American Journal of Clinical Hypnosis, 37*, 95–106.

Kirsch, I., & Lynn, S. J. (1995). The altered state of hypnosis: Changes in the theoretical landscape. *American Psychologist, 10*, 846.

Kirsch, I., & Lynn, S. J. (1997). Hypnotic involuntariness and the automaticity of everyday life. *American Journal of Clinical Hypnosis, 40*, 329–348.

Kirsch, I., & Lynn, S. J. (1999). The automaticity of behavior in clinical psychology. *American Psychologist, 54*, 504–575.

Lynn, S. J. (1997). Automaticity and hypnosis: A sociocognitive account. *International Journal of Clinical and Experimental Hypnosis, 45*, 239–250.

Lynn, S. J., & McConkey, K. M. (1998). *Truth in memory*. New York: Guilford Press.

Lynn, S. J., & Sivec, H. (1992). The hypnotizable subject as creative problem solving agent. In E. Fromm & M. Nash (Eds.), *Contemporary perspectives in hypnosis research* (pp. 292–333). New York: Guilford Press.

McConkey, K. M. (1991). The construction and resolution of experience and behavior in hypnosis. In S. J. Lynn & J. W. Rhue (Eds.), *Theories of hypnosis: Current models and perspectives* (pp. 542–563). New York: Guilford Press.

Mesmer, F. A. (1980). *Mesmerism: A translation of the original scientific and medical writings of F. A. Mesmer* (G. Block, Trans.). Los Altos, CA: W. Kaufmann.

Micale, M. (1985). The Salpêtrière in the age of Charcot: An institutional perspective on medical history in the late nineteenth century. *Journal of Contemporary History, 20*, 703–731.

Micale, M. (1995). *Approaching hysteria*. Princeton, NJ: Princeton University Press.

Midelfort, H. C. (2005). *Exorcism and enlightenment: Johann Joseph Gassner and the demons of eighteenth-century Germany.* New Haven, CT: Yale University Press.

Murray, H. A. (1938). *Explorations in personality: A clinical study of fifty men in college.* New York: Oxford University Press.

Nash, M. R. (ed.) (2002). Mesmer, Franklin, and the Royal Commission [50th Anniversary Special Issue]. *International Journal of Clinical and Experimental Hypnosis, 50*(4).

Orne, M. T. (1959). The nature of hypnosis: Artifact and essence. *Journal of Abnormal Psychology, 58,* 277–299.

Orne, M. T. (1979). On the simulating subject as a quasi-control group in hypnosis research: What, why, and how? In E. Fromm & R. Shor (Eds.), *Hypnosis: Developments in research and new perspectives* (2nd ed., pp. 519–565). Chicago: Aldine.

Pattie, F. A. (1937). The genuineness of hypnotically produced anesthesia of the skin. *American Journal of Psychology, 49,* 435–443.

Pattie, F. A. (1956). Mesmer's medical dissertation and its debt to Mead's *de imperio solis ac lunae. Journey of the History of Medicine and Allied Sciences, 11,* 275–287.

Pattie, F. (1994). *Mesmer and animal magnetism: A chapter in the history of medicine.* Hamilton, NY: Edmonston.

Pinnell, C. A., & Covino, N. A. (2000). Empirical findings on the use of hypnosis in medicine: A critical review. *International Journal of Clinical and Experimental Hypnosis, 48,* 170–194.

Pintar, J., & Lynn, S. J. (2008). *Hypnosis: A Brief history.* Oxford, England: Wiley-Blackwell.

Poyen, C. (1837). *Progress of animal magnetism in New England.* Boston: Weeks, Jordan, and Co.

Sarbin, T. R., & Coe, W. C. (1972). *Hypnosis: A social psychological analysis of influence communication.* New York: Holt, Rinehart & Winston.

Sheehan, P. W. (1991). Hypnosis, context, and commitment. In S. J. Lynn & J. W. Rhue (Eds.), *Theories of hypnosis: Current models and perspectives* (pp. 520–541). New York: Guilford Press.

Spanos, N. P. (1982). Hypnotic behavior: A cognitive, social psychological perspective. *Research Communication in Psychology, Psychiatry, & Behavior, 7,* 199–213.

Spanos, N. P. (1991). A sociocognitive approach to hypnosis. In S. J. Lynn & J. W. Rhue (Eds.), *Theories of hypnosis: Current models and perspectives* (pp. 324–361). New York: Guilford Press.

Spanos, N. P., & Chaves, J. F. (1989). *Hypnosis: The cognitive–behavioral perspective.* Amherst, NY: Prometheus Books.

Spanos, N. P., & Chaves, J. F. (1991). History and historiography of hypnosis. In S. J. Lynn & J. W. Rhue (Eds.), *Theories of hypnosis: Current models and perspectives* (pp. 43–92). New York: Guilford Press.

Taves, A. (1999). *Fits, trances, and visions: Experiencing religion and explaining experience from Wesley to James.* Princeton, NJ: Princeton University Press.

Wagstaff, G. F. (2001). Different approaches to hypnosis. *Psychology Review, 7,* 2–5.

White, R. W. (1941). A preface to a theory of hypnotism. *Journal of Abnormal and Social Psychology, 36,* 477–505.

Winter, A. (1998). *Mesmerized: Powers of mind in Victorian Britain.* Chicago: University of Chicago Press.

Woody, E. Z., & Bowers, K. S. (1994). A frontal assault on dissociated control. In S. J. Lynn & J. W. Rhue (Eds.), *Dissociation: Clinical and theoretical perspectives* (pp. 52–79). New York: Guilford Press.

Woody, E., & Farvolden, P. (1998). Dissociation in hypnosis and frontal executive function. *American Journal of Clinical Hypnosis, 40,* 206–215.

3

HYPNOTIZABILITY MATTERS: THE WHAT, WHY, AND HOW OF MEASUREMENT

AMANDA J. BARNIER AND JAMES R. COUNCIL

Although assessment sets clinical psychology apart from other mental health professions, virtually no attention has been given to the use of hypnotizability scales in clinical assessment. Out of 19 chapters in the *Casebook of Clinical Hypnosis* (Lynn, Kirsch, & Rhue, 1996), for example, only the chapters by Spiegel, Barabasz, and Barabasz and by Horevitz reported a formal hypnotizability assessment. Similarly, a survey by Barnier and McConkey (2004) of experimental and clinical empirical articles published in the *International Journal of Clinical and Experimental Hypnosis* from 1992 to 2003 revealed that clinical researchers were much less likely to use formal assessment than laboratory researchers; 82% of published articles that did not report a formal hypnotizability measure involved clinical research. Finally, a survey of practitioners by Cohen (1989) indicated that of those who used hypnosis, less than 10% routinely assessed hypnotizability with standardized tests. These data are disappointing, given the clinical significance of hypnotizability. As we contend in this chapter, the initial assessment is critical to achieving success in hypnotherapy.

If practitioners were aware of the clinical significance of hypnotizability, they might be more likely to assess this important individual difference. Hypnosis scales are relatively quick and easy to administer, score, and interpret, and require little training to administer. Their reliabilities are as good as those of any other psychological measure, including IQ tests. Their validity is also good; hypnotizability tests measure the tasks and experiences traditionally associated with the domain of hypnosis. The availability of psychometrically sound measures of hypnotizability has permitted an impressive body of research and the general recognition that hypnosis is a valid and important area of scientific inquiry.

Individual differences in hypnotizability are approximately normally distributed in the population (i.e., as indexed by large norming samples of hypnotizability measures; for a review, see Barnier & McConkey, 2004) and are temporally stable. Most important, these differences are diagnostically useful. For instance, it is widely accepted that high hypnotizability is virtually essential for a diagnosis of dissociative identity disorder (American Psychiatric Association, 1994; Frischholz & Braun, 1991; see also chap. 17, this volume). Hypnotic suggestibility has been shown to relate to other psychiatric syndromes as well, including eating disorders and phobias (e.g., Crawford & Barabasz, 1993; Pettinati, Horne, & Staats, 1985). Hypnosis scales also predict a number of clinically meaningful variables, including the effectiveness of hypnotherapy with such disorders as obsessive–compulsive disorder, obesity, and phobias (Kirsch, Montgomery, & Saperstein, 1995), as well as the instantiation of false memories following leading suggestions (Barnier & McConkey, 1992). Even when hypnosis is not used in treatment, hypnotizability scores may relate significantly to therapy outcomes. Hypnotic assessment can thus provide valuable clinical observations, experiences, and intuitions for both the client and therapist. It allows the therapist to observe an individual's responses to hypnosis under standard conditions and allows clients to explore a range of hypnotic experiences.

In this chapter we (a) summarize the development of standardized hypnotizability scales and highlight the features of current scales; (b) review the relationship between hypnotizability, psychopathology, and treatment; and (c) provide guidance to practitioners for incorporating hypnotizability measures into their clinical work. In other words, in this chapter we cover the what, why, and how of hypnotizability assessment.

WHAT IS HYPNOTIZABILITY ASSESSMENT?

Hypnosis has been defined as

A process in which one person, designated the *hypnotist*, offers suggestions to another person, designated the *subject*, for imaginative experiences entailing alterations in perception, memory, and action. In the classic case, these experiences are associated with a degree of subjective conviction bordering on delusion and an experienced involuntariness bordering on compulsion. As such, the phenomena of hypnosis reflect alterations in consciousness that take place in the context of a social interaction. (Kihlstrom, 2008, p. 21)

Hypnotizability has been defined as "the capacity to produce those effects generally considered to be 'hypnotic'" (Weitzenhoffer, 1997, p. 128). So the best way to measure it is to test whether people actually show hypnotic effects, by taking "samples of hypnotic performance under standard conditions of induction and testing" (Hilgard, 1965, p. 69). Thus, if a clinician wishes to assess hypnotic ability, he or she must do hypnosis. Almost all hypnotizability measures involve administering a standard induction procedure, suggesting a number of hypnotic experiences, and scoring responses according to predetermined pass/fail criteria. Although hypnotizability can be operationally defined simply as the total score on such a measure, this score can provide clinically valuable information about the person. (For a discussion of the identification and characteristics of the highly hypnotizable person, see Barnier & McConkey, 2004.)

The Path to Modern Hypnotizability Measurement

Mesmer and his students described the stages of hypnosis and recognized that relatively few people could reach the deepest stages (Edmonston, 1986). As animal magnetism gave way to neurophysiology in 19th-century explanations of hypnosis, conceptions of hypnosis took on a strong medical orientation. In particular, research and practice by such prominent figures as James Braid and Jean-Martin Charcot resulted in a catalog of hypnotic phenomena that mimicked the symptoms of neurological disorders (see chap. 2, this volume). These "symptoms" were believed to mark successive stages of hypnosis and were used informally to gauge individual differences in hypnotizability. They were later institutionalized in formal measures and remain with us as, for instance, the amnesia, anosmia, catalepsy, and hallucination items on the Stanford scales and other major contemporary measures (Spanos & Chaves, 1991).

19th-Century Measures

The idea that hypnosis occurs in successive stages, combined with Braid's concept of hypnosis as sleep, paved the way for early scales that rated levels of hypnotic depth (Hilgard, Weitzenhoffer, Landes, & Moore, 1961). Around 1890, Liebeault and Bernheim developed scales that rated progressive levels of hypnotic "depth." These were based on the assumption that suggestions of varying difficulty could discriminate between people who are able to achieve different levels of hypnotic depth (Weitzenhoffer, 1953). These scales lacked standard procedures, and ratings tended to be based on classes of events rather than on specific tests. Nevertheless, a number of large samples yielded distributions of hypnotic responsivity that are in fairly good agreement with findings from modern scales (Hilgard et al., 1961).

20th-Century Measures

The next significant developments occurred in the 1930s and 1940s, when a number of scales were published. The most important were scales by Davis and Husband (1931); Barry, MacKinnon, and Murray (1931); and Friedlander and Sarbin (1938). The Davis-Husband Scale (Davis & Husband) was practical and covered a wide range of hypnotic behaviors. However, it did not meet even minimal standards for scientific acceptability (Barber, 1969; Weitzenhoffer, 1953). Like its 19th-century predecessors, this scale assigned ratings of hypnotic depth on the basis of the appearance of classes of responses thought to indicate various levels of hypnotic depth. Although the Davis-Husband Scale was used in many studies of hypnotizability, it had no standard induction procedure, nor did it specify standard test suggestions or explicit criteria to determine whether suggestions were passed or failed. The Friedlander-Sarbin Scale combined features of both the Davis-Husband Scale and a six-item scale by Barry et al.. The Friedlander-Sarbin Scale was much better for research because it used standard procedures, items, and scoring. These included a scripted-out induction procedure and a specific set of test suggestions with standardized scoring criteria (Friedlander & Sarbin). The researcher scored each item as it was presented.

The Stanford Scales

In 1957, Ernest Hilgard, Andre Weitzenhoffer, and their colleagues at Stanford University began a major study of hypnotic responsivity that made Stanford one of the foremost centers for hypnosis research in the world. Initially, they used a modification of the Friedlander-Sarbin Scale. However, it soon became evident that they needed a new measure because the Friedlander-Sarbin scale yielded a bimodal distribution and too many extremely low scores (Hilgard et al., 1961).

Stanford Hypnotic Susceptibility Scale, Forms A and B. Weitzenhoffer and Hilgard refined and expanded the Friedlander-Sarbin Scale, adding easier items to spread the distribution of scores. They also simplified the scoring. The result was the Stanford Hypnotic Susceptibility Scale, Forms A and B (SHSS:A and B; Weitzenhoffer & Hilgard, 1959). Although these scales are no longer widely used (see Barnier & McConkey, 2004), two of the most important and widely used current scales are derived from the SHSS:A and B and share many items: the Stanford Hypnotic Susceptibility Scale, Form C (SHSS:C; Weitzenhoffer & Hilgard, 1962) and the Harvard Group Scale of Hypnotic Susceptibility, Form A (HGSHS:A; Shor & Orne, 1962).

Forms A and B of the SHSS are essentially equivalent, with only slight changes in wording and procedure. The two alternate forms allow repeated measurement without contamination from practice effects. The scales begin with a test of waking suggestibility—a suggestion before the hypnotic induction for the participant to experience his or her body as swaying and falling—which serves to introduce the experience of responding to suggestions. The hypnotic induction procedure consists of repeated suggestions for relaxation, drowsiness, and eye closure. The induction is read verbatim, and the experimenter is not allowed to deviate from the scripted procedure. Following the script is extremely important even if it seems constrictive, because standard procedures are essential for reliable measurement.

Participants score one point if they pass the waking suggestibility item and one point if they close their eyes before a direct command to do so during the induction. After the induction, the hypnotist administers 10 additional suggestions: (a) hand lowering, in which the hypnotist asks the participant to hold out his or her arm and suggests that the arm is becoming heavier and heavier (ideomotor); (b) arm immobilization, in which the hypnotist suggests that the participant's arm is too heavy to move and challenges him or her to lift it (challenge); (c) finger lock, in which the hypnotist asks the participant to interlock his or her fingers, suggests that they cannot be pulled apart, and challenges him or her to try (challenge); (d) arm rigidity, in which the hypnotists asks the participant to extend his or her arm, suggests that it cannot bend, and challenges him or her to bend the arm (challenge); (e) moving hands, in which the hypnotist asks the participant to hold his or her arms in front of them 12 inches apart and suggests that the hands will move together (ideomotor); (f) verbal inhibition, in which the hypnotist suggests that the participant cannot say his or her name and challenges them to try (challenge); (g) hallucination, in which the hypnotist suggests that a fly is buzzing around the participant (cognitive–delusory); (h) eye catalepsy, in which the hypnotist suggests that the participant's eyes are tightly closed and challenges him or her to open them (challenge); (i) posthypnotic suggestion, in which the hypnotist suggests that after hypnosis the participant will perform a behavioral act when he or she hears a cue (ideomotor/cognitive–delusory); and (j) posthypnotic amnesia, in which the hypnotist suggests that after hypnosis the participant will be unable to remember the events of hypnosis (cognitive–delusory).

As noted in this list, these suggestions are of three main types: *ideomotor suggestions*, which involve ideas becoming actions; *challenge suggestions*, which suggest a state of affairs and then invite the participant to challenge it; and *cognitive–delusory suggestions*, which involve alterations in perception, emotion, action, or memory. These types are consistent with factor analyses of hypnotizability measures (e.g., Balthazard & Woody, 1985; Woody, Barnier, & McConkey, 2005). Easy and difficult items are interspersed so that participants can be tested on a wide range of responses without experiencing too many consecutive failures. Each item is scored as pass (1 point) or fail (0 points) according to defined criteria. For example, the hand-lowering item is passed if the participant's arm lowers by at least 6 inches at the end of 10 seconds. Together, the scores for the 12 items are summed to generate a total score ranging from 0 to 12.

Hilgard's (1965) norms indicate slightly skewed distributions of scores on the SHSS:A and B, with many more participants scoring at the low end of the range than at other levels. Hilgard's data also suggest that the distribution is bimodal, with the smaller mode among the more highly responsive participants. Internal consistency and test–retest reliability, even after long intervals, appear to be good (Hilgard, 1965; Piccione, Hilgard, & Zimbardo, 1989).

Stanford Hypnotic Susceptibility Scale, Form C. The content of the SHSS:A and B consists predominantly of simple ideomotor and challenge items, so these scales are not especially sensitive to differences among the most responsive participants (Hilgard, 1965; Perry, Nadon, & Button, 1992; Woody, Barnier, & McConkey, 2005). The Stanford group addressed this shortcoming by developing the SHSS:C (Weitzenhoffer & Hilgard, 1962). Although the SHSS:C retains the same format and number of items as the SHSS:A and B, it includes new, more difficult, cognitive–delusory items that assess the participant's ability to experience distortions of perception and memory during hypnosis. The SHSS:C also differs from the SHSS:A and B in presenting the items in approximate order of increasing difficulty, as a *graded difficulty* or *achievement after practice* scale (Hilgard, 1965; see also Barnier & McConkey, 2004).

The SHSS:C retains the following six items from the SHSS:A: hand lowering, moving hands apart, mosquito hallucination, arm rigidity, arm immobilization, and posthypnotic amnesia. The six new items include the following: (a) taste hallucination, in which the hypnotist suggests that the participant will experience a sweet taste and then a sour taste in his or her mouth (cognitive–delusory); (b) dream, in which the hypnotist suggests that for the next few minutes the participant will have a "dream" about hypnosis (cognitive–delusory); (c) age regression, in which the hypnotist suggests that the participant is going back in time to an experience in school at about 10 years of age and then to an earlier experience at about 7 years of age (cognitive–delusory); (d) anosmia to ammonia, in which the hypnotist suggests that the participant can no longer smell and challenges him or her to take a sniff from a bottle of undiluted ammonia (cognitive–delusory); (e) hallucinated voice, in which the hypnotist suggests that the participant will be asked several questions over a (nonexistent) intercom by a (nonexistent) person in the next room (cognitive–delusory); and (f) negative visual hallucination, in which the hypnotist places three small boxes on a table in front of the participant, suggests that there are only two boxes, and asks the participant to open his or her eyes and to describe the boxes he or she sees (cognitive–delusory; see the published scales for more details of administration and scoring; see also, Barnier & McConkey, 2004).

Normative data reported by Hilgard (1965) indicated that the SHSS:C is internally consistent (K-R 20 = .85) and correlates well with the SHSS:A ($r = .72$). The addition of the new cognitive–delusory items makes the scale more difficult than the SHSS:A. Whereas 10% of participants obtain scores of 11 or 12 on the SHSS:A, only 5% obtain such high scores on the SHSS:C (Hilgard, 1965). Because, compared with the HGSHS:A, the SHSS:C has a greater number of the more difficult, cognitive items thought to be characteristic of only highly hypnotizable people, the SHSS:C is a particularly good scale for identifying and/or confirming high hypnotic ability. The greater cognitive content also seems to make the SHSS:C correlate more highly with personality questionnaires than do other hypnosis scales (Balthazard & Woody, 1992; Hilgard, 1978–1979). Although the SHSS:C is currently out of print, it can be downloaded from John Kihlstrom's Web site at the University of California, Berkeley (http://socrates.berkeley.edu/~kihlstrm/hypnosis_research.htm).

Variations on the Stanford Theme

The Stanford scales have been enormously influential because of their superior psychometric characteristics. However, the scales were primarily designed for research use with individual participants, and they have been adapted to various populations and applications. The best-known adaptation is the Harvard Group Scale of Hypnotic Susceptibility, Form A (Shor & Orne, 1962). Other variations include brief scales for use in clinical settings, scales designed to yield more differentiated descriptions of hypnotic ability, and scales for children.

Group Adaptations. The HGSHS:A (Shor & Orne, 1962), a group adaptation of the SHSS:A, was developed at Harvard University by Ronald Shor and Emily Carota Orne. It can be administered to many participants in a single session, which allows more efficient data collection for researchers. After the 12 test suggestions have been administered and hypnosis is terminated, participants report on their behavioral responses in a test booklet using a forced-choice method. Psychometrically, the HGSHS:A is on a par with the SHSS:A (Hilgard, 1965). Perry et al. (1992) cautioned that it is best used as a screening device because it may misclassify a participant's level of hypnotic responsivity. International norms for the HGSHS:A (i.e., American, Australian, Canadian, Danish, Finnish, German, Italian, and Spanish) are available and indicate that the scores are in good agreement across cultural and language groups (for a review, see Barnier & McConkey, 2004). These data also indicate no evidence of bimodality and a much less positive skew than Hilgard's (1965) norms for the SHSS:A, as noted previously. It is likely that changes in attitudes and preconceptions about hypnosis have influenced distributions of scores over the past 20 to 30 years. Although the HGSHS is currently out of print, a copy can be downloaded from John Kihlstrom's Web site at the University of California, Berkeley (http://socrates.berkeley.edu/~kihlstrm/hypnosis_research.htm).

Another group scale, the *Waterloo-Stanford Group C* (WSGC; Bowers, 1993, 1998), is an adaptation of the SHSS:C. It has been fully documented in the two cited articles, including copies of the manual and response booklet included in Bowers (1998). Normative data and a comparison with the SHSS:C were presented by Bowers (1993). The WSGC is similar to the SHSS:C, although it is self-scoring and some items have been adapted for easier group presentation. The normative and comparative data are in good agreement with the SHSS:C.

Brief Clinical Scales. Two major problems with using the Stanford scales clinically are the time required for administration and the need to make arm and hand movements while in a seated position. In addition, challenge suggestions may lead to failure experiences; that is, if participants fail to overcome the suggestion, they may feel out of control; if they do overcome the suggestion, they have failed to respond successfully (see Frankel, 1978–1979).

The *Stanford Hypnotic Clinical Scale for Adults* (SHCS:A; Morgan & Hilgard, 1978–1979a) is a brief scale that conforms closely to the standard Stanford scale format, although it addresses the problems noted previously. The correlation with the SHSS:C is $r = .72$. The SHCS:A requires 20 minutes to administer and is suitable for patients with limited movement. After a standard induction, five test suggestions modified from the SHSS:A and B and the SHSS:C are administered. These items were chosen to maximize the likelihood of having successful hypnotic experiences and for their potential to elicit clinically useful information. *Moving hands together* is an easy ideomotor item that introduces the patient to the idea of responding to suggestions. The *dream* item is a relatively easy cognitive–delusory item that can reveal a variety of contents but is especially useful for determining a patient's attitude toward hypnosis. *Age regression*, another cognitive–delusory item, may reveal important information about a patient's childhood but should be used with caution if patients have experienced traumatic childhood events. The *posthypnotic suggestion* (i.e., clearing the throat or coughing), a combination ideomotor/cognitive–delusory item, indicates whether the patient can continue to respond to suggestions after formal hypnosis is terminated. Finally, *posthypnotic amnesia*, a cognitive–delusory item, may yield useful information for working with both memory and pain. Barnier and McConkey's (2004) survey indicated that when a hypnotizability scale was used in clinical research, the SHCS:A was the scale of choice. The SHCS:A can be found in its entirety in Hilgard and Hilgard (1975).

Another clinical scale from the Stanford group is the *Stanford Hypnotic Arm Levitation and Test* (SHALIT; Hilgard, Crawford, & Wert, 1979). This is not truly a Stanford scale because it relies on only one ideomotor suggestion, arm levitation. However, the scale correlates significantly with both the SHSS:A ($r = .63$) and the SHSS:C ($r = .52$). Because the SHALIT takes only 6 minutes to administer, it may be useful in limited circumstances as a brief screening measure. In addition to objective scoring by the experimenter, participants self-report on both their hypnotic depth and hypnotic involuntariness.

In addition to the brief Stanford variations, other brief standardized hypnosis scales have been developed for use in both clinical and research settings. We review these when we consider hypnosis scales derived from different orientations.

Hypnotic Profile Scales. To answer the need for a scale to differentially assess the abilities of good hypnotic subjects, Weitzenhoffer and Hilgard (1963, 1967) developed the *Stanford Profile Scales of Hypnotic Susceptibility, Forms I and II* (SPS:I and II). Both forms are administered for a complete assessment. In contrast to the other Stanford scales, the purpose is not to obtain a single global score but rather a profile of hypnotic abilities. The six major subscales indicate performance on agnosia and cognitive distortions, positive hallucinations, negative hallucinations, dreams and regressions, amnesia and posthypnotic compulsion, and loss of motor control. Norms for these scales were based on high scorers from a sample screened on the SHSS:A. Unfortunately, the SPS:I and II have not been used widely or systematically, even though they sensitively measure abilities that are potentially of great clinical utility (McConkey & Barnier, 2004).

Children's Scales. Two extensions of the Stanford scales are designed for use with children and adolescents. The Children's Hypnotic Susceptibility Scale (London, 1963) uses a wide range of items taken from the SHSS:A and B as well as from the SPS:I and II. The scale has two parts, progressing from easier ideomotor and challenge items in Part I to more difficult cognitive-delusory items in Part II. There are two forms: one for children (ages 5–12 years) and one for adolescents (ages 13–16 years). The two forms are identical in content but differ by using age-appropriate wording.

Like the adult version, the *Stanford Hypnotic Clinical Scale for Children, Forms A and B* (SHCS:C; Morgan & Hilgard, 1978–1979b) is a brief scale with clinically useful content. Form B is suitable for younger children, 4 to 8 years. With younger or anxious participants, the scale can be administered with eyes open and imagination instructions rather than a hypnotic induction. It correlates well ($r = .67$) with an adaptation of the SHSS:A for children.

Scales Reflecting Other Theoretical Orientations

Although the Stanford scales were intended to be theoretically neutral, they still reflect Hilgard's (1974, 1991) theoretical framework. Thus, they include an induction as an integral component and suggestions for "classic" hypnotic phenomena. Suggestions also became increasingly cognitive with the SHSS:C reflecting Hilgard's developing view of hypnosis as essentially dissociative (Hilgard, 1973, 1974). Other researchers and clinicians have developed alternative measures of hypnotizability. We review these scales next.

Barber Suggestibility Scale. The Barber Suggestibility Scale (BSS; Barber, 1965) was designed from a strongly behavioral perspective to focus on the antecedents, behaviors, and consequences of hypnotic suggestions. It was designed mostly for research and can be administered with or without a hypnotic induction. The BSS consists of eight items (across the three item types): arm lowering (ideomotor), arm levitation (ideomotor), hand lock (challenge), thirst hallucination (cognitive–delusory), verbal inhibition (challenge), body immobility (challenge), posthypnotic-like response (ideomotor/cognitive–delusory), and selective amnesia (cognitive–delusory). The experimenter scores the test responses on the basis of both observation of objective behavior and an inquiry about subjective experiences. Although the BSS is no longer widely used (Barnier & McConkey, 2004), it is briefer than the Stanford scales (taking less than half an hour to administer and score) and has good reliability and validity. Barber (1965) provided detailed norms and psychometric data on the BSS. Test–retest correlations are in the .80s, and internal consistencies are in the same range under both waking and hypnotic induction conditions. The BSS can be found in its entirety in Barber (1969).

Carleton University Responsiveness to Suggestion Scale. The Carleton University Responsiveness to Suggestion Scale (CURSS; Spanos, Radtke, Hodgins, Bertrand, Stam, & Dubreuil, 1983) was developed from a cognitive–behavioral perspective as an alternative to the Stanford scales. This scale takes less than 15 minutes to administer and can be used with either groups or individuals. The seven test suggestions (across the three item types) are arm rising (ideomotor), arms moving apart (ideomotor), arm catalepsy (challenge), arm immobility (challenge), auditory hallucination (cognitive–delusory), visual hallucination (cognitive–delusory), and amnesia (cognitive–delusory). Like the HGSHS:A, the CURSS is self-scored by participants after the hypnotic experience. The CURSS has a unique scoring system, which includes both overt and subjective responses. The objective score (CURSS:0) is the number of suggestions to which the participant makes an overt behavioral response. The subjective score (CURSS:S) is a self-report rating on a 4-point scale of the degree to which the participant experienced each suggestion. Objective involuntariness (CURSS:0I) combines ratings of passing each suggestion behaviorally and experiencing the behavior as occurring involuntarily. Comparing these scores provides an indication of the degree to which participants voluntarily complied with the suggestions, in contrast to genuinely experiencing the suggested effects.

The CURSS has good reliability and relates satisfactorily to other standardized hypnosis scales (Spanos et al., 1983; Spanos, Radtke, Hodgins, Stam, & Bertrand, 1983). However, the scores have a severe positive skew with as many participants scoring in the low range as in the medium and high combined. Unfortunately, the CURSS remains unpublished, and thus it has been used far less often than the Stanford scales (Barnier & McConkey, 2004).

Creative Imagination Scale. The Creative Imagination Scale (CIS; Barber & Wilson, 1978–1979; Wilson & Barber, 1978) was developed by Barber as a permissive alternative to the more authoritarian BSS and Stanford scales. It is appropriate for both clinical and research applications. The CIS does not use a hypnotic induction procedure, although it can be used with one. Instead, it uses guided imagination instructions to help participants experience the suggested effects. The 10 suggestions (across the three item types) include experiences of arm heaviness (ideomotor), hand levitation (ideomotor), finger anesthesia (cognitive–delusory), water hallucination (i.e., imagining drinking water; cognitive-delusory), olfactory-gustatory hallucination (cognitive–delusory), music hallucination (cognitive–delusory), temperature hallucination (i.e., hand warming; cognitive–delusory), time distortion (cognitive–delusory), age regression (cognitive–delusory), and mind–body relaxation (ideomotor/cognitive–delusory). After the last suggestion, participants use Likert scales to compare each suggested experience with a similar real experience. The CIS has acceptable reliability (test–retest $r = .82$) and correlates significantly with the BSS, HGSHS:A, SHSS:C, and measures of imaginative ability (Council, Kirsch, Vickery, & Carlson, 1983). Because the CIS is nonauthoritarian and presents suggestions as experiences under the participant's control, it may be particularly useful for work with persons who are apprehensive about hypnosis or fearful of losing control.

Diagnostic Rating Scale. The Diagnostic Rating Scale (DRS; Orne & O'Connell, 1967) differs from all the scales discussed thus far in that, like the earlier Davis-Husband Scale, the DRS estimates individuals' hypnotizability on the basis of their response to a flexible array rather than to a standardized set of hypnotic suggestions. Also, rather than using strict pass/fail criteria, the DRS relies on clinical observations of responses. Although formal normative and standardization information is not available for this scale, Hilgard (1978–1979) provided approximate norms. The DRS has not been widely used or systematically investigated (Barnier & McConkey, 2004) perhaps because the scale's flexible administration requires a trained researcher or clinician who can make judgments about which hypnotic suggestions to include and then appropriately interpret the resulting responses. However, for a trained clinician, the DRS is a powerful way to index a person's hypnotic profile across a range of clinically relevant suggestions (McConkey & Barnier, 2004).

Hypnotic Induction Profile. The Hypnotic Induction Profile (HIP; Spiegel & Spiegel, 1978) was developed in a clinical setting for clinical applications, although its authors have always stressed the importance of empirical validation. It takes less than 10 minutes to administer but is said to be a rich source of clinically relevant information. The most unique and controversial aspect of the HIP is its *eye-roll test*, hypothesized to be a physiological indicator of hypnotizability (Spiegel & Spiegel, 1978). The eye-roll score is based on how high a participant can roll his or her eyes upward and is measured by the amount of sclera visible between the bottom of the iris and the lower eyelid. Although research findings are mixed, most find no relationship between the eye roll and other measures of hypnotizability (Perry et al., 1992). The rest of the HIP is scored on the basis of responses to a procedure that combines a hypnotic induction and the single ideomotor item, arm levitation. Degree of arm levitation is objectively scored and combined with other ratings, including posthypnotic arm levitation and subjective ratings obtained after hypnosis. Interrater reliability, internal consistency, and test–retest reliabilities of the induction score are equivalent to those of other standard scales (Spiegel & Spiegel). HIP scores (combining eye roll and arm levitation) correlate at low but significant levels with both the SHSS:A and SHSS:C (Perry et al.; Sheehan & McConkey, 1982). Proponents of the HIP report that it has great clinical utility and can be administered with minimal obtrusiveness in clinical settings. Herbert and David Spiegel's (1978) volume *Trance and Treatment* presents a detailed discussion of the HIP and its integration into clinical practice.

From this review it should be clear that the field of hypnosis offers a broad range of hypnotizability measures to the practitioner: long or short, for adults or for children, more standardized or more tailored, and appropriate across cultures and languages. Most have excellent psychometric properties. In the next section, we discuss the clinical significance of hypnotizability.

WHY SHOULD HYPNOTIZABILITY BE ASSESSED?

In this section, we discuss how hypnotizability relates to specific disorders and to the outcomes of both hypnotic and nonhypnotic treatments.

Hypnotizability and Psychopathology

The clinical literature indicates that hypnotizability may be related to various psychopathologies. In particular, extreme high hypnotizability, or suggestibility, has been seen as a core component of personality disorders and other chronic conditions. Although modern theory and research have depathologized hypnotizability, researchers who study clinical samples (e.g., Spiegel & Spiegel, 1978), still report that high hypnotizability is associated with a set of core personality characteristics often associated with psychopathology.

The Grade 5 Syndrome

The label *Grade 5* derives from the highest score (5) that one can obtain on the HIP (Spiegel, 1974; Spiegel & Spiegel, 1978). These individuals profoundly experience the classic hypnotic phenomena when formally assessed. In everyday life, Grade 5 individuals are extremely trusting, uncritical, illogical, extremely responsive to external forces, have dissociative tendencies that make them feel out of control of their behavior, and are easily manipulated and drawn into destructive relationships. According to Spiegel and Spiegel (1978), Grade 5 individuals present clinically with classic hysterical symptoms, including conversion reactions, dissociative episodes, and inappropriate sexual behavior.

The Fantasy-Prone Personality

On the basis of interviews with a sample of highly hypnotizable persons, Wilson and Barber (1981) described a personality syndrome they labeled *fantasy-proneness*. These individuals spend a majority of their time daydreaming and fantasizing, and their fantasies are extremely vivid, "as real as real." Although Wilson and Barber did not report significant psychopathology in their fantasy-prone group, Rhue and Lynn (1987) found clear signs of maladjustment in another sample of high fantasizers. They obtained mean scores on MMPI scales 8 (Schizophrenia) and 9 (Hypomania) that were clinically elevated and significantly higher than those of control participants. A conservative interpretation of these results suggests that fantasy proneness is associated with unconventional thinking, willingness to report unusual experiences, and strong fantasy involvements. Rhue and Lynn also identified a subset of fantasizers whose profiles and psychiatric histories indicated significant maladjustment, and who reported that they were likely to have been physically abused during childhood. High fantasizers also report having significantly more guilty–dysphoric daydreams than medium and low fantasizers (Council & Huff, 1990), indicating that the content of fantasy-prone persons' daydreams may not be as uniformly gratifying as Wilson and Barber (1981) suggested.

The Amnesia-Prone Personality

Barrett (1996) and Barber (1999) described another type of highly hypnotizable person. *Amnesia-prone* individuals are prone to exhibit spontaneous posthypnotic amnesia and to respond profoundly to suggested posthypnotic amnesia. In contrast to the other types, they require a lengthy hypnotic induction. Once hypnotized, although highly responsive to suggestions, they appear lethargic and subdued. When hypnosis is terminated, these people are confused, drowsy, and cannot remember their experiences during hypnosis. The hypnotic experiences of amnesia-prone persons are qualitatively different as well. Although fantasy-prone individuals remember their hallucinatory experiences and can accept that they were suggested effects, amnesia-prone individuals do not remember suggestions to hallucinate and typically believe that their hallucinations were real events (Barber, 1999; Barrett, 1996). They are also highly responsive to suggested psychosomatic effects, both in and out of hypnosis.

The characteristics of amnesia-prone individuals have great clinical significance. They are not fantasizers; their daydreams and imaginings are mundane, constricted, and soon forgotten (Barber, 1999). They are quite forgetful in general, failing to remember even salient recent events. In addition, they commonly report having *blank states*, in which they are unaware of any mental contents or processes. In general, these individuals were physically and/or sexually abused as children (Barber, 1999).

Hypnotizability and Specific Syndromes

The Diagnostic and Statistical Manual of Mental Disorders (4th ed.; *DSM–IV*; American Psychiatric Association, 1994) relates high hypnotizability to several diagnostic categories: Dissociative Amnesia, Dissociative Fugue, Dissociative Identity Disorder, and Depersonalization Disorder. The *DSM–IV* also states that hypnosis can be useful in differentiating conversion disorder from malingering, because hypnosis will relieve symptoms for patients with conversion disorder but not for malingerers.

It should also be noted that excellent hypnotic subjects are at risk of misdiagnosis. Studies of the fantasy-prone personality (Lynn & Rhue, 1986; Wilson & Barber, 1981) and the Grade 5 syndrome (Spiegel, 1974) suggest that highly hypnotizable individuals may be at risk of misdiagnosis because of their experiences of vivid, involuntary hallucinations and reports of unusual thoughts and experiences. Their extreme vulnerability to social influence can even lead them to adopt the symptoms of other psychiatric disorders when institutionalized (Spiegel, 1974). In one study, Bliss, Larson, and Nakashima (1983) examined 45 psychiatric inpatients reported to have auditory hallucinations, most of whom had been diagnosed with some form of schizophrenia; 60% were found to be excellent hypnotic subjects.

Dissociative Identity Disorder

Dissociative identity disorder (DID), previously referred to as multiple personality disorder, is strongly identified with high hypnotizability. Hypnosis has figured prominently in the diagnosis and treatment of well-known cases of multiple personality, including those of Sally Beauchamp (Prince, 1906) and Eve (Thigpen & Cleckley, 1957). Nevertheless, diagnosing dissociative disorders is tricky. Genuine DID cases may be misdiagnosed as other disorders, particularly schizophrenia, because these excellent hypnotic subjects are prone to displaying hallucinations, delusions, and bizarre behaviors (Bliss, 1983, 1986; Bliss et al., 1983). Hypnosis may be quite useful in the differential diagnosis of DID. Typically, patients with DID score among the top 10% on standardized measures of hypnotizability, significantly higher than comparison groups (Bliss, 1983, 1986; Frischholz & Braun, 1991). Frischholz and Braun reported that, on the SHSS:C amnesia item, individuals with DID recalled fewer items during amnesia and remembered more items after the reversibility cue was administered than did those without DID and patients with other diagnoses.

Posttraumatic Stress Disorder

Dissociation and hypnotizability are important components of posttraumatic stress disorder (PTSD). *DSM–IV* criteria for PTSD include vivid reexperiencing of traumatic events, amnesia, depersonalization, and emotional numbing. Spiegel, Hunt, and Dondershine (1988) and Stutman and Bliss (1985) found that Vietnam veterans diagnosed with PTSD were significantly more hypnotizable than veterans without PTSD or psychiatric patients with other diagnoses. Stutman and Bliss raised a "chicken or the egg" question about this relationship: Does trauma enhance hypnotizability, or does high hypnotizability predispose a person to develop PTSD after a traumatic experience? Unfortunately, no prospective studies have been conducted to determine whether high hypnotizability is a risk factor for PTSD. Butler, Duran, Jasiukaitis, Koopman, and Spiegel (1996) proposed a diathesis–stress model involving two continuous factors, hypnotizability and traumatic experience. Whereas a severe traumatic experience, such as rape, could trigger PTSD symptoms in almost anyone, a highly hypnotizable person could develop posttraumatic symptomatology after a much less intense experience.

Phobias

In a seminal paper, Frankel and Orne (1976) related hypnotizability to phobic behavior; phobic patients were significantly more hypnotizable than a control sample, and those with multiple phobias were more hypnotizable than those with a single phobia. The finding of higher hypnotizability in individuals with phobias has been replicated in five studies (Foenander, Burrows, Gerschman, & Horne, 1980; Gerschman, Burrows, & Reade, 1987; Gerschman, Burrows, Reade, & Foenander, 1979; John, Hollander, & Perry, 1983; Kelly, 1984). Gerschman et al. (1987) and Kelly, Brown, and

Crawford (1986), studying a nonclinical sample of college women, supported the finding that individuals with multiple phobias were more hypnotizable and found that reporting intense fears on a fear survey was related to high hypnotizability. Crawford and Barabasz (1993) explained the relationship between hypnotizability and phobias in terms of a highly hypnotizable person's tendency to become intensely absorbed in memories of an initial fearful experience, resulting in phobic avoidance. On the basis of Hilgard's (1974, 1991) neodissociation theory, Crawford and Barabasz also suggested that memories of the fear could be dissociated from awareness, resulting in behavior that seems to exist without self-control or awareness.

Eating Disorders

Pettinati, Horne, and Staats (1985) reported that female psychiatric patients with bulimia nervosa were highly hypnotizable, but those with anorexia nervosa scored in the middle range. Barabasz (1991) also found that bulimic women and girls were significantly more hypnotizable than nonbulimic controls. Pettinati et al. reported a trend in the anorexic group for purgers (i.e., those who controlled their weight through vomiting or laxatives) to be more hypnotizable than abstainers (i.e., those who controlled their weight by refusing to eat). These results are consistent with clinical impressions that persons with bulimia are more apt to feel a loss of control over their behavior and that binging and purging may take place in a dissociated, hypnotic-like state. Likewise, Groth-Marnat and Schumaker (1990) found that hypnotizability was associated with negative attitudes toward eating and fear of becoming overweight. They interpreted these results as indicating that high hypnotizability may facilitate the adoption of extreme attitudes and perceptual distortions related to one's body.

Overall, clinical research indicates a variety of meaningful relationships between hypnotizability and various symptoms and disorders. In some cases, such as the Grade 5 syndrome (Spiegel, 1974), the relationships are largely based on clinical impressions and do not have strong empirical validation. However, other findings, such as the link between hypnotizability and dissociative disorders, phobias, and eating disorders, have been confirmed in multiple studies.

Hypnotizability and Treatment Outcomes

Hypnotizability relates not only to psychopathology but also to treatment outcomes. Most of the relevant research has focused on the outcomes of hypnotic interventions, but some studies have shown that hypnotizability can even predict the outcome of nonhypnotic therapeutic interventions. The strongest evidence that hypnotizability predicts successful treatment comes from research on hypnosis for pain relief. Ernest and Josephine Hilgard deserve much of the credit for exciting research interest in this area through their well-run laboratory and clinical studies. See their book, *Hypnosis in the Relief of Pain* (Hilgard & Hilgard, 1975), for a description of the research and applications. Subsequent research, reviewed by Brown (1992), has expanded their findings on acute pain to chronic pain, headache, and painful medical procedures.

Noting that hypnotizability predicts the outcome of hypnotic treatments for pain, warts, and asthma but not for cigarette smoking, Perry, Gelfand, and Marcovitch (1979) proposed that the degree of volition involved in a problem behavior, as well as the motivation for change, may account for the relative differences in the efficacy of hypnotherapy. Take, for instance, the differences between pain and smoking. Even though smoking has severe health consequences, the act of lighting up a cigarette is self-initiated and leads to an enjoyable experience. Many smokers are not motivated to quit. In contrast, the vast majority of people do not enjoy pain, do not seek or initiate painful experiences, and are highly motivated for the pain to stop. Whereas hypnotic interventions for pain and other nonvolitional disorders attempt to decrease the unpleasantness of an unwanted experience, hypnotic interventions for smoking attempt to decrease the pleasantness of a desired experience.

Wadden and Anderton's (1982) extensive review of the research literature supported Perry et al.'s (1979) proposal: Hypnotizability is significantly related to the success of hypnotic interventions for nonvoluntary afflictions such as pain, warts, and asthma but not for self-initiated problems such as addictions and overeating. A decade later, Brown (1992) came to a similar conclusion in his review of subsequent clinical hypnosis research and added more nonvolitional problems to the list of targets for hypnotic treatment. However, Brown also cited findings that hypnotizability may affect outcomes of interventions for volitional problems such as smoking and weight control. Although hypnotic ability seems unrelated, or at least significantly less related, to the outcome of hypnotic treatments for volitionally based disorders, this does not mean that hypnosis is ineffective for such problems. Kirsch, Montgomery, and Sapirstein (1995), in a meta-analysis of 18 studies, showed that adding hypnosis to cognitive–behavioral therapy (CBT) substantially enhanced treatment outcome.

Hypnotizability and Nonhypnotic Therapies

Although relatively few studies have examined how hypnotizability relates to the outcomes of nonhypnotic interventions, results indicate that assessing hypnotizability can be valuable even when nonhypnotic interventions are planned. Some of the first studies investigating this question found a correlation between hypnotic ability and pain reduction with nonhypnotic techniques such as biofeedback and cognitive restructuring (Andreychuk &

Skriver, 1975; Spanos, Radtke-Bodorik, Ferguson, & Jones, 1979). Results for acupuncture analgesia have been mixed. Katz, Kao, Spiegel, and Katz (1974) reported a direct relationship with hypnotizability, but two other studies did not support these findings (Knox, Gekoski, Shum, & McLaughlin, 1981; Stern, Brown, Ulett, & Sletten, 1977).

Hypnotizability has also been found to potentiate nonhypnotic therapy for psychological disorders. For instance, Nace, Warwick, Kelley, and Evans (1982) assessed hypnotizability prior to the initiation of psychotherapy and kept therapists blind to their clients' levels of hypnotic ability. This study was notable for including a variety of disorders and therapy approaches as well as multiple therapists. Nace et al. found that highly hypnotizable individuals showed positive change more quickly after brief psychotherapy. Although low hypnotizable participants caught up over 6 months posttherapy, both groups maintained their gains.

Bowers and LeBaron (1986) suggested that therapeutic outcomes may correlate with hypnotic ability to the extent that the therapy procedures resemble hypnosis. For example, many cognitive–behavioral techniques involving imagery and relaxation could easily be labeled *hypnosis* with little or no change in procedures. Even though CBT has been proven effective with a wide range of problems and clients, labeling it *hypnosis* might potentiate its effects for more hypnotizable clients. Bowers and LeBaron (1986) cited additional data indicating that subtle cues can activate hypnotic ability. Even a casual mention of hypnosis during a phone call soliciting research participation was enough to activate a hypnotizability effect in a subsequent session even though hypnosis was not actually used in the research session.

The available data show that hypnotizability is clinically significant. Hypnotizability relates to personality profiles as well as to psychopathology. It is a formal (or informal) diagnostic criterion for some clinical disorders and, in some cases, an important basis for differential diagnosis. Hypnotizability also predicts treatment outcome. Although these effects are strongest for hypnotic treatment of nonvolitional disorders, they can extend to hypnotic treatment of volitional disorders and nonhypnotic treatment of a range of disorders. Given the potential importance of hypnotizability, in the final section we offer guidance to practitioners for incorporating hypnotizability measures into their clinical work.

HOW SHOULD HYPNOTIZABILITY BE CLINICALLY ASSESSED?

Hypnotizability measures provide information about a personality variable that is related to both the diagnosis and treatment of particular clinical problems. Assessing hypnotizability also offers the chance for the clinician to engage with the client in a relatively structured and safe interaction while collecting data about the person's hypnotic, imaginative, relaxation, and other clinically relevant abilities. However, there are some potential disadvantages of hypnotizability measurement. Some measures are time consuming and provide more data than a typical clinician would need. Other measures, or specific items within measures, may be inappropriate for certain clients. For instance, medical patients with restricted movement may find ideomotor suggestions beyond their physical abilities, highly anxious people may find the need to "relinquish control" threatening, and clients who have experienced traumatic childhood events may find age regression or posthypnotic amnesia items upsetting. All of these issues can be dealt with through careful selection of appropriate measures and items and by skillful rapport building and fully informed consent.

One significant challenge of hypnotizability assessment that needs to be managed well is the potential for low scores to generate a sense of failure and negative treatment expectations. When assessed with standardized scales, 10% to 15% of individuals will experience virtually nothing, despite motivation and their best efforts (e.g., Barnier & McConkey, 2004). One way to avoid such a reaction is to present hypnosis and the hypnotizability measure as an "opportunity for relaxation and imagination" rather than as an exercise in passing or failing. Indeed, many of the Stanford scale scripts incorporate language that helps the participant to interpret a "failure" (i.e., as defined by the behavioral criterion) in a positive light or simply as a function of individual differences. For example, with the SHSS:C hand lowering item, if the participant's hand has not fallen to criterion for passing, the hypnotist says, "That's good. . . . You probably experienced much more heaviness and tiredness in your arm than you would have if you had not concentrated on it and had not imagined something trying to force it down." That is, the participant's attention is drawn to what he or she experienced rather than to what he or she did not. Thus, a client may be completely unaware of "failing" the item.

Another way to avoid a negative reaction to a low score is to use a *graded difficulty* test (e.g., SHSS:C, DRS; Orne & O'Connell, 1967; Weitzenhoffer & Hilgard, 1962) and to stop if a participant fails two consecutive items. In these hypnotizability measures, the test suggestions are ordered roughly in terms of difficulty. If a participant passes the earlier easy items but then fails the next two, one can safely assume that he or she will fail the remaining more difficult items.

Selecting a Measure

Given that hypnotizability measures are a useful part of a practitioner's toolkit, which measure should the clinician choose? In the clinical context, practitioners will be most interested in the level of hypnotic ability that predicts and/or maximizes treatment success. They will be looking for a measure that identifies hypnotic responses and cognitive abilities that are related to and benchmarked to clinical utility (Barber, 1993).

It is important to understand the major types of scales available and their main purpose. Most hypnotizability scales can be categorized in one of three ways, as either (a) behavioral hypnotic scales, which are labeled *hypnotic*, involve a standard induction , and emphasize behavior over experience; (b) behavioral scales of suggestibility, which measure responsiveness to suggestion with or without an induction procedure; or (c) clinical scales, which index clinically useable hypnotic capacity (Stern, Spiegel, & Nee, 1978–1979). In general, hypnotizability scales have three major uses: (a) formal hypnotizability assessment in the laboratory, (b) selection of particular participants for additional testing or research, and (c) assessment of clinically relevant hypnotic ability. Many of the scales have more than one purpose. For instance, the DRS (Orne & O'Connell, 1967) is a flexible scale that can be used for assessment, selection, and clinical measurement (for a summary of the type, design, purpose, items, induction, and scoring of current measures, see Barnier & McConkey, 2004, Table 2.1; for a detailed summary of a number of these measures, see Sheehan & McConkey, 1982). There are several issues to consider when selecting a scale.

Who Is Being Assessed?

Depending on whether the client is an adult, an adolescent, an older child, or a younger child, the clinician should choose an age-appropriate measure and form (e.g., SHCS:A vs. SHCS:C, Forms A and B; Morgan & Hilgard, 1978–1979a). If the client has never been exposed to hypnosis, one might choose a different measure than if the client has experienced hypnosis before. In the research setting, the participant's first exposure to hypnosis is typically via the nonthreatening and nonpersonal HGSHS:A (Shor & Orne, 1962). Many researchers then "confirm" hypnotizability with the more difficult SHSS:C (Weitzenhoffer & Hilgard, 1962), which has more personal content (e.g., dream, age regression). Finally, if the client has issues with personal control or authority, the clinician might choose a more permissive scale such as the CIS (Wilson & Barber, 1978). Alternatively, if the client has transference issues, one might choose a scale that follows a set, relatively nonpersonal administration, such as one of the Stanford scales, which may help to maintain interpersonal distance between therapist and client. This is partly an issue of rapport, which is a central aspect of hypnosis and the hypnotic interaction.

How Much Time Is Available?

As indicated earlier, standardized scales vary in length from 6 min (SHALIT; Hilgard et al., 1979) to over 1 hour (SHSS:A & B; SHSS:C, SPS:I & II; HGSHS:A). Additional time should be allowed for informed consent procedures; for measuring, discussing, and addressing the participant's attitudes and expectancies about hypnosis; as well as for assessing subjective responses to hypnosis.

In general, there is a trade-off between, on the one hand, hypnotizability scale length and administration time and, on the other hand, information gathered and the scale's psychometric properties. For example, the SHALIT (Hilgard et al., 1979) includes just one item (i.e., arm levitation) and takes only 6 min to administer. Although brief, it provides information about only one relatively simple direct motor item. In contrast, the SHCS:A includes five items and takes approximately 20 min to administer, but provides a greater range of clinically useful information.

What Kinds of Hypnotic Abilities Need To Be Measured?

This issue relates to the previous one in the sense that, obviously, not all hypnotizability scales measure precisely the same thing; they all measure an underlying general factor of hypnotizability. But not all scales are equally good measures of the ability to experience particular hypnotic events. From a sophisticated statistical analysis of a large set of HGSHS:A and SHSS:C data, Woody et al. (2005) identified four component factors (i.e., subscales) that generally overlap with the three item types indicated earlier: direct motor, motor challenge, cognitive–delusory, and posthypnotic amnesia. Although these building blocks of hypnotic responding were all related to a general hypnotizability factor, they were differentially related to participants' responses to a new set of hypnotic suggestions in subsequent hypnosis experiments. For instance, the ability of a participant to respond successfully to a hypnotic suggestion for color hallucination was predicted only by his or her earlier score on the cognitive–delusory items of the HGSHS:A and SHSS:C, and not by his or her scores on the direct motor, motor challenge, and posthypnotic amnesia items of these scales (Woody et al., 2005).

One inference from the analysis by Woody et al. (2005) is that certain complicated hypnotic responses—the sorts of abilities and experiences that clinicians may be most interested in, including age regression, negative hallucinations (e.g., analgesia), posthypnotic responding, and posthypnotic amnesia—may best be predicted by subscales of hypnotizability measures and not by the total scores. More important for the present discussion, some hypnotizability scales do not include the kinds of items needed to predict these clinically relevant responses. For example, in the experimental domain, we say that the HSGSH:A does not have much *top*. By that we mean that the HGSHS:A includes many easy, direct motor and motor challenge items but not enough difficult, cognitive–delusory items. So, compared with the SHSS:C, the HGSHS:A does not assess cognitive–delusory ability well at all. If a researcher is interested in a particular form of cognitive–delusory ability, given the findings of Woody et al. (2005), he or she should use a scale with cognitive–delusory items. The same principle follows for clinical assessment; if a clinician is interested in a certain sort of clinically useful hypnotic ability, he or she should chose a scale that includes items that measure it.

Finally, although a clinician may be more likely to chose a clinical scale or a multipurpose scale that provides clinically relevant assessment, be aware that "laboratory" scales, such as the SHSS:A and B, SHSS:C, and SPS:I and II, include a large set of verbatim hypnotic suggestions, all with published norms and pass percentages for items. For example, the HGSHS:A (Shor & Orne, 1962) contains verbatim wording for posthypnotic suggestion and posthypnotic amnesia items; norming data indicate that approximately 26% and 46% of people pass these items, respectively (McConkey et al., 1996). The SHSS:C (Weitzenhoffer & Hilgard, 1962) contains verbatim wording for an age regression item; norming data indicate that approximately 43% of people pass this item. Thus, these scales are a rich source of hypnotic items, which can be adapted to clinical assessment (e.g., by inserting them into a flexible measure such as the DRS; Orne & O'Connell, 1967) or following assessment in therapy.

Setting the Stage and Administering the Scale

Once a clinician has decided to assess hypnotizability and has chosen a measure, all that remains is to set the stage and to administer the scale. To set the stage, one first needs to obtain informed consent. Informed consent involves explaining exactly what will happen during hypnosis and informing the participant that hypnosis can be stopped at any time. In our view, the notion that a hypnotized person loses total control to the hypnotist is an unfortunate myth (i.e., the *Svengali myth*; Kihlstrom, 2008; see also Green, Page, Rasekhy, Johnson, & Bernhardt, 2006). However, there has been controversy and conflicting research findings on this issue dating back over the past 100 years and more, mostly concerning whether hypnotized persons can be induced to perform harmful or antisocial acts (Barber, 1969; Golden, 1986).

On the basis of our research and practice, we believe that people do not become mindless automatons controlled by the hypnotist (e.g., Barnier, Dienes, & Mitchell, 2008). Although other researchers and clinicians may hold different views (e.g., chaps 2, 4, and 5, this volume), in our experience, explaining to clients that the element of control in hypnosis belongs to them, and that the clinician's job is to simply guide them along, tends to result in more desirable outcomes. We also believe that clients who are told that they are in control of their hypnotic experiences and can stop at any time, will be more comfortable in responding to the limit of their ability.

The issue of informed consent is related to attitudes and expectancies, which are addressed next. People bring to the hypnotic setting strong cultural views and attitudes about hypnosis, which are influenced by exaggerated representations in the popular media. For instance, Green et al. (2006) surveyed university students in Australia, Germany, the United States, and Iran and reported both positive and negative beliefs and attitudes. Across these national groups, 55% of respondents found the whole idea of becoming hypnotized an attractive prospect, but 50% agreed that they had some apprehensions about hypnosis and being hypnotized. Of most relevance, 44% of respondents, and 71% from Iran, agreed with the statement that "a hypnotized person is robotlike and goes along with whatever the hypnotist suggests"; 70% agreed that "hypnosis is an altered state of consciousness, quite different from normal waking consciousness"; and only 29% agreed that "the experience of hypnosis depends on the ability of the subject, not on the ability of the hypnotist" (Green et al., 2006).

These sorts of beliefs and attitudes influence hypnotizability. Positive attitudes are necessary but not sufficient for hypnotic responding (Barnier & McConkey, 2004; Spanos, Brett, Menary, & Cross, 1987). People with negative or fearful attitudes toward hypnosis are almost always less hypnotizable, whereas those with positive, accepting attitudes may be high, medium, or low in hypnotizability. There are a number of pen-and-paper measures that index attitudes, expectancies, and rapport. These include (a) the 14-item Attitudes Toward Hypnosis scale by Spanos et al. (1987), which indexes (across three subscales) positive beliefs about hypnosis, beliefs about the mental stability of hypnotizable people, and an absence of fear concerning hypnosis; (b) McConkey's (1986) 21-item Opinions About Hypnosis scale, which indexes peoples' beliefs about hypnosis as an altered state of consciousness; and (c) Nash and Spinler's (1989) 20-item Archaic Involvement Measure, which indexes participants' perception of the power of the hypnotist, positive emotional bond to the hypnotist, and fear of negative appraisal.

Once the stage is set, the hypnotizability scale can be administered. Administration has two important aspects. First, one must follow the procedures exactly. The value of a standardized scale comes from its standardized procedure. In other words, for a number of scales, it is important to follow the hypnosis script and scoring instructions. Second, it is extremely useful to collect converging data about the participant's hypnotic responses. Most hypnotizability scales focus on what the participant does or says in response to each item. One major assumption of hypnotizability scales is that behavior is a valid indicator of underlying experience. For instance, if a participant swats at the air in response to the HGSHS:A fly hallucination item, we assume that he or she heard or felt the fly buzzing around his or her head. But there are two possible mismatches. Perhaps the participant swatted the air because he or she felt compelled to, not because he or she heard the fly. In this case, the participant shows the behavior and passes the behavioral criterion in the absence of a genuine experience; hypnotizability scores overestimate his or her ability. Alternatively, perhaps the participant does not swat the air but still hears and feels the fly. In this case, he or she has a genuine experience but does not show the behavior, and the hypnotizability score underestimates his or her ability.

There are a number of ways of finding out what the participant is feeling and thinking during hypnosis. A few hypnotizability scales, such as the CURSS (Spanos, Radtke, Hodgins, Bertrand, Stam, & Dubreuil, 1983), ask participants after hypnosis to rate how their hypnotic responses felt: whether they felt real and whether they were involuntary. These scales generate objective as well as subjective hypnotizability scores. Other scales, such as the Stanford scales, have similar subjective questions in addition to the standardized behavioral measure (Kirsch, Council, & Wickless, 1990; Kirsch, Milling, & Burgess, 1998). The two disadvantages of this method are, however, that the ratings are retrospective (i.e., after hypnosis is over) and that they subjectively average quite complex experiences.

One alternative is to conduct an in-depth posthypnotic inquiry into the participant's hypnotic experiences. Sheehan and McConkey (1982) developed the Experiential Analysis Technique (EAT), which can easily be adapted for clinical use. In this procedure, the hypnosis session is video recorded. Later (sometimes with an independent interviewer), participants watch the video of their hypnosis session and are invited to talk about their hypnotic experiences as they watch the tape. This procedure yields interesting and important information about exactly how people interpret hypnotic suggestions and how they construct their hypnotic experiences. For example, McConkey, Glisky, and Kihlstrom (1989) used this procedure to interview two excellent hypnotic participants after their hypnosis sessions. During hypnosis, they received suggestions for difficult cognitive–delusory items, such as positive and negative visual hallucination, anesthesia, and posthypnotic amnesia. The EAT interview revealed that these two talented hypnotic participants interpreted and processed the suggestions in different ways, one passively and one actively. Practitioners can adapt these laboratory techniques of rating scales and interview to explore their clients' private experiences of hypnosis and hypnotizability.

CONCLUSION

Modern hypnotizability scales are important and powerful tools. They provide a setting for practitioner and client to engage in an often relaxing, enjoyable, and rapport-building interaction. They give clients an empowering opportunity to harness skills and abilities that they can use in the therapeutic process as well as in their daily lives. Most important, hypnotizability scales, thanks to their excellent psychometric properties, provide reliable and valid information about clinically significant behaviors and experiences. Learning to assess hypnotizability should be standard training for clinical psychologists.

REFERENCES

American Psychiatric Association. (1994). *Diagnostic and statistical manual of mental disorders* (4th ed.). Washington, DC: Author.

Andreychuk, T., & Skriver, O. (1975). Hypnosis and biofeedback in the treatment of migraine. *International Journal of Clinical and Experimental Hypnosis, 23*, 172–183.

Balthazard, C. G., & Woody, E. Z. (1985). The "stuff" of hypnotic performance: A review of psychometric approaches. *Psychological Bulletin, 98*, 283–296.

Balthazard, C. G., & Woody, E. Z. (1992). The spectral analysis of hypnotic performance with respect to "absorption." *International Journal of Clinical and Experimental Hypnosis, 40*, 21–43.

Barabasz, M. (1991). Hypnotizability in bulimia. *International Journal of Eating Disorders, 10*, 117–120.

Barber, J. (1993). The clinical role of responsivity tests: A master class commentary. *International Journal of Clinical and Experimental Hypnosis, 41*, 165–168.

Barber, T. X. (1965). Measuring "hypnotic-like" suggestibility with and without "hypnotic induction": Psychometric properties, norms, and variables influencing response to the Barber Suggestibility Scale (BSS). *Psychological Reports, 16*, 809–844.

Barber, T. X. (1969). *Hypnosis: A scientific approach*. New York: Van Nostrand Reinhold.

Barber, T. X. (1999). Hypnosis: A mature view. *Contemporary Hypnosis, 16*, 123–127.

Barber, T. X., & Wilson, S. C. (1978–1979). The Barber Suggestibility Scale and the Creative Imagination Scale: Experimental and clinical applications. *American Journal of Clinical Hypnosis, 21*, 84–108.

Barnier, A. J., Dienes, Z., & Mitchell, C. A. (2008). How hypnosis happens: New cognitive theories of hypnotic responding. *The Oxford handbook of hypnosis: Theory, research and practice* (pp. 141–177). Oxford: Oxford University Press.

Barnier, A. J., & McConkey, K. M. (1992). Reports of real and false memories: The relevance of hypnosis, hypnotizability, and context of memory test. *Journal of Abnormal Psychology, 101*, 521–527.

Barnier, A. J., & McConkey, K. M. (2004). Defining and identifying the highly hypnotisable person. In M. Heap, R. Brown, & D. Oakley (Eds.), *High hypnotisability: Theoretical, experimental and clinical issues* (pp. 30–60). London: Brunner-Routledge.

Barry, H., MacKinnon, D. W., & Murray, H. A., Jr. (1931). Studies on personality: Hypnotizability as a personality trait and its typological relations. *Human Biology, 13*, 1–36.

Barrett, D. (1996). Fantasizers and dissociaters: Two types of high hypnotizables, two different imagery styles. In R. G. Kunzendorf, N. P. Spanos, & B. Wallace (Eds.), *Hypnosis and imagination* (pp. 123–135). Amityville, NY: Baywood Publishing.

Bliss, E. L. (1983). Multiple personalities, related disorders and hypnosis. *American Journal of Clinical Hypnosis, 26*, 114–123.

Bliss, E. L. (1986). *Multiple personality, allied disorders and hypnosis*. New York: Oxford University Press.

Bliss, E. L., Larson, E. M., & Nakashima, S. R. (1983). Auditory hallucinations and schizophrenia. *Journal of Nervous and Mental Disease, 171*, 30–33.

Bowers, K. S. (1993). The Waterloo-Stanford Group C (WSGC) scale of hypnotic susceptibility: Normative and comparative data. *International Journal of Clinical and Experimental Hypnosis, 41*, 35–46.

Bowers, K. S. (1998). Waterloo-Stanford Group Scale of Hypnotic Susceptibility, Form C: Manual and response booklet. *International Journal of Clinical and Experimental Hypnosis, 46*, 250–268.

Bowers, K. S., & LeBaron, S. (1986). Hypnosis and hypnotizability: Implications for clinical intervention. *Hospital and Community Psychiatry, 37*, 457–467.

Brown, A., & Crawford, H. (1986). Hypnotizability, intense fears, and eating disorder patterns: Tapping similar underlying cognitive processes. *International Journal of Clinical and Experimental Hypnosis, 34*, 275.

Brown, D. (1992). Clinical hypnosis research since 1986. In E. Fromm & M. R. Nash (Eds.), *Contemporary hypnosis research*. New York: Guilford Press.

Butler, L. D., Duran, R. E., Jasiukaitis, P., Koopman, C., & Spiegel, D. (1996). Hypnotizability and traumatic experience: A diathesis–stress model of dissociative symptomatology. *American Journal of Psychiatry, 153*, 42–63.

Cohen, S. B. (1989). Clinical uses of measures of hypnotizability. *American Journal of Clinical Hypnosis, 32*, 4–9.

Council, J. R., & Huff, K. D. (1990). Hypnosis, fantasy activity, and reports of paranormal experiences in high, medium, and low fantasizers. *British Journal of Experimental and Clinical Hypnosis, 7*, 9–15.

Council, J. R., Kirsch, I., Vickery, A. R., & Carlson, D. (1983). "Trance" versus "skill" hypnotic inductions: The effects of credibility, expectancy, and experimenter modeling. *Journal of Consulting and Clinical Psychology, 51*, 432–440.

Crawford, H. J., & Barabasz, A. F. (1993). Phobias and intense fears: Facilitating their treatment with hypnosis. In S. J. Lynn, I. Kirsch, & J. W. Rhue (Eds.), *Handbook of clinical hypnosis* (pp. 311–338). Washington, DC: American Psychological Association.

Davis, L. W., & Husband, R. W. (1931). A study of hypnotic susceptibility in relation to personality traits. *Journal of Abnormal and Social Psychology, 26*, 175–182.

Edmonston, W. E. (1986). *The Induction of hypnosis.* New York: Wiley.

Foenander, G., Burrows, G. D., Gerschman, J. A., & Horne, D. J. de L. (1980). Phobic behavior and hypnotic susceptibility. *Australian Journal of Clinical and Experimental Hypnosis, 8*, 41–46.

Frankel, F. H. (1978–1979). Scales measuring hypnotic responsivity: A clinical perspective. *American Journal of Clinical Hypnosis, 21*, 208–218.

Frankel, F. H., & Orne, M. T. (1976). Hypnotizability and phobic behavior. *Archives of General Psychiatry, 33*, 1259–1261.

Friedlander, J. W., & Sarbin, T. R. (1938). The depth of hypnosis. *Journal of Abnormal and Social Psychology, 33*, 453–475.

Frischholz, E. J., & Braun, B. G. (1991, August). *Diagnosing dissociative disorders: New methods.* Paper presented at the meeting of the American Psychological Association, San Francisco, CA.

Gerschman, J. A., Burrows, G. D., & Reade, P. C. (1987). Hypnotizability and dental phobic disorders. *International Journal of Psychosomatics, 33*, 42–47.

Gerschman, J. A., Burrows, G. D., Reade, P. C., & Foenander, G. (1979). Hypnotizability and the treatment of dental phobic behavior. In G. D. Burrows & D. R. Collison (Eds.), *Hypnosis* (pp. 33–39). Amsterdam: Elsevier.

Golden, W. H. (1986). Can hypnotized patients be persuaded to do almost anything? In B. Zilbergeld, M. G. Edelstien, & D. L. Araoz (Eds.), *Hypnosis questions and answers* (pp. 470–476). New York: Norton.

Green, J. P., Page, R. A., Rasekhy, R., Johnson, L., & Bernhardt, S. E. (2006). Cultural views and attitudes about hypnosis: A survey of college students across four countries. *International Journal of Clinical and Experimental Hypnosis, 54*, 263–280.

Groth-Marnat, G., & Schumaker, J. F. (1990). Hypnotizability, attitude toward eating, and concern with body size in a female college population. *American Journal of Clinical Hypnosis, 32*, 194–200.

Hilgard, E. R. (1965). *Hypnotic susceptibility.* New York: Harcourt, Brace & World.

Hilgard, E. R. (1973). The domain of hypnosis, with some comments on alternative paradigms. *American Psychologist, 28*, 972–982.

Hilgard, E. R. (1974). Toward a neodissociation theory: Multiple cognitive controls in human functioning. *Perspectives in Biology and Medicine, 17*, 301–316.

Hilgard, E. R. (1978–1979). The Stanford Hypnotic Susceptibility Scales as related to other measures of hypnotic responsiveness. *American Journal of Clinical Hypnosis, 21*, 68–82.

Hilgard, E. R. (1991). A neodissociation interpretation of hypnosis. In S. J. Lynn & J. W. Rhue (Eds.), *Theories of hypnosis: Current models and perspectives* (pp. 83–104). New York: Guilford Press.

Hilgard, E. R., Crawford, H. J., & Wert, A. (1979). The Stanford Hypnotic Arm Levitation Induction and Test (SHALIT): A six minute hypnotic induction and measurement scale. *International Journal of Clinical and Experimental Hypnosis, 27*, 111–124.

Hilgard, E. R., & Hilgard, J. R. (1975). *Hypnosis in the relief of pain*. Los Altos, CA: W. Kaufmann.

Hilgard, E. R., Weitzenhoffer, A. M., Landes, J., & Moore, R. K. (1961). The distribution of susceptibility to hypnosis in a student population: A study using the Stanford Hypnotic Susceptibility Scale. *Psychological Monographs, 75*, 1–22.

John, R., Hollander, B., & Perry, C. (1983). Hypnotizability and phobic behavior: Further supporting data. *Journal of Abnormal Psychology, 92*, 390–392.

Katz, R. L., Kao, C. Y., Spiegel, H., & Katz, G. J. (1974). Pain, acupuncture, hypnosis. *Advances in Neurology, 4*, 819–825.

Kelly, S. F. (1984). Measured hypnotic response and phobic behavior: A brief communication. *International Journal of Clinical and Experimental Hypnosis, 32*, 1–5.

Kihlstrom, J. F. (2008). The domain of hypnosis, revisited. In M. R. Nash & A. J. Barnier (Eds.), *Oxford handbook of hypnosis: Theory, research and practice* (pp. 21–52). Oxford, England: Oxford University Press.

Kirsch, I., Council, J. R., & Wickless, C. (1990). Subjective scoring for the Harvard Group Scale of Hypnotic Susceptibility, Form A. *International Journal of Clinical and Experimental Hypnosis, 38*, 112–124.

Kirsch, I., Milling, L. S., & Burgess, C. A. (1998). Experiential scoring for the Waterloo-Stanford Group C Scale. *International Journal of Clinical and Experimental Hypnosis, 46*, 269–279.

Kirsch, I., Montgomery, G., & Sapirstein, G. (1995). Hypnosis as an adjunct to cognitive behavioral psychotherapy: A meta-analysis. *Journal of Consulting and Clinical Psychology, 63*, 214–220.

Knox, V. J., Gekoski, W. L., Shum, K., & McLaughlin, D. M. (1981). Analgesia for experimentally induced pain: Multiple sessions of acupuncture compared to hypnosis in high- and low-susceptible subjects. *Journal of Abnormal Psychology, 90*, 28–34.

London, P. (1963). *Children's Hypnotic Susceptibility Scale*. Palo Alto, CA: Consulting Psychologists Press.

Lynn, S. J., Kirsch, I., & Rhue, J. W. (Eds.). (1996). *Casebook of clinical hypnosis*. Washington, DC: American Psychological Association.

Lynn, S. J., & Rhue, J. W. (1986). The fantasy-prone person: Hypnosis, imagination, and creativity. *Journal of Personality and Social Psychology, 51*, 404–408.

McConkey, K. M. (1986). Opinions about hypnosis and self-hypnosis before and after hypnotic testing. *International Journal of Clinical and Experimental Hypnosis, 34*, 311–319.

McConkey, K. M., Glisky, M. L., & Kihlstrom, J. F. (1989). Individual differences among hypnotic virtuosos: A case comparison. *Australian Journal of Clinical and Experimental Hypnosis, 17*, 131–140.

McConkey, K. M., & Barnier, A. J. (2004). The highly hypnotisable person: Unity and diversity in behaviour and experience. In M. Heap, R. Brown, & D. Oakley (Eds.), *The highly hypnotisable person: Theoretical, experimental and clinical issues* (pp. 61–84). London: Brunner-Routledge.

Morgan, E., & Hilgard, J. R. (1978–1979a). The Stanford Hypnotic Clinical Scale for adults. *American Journal of Clinical Hypnosis, 21*, 134–147.

Morgan, E., & Hilgard, J. R. (1978–1979b). The Stanford Hypnotic Clinical Scale for children. *American Journal of Clinical Hypnosis, 21*, 148–169.

Nace, E. P., Warwick, A. M., Kelley, R. L., & Evans, F. J. (1982). Hypnotizability and outcome in brief psychotherapy. *Journal of Clinical Psychiatry, 43*, 129–33.

Nash, M. R., & Spinler, D. (1989). Hypnosis and transference: A measure of archaic involvement with the hypnotist. *International Journal of Clinical and Experimental Hypnosis, 37*, 129–144.

Orne, M. T., & O'Connell, D. N. (1967). Diagnostic ratings of hypnotisability. *International Journal of Clinical and Experimental Hypnosis, 15*, 125–133.

Perry, C., Gelfand, R., Marcovitch, P. (1979). The relevance of hypnotic susceptibility in the clinical context. *Journal of Abnormal Psychology, 88*, 592–603.

Perry, C., Nadon, R., & Button, J. (1992). The measurement of hypnotic ability. In E. Fromm & M. R. Nash (Eds.), *Contemporary hypnosis research* (pp. 459–490). New York: Guilford Press.

Pettinati, H. M., Horne, R. L., & Staats, J. S. (1985). Hypnotizability in patients with anorexia nervosa and bulimia. *Archives of General Psychiatry, 42*, 1014–1016.

Piccione, C., Hilgard, E. R., & Zimbardo, P. G. (1989). On the degree of stability of measured hypnotizability over a 25-year period. *Journal of Personality and Social Psychology, 56*, 289–295.

Prince, M. (1906). *The dissociation of a personality*. New York: Longmans, Green.

Rhue, J. W., & Lynn, S. J. (1987). Fantasy proneness: Developmental antecedents. *Journal of Personality, 55*, 121–137.

Sheehan, P. W., & McConkey, K. M. (1982). *Hypnosis and experience: The exploration of phenomena and process*. Hillsdale, NJ: Erlbaum.

Shor, R. E., & Orne, E. C. (1962). *The Harvard Group Scale of Hypnotic Susceptibility, Form A*. Palo Alto, CA: Consulting Psychologists Press.

Spanos, N. P., Brett, P. J., Menary, E. P., & Cross, W. P. (1987). A measure of attitudes toward hypnosis: Relationships with absorption and hypnotic susceptibility. *American Journal of Clinical Hypnosis, 30,* 139–150.

Spanos, N. P., & Chaves, J. F. (1991). History and historiography of hypnosis. In S. J. Lynn & J. W. Rhue (Eds.), *Theories of hypnosis: Current models and perspectives* (pp. 43–78). New York: Guilford Press.

Spanos, N. P., Radtke-Bodorik, H. L., Ferguson, J. D., & Jones, B. (1979). The effects of hypnotic susceptibility, suggestions for analgesia, and the utilization of cognitive strategics on the reduction of pain. *Journal of Abnormal Psychology, 88,* 282–292.

Spanos, N. P., Radtke, H. L., Hodgins, D. C., Bertrand, L. D., Stam, H. J., & Dubreuil, D. L. (1983). The Carleton University Responsiveness to Suggestion Scale: Stability, reliability, and relationships with expectancy and "hypnotic experiences." *Psychological Reports, 53,* 555–563.

Spanos, N. P., Radtke, H. L., Hodgins, D. C., Bertrand, L. D., Stam, H. J., & Moretti, P. (1983). The Carleton University Responsiveness to Suggestion Scale: Relationship with other measures of hypnotic susceptibility, expectancies, and absorption. *Psychological Reports, 53,* 723–734.

Spanos, N. P., Radtke, H. L., Hodgins, D. C., Stam, H. J., & Bertrand, L. D. (1983). The Carleton University Responsiveness to Suggestion Scale: Normative data and psychometric properties. *Psychological Reports, 53,* 523–535.

Spiegel, H. (1974). The Grade 5 syndrome: The highly hypnotizable person. *International Journal of Clinical and Experimental Hypnosis, 22,* 303–319.

Spiegel, D., Hunt, T., & Dondershine, H. E. (1988). Dissociation and hypnotizability in posttraumatic stress disorder. *American Journal of Psychiatry, 145,* 301–305.

Spiegel, H., & Spiegel, D. (1978). *Trance and treatment: Clinical uses of hypnosis.* New York: Basic Books.

Stern, D. B., Spiegel, H., & Nee, J. C. M. (1978–1979). The Hypnotic Induction Profile: Normative observations, reliability and validity. *American Journal of Clinical Hypnosis, 21,* 109–133.

Stern, J. A, Brown, M., Ulett, A., & Sletten, L. (1977). A comparison of hypnosis, acupuncture, morphine, Valium, Aspirin, and placebo in the management of experimentally induced pain. *Annals of the New York Academy of Sciences, 296,* 175–193.

Stutman, R. K., & Bliss, E. L. (1985). Posttraumatic stress disorder, hypnotizability, and imagery. *American Journal of Psychiatry, 141,* 741–743.

Thigpen, C. H., & Cleckley, H. M. (1957). *The three faces of Eve.* New York: McGraw-Hill.

Wadden, T. A., & Anderton, C. H. (1982). The clinical use of hypnosis. *Psychological Bulletin, 91,* 215–243.

Weitzenhoffer, A. M. (1953). *Hypnotism: An objective study in suggestibility.* New York: Wiley.

Weitzenhoffer, A. M. (1997). Hypnotic susceptibility: A personal and historical note regarding the development and naming of the Stanford scales. *International Journal of Clinical and Experimental Hypnosis, 45,* 126–143.

Weitzenhoffer, A. M., & Hilgard, E. R. (1959). *Stanford Hypnotic Susceptibility Scales, Forms A and B.* Palo Alto, CA: Consulting Psychologists Press.

Weitzenhoffer, A. M., & Hilgard, E. R. (1962). *Stanford Hypnotic Susceptibility Scales, Form C.* Palo Alto, CA: Consulting Psychologists Press.

Weitzenhoffer, A. M., & Hilgard, E. R. (1963). *Stanford Profile Scales of Hypnotic Susceptibility: Forms I and II.* Palo Alto, CA: Consulting Psychologists Press.

Weitzenhoffer, A. M., & Hilgard, E. R. (1967). *Revised Stanford Profile Scales of Hypnotic Susceptibility: Forms I and II.* Palo Alto, CA: Consulting Psychologists Press.

Wilson, S. C., & Barber, T. X. (1978). The Creative Imagination Scale as a measure of hypnotic responsiveness: Applications to experimental and clinical hypnosis. *American Journal of Clinical Hypnosis, 20,* 235–249.

Wilson, S. C., & Barber, T. X (1981). Vivid fantasy and hallucinatory abilities in the life histories of excellent hypnotic subjects ("somnambules"): Preliminary report with female subjects. In E. Klinger (Ed.), *Imagery: Vol. 2. Concepts, results, and applications* (pp. 133–152). New York: Plenum Press.

Woody, E. Z., Barnier, A. J., & McConkey, K. M. (2005). Multiple hypnotizabilities: Differentiating the building blocks of hypnotic response. *Psychological Assessment, 17,* 200–211.

4

PSYCHOPHYSIOLOGICAL FOUNDATIONS OF HYPNOSIS AND SUGGESTION

DAVID A. OAKLEY AND PETER W. HALLIGAN

The 16-year period since the previous edition of this handbook (Rhue, Lynn, & Kirsch, 1993) has witnessed a rapid growth in psychophysiological studies of hypnosis. A number of general reviews have appeared (Barabasz & Barabasz, 2007; Lynn, Kirsch, Knox, Fassler, & Lilienfeld, 2007; Oakley, 2008; Oakley & Halligan, 2009; Rainville & Price, 2003; Ray & De Pascalis, 2003; Raz & Shapiro, 2002, Spiegel, 2003) together with some thoughtful theoretical and integrative papers (e.g., Barnier & McConkey, 2003; Burgess, 2007; De Pascalis, 2007; Killeen & Nash, 2003; Ray & Tucker, 2003; Raz, 2005; Woody & Szechtman, 2003). In this chapter we review some of the major developments. We begin by addressing some general issues relating to the nature of hypnosis itself that are relevant when considering hypnosis from a neurocognitive perspective. We then discuss a range of study designs that are now possible given recent developments in brain imaging technology. There follows a review of recent electroencephalography (EEG), positron emission tomography (PET), and functional magnetic resonance imaging (fMRI) studies that explore brain activity associated with hypnotic induction and with specific suggestions, such as those resulting in changes in vision, pain, relaxation, movement, and hearing. Finally, we discuss general conclusions about the brain and the processes of hypnosis and suggestion based on these studies and consider some implications for their clinical use.

GENERAL ISSUES

Historically, there has been a long-standing divergence of views concerning the nature of hypnosis, often polarized as the *state versus nonstate* debate. This centers on the critical issue of whether the process of becoming hypnotized produces a distinctive behavioral *state* (i.e., trance), which is in turn characterized by a unique neural *signature* (i.e., brain or cognitive activity). A second issue concerns whether traditional induction procedures are necessary for achieving this state of hypnosis. As Burgess (2007) pointed out, the answer to the question of whether hypnosis constitutes a state largely depends on how such a state is operationalized, namely, as a subjectively reportable "natural variation" in the stream of wakeful consciousness or one that involves a more radical change in brain function (i.e., what Burgess terms a *meta-state*), similar to the way that REM sleep is considered a meta-state with its own distinctive physiological and psychological characteristics.

It is probably fair to say that those who propose the state view assume that there is some form of distinctive underlying neural meta-state (e.g., Bowers, 1992; Gruzelier 1998; Hilgard, 1977; Orne, 1959; Rainville, Hofbauer, Paus, Duncan, Bushnell, & Price, 1999; Weitzenhoffer, 2000), although there is little consensus as to the precise nature of this state. In this chapter, we review evidence of distinctive (i.e., time-locked) psychophysiological changes associated with hypnosis and evidence of characteristic brain-related changes accompanying congruent behavioral and subjective reports, all of which would support the use of a meta-state label. The shorthand term that best captures this distinctive mental state is *trance*, a state characterized by mental changes, such as an increased sense of absorption or mental focus, though these may also be facets of other more mundane mental states. Finally, a related and growing issue is the extent to which this hypothesized state relates to the neurocognitive processes underpinning suggestion.

For consistency, in this chapter we use the term *hypnosis* to describe the putative trance state following an induction procedure, which we argue is distinct from suggestion. Supporting this distinction is the well-established observation that individuals responsive to suggestions used in hypnotizability tests also tend to respond whether or not they have been exposed to a hypnotic induction procedure (e.g., Braffman & Kirsch, 1999). Some definitions of hypnosis, however, make *suggestion* a defining feature (see Oakley, 2008, for further discussion). That is, hypnosis is defined by a subject's responsiveness to specific sorts of suggestion whether or not a formal hypnotic induction procedure is used (e.g., Green, Barabasz, Barrett, & Montgomery, 2005). However, as Kihlstrom (2003) pointed out, if hypnosis is identified primarily with the effects of suggestion, there is little chance of finding a unique hypnotic signature. Some have argued for this reason that searching for neural correlates while participants are responding to suggestions is potentially more fruitful (e.g., Boly, Faymonville, Vogt, Maquet, & Laureys, 2007).

Depending on what effects are suggested, brain activations may differ in a number of ways, including lateralization (Jasiukaitis, Nouriani, Hugdahl, & Spiegel, 1997). Patterns of brain activation associated with suggestions given in hypnosis to see a gray-scale stimulus in color, for example (Kosslyn, Thompson, Constantini-Ferrando, Alpert, & Spiegel, 2000), are different from those associated with a suggestion that leads the subject to report hearing a hallucinated voice (Szechtman, Woody, Bowers, & Nahmias, 1998). Even when the suggested effect is similar, the associated brain activity may be different depending on the type of suggestion used. Suggestions that impair an individual's ability to report a visually presented stimulus, for instance, may result in reduced amplitude in a key component of subsequent brain activity if the suggestion is that their view is being blocked by the presence of a physical object, such as a cardboard box, but lead to an increase in amplitude if it is suggested that they have simply lost the ability to see the stimulus (Barabasz, Barabasz, Jensen, Calvin, Trevisan & Warner, 1999). Consequently, many who equate hypnosis with suggested effects have taken this to imply the absence of a unique neural signature for hypnosis. This in turn has led some to view the pursuit of a "special state" or trance as irrelevant, on both theoretical and pragmatic grounds, given the absence of a widely recognized or agreed on behavioral marker (for further discussion of this issue, see Kirsch & Lynn, 1995; Lynn et al., 2007). The failure to find such a marker, however, may simply reflect a historical lack of sophisticated recording equipment and data analysis, as De Pascalis (1999) indicated in connection with EEG exploration of hypnosis. In view of recent developments in neurophysiological recording, we will, as urged by Kirsch and Lynn and, more recently, Kallio and Revonsuo (2003), return to the relationship between hypnotic state (assuming one exists) and the neural patterns evoked by suggestion.

The question of whether being hypnotized is itself associated with a distinctive brain pattern is particularly salient when neuroimaging techniques are involved because they frequently depend on an identifiable *resting* brain state on which to base comparisons. If there are recognizable changes in brain activity associated with hypnosis, it raises the related issue of examining the cognitive changes that accompany them. Possible contenders for the latter include increased absorption, mental calming, focusing of attention (especially inward), relaxation, time distortion, and changes in affect and volitional control (Lynn et al., 2007; Naish, 2007; Oakley, 2008; Ott, 2007;

Pekala & Kumar, 2007; Rainville & Price, 2003). However, studies such as that by Bányai and Hilgard (1976) indicate that relaxation is not an essential component of hypnosis. In addition, we, along with other contributors to this volume, also exclude loss of control as one of the defining features of hypnosis.

RESEARCH METHODS AND DESIGN

Much of the recent research into the neuropsychophysiology of hypnosis has been driven by the development and refinement of brain imaging techniques such as EEG, PET, fMRI, and magnetoencephalography (MEG; for an overview, see Ray & Oathes, 2003).

EEG is probably the most established technique, capable of detecting underlying brain changes via electrical activity, usually recorded by electrodes placed on the scalp. The output is analyzed either in terms of its frequency—identified as *theta* (4–8 Hz), *alpha* (8–13 Hz), *beta* (17–30 Hz), and *gamma* (30–60 Hz)—or as a waveform derived from the averaged patterns of activity following the repetitive occurrence of a stimulus event. The waveform is referred to as an *event-related potential* (ERP), whose positive- and negative-going peaks are identified according to the time in milliseconds that they follow the stimulus event. Hence, a positive-going peak at 300 ms latency is labeled the *P300*.

The most recent developments in EEG technique have focused on increasingly sophisticated forms of signal analysis (Burgess, 2007). MEG, a more recently developed technology, uses the magnetic fields produced by electrical activity in the brain to provide better spatial resolution and higher temporal resolution than EEG for underlying neuronal activity using a large number of *superconducting quantum interference devices* (SQUIDs), sensors capable of reading extremely sensitive changing magnetic fields from the surface of the head. We are not aware of any hypnosis studies involving MEG.

PET and fMRI techniques are based on the fact that blood flow in different brain areas varies in relation to the degree of local or regional activity. These changes are monitored in a PET scanner using gamma ray detection systems following injection or inhalation of a radioactive tracer by the participant. The fMRI technique makes use of the fact that oxygenated blood has different magnetic properties to deoxygenated blood; the difference between the two can be taken as an indication of the intensity of metabolic activity in particular sets of neurons when blood flows through them. In fMRI, the participant's head is enclosed in a large external magnet that creates a strong magnetic field where the variations in blood flow are recorded. Because fMRI is less invasive than PET and offers better temporal and spatial resolution of brain activity, it has gradually become the method of choice for most cognitive brain neuroimaging studies.

Potential disadvantages of fMRI are the associated noise and, as with PET, the need to partially enclose and restrain the participant in the tube of the scanner. There is evidence however, that hypnotized individuals tolerate the often lengthy fMRI procedures well and that neither depth of hypnosis nor the ability to respond to suggestions is compromised by the scanning environment (Oakley, Deeley, & Halligan, 2007). Although offering the advantages of increased spatial resolution, neither PET nor fMRI can match the superior temporal resolution of EEG and MEG. However, new technologies such as magnetic source imaging (MSI; e.g., Simos et al., 2000) combine the strengths of both MRI and MEG procedures and, together with other sophisticated forms of MRI, such as functional diffusion tensor imaging (fDTI; e.g., Guye et al., 2003), could provide further insights regarding the psychophysiological basis of trance and suggestion.

However, most imaging studies involving hypnosis tend to use it as a tool to investigate other cognitive or perceptual conditions (*instrumental research*), and only relatively few studies have explicitly set out to explore the neural basis for hypnosis and suggested hypnotic phenomena in their own right (*intrinsic research;* for further discussion of the instrumental/intrinsic distinction, see Barnier & McConkey, 2003; Oakley, 2006, 2008; Reyher, 1962).

Irrespective of whether studies have been instrumental or intrinsic in focus, experimental neuroscience requires the research questions to be clearly framed for its (increasingly expensive) techniques to provide useful answers. The examples that follow illustrate the importance of clarifying the experimenters' aims, identifying relevant variables, and reviewing experimental design when assessing studies exploring the neurophysiology of hypnosis (for further discussion on ideal designs in hypnosis research, see Lynn et al., 2007, and Kallio & Revonsuo, 2003).

It may be helpful to reiterate at this point that we are using the term *hypnosis* as a label for the mental state (i.e., trance) that is presumed to result from the administration of a hypnotic induction procedure; we distinguish this from the effects of suggestion. Suggestions may be given without hypnosis, traditionally labeled *waking suggestions;* or in hypnosis, commonly described as *hypnotic suggestions*. Figure 4.1 shows the most basic experimental designs needed to address the effects of a hypnotic induction procedure (i.e., trance) and/or those of suggestion, including the relationship between them. It is not seriously contested that suggestion following a hypnotic induction produces "real" changes at the levels of subjective experience as well as time-congruent brain activity. What remains unresolved, however, is whether different or similar effects are produced by suggestion with or without a hypnotic induction. Equally, there is no consensus as to the subjective and brain-level

	No Hypnosis	Hypnosis
No Suggestion	A Normal alert state	B Neutral hypnosis
Suggestion	C Waking suggestion	D Hypnotic suggestion

Figure 4.1. Basic 2 × 2 design for studies primarily interested in hypnosis, suggestion, and their interactions. "Hypnosis" denotes where the label *hypnosis* has been
used and a hypnotic induction procedure employed. "No Hypnosis" denotes where
the procedure has not been labeled *hypnosis* and no hypnotic induction has been
used. "Suggestion" denotes where a suggestion intended to elicit changes in sensory, motor, or cognitive function has been given, and "No Suggestion" denotes
where no such suggestion has been given. The contents of the Cells A, B, C, and D
are labels that have commonly been applied to the four resulting conditions.

changes that accompany the hypnotic induction procedure in the absence of
suggestions.

In Figure 4.1, in the *no-hypnosis* condition, the procedure is not labeled
hypnosis and no induction procedure is given. In the *hypnosis* condition, the
procedure is identified as hypnosis and an induction procedure used. For con-
venience, the effects of expectancy created by labeling the situation as hypnosis, and the inclusion of an induction procedure as the hypnosis condition,
are conflated, though it is clear that both expectancy and labeling are important variables (Gandhi & Oakley, 2005). More sophisticated designs could
separate these two components. The *suggestion* condition is one in which a
suggestion intended to elicit specific changes in sensory, motor, or cognitive
function is given; in the *no-suggestion* condition, this does not occur. Cell A in
this figure is thus the "normal," waking (nonhypnotized) alert state. Cell B
is the condition we have identified as hypnosis and has also been called *neutral hypnosis* or *anesis* (Edmonston, 1991; Kallio & Revonsuo, 2003). Cell C
corresponds to giving a waking suggestion and Cell D a hypnotic suggestion.
It is of course essential that the wording of each suggestion is identical in
Conditions C and D (Braffman & Kirsch, 1999; Hull, 1933).

A comparison of Cells A and B is the most direct means of identifying changes attributable to the hypnotic induction procedure; comparing
Cells C and D would potentially reveal any difference in the responses to suggestion that may be attributable to the hypnosis state. In the absence of a difference between C and D, however, there is the possibility that the presence
of a suggestion in C may have caused highly hypnotizable individuals to

slip accidentally into hypnosis: the phenomenon of *spontaneous hypnosis* (Barabasz, 2005). This is a major reason why this 2 × 2 design has been avoided in some of the more recent hypnosis literature (see Kosslyn et al., 2000), although the need for it was identified many years ago (see, e.g., Hull, 1933; Hull & Huse, 1930). Whether people "slip" into hypnosis is, as earlier researchers realized, an empirical question. If they do not, brain activity in Conditions C and D should be found to be different, but we would expect to see some activity in common for B and D if the hypnosis condition is relevant. Equally, if there is a uniquely hypnotic state and individuals really do slip into it accidentally, Conditions C and D should share these same activities, attributable to hypnosis, which should also be present in B and absent only in Condition A. The following studies illustrate the design outlined in Figure 4.1.

In an instrumental hypnosis study, Deeley et al. (2008) investigated the normal resting state of brain activity (i.e., *default mode*) when individuals were engaged in a low-demand cognitive task (see Figure 4.2). Brain activity was measured before, during, and after hypnosis while the participants were passively watching an alternating checkerboard display. The study showed that the resting brain state was different in the no-hypnosis condition (Cell A) compared with the hypnosis condition (Cell B), and identified engagement in spontaneous conceptual thought as a significant component of the normal default mode condition. This outcome is also consistent with the view that the hypnotic induction procedure is associated with a durable state change and that reduced conceptual thought is a feature of neutral hypnosis. The study claims nothing about the relationship of this state to suggestion, nor

	No Hypnosis	Hypnosis
No Suggestion	A Normal rest state	B Neutral hypnosis rest state
Suggestion	C	D

Figure 4.2. Design of a study by Deeley, Oakley, Giampietro, et al. (2008) to study the normal default mode of brain activity. "Hypnosis" denotes where the label *hypnosis* has been used and a hypnotic induction procedure employed. "No Hypnosis" denotes where the procedure has not been labeled *hypnosis* and no hypnotic induction has been used. "Suggestion" denotes where a suggestion intended to elicit changes in sensory, motor, or cognitive function has been given, and "No Suggestion" denotes where no such suggestion has been given. The contents of the Cells A and B are labels based on the descriptions used by the authors to identify the conditions they used.

does it exclude the possibility that hypnosis has features in common with other mental states that also differ from the normal resting state.

Figure 4.3 shows the two conditions (B and D) used in another instrumental study by Halligan, Athwal, Oakley, and Frackowiak (2000) in which a hypnotically suggested left leg paralysis was used as an analogue for conversion ("hysterical") paralysis. With the right leg as the control, lateralized brain changes were found that were associated with the paralysis suggestion and that were similar to those reported earlier in a conversion disorder patient with comparable leg paralysis (Marshall, Halligan, Fink, Wade, & Frackowiak, 1997). In contrast to the previous example, this study did not inform us about hypnosis per se, as there was no comparison possible between hypnosis and no-hypnosis conditions (e.g., A vs. B).

The experimental design shown in Figure 4.1 is constrained in that it does not address other important questions, such as how similar hypnotically suggested effects are to actual experiences. Does a suggested experience of being touched on the back of the hand, for example, produce the same activity in relevant brain areas as actually being touched? A related question is whether imagined experiences are similar in neural activation terms to suggested experiential changes. Does imagining being touched on the hand, for example, produce a similar neural effect to a suggested experience of the same touch, and, in turn, what is the relation of both of these to the effects of experiencing an actual touch? More important, are these actual, suggested, and imagined effects different when in the hypnosis compared with a no-hypnosis

	No Hypnosis	Hypnosis
No Suggestion	A	B Normal leg
Suggestion	C	D Paralyzed leg

Figure 4.3. Design of a study by Halligan, Athwal, Oakley, and Frackowiak (2000) to study hypnotic paralysis as an analogue for unilateral lower limb conversion disorder. "Hypnosis" denotes where the label *hypnosis* has been used and a hypnotic induction procedure employed. "No Hypnosis" denotes where the procedure has not been labeled *hypnosis* and no hypnotic induction has been used. "Suggestion" denotes where a suggestion intended to elicit changes in sensory, motor, or cognitive function has been given, and "No Suggestion" denotes where no such suggestion has been given. The contents of the Cells B and D are labels based on the descriptions used by the authors to identify the conditions they used.

condition? Figure 4.4 places these variables into a 2 × 4 design, though clearly more variants are possible.

Again, the questions that can be addressed depend crucially on which cells are completed for any given experiment. Examples of two studies are given in Figures 4.5 and 4.6 and illustrate what can and what cannot be concluded from their results. Figure 4.5 summarizes the experimental and control conditions (i.e., Cells B, D, F, and H) in an instrumental study reported by Derbyshire, Whalley, Stenger, and Oakley (2004) that used suggestion in hypnosis to create "an experience of pain in the absence of any noxious stimulus" (p. 392) as an analogue of clinical functional pain conditions. In addition to having provided insights into functional pain, this

	No Hypnosis	Hypnosis
No Suggestion	A Normal alert state	B Neutral hypnosis
Suggestion	C Waking suggestion	D Hypnotic suggestion
Imagination	E Waking imagination	F Hypnotic imagination
Stimulation	G Normal experience of the real thing	H Hypnotic experience of the real thing

Figure 4.4. A 2 × 4 design for studies interested in hypnosis, suggestion, imagination, external stimulation, and their interactions. "Hypnosis" denotes where the label *hypnosis* has been used and a hypnotic induction procedure employed. "No Hypnosis" denotes where the procedure has not been labeled *hypnosis* and no hypnotic induction has been used. "Suggestion" denotes where a suggestion intended to elicit changes in sensory experience has been given, and "No Suggestion" denotes where no such suggestion has been given. "Imagination" denotes where the participant has been instructed to imagine experiencing the change suggested in the suggestion condition. "Stimulation" denotes where an actual stimulus is presented, creating a sensory experience corresponding to that suggested in the suggestion condition. The contents of Cells A to H are descriptive labels for the eight resulting conditions.

	No Hypnosis	Hypnosis
No Suggestion	A	B Neutral hypnosis rest state
Suggestion	C	D Hypnotically induced pain
Imagination	E	F Imagined pain
Stimulation	G	H Physically induced pain

Figure 4.5. Design of a study by Derbyshire, Whalley, Stenger, and Oakley (2004) to investigate suggested and imagined heat pain compared with pain produced by an actual heat stimulus with participants in hypnosis in all conditions. "Hypnosis" denotes where the label *hypnosis* has been used and a hypnotic induction procedure employed. "No Hypnosis" denotes where the procedure has not been labeled *hypnosis* and no hypnotic induction has been used. "Suggestion" denotes where a suggestion intended to elicit changes in sensory experience has been given, and "No Suggestion" denotes where no such suggestion has been given. "Imagination" denotes where the participant has been instructed to imagine experiencing the change suggested in the suggestion condition. "Stimulation" denotes where an actual stimulus is present, creating a sensory experience corresponding to that suggested in the suggestion condition. The contents of Cells B, D, F, and H are labels based on the descriptions used by the authors to identify the conditions they used.

study revealed the relative neural signatures associated with hypnotically suggested and imagined pain but said little about hypnosis per se because no hypnosis/no-hypnosis comparisons were possible. In particular, the study showed that a hypnotically suggested pain experience activated similar brain areas as a physically presented pain stimulus but that imagining the effects of the same stimulus in hypnosis did not. The study did not address the possible effects of the same pain suggestions and imagery on brain activity outside hypnosis.

In an intrinsic study, Kosslyn et al. (2000) used Conditions D, E, G, and H to "determine whether hypnosis can modulate color perception" (p. 1279;

	No Hypnosis	Hypnosis
No Suggestion	A	B
Suggestion	C	D Hallucinate color
Imagination	E Remember and visualize color	F
Stimulation	G Perceive color veridically	H Perceive color veridically

Figure 4.6. Design of a study by Kosslyn, Thompson, Constantini-Ferrando, Alpert, and Spiegel (2000) that investigated the effect of a suggestion given in hypnosis to experience color in a gray-scale stimulus display and an instruction to imagine the corresponding color change when not hypnotized, compared with actual viewing of a colored display. "Hypnosis" denotes where the label *hypnosis* has been used and a hypnotic induction procedure employed. "No Hypnosis" denotes where the procedure has not been labeled *hypnosis* and no hypnotic induction has been used. "Suggestion" denotes where a suggestion intended to elicit changes in sensory experience has been given, and "No Suggestion" denotes where no such suggestion has been given. "Imagination" denotes where the participant has been instructed to imagine experiencing the change suggested in the suggestion condition. "Stimulation" is where an actual stimulus is presented, creating a sensory experience corresponding to that suggested in the suggestion condition. The contents of the Cells D, E, G, and H are labels based on the descriptions used by the authors to identify the conditions they used.

see Figure 4.6). The study provided useful information about hallucinated and imagined color, although, again, nothing directly about the role of hypnosis, per se, in producing the suggested effects (because the relevant conditions corresponding to Cells C and F were not included in the design). In particular, it was seen that suggestions to hallucinate color into a gray-scale stimulus in hypnosis activated the same color processing areas in both brain hemispheres as when actually perceiving the colored stimulus, whereas the mental imagery condition (e.g., "remember and visualize color") in the no-hypnosis condition produced the activation only on the right side. What this study did not tell us, however, is whether the same bilateral activations of color processing areas would have been found if the hallucination suggestions had been given in the no-hypnosis condition. Comparison G and H had the potential to reveal hypnosis related effects but none were detected, suggesting that, in the absence of specific suggestions, hypnosis does not affect the processing of color information.

In the next section we review the research literature on the neurophysiology of hypnosis and suggestion, with reference to Figures 4.1 through 4.6. Before doing so, we should note that it is traditional to classify participants in hypnosis studies as being either *high hypnotizable* or *low hypnotizable* on the basis of their scores on standard hypnotic susceptibility tests, such as the Harvard Group Scale of Hypnotic Susceptibility (Shor & Orne, 1962) or the Stanford Hypnotic Susceptibility Scale (Weitzenhoffer & Hilgard, 1962). These tests measure *hypnotizability* as the quantifiable degree to which individuals respond to a series of suggestions following a hypnotic induction procedure. Given that we separated hypnosis (i.e., trance) and suggestion, this is not entirely consistent with the definition of hypnosis adopted here. In our formulation, hypnotizability refers to the ease with which participants enter a hypnotic (i.e., trance) state and/or the extent to which they experience it. Alternatively, insofar as the hypothesized hypnotic state facilitates responding to suggestion, we might, as Braffman and Kirsch (1999) argued, consider the magnitude of the change in suggestibility from the nonhypnotized to the hypnotized state as reflecting an individual's hypnotizability. However, for consistency with the experimental literature, we continue to use the labels *high hypnotizable* and *low hypnotizable* as well as related terms, such as *hypnotizability*, in the traditional way to refer to scores on standardized hypnotic susceptibility tests. It is also important to note that the studies considered next mainly involved participants who were high hypnotizable, preselected using standard hypnotizability scales; this should be kept in mind when attempting to generalize from particular experimental findings (see Horton & Crawford, 2004; Lynn et al., 2007).

STUDIES OF HYPNOSIS

Studies in this section address the possibility that the effects of the hypnotic induction procedure per se are associated with distinct patterns of psychoneurophysiological activity. That is, they have explored the condition of hypnosis, or trance, as we defined it earlier, in the absence of targeted suggestions. As noted earlier, this condition has also been labeled *neutral hypnosis* (Edmonston, 1991; Kallio & Revonsuo, 2003).

Electroencephalography Studies

The experiments in this first group are longitudinal in that they looked for systematic changes across the time course of the hypnotic induction process, for which the high temporal resolution of EEG techniques is well-suited. An important series of longitudinal studies reviewed by Gruzelier (1998) used a traditional relaxation-based induction procedure with eye fixation followed by suggestions of relaxation and eye closure, which in turn were followed by imagery associated with deep relaxation and a dreamlike experience. Combining this induction procedure with a series of behavioral measures and EEG recording techniques, Gruzelier argued for a three-stage model of the hypnotic induction process. The first stage corresponds to *sensory fixation and concentration* in which thalamocortical networks engage left-sided fronto-limbic focused attentional systems. This is followed by a *release or "letting go"* stage, which is characterized by suspension of reality testing and critical evaluation involving "the handing over of executive and planning functions to the hypnotist,"(p. 5) and which is mediated by fronto-limbic inhibitory systems. The final stage is one of *relaxed, passive imagery*, which is accompanied by an increase in more posterior, predominantly right-sided, cortical activity. A strength of this aggregate approach is that it uses a clearly specified and standardized induction procedure that allows for the organization of a large amount of neuropsychophysiological evidence into a consistent framework. It has also allowed the identification of differences that can be attributed to hypnotizability. In particular, individuals who are low hypnotizable appear to find difficulty in engaging left frontal attentional control systems and fail to display the inhibitory processes associated with the letting go stage. It remains to be seen to what extent other types of induction procedures, perhaps those that do not include relaxation suggestions, follow similar neurophysiological progressions. In particular, it is not yet clear how consistent the appearance of frontal inhibition is when other types of suggestion are given concurrently with the induction (Wagstaff, 2000). It is also worth noting here that, consistent with Gruzelier's model, Dietrich (2003) proposed that deregulation of prefrontal cortex activity is a common feature in altered states of consciousness, such as those seen in meditation and daydreaming as well as hypnosis (i.e., the *transient hypofrontality hypothesis*).

A related approach has been developed in a systematic program of research by De Pascalis (1999, 2007) based on the view that a particular frequency of brain wave activity detected by EEG recording is the physiological marker of *focused arousal* (De Pascalis, 1999). Specifically, it was suggested that brain activity in the gamma frequency range (i.e., around 40 Hz) could be equated with the sort of *attentional focusing*, or absorption, commonly regarded as a central product of the hypnotic induction procedure. This view was later extended to encompass neurophysiological theories of consciousness by proposing that brain activity in the gamma frequency range provides a means of integrating mental experience, as a sort of "carrier wave" that binds together activity in disparate brain areas to form a coherent whole. Gamma frequency coherence has been used to explain a range of processes, from how activity in dispersed individual neurons may be bound together into integrated representations of objects to how diverse representations can be bound into a single experience of consciousness (De Pascalis, 2007). Because hypnosis seems to involve the ability to exclude irrelevant stimuli and to focus attention on a more limited set of mental activities, it has been argued that this might be reflected in increased levels of gamma EEG activity following a hypnotic induction procedure (De Pascalis, 1999). It might also account for an increased capacity in individuals who are high hypnotizable to deploy synchronized gamma activity in selectively binding together dispersed neural activities into coherent subjective experiences.

Two studies from this series are particularly relevant to the question of the neurophysiological accompaniments of a hypnotic induction procedure. De Pascalis and Penna (1990) used the induction from a standard hypnotic susceptibility scale, commencing with an eyes-open stage followed by eye closure and relaxation suggestions along with test items from the scale, including age regression and a hypnotic dream. The main finding was that in the early part of the induction, participants who were high hypnotizable showed increased gamma band activity in both hemispheres compared with a baseline no-hypnosis condition. As induction progressed, however, this activity decreased over the left hemisphere and increased over the right. Participants who were low hypnotizable, in contrast, showed reductions over both hemispheres. Using similar hypnosis procedures, De Pascalis (1993) again reported that participants who were high hypnotizable showed greater amplitude gamma activity (at frontal, central, posterior recording sites) during the induction process compared with participants who were low susceptible; this difference was also present in the prehypnosis resting condition. During the later hypnotic dream section of the procedure, the gamma band activity in the individuals who were high hypnotizable was greater in the right hemisphere, in particular in posterior areas. An incidental finding was that EEG activity in the closely related beta range was greater in the left hemisphere compared with the right early in the induction process but that the left hemisphere activity subsequently diminished to be more similar to that in the right hemisphere. De Pascalis (2007) concluded that the results of both studies are consistent with Gruzelier's (1998) model of hypnosis with its emphasis on progressive shifting of activity from the left to the right hemisphere and involving a process of frontal cortical inhibition.

A similar case to that of gamma activity has been explored for much slower frequency brain activity in the alpha and theta bands (Crawford & Gruzelier, 1992; Williams & Gruzelier, 2001). Theta activity in particular has been proposed as a diagnostic feature of the progression from a nonhypnotized to a hypnotized state; high levels of theta activity have been identified as a strong indicator of hypnotizability (Graffin, Ray, & Lundy, 1995; Horton & Crawford, 2004; Ray, 1997; Sabourin, Cutcomb, Crawford, & Pribram, 1990). Although these are interesting relationships, it is not clear whether they depend on depth of hypnotic trance, on relaxation, or on cognitive factors, such as focusing on verbal instructions (Graffin et al. 1995; Lynn et al., 2007). In an attempt to address some of these questions, Williams and Gruzelier (2001) analyzed EEG activity in more narrowly defined alpha and theta bands before, during, and after hypnosis in two groups of participants who were either high or low hypnotizable. They found no differences between groups in theta activity before or during hypnosis, though theta activity remained elevated in the participants who were high hynotizable after termination of hypnosis. In contrast, alpha activity increased during hypnosis in participants who were high hypnotizable compared with before or after hypnosis, whereas the converse pattern was seen in the participants who were low hypnotizable. Participants who were high hypnotizable also showed significantly higher levels of alpha activity overall compared with those who were low hypnotizable. Williams and Gruzelier concluded from their data that theta activity is an index of relaxation, whereas alpha activity is more closely related to hypnotizability and hypnosis per se.

Positron Emission Tomography and Functional Magnetic Resonance Imaging Studies

This second group of studies focused primarily on hypnosis as the "end-state" of the hypnotic induction process. The issue is whether the verbal instructions given to participants during hypnotic induction and deepening procedures create a qualitatively distinct brain state (that mirrors the observable trance behaviors) compared with a nonhypnosis condition. In Figure 4.1, the appropriate comparison is Cell A versus Cell B. (An example of a study that compares data in these two cells is given in Figure 4.2.) It is important that the administration of a hypnotic induction procedure is the only independent variable and that any ancillary task carried out in the two conditions is the same. Of seven studies that addressed this issue, three are of limited relevance because they confounded the induction of trance with other task demands (Faymonville et al., 2000; Grond, Pawlik, Walter, Lesch, & Heiss, 1995; Maquet et al., 1999), but five meet the minimal criteria for separating trance condition and general task demands (Crawford, Gur, Skolnick, Gur, &

Benson, 1993; Deeley et al., 2008; Egner, Jamieson, & Gruzelier, 2005; Rainville, Hofbauer, Bushnell, Duncan, & Price, 2002; Rainville et al., 1999).

The three studies that are difficult to interpret from a neutral trance perspective all used PET. In the first of these, Grond et al. (1995) contrasted brain states in resting wakefulness with hypnosis. The hypnosis condition, however, involved an induction procedure that included suggestions for catalepsy. The underactivation in visual cortex and relative overactivation in sensorimotor areas reported in the hypnosis condition could therefore be most easily explained in terms of the different task demands in the two conditions rather than being indicative of trance itself.

Maquet et al. (1999) explored brain activations in two hypnosis conditions compared with an alert nonhypnosis condition. In addition to an induction procedure, one hypnosis condition involved participants in revivification of positive life experiences and, in the other, color hallucinations. In the nonhypnosis condition, participants listened to autobiographical information and engaged in related imagery. No significant differences in brain activity activations were found in the two hypnosis conditions, but both revealed widespread increases in activation in visual, motor, and parietal areas compared with the alert condition. Again, these differences are as likely to be due to the differing task demands in the no hypnosis and the hypnosis conditions as they are to be due to the presence or absence of trance.

The third of these studies (Faymonville et al., 2000) compared a nonhypnotic resting state with an autobiographical imagery condition and a hypnosis condition consisting of an induction procedure plus a reexperiencing of autobiographical memories. Activation of right extrastriate cortex and anterior cingulate cortex was greater in the hypnosis condition compared with the other two. Concurrent heat–pain stimulation was common to all three conditions; it was found that pain ratings were lower in the hypnosis condition. The observed differences in activation in the hypnosis and no-hypnosis conditions again seem plausibly explainable by the differing task demands in all three conditions rather than being the effects of the hypnotic induction procedure or the presence of trance. The difference in anterior cingulate cortex activity, for instance, is consistent with the variations in pain experience between the three conditions (Rainville, Duncan, Price, Carrier, & Bushnell, 1997). Similarly, other studies have shown clear brain activation differences between imagining and reexperiencing the same events even within hypnosis (Derbyshire et al., 2004; Szechtman et al., 1998).

The remaining five studies provide the basis for a more direct evaluation of the effects of trance. Two of them, Rainville et al. (1999) and Rainville et al. (2002), used data drawn from earlier PET studies investigating the effect of suggestion on pain affect and pain intensity (Hofbauer, Rainville, Duncan, & Bushnell, 2001; Rainville et al., 1997). The two conditions of interest in Rainville et al. (1999) are a prehypnosis baseline and a hypnosis alone condition in both of which the participant's left hand was immersed in water that varied in temperature. The baseline condition was one of restful wakefulness with eyes closed, and the hypnosis condition differed only in that it followed a hypnotic induction procedure that also involved eye closure and relaxation. The most notable hypnosis-related effect was widespread activation in occipital regions, which seems likely to be linked to the spontaneous engagement in vivid visual imagery reported by a number of participants in the hypnosis condition. A second area of hypnosis-related activity increase was in the right anterior cingulate cortex, though it was in a different location to that identified earlier by Rainville et al. (1997) as an area associated with processing the aversive components of pain, thus indicating that hypnosis and the pain areas within the anterior cingulate cortex are different. In contrast, decreased activity was seen in posterior parietal sites in the hypnosis condition, which is consistent with the decrease in attention to extraneous stimuli and general body-sense awareness that participants in hypnosis frequently report.

The second of these reports (Rainville et al., 2002), using similar experimental procedures, confirmed the earlier findings but also took subjective ratings that allowed researchers to correlate brain changes specifically associated with absorption and with relaxation. We consider relaxation to be a suggested effect, and we return to this in a later section. For absorption, however, areas of increased brain activation included upper pons, thalamus, rostral areas of right anterior cingulate cortex, prefrontal cortex (especially right ventro-lateral frontal cortex, right inferior frontal cortex, and anterior insula), and right inferior parietal lobule. Rainville et al. (2002) identified these areas as an *executive attentional network* associated with the general regulation of attentional processes and error detection as well as with monitoring conflict and the difficulty of task performance. This study also reported a negative correlation between absorption and activity in the left and right lateral parietal cortices, which may reflect the decreased monitoring of external sources of information and reduced spatio-temporal monitoring that is often reported by hypnotized individuals.

In an early study, described in more detail later, Crawford et al. (1993) used cerebral blood flow measurements to compare brain activity during "rest" states in both hypnosis and no-hypnosis conditions. They found significantly higher levels of cortical activation overall in the hypnosis resting condition compared with the "awake" resting condition, which they took to support the view that "hypnosis takes effort" and that even when hypnotized individuals show signs of physical relaxation during hypnosis, "they are cognitively alert and activating their supervisory, attentional control system" (p. 191).

In a more recent study investigating the correlates of neutral hypnosis, Deeley et al. (2008) used fMRI to compare brain activity both in and out of hypnosis. To standardize task demands, participants were asked to monitor a flashing checkerboard display in both conditions. The hypnotic induction procedure used was derived from the three-step model described by Gruzelier (1998) and included relaxation suggestions and dreamlike imagery (Oakley et al., 2007). In addition, subjective hypnotic depth measurements were taken from the participants in each condition. Correlational analyzes showed depth-related increases in brain regions involved in working memory and the maintenance of attention. It is of interest to note that a negative relationship was found between hypnotic depth and activity in left medial frontal gyrus, bilateral parahippocampal gyri, and left posterior cingulate gyrus, which have been identified as components of the default mode of brain activity that is present when task demands are low (Gusnard & Raichle, 2001). This suggests that the default mode following a hypnotic induction procedure is different from that in a nonhypnotized state. In particular, subjective accounts of mental state changes indicated that an important component of this is a reduction in the incidence of spontaneous conceptual thought that characterizes default mode activity outside hypnosis.

An interesting study by Egner et al. (2005) involving both fMRI and EEG techniques introduced the Stroop Color–Word Interference Test (Stroop, 1935) as the common task in their hypnosis and no-hypnosis conditions. This enabled them to investigate the effects of hypnotic induction on conflict monitoring and cognitive control processes inherent in the Stroop test. The hypnotic induction procedure avoided references to relaxation, heaviness, or sleep, and no suggestions were given that related to performance on the Stroop test. Conflict-related mental processes, reflected in increased activity in anterior cingulate cortex, increased during the Stroop test in hypnosis. In contrast, the hypnotic induction procedure was not associated with any changes in cognitive control, which are typically mediated by left frontal cortex. These changes are compatible with earlier studies that have found a deterioration in performance on Stroop tests, as shown in increased color naming response times, following a hypnotic induction procedure in the absence of performance related suggestions (Jamieson & Sheehan, 2004; Sheehan, Donovan, & MacLeod, 1988). A particular strength of the Egner et al. study is that they compared the performance of participants who were high and low hypnotizable and found that the increase in conflict-related activity during the Stroop test following the hypnotic induction procedure was present only in the high hypnotizable group. The authors concluded that following a hypnotic induction procedure in participants who were high hypnotizable, there is a decoupling of the link that is normally present between conflict monitoring, associated with anterior cingulate cortex, and cognitive control functions mediated by left lateral frontal cortex. Consistent with this conclusion, they showed, using EEG data collected separately, decreased gamma band coherence between frontal midline and left lateral scalp sites in the high hypnotizable group. In contrast to the widespread assumption that hypnosis is associated with a general increase in focusing of attention, Egner et al. pointed out that some aspects of attentional processing may be impaired following a hypnotic induction, at least in individuals who are high hypnotizable.

A related and potentially important consideration, especially in the context of instrumental neuroimaging studies, is whether the trance state itself, in the absence of targeted suggestions, influences normal processing of sensory information or execution of motor actions. That is, does the hypnotic end state alter sensorimotor function? Deeley et al. (2008a) used fMRI to explore brain activity when participants were listening to spoken words or viewing a checkerboard display either during hypnosis or when not hypnotized. There were no significant differences in brain activity when processing visual information in these two conditions although an increase in activity in auditory cortical areas during hypnosis was observed. The authors concluded that the latter finding could be interpreted as an increase in attention to the spoken words implicit in the induction procedure itself but that the data were consistent with the view that hypnosis, per se, does not directly affect sensory processing. Though this is the only report to date to address this question directly, incidental observations from other studies support this view. Several authors have noted that hypnotic induction without specific suggestions for altered perception has no significant effect on reported pain experience or on pain-related patterns of brain activity (Crawford et al., 1993; Hofbauer, Rainville, Duncan, & Bushnell, 2001; Rainville et al., 1997; Rainville et al., 1999; Rainville et al., 2002). Similarly, Kosslyn et al. (2000) found no effect of the induction of hypnosis on activity in brain areas concerned with color processing unless explicit suggestions were given. Normal patterns of brain activity have been reported when hypnotized subjects are preparing to move in hypnotic paralysis and feigning conditions (Oakley, Ward, Halligan, & Frackowiak, 2003; Ward, Oakley, Frackowiak, & Halligan, 2003).

Conclusions

A consensus has emerged from the longitudinal EEG studies that a systematic shift in brain activity can be seen from the left hemisphere to the right as hypnotic induction progresses; this pattern is consistent with a descriptive model of the process based on a range of experimental psychoneurophysiological data (De Pascalis, 2007; Gruzelier, 1998). However, both De Pascalis (2007) and Gruzelier used similar relaxation-based induction procedures, including a final dream sequence. This raises the question of whether the patterns they observed are related to hypnosis (i.e., trance) per se or to the particular induction procedure and associated suggestions that they used. Continuing work on other EEG frequencies using more refined analysis seems to indicate that alpha band activity shows promise as a marker of the hypnotic state or trance per se, whereas theta band activity, once a strong contender for that role, may be more closely related to the relaxation that commonly accompanies traditional forms of hypnotic induction.

Taking an overview of those end-state studies that directly address the question of neutral hypnosis, brain activation patterns have been identified that are broadly congruent with the subjective accounts individuals provide for their experience of hypnosis. In particular, decreased attention to external stimuli, reduced general body sense awareness (Rainville et al., 1999), greater absorption (Rainville et al., 2002), and a reduction in spontaneous conceptual thought (Deeley et al., 2008) have all been identified. Similarly, Egner et al. (2005) showed an apparently spontaneous disconnection between activity in brain areas mediating conflict monitoring and cognitive control that is consistent with independent prior observations of impaired performance in the Stroop test (Stroop, 1935) following a hypnotic induction in individuals who are high hypnotizable. Again, it is important to bear in mind that, with the exception of Egner et al., the induction procedures used in these end-state studies have included relaxation suggestions. Given that traditional induction procedures typically incorporate relaxation suggestions, relaxation may be thought of as an integral part of these procedures but, as argued earlier, not as an essential component of neutral hypnosis, trance, or hypnosis per se. Finally, on the basis of what little evidence there is from one study (Deeley et al., 2008a) and a number of incidental findings, more fundamental sensory and motor control processes do not seem to be discernibly affected by the induction of hypnosis (i.e., trance) in the absence of targeted suggestions.

Overall, viewed singly or in combination, the changes in brain activity associated with neutral hypnosis or trance do not as yet meet Burgess's (2007) criteria for hypnosis to be considered a distinctive meta-state. However, they do give neuropsychological credibility to subjective accounts of what it is like to be in a hypnotic trance, and this is important. There is clearly a need for further studies designed specifically to examine the neural mechanisms underlying the subjective changes brought about by a range of different induction procedures, especially those not involving relaxation suggestions. A potentially productive alternative longitudinal approach would be to use neuroimaging (i.e., particularly event related fMRI , MEG, or a combination of the two) to track the process of hypnotic induction, deepening, and deinduction sequentially over time along the lines of Gruzelier's (1998) model.

From a clinical perspective, therapists and others can use these data to inform clients that although hypnosis is not an "altered state of consciousness" such as that which accompanies REM sleep, it does represent a different baseline state compared with simple eyes-closed restfulness. In other words, hypnosis has a different default mode and there are clearly identifiable brain changes corresponding to this mental state. The commonly used analogy that hypnosis is not unlike other everyday states with some similarities to other focused, absorbed (i.e., trancelike) states, such as daydreaming or reading a good book, fits well with the data we have reviewed. For clinicians, it is reassuring that the behavioral and subjectively identifiable state achieved has a potentially demonstrable neurophysiological signature and that this state is potentially independent of, though may interact with, suggestion, a topic we turn to in the next section.

STUDIES OF SUGGESTION

Although our focus here lies with the neurophysiology of suggestion in relation to hypnosis, the topic of suggestion is much broader and includes phenomena variously labeled as primary and secondary suggestibility, direct and indirect suggestibility, interrogative suggestibility, compliance, and placebo effects (Polczyk & Pasek, 2006; Schumaker, 1991). The context in which suggestibility is measured is critically important. Braffman and Kirsch (1999) argued that responsiveness to the sort of suggestions conventionally associated with the domain of hypnosis and measured by standard tests such as the Harvard Group Scale of Hypnotic Susceptibility (Shor & Orne, 1962) should be described as *hypnotic suggestibility* when it is preceded by a hypnotic induction procedure (i.e., Cell D in Figure 4.1) and as *imaginative suggestibility* when it is not (i.e., Cell C).

Effects of Suggestion in Hypnosis

These studies have combined suggestion with hypnosis but have not made it their main concern to compare this condition with the effects of the same suggestion outside hypnosis. In terms of Figure 4.1, studies in this group can be categorized as having a primary interest in the effects of suggestion by comparing B versus D (an example is given in Figure 4.3) or A versus D, and sometimes with the addition of other comparisons such as F and H in Figure 4.4 (an example of this is shown in Figure 4.5).

Electroencephalography Studies

There is a substantial literature demonstrating that hypnotically suggested changes influence the amplitude of ERPs. This has been shown, for example, for visually presented stimuli (De Pascalis, 1994; Jasiukaitis, Nouriani, & Spiegel, 1996; Spiegel & Barabasz, 1988; Spiegel, Cutcomb, Ren, & Pribram,

1985), auditory stimuli (Barabasz, 2000), olfactory stimuli (Barabasz & Lonsdale, 1983), pain (Croft, Williams, Haenschel, & Gruzelier, 2002; De Pascalis & Cacace, 2005; De Pascalis, Cacace & Massicolle, 2004), and memory (LaBerge & Zimbardo, 1999). The following sections provide a selective review that illustrates some of the findings that have emerged.

Vision and Olfaction-Related Suggestions. Though there is a clear suggestion-related effect on ERPs in hypnotized individuals, early results were inconsistent with regard to the direction of change observed. Spiegel et al. (1985), for example, demonstrated significant amplitude reductions in highly hypnotizable participants in the P300 component of a visual ERP following a suggestion intended to reduce visual awareness. However, with an apparently similar procedure that instead used suggestions of reduced responsiveness to the sense of smell, Barabasz and Lonsdale (1983) found an increase in the P300 of an olfactory ERP. One possible explanation offered for this disparity was that it was the product of the type of suggestion given rather than any other difference, such as the sensory modality involved (Spiegel & Barabasz, 1988). Specifically, Spiegel et al. used the *positive obstructive* suggestion that a hallucinated cardboard box was blocking the participant's direct view of the visual stimulus display, whereas Barabasz and Lonsdale gave the *negative obliterating* suggestion that the participants had completely lost the sense of smell. This explanation was strongly supported by later research.

Barabasz et al. (1999) compared the ERP effects, in participants who were high hypnotizable, of giving suggestions for obstructive visual and auditory hallucinations (e.g., the suggested presence of either a cardboard box blocking the computer screen or of wearing sound-attenuating earplugs) with negative obliterating suggestions (e.g., the suggestion of travelling through a dark nebula in space where one could see nothing at all, or of becoming completely unable to hear following the experimenter saying the words "Deaf, deaf"). Consistent with the hypothesis, P300 amplitudes were reduced during the positive obstructive hallucinations but were higher when they were experiencing the effects of the negative obliterating suggestions in both visual and auditory modalities. One explanation that has been offered for this difference is that, in the positive obstructive condition, some residual ability to detect the target stimulus is congruent with the suggestion given (e.g., light being seen around the box, some sound getting past the earplugs). In the negative obliteration condition, however, any such residual sensory ability, however faint, is incongruent with the suggested effect of complete sensory loss and causes a reaction of surprise, which is thought to be responsible for the elevated amplitude of the P300 component of the ERP in this condition (for a fuller discussion, see Barabasz & Barabasz, 2007).

Pain-Related Suggestions. Several EEG-related studies have looked at hypnotically suggested analgesia. Croft et al. (2002), for example, used painful electrical stimuli and at prefrontal sites identified gamma band activity originating in anterior cingulate cortex (ACC) that predicted subjective pain ratings under normal control conditions. This predictive relationship was lost during hypnosis and hypnotic analgesia in participants who were high hypnotizable but was not altered by hypnosis procedures in participants who were low hypnotizable. This was seen as evidence for hypnosis disrupting frontal attentional systems involving the ACC and is consistent with impaired attentional control as reflected in poorer performance on the Stroop test (Stroop, 1935) after hypnotic induction procedures (Jamieson & Sheehan, 2004; Kaiser, Barker, Haenschel, Baldeweg, & Gruzelier, 1997; Nordby, Hugdahl, Jasiukaitis, & Spiegel, 1999). Similarly, De Pascalis and Cacace (2005) and De Pascalis et al. (2004) recorded gamma frequency patterns relating to painful electrical stimuli and found that compared with a painful control condition participants who were high hypnotizable showed reduced activity over frontal and central scalp locations during focused analgesia produced by an obstructive hallucination in hypnosis and with a posthypnotic suggestion. These changes again corresponded with reductions in subjective pain ratings. This outcome is similar to the ERP studies mentioned earlier that have shown blocking of visual and auditory stimulus perception and reduction in the P300 by obstructive hallucinations. On the basis of these more recent studies, De Pascalis (2007) suggested that obstructive hallucinations may create inhibitory processes in the brain capable of modulating early perceptual processing.

Positron Emission Tomography and Functional Magnetic Resonance Imaging Studies

With the exception of Rainville et al. (2002), all of the evidence reviewed in this section originates from the instrumental use of hypnosis, in that researchers were primarily interested in using the suggested effects to explore or to provide an experimental model for some other psychological process or clinical condition. As such, the hypnosis condition is common to all cells in the design matrix. The decision to use a combination of hypnosis with suggestion rather than simply using the suggestion on its own is commonly pragmatic and driven by the explicit, or more usually implicit, belief that this combination maximizes the effects of the suggestion, though this assumption has rarely been tested experimentally.

Relaxation-Related Suggestions. There is sufficient evidence from studies of *active–alert hypnosis* (Bányai & Hilgard, 1976; Bányai, Zseni & Túry, 1993; Cardeña, Alarcon, Capafons, & Bayot, 1998; Fellows & Richardson, 1993; Wark, 2006) to consider relaxation to be a suggested effect rather than an essential component of trance (Oakley, 2008). The only study that has information relating to the specific effects of relaxation suggestions is Rainville et al. (2002), who used PET to compare a normally relaxed resting condition before a hypnotic induction with the state of increased relaxation in hypnosis (i.e., Cells A and D in Figure 4.1). With increasing levels of reported relaxation, they found reduced activity in midbrain and thalamic areas involved in the regulation of cortical arousal and wakefulness and related reductions in activation of somatosensory areas and insula. Reflecting the heterogeneity of functions in the cingulate area, positive correlations were found with relaxation and activity in posterior regions of right anterior cingulate cortex close to, but separate from, absorption-specific activation sites. Increased activations related to relaxation bilaterally were also found in precentral gyrus and in occipital cortex, the former possibly reflecting the involvement of motor and premotor areas in achieving the relaxation response and the latter in the engagement with vivid visual imagery and reliving experiences that subjects commonly report in hypnosis

Movement-Related Suggestions. In the first of a short series of studies investigating possible models of conversion disorder, Halligan et al. (2000) used suggestion of left leg paralysis in a single participant and found, using PET, increased activations in right anterior cingulate cortex and right orbitofrontal cortex during attempted movement of the affected leg (see Figure 4.3). They interpreted these activations as representing inhibitory processes that served to prevent the final execution of the motor response. The same pattern of activation had previously been reported by Marshall et al. (1997) in a patient with conversion paralysis of her left leg, suggesting that similar underlying processes might be involved (see also Athwal, Halligan, Fink, Marshall, & Frackowiak, 2001). More recently, in a group study combining fMRI with suggested paralysis of the right upper limb, a similar pattern emerged, with increased activation in anterior cingulate gyrus and superior frontal gyrus when participants attempted to move the "paralyzed" limb (Deeley et al., 2008b).

In all of these studies, there was clear evidence of motor area activation when participants were preparing to make a movement in both the paralyzed and normal limbs, indicating that the suggestion-based inhibition was not of the intention to move but rather of the attempt to execute the movement. A related study by Ward et al. (2003) compared a hypnotically suggested left leg paralysis with feigning the same paralysis in hypnosis. They found that the hypnotic paralysis was associated with increased activation in right orbitofrontal cortex, whereas the increased activity associated with feigning was in left ventrolateral prefrontal cortex and right posterior cortex. This is a good indication that the activations seen during hypnotically suggested paralysis in the previous studies in the series are unlikely to be the products of malingering or faking (see also Oakley et al., 2003).

In a related study by Blakemore, Oakley, and Frith (2003) investigating the phenomenon of alien control of movement seen in clinical conditions such as schizophrenia and acquired brain damage, hypnotized participants in a PET scanner experienced upward arm movements that were either intentionally produced by the participants themselves, passively produced using a pulley device, or produced by suggestion (i.e., they were ideomotor arm levitations). The intentional and suggested arm movements, but not the passive movements, were accompanied by expected activations in corresponding voluntary motor areas. Passive movements produced by the pulley were distinctive in that they were accompanied by activations in bilateral cerebellum and parietal cortex that are typically generated in response to limb movement caused by an external agency. It is notable that these same activations were also seen in the suggested movement, which is congruent with it being experienced as a truly passive or "alien" movement.

Hearing-Related Suggestions. In another PET study relating to symptoms typical of schizophrenia, Szechtman et al. (1998) tested hypnotized participants while they were listening to a tape recorded message, hallucinating the same message in response to suggestion, or imagining hearing the same message "as vividly as possible." They found distinctive activations of right anterior cingulate cortex in the listening and hallucinating conditions, which were related to clarity and externality ratings of the experience. This did not occur in the baseline condition or when instructed to imagine hearing the spoken message. Again, this underlines the virtual reality aspect of the hypnotically suggested experience compared with imagining it. Because the activity of anterior cingulate cortex also correlates with measures of auditory hallucination in schizophrenics, a strong case can be made for common mechanisms and that hypnotically suggested hallucinations could be used as a viable experimental model for the clinical symptom.

Pain-Related Suggestions. In another study exploring analogues for functional, or "medically unexplained" clinical problems, Derbyshire et al. (2004) used fMRI to compare brain activations during the experience of externally produced heat pain, hypnotically suggested heat pain, and imagined heat pain (see Figure 4.5). They found similar activation patterns in classic pain areas such as thalamus, anterior cingulate, insula, prefrontal, and parietal cortices during both the physically and hypnotically induced pain. Little activation of any of these areas was seen in the imagined pain condition. This outcome clearly demonstrates not only the possibility of a functional pain but also that it can be accepted as subjectively real and not simply imagined. Raij, Numminen, Narvanen, Hiltunen, and Hari (2005) replicated these findings in a similar fMRI study using laser-generated pain.

In the first of two linked studies examining the brain mechanisms underlying pain perception, participants experienced a rest condition and a suggestion condition during PET scanning (Rainville et al., 1997). In both conditions, painfully hot stimulation was delivered via a water bath to the left hand but was accompanied in the experimental condition by suggestions to increase or decrease the subjective unpleasantness of the stimulus without affecting its intensity. Both conditions were accompanied by activations in established pain processing areas (anterior cingulate cortex, rostral insula, and somato-sensory cortex), but in the suggestion condition, activity in anterior cingulate cortex was modulated in accordance with the direction of the suggested change in pain affect. Following this, Hofbauer et al. (2001) replicated the previous study but changed the suggestions to create experiences of reduced or increased pain intensity rather than pain unpleasantness. This time, significant modulation of brain activation related to the direction of suggested change was seen in primary somatosensory cortex but not in anterior cingulate cortex. These two studies not only add significantly to our understanding of brain mechanisms underlying various aspects of pain experience but also show that direct suggestions given after hypnotic induction can produce clear and predictable changes in brain areas related to the suggested effects.

In addition to these studies, there is also a small group of hypnosis studies that have added to our general understanding of the intriguing relationship between the subjective experience of position and movement in phantom limbs and the experience of phantom limb pain (Oakley, Gracey-Whitman, & Halligan, 2002; Ramachandran & Hirstein, 1998). In the earliest of these studies, Ersland et al. (1996) showed using fMRI that following a hypnotic induction procedure, a patient who had lost his right arm just above the elbow was able to respond to suggestions to experience tapping of the fingers of his phantom right arm and that these subjective movements were accompanied by appropriate activations of left motor cortex. In a similar study using PET, Willoch et al. (2000) extended these observations in a group of upper limb amputees who received a series of suggestions following a hypnotic induction procedure to create movements and resting positions of the phantom limb that were either comfortable or uncomfortable. The suggested phantom limb movements were accompanied by appropriate activations in contralateral somato-sensory areas; painful movements or positions were accompanied by activations in brain areas, such as anterior cingulate cortex, normally associated with pain processing. The same group subsequently reported similar PET findings in the context of a more detailed clinical description of two cases of phantom limb pain (Rosen, Willoch, Bartenstein, Berner, & Rosjo, 2001).

Stroop-Related Suggestions. In a study combining fMRI and ERP techniques, Raz, Fan, and Posner (2005) demonstrated a striking significant effect when participants responded to the classic Stroop test (Stroop, 1935) using the suggestion that the visually presented color words would become meaningless. The result in participants who were high hypnotizable, but not in participants who were low hypnotizable, was that color words no longer produced the usual interference when subjects were asked to report the ink color in which the word was printed and when the two were in conflict. Compared with a no-suggestion condition, the reduction in Stroop interference in the high hypnotizable group was accompanied by reduced activity in anterior cingulate and in occipital cortical areas, which is consistent with the role of these areas in monitoring cognitive conflict and in processing visually presented stimuli, respectively. A unique aspect of this study was that a posthypnotic suggestion was used. That is, the suggestion was given in hypnosis to take effect after the termination of hypnosis and all Stroop testing was carried out when participants were no longer hypnotized.

We have included the Raz et al. (2005) study in this section, though some aspects of its design make it difficult to categorize with certainty. In particular, the experimental conditions at the time of testing correspond to Cells A and C on the left side of Figure 4.1 unless it is assumed that when carrying out the posthypnotic suggestion, the participant briefly reenters the hypnotic state that was involved in setting it up. It is not necessary to make the latter assumption, however, because a more recent study by Raz, Kirsch, Pollard, and Nitkin-Kaner (2006) showed that equivalent Stroop reduction effects could be produced irrespective of whether hypnosis was used to establish the suggested effect. As the authors concluded, this clearly indicated that the effect was "[due to] suggestion rather than hypnosis" (p. 93).

General Processes in Suggestion. Rainville et al. (1999) carried out an extended reanalysis of data acquired in two of the conditions included in an earlier report (Rainville et al., 1997). One condition was hypnosis alone, and the other was hypnosis plus suggestion of increase or decrease in the subjective unpleasantness of painful stimuli (i.e., a comparison of Cells B and D in Figure 4.1). They were able to isolate the brain activity relating to the presence of suggestion itself irrespective of the presence of painful stimulation, which was common to both conditions, and irrespective of the specific effects of the suggestions on pain experience. Main effects attributable to suggestion, per se, were found in the frontal lobes, with strong activations seen in the left inferior frontal gyrus and left dorsolateral areas, which the authors suggested reflected internal verbal rehearsal of the suggestions or the process of holding them in working memory during the scan.

Prefrontal cortical areas have also been implicated in monitoring external events or reality testing, with right frontal areas being concerned with external monitoring and the left frontal lobe possibly involved in internal reinterpretation of that external reality. Frontal cortical activation may thus be common to all situations in which suggestions are used to attempt to alter the meaning of perceptual events, though it is important to note that both suggestions in this study related to pain affect modulation. The interesting observation that some parietal areas showed increased responses in the presence of suggestion but decreases in the hypnosis alone condition indicates that the effects of some suggestions may override changes in brain activity attributable to neutral hypnosis.

Effects of Hypnosis and Suggestion

The three studies in this section all involve PET or fMRI and look at the interaction between hypnosis (i.e., trance) and suggestion. The main focus of these studies, however, is again on the effects of suggestion rather than on the effects of hypnosis. Their defining feature is that they include potential comparisons between matching cells in the left-hand and right-hand columns of Figures 4.1 and A versus B, C versus D, E versus F, or G versus H, ideally with the main focus on the comparison between Cells C and D. An example of a study in this group is shown as Figure 4.6. The comparison A versus B was considered separately in an earlier section.

Pain-Related Suggestions

In an early, well-designed study that included comparisons of the same suggestion with and without hypnosis (Cells C and D), Crawford et al. (1993) used the 133Xe inhalation technique (a precursor to the use of PET for research purposes) to measure differential regional cortical blood flow. The five participants who were high hypnotizable showed significant reductions in subjectively reported ischemic pain when given analgesia suggestions without hypnosis but significantly greater reductions with the same suggestions in hypnosis. Taking overall measures of cerebral blood flow, analgesia-related increases in cortical activity were also found to be greater in the hypnosis condition compared with the no-hypnosis condition. Further analysis revealed that successful hypnotic analgesia for ischemic pain was associated with significant bilateral activation of orbitofrontal cortex, which was interpreted as supporting the involvement of an anterior supervisory attentional system engaged in selectively inhibiting thalamocortical activity. Cerebral blood flow increases were also seen in somatosensory cortical areas when hypnotized participants were experiencing pain, and further increases in these areas were found during hypnotic analgesia. The second of these somatosensory cortex activations is difficult to interpret, especially in the light of the later observations of Hofbauer et al. (2001), who found a decrease in activation of somatosensory cortex with hypnotic analgesia.

Derbyshire, Whalley, and Oakley (2009) used suggestions based on a *pain-dial* paradigm to increase and decrease subjective pain levels in fibromyalgia patients during fMRI scanning. Participants received the same suggestions outside hypnosis and following a hypnotic induction procedure (i.e., comparing C with D). Subjective reports of the amount of suggested change in pain experienced were not significantly different in the two conditions, though the participants reported experiencing significantly more control over their pain in the hypnosis condition. In both conditions, widespread areas of the midbrain, cerebellum, thalamus, midcingulate cortex, primary and secondary sensory cortex, inferior parietal cortex, prefrontal cortex, and insula showed changing levels of activation corresponding to the intensity of the subjectively reported pain experience. However, the brain activations were much weaker overall in the nonhypnosis condition, with significant attenuation of the suggested effects observed in the thalamus and insula and in prefrontal and sensory cortices. This indicates that, at the level of brain activity at least, there appear to be significant differences in the effectiveness of suggestions depending on whether they are administered after a hypnotic induction procedure, even when these differences are not evident at the level of subjective report.

Color Vision-Related Suggestions

Kosslyn et al. (2000) reported a PET study in which participants were presented with colored or equivalent gray-scale versions of square-patterned stimuli. Testing was carried out either without hypnosis or following a hypnotic induction procedure; participants viewed the two sets of stimuli for some of the time in each condition exactly as they were presented. In the hypnosis condition, they were also given a *visual hallucination task* in which it was suggested that they could drain away the color from the colored stimulus or add color into the gray-scale stimuli and see the stimulus in its other form. In the comparable no-hypnosis condition they were asked to remember and visualize the same color transformations as a mental imagery control for the hypnosis condition. (This experimental design is summarized in Figure 4.6.) Kosslyn et al. found increased activation in cortical color-processing areas (fusiform gyrus) bilaterally when viewing color either veridically or following a suggested color hallucination in the hypnosis condition. In the no-hypnosis imagination condition, however, the increased fusiform area activation was seen only on the right. This seems clear evidence that a suggested color hallucination experienced as real creates a relevant activation of color processing areas in the brain, though this particular experimental design does not allow us to decide whether the hypnotic induction procedure was important in producing this outcome. The study also confirms that when participants are asked to imagine a perceptual event, in this case outside hypnosis, the associated brain activations are not the same as those produced by the event itself. Analysis of data from the two matching cells (G and H) revealed no differences in brain activation that could be attributed to hypnosis, per se.

Conclusions

Collectively, the converging evidence reviewed in this section provides impressive proof that suggestions following a hypnotic induction produce effects that are both real in terms of subjective experience and in the concurrent activation of relevant brain areas. The effects are also highly specific, with different brain areas being activated if, for instance, a pain-related suggestion concerns the unpleasantness, as opposed to the intensity, of the noxious stimulus (Rainville et al., 1997). For clinicians, this means that not only is the wording of suggestions important but that suggestions can also be targeted with precision to produce specific changes that are of maximal clinical relevance. In addition, the neuroimaging evidence showing that relevant brain-based changes correspond to the suggestions given is particularly helpful when proposing a psychological intervention such as hypnosis to a client who is experiencing what he or she perceives to be a wholly physical, bodily-related problem, such as pain or gastrointestinal disorder, and is consequently resistant to the idea of psychological treatment. Related to this, there is also strong evidence that presenting symptoms such as pain, paralysis, alien movement, and disturbances in visual processing can be functional and that experimental models of them can be created using suggestion in hypnosis. This, in turn, can have implications for the treatment of symptoms that are believed to be functional, such as those seen in conversion disorders (Oakley, 1999, 2001). Likewise, some studies have shown that whereas experiencing a stimulus-based perceptual change and experiencing a corresponding suggested change produce similar brain activation patterns, imagining the same event is not accompanied by "as real" brain changes, whether the imagination condition is in hypnosis (Derbyshire et al., 2004; Szechtman et al., 1998) or outside hypnosis (Kosslyn et al., 2000). There is also evidence that a suggested phenomenon (e.g., leg paralysis) is mediated within the brain differently from simulation or malingering of the same symptoms (Ward et al., 2003). Collectively, these findings provide a compelling evidential base for accepting as real many functionally presented (or medically unexplained) symptoms previously considered or explained away as merely imaginary or as malingering.

In addition to providing a rationale for the client, it is important for the clinician to understand that quite subtle differences in the form of words used can change the experience the client has from one of "virtual reality" to one of "imagination." Asking a hypnotized phobic patient, for instance, to imagine looking at a spider in the corner of the room will produce a different subjective experience and, on the evidence we have so far, a much-reduced response in relevant brain areas compared with saying, "Look in the corner of the room and you will see a spider." The latter will arguably create a virtual or proximal reality experience that can serve as an in vivo context for a therapeutic intervention such systematic desensitization, with likely improvements in efficacy (e.g., Walters & Oakley, 2003). ERP studies also illustrate the importance of the use of language in suggestions for experiential change. In particular, suggestions that leave room for the suggested effect to be partial, albeit still profound, rather than absolute may have a greater capacity for producing the subjective effect in combination with a congruent brain effect (e.g., Barabasz et al. 1999).

What is less clear from these reviewed findings is the extent to which these suggested effects and, in particular, their brain-level counterparts, rely on the prior induction of hypnosis. There is little empirical evidence available to address this question, but Crawford et al. (1993) found that an analgesia suggestion produced a greater reduction in reported pain when given in hypnosis, compared with a no-hypnosis condition, and that this was reflected in corresponding differences in associated levels of cortical activation. Derbyshire et al. (2009) also made the direct comparison between the same pain modulation suggestion under hypnosis and no-hypnosis conditions and found that, though in their study there was little difference in the degree of subjective change reported in the two conditions, there was a greater sense of control in the hypnosis condition and a much more profound change in congruent brain activity. Both of these studies support the view that the prior induction of hypnosis is a clinically helpful strategy. Derbyshire et al. also raised the intriguing possibility that, in some situations at least, the subjective account may be more influenced by compliance effects outside hypnosis than when the individual is hypnotized.

GENERAL CONCLUSIONS

Much of the recent brain imaging-related research into hypnosis thus far appears to confirm the involvement of an executive system, involving activation of structures from the brainstem to frontal cortex, many of which regulate attentional processes to produce a state of focused attention, absorption, and reduced conceptual thought, accompanied by a reduction in parietal–cortical activity corresponding to the process of disattending to external, including body-related, stimuli. It is worth noting that the brain structures implicated are all those that might be expected to be involved, given the content of the behavioral and subjective reports. Thus hypnosis (i.e., trance) appears to be a perfectly natural engagement of selective brain regions in the sense of recruiting normal brain processes, many of which are actively engaged when pursuing many other everyday cognitive tasks. There is more literature on the effects of suggestion in hypnosis that shows consistently that these effects are highly specific and produce changes in brain activity in areas of the brain that are known to be involved in the sensory, motor, and cognitive processes targeted by the suggestion. There is a need for more direct comparisons of the effects of exactly the same suggestion under both hypnotic and nonhypnotic conditions to elucidate the necessity for the hypnotic induction in producing these effects.

In more general terms, it is evident from the research reviewed in this chapter on both hypnosis (i.e., trance) and the effects of suggestion that ACC is ubiquitously mentioned. Modulation of ACC activity has been described, for example, in the context of hypnotically induced pain (Derbyshire et al., 2004), the affective component of pain (Rainville et al., 1997), phantom limb pain (Willoch et al., 2000), analgesia (Croft et al., 2002), relaxation (Rainville et al., 2002), absorption (Rainville, 2002), conflict monitoring (Egner et al., 2005; Raz et al., 2005), hypnotic paralysis (Deeley et al., 2007a; Halligan et al., 2000), and auditory hallucination (Szechtman et al., 1998). This raises the question of whether ACC is specifically involved in the general process of generating hypnosis or of implementing suggestion, or whether this simply reflects the diversity of functions within the ACC that are also tapped in different ways by the specific suggestions and induction procedures that have been used. Regarding suggestion, evidence from Rainville et al. (1999) indicated that frontal cortical areas are the most likely candidates for having a more general role. Recent reviews have explored the potential role of ACC in hypnosis (e.g., Jamieson & Woody, 2007; Ray & Tucker, 2003), but whatever brain areas are involved at an executive level, specific semantic and memorial systems must presumably be engaged for the effects of suggestion to become experienced.

Recent advances in paradigm design and combined uses of EEG, PET, and fMRI provide a fresh opportunity to look again at the question of a distinct hypnotic state and to explore the relationship of that state to suggestion. We anticipate that further refinements in imaging technologies (e.g., MEG, MSI, fDTI), and experimental designs will offer a greater understanding of both hypnosis and the wider aspects of modulating conscious awareness.

REFERENCES

Athwal, B. S., Halligan, P. W., Fink, G. R., Marshall, J. C., & Frackowiak, R. S. J. (2001). Imaging hysterical paralysis. In P. W. Halligan, C. Bass, & J. C. Marshall (Eds.), Contemporary approaches to the study of hysteria: Clinical and theoretical perspectives (pp. 216–234). Oxford, England: Oxford University press.

Bányai, E. A., & Hilgard, E. R. (1976). A comparison of active–alert hypnotic induction with traditional relaxation induction. Journal of Abnormal Psychology, 85, 218–224.

Bányai, E. I., Zseni, A., & Túry, F. (1993). Active–alert hypnosis in psychotherapy. In J. W. Rhue, S. J. Lynn, & I. Kirsch (Eds.), Handbook of clinical hypnosis (pp. 217–290). Washington, DC: American Psychological Association.

Barabasz, A. (2000). EEG markers of alert hypnosis: The induction makes a difference. *Sleep and Hypnosis, 2*, 164–169.

Barabasz, A. F. (2005). Whither spontaneous hypnosis: A critical issue for practitioners and researchers. *American Journal of Clinical Hypnosis, 48*, 91–97.

Barabasz, A., & Barabasz, M. (2007). Hypnosis and the brain. In M. R. Nash, & A. J. Barnier (Eds.), *The Oxford handbook of hypnosis* (pp. 337–363). Oxford, England: Oxford University Press.

Barabasz, A., Barabasz, M., Jensen, S., Calvin, S., Trevisan, M., & Warner, D. (1999). Cortical event-related potentials show the structure of hypnotic suggestions is crucial. *International Journal of Clinical and Experimental Hypnosis, 47*, 5–22.

Barabasz, A., & Lonsdale, C. (1983). Effects of hypnosis on P300 olfactory evoked potential amplitudes. *Journal of Abnormal Psychology, 92*, 520–525.

Barnier, A. J., & McConkey, K. M. (2003). Hypnosis, human nature, and complexity: Integrating neuroscience approaches into hypnosis research. *International Journal of Clinical and Experimental Hypnosis, 51*, 282–308.

Blakemore, S-J., Oakley, D. A., & Frith, C. D. (2003). Delusions of alien control in the normal brain. *Neuropsychologia, 41*, 1058–1067.

Boly, M., Faymonville, M-E., Vogt, B. A., Maquet, P., & Laureys, S. (2007). Hypnotic regulation of consciousness and the pain neuromatrix. In G. A. Jamieson (Ed.), *Hypnosis and conscious states: The cognitive neuroscience perspective* (pp. 15–27). Oxford, England: Oxford University Press.

Bowers, K. S. (1992). Imagination and dissociation in hypnotic responding. *International Journal of Clinical and Experimental Hypnosis, 40*, 253–275.

Braffman, W., & Kirsch, I. (1999). Imaginative suggestibility and hypnotizability: An empirical analysis. *Journal of Personality and Social Psychology, 77*, 578–587.

Burgess, A. (2007). On the contribution of neurophysiology to hypnosis research: Current state and future directions. In G. A. Jamieson (Ed.), *Hypnosis and conscious states: The cognitive neuroscience perspective* (pp. 195–219). Oxford, England: Oxford University Press.

Cardeña, E., Alarcon, A., Capafons, A., & Bayot, A. (1998). Effects on suggestibility of a new method of active–alert hypnosis: Alert hand. *International Journal of Clinical and Experimental Hypnosis, 46*, 280–294.

Crawford, H. J., Gur, R. C., Skolnick, B., Gur, R. E., & Benson, D. M. (1993). Effects of hypnosis on regional cerebral blood flow during ischemic pain with and without suggested hypnotic analgesia. *International Journal of Psychophysiology, 15*, 181–195.

Croft, R. J., Williams, J. D., Haenschel, C., & Gruzelier, J. H. (2002). Pain perception, hypnosis, and 40Hz oscillations. *International Journal of Psychophysiology, 46*, 101–108.

Deeley, Q., Oakley, D. A., Giampietro, V., Brammer, M. J., Williams, S. C. R., Toone, B., & Halligan, P. W. (2008). *Modulating the default mode of brain function: Evidence from hypnosis and functional MRI.* Manuscript submitted for publication.

Deeley, Q., Oakley, D. A., Toone, B., Giampietro, V., Brammer, M. J., Williams, S. C. R., & Halligan, P. W. (2008a). *Does hypnosis affect visual and auditory processing? An fMRI study.* Manuscript in preparation.

Deeley, Q., Oakley, D. A., Toone, B., Giampietro, V., Brammer, M. J., Williams, S. C. R., & Halligan, P. W. (2008b). *The functional anatomy of suggested limb paralysis.* Manuscript submitted for publication.

De Pascalis, V. (1993). EEG spectral analysis during hypnotic induction, hypnotic dream, and age regression. *International Journal of Psychophysiology, 15,* 153–166.

De Pascalis, V. (1994). Event-related potentials during hypnotic hallucinations. *International Journal of Clinical and Experimental Hypnosis, 42,* 39–55.

De Pascalis, V. (1999). Psychophysiological correlates of hypnosis and hypnotic susceptibility. *International Journal of Clinical and Experimental Hypnosis, 47,* 117–143.

De Pascalis, V. (2007). Phase-ordered gamma oscillations and the modulation of hypnotic experience. In G. A. Jamieson (Ed.), *Hypnosis and conscious states: The cognitive neuroscience perspective* (pp. 67–89). Oxford, England: Oxford University Press.

De Pascalis, V., & Cacace, I. (2005). Pain perception, obstructive imagery and phase-ordered gamma oscillations. *International Journal of Psychophysiology, 56,* 157–169.

De Pascalis, V., Cacace, I., & Massicolle, F. (2004). Perception and modulation of pain in waking and hypnosis: Functional significance of phase-ordered gamma oscillations. *Pain, 112,* 27–36.

De Pascalis, V., & Penna, P. M. (1990). 40 Hz EEG activity during hypnotic induction and hypnotic testing. *International Journal of Clinical and Experimental Hypnosis, 38,* 125–138.

Derbyshire, S. W. G., Whalley, M. G., & Oakley, D. A. (2009). Fibromyalgia pain and its modulation by hypnotic and nonhypnotic suggestion: An fMRI analysis. *European Journal of Pain, 13,* 542–550.

Derbyshire, S. W. G., Whalley, M. G., Stenger, V. A., & Oakley, D. A. (2004). Cerebral activation during hypnotically induced and imagined pain. *NeuroImage, 23,* 392–401.

Dietrich, A. (2003). Functional neuroanatomy of altered states of consciousness: The transient hypofrontality hypothesis. *Consciousness and Cognition, 12,* 321–256.

Edmonston, W. E. (1991). Anesis. In S. J. Lynn & J. W. Rhue (Eds.), *Theories of hypnosis: Current models and perspectives* (pp. 197–237). New York: Guilford Press.

Egner, T., Jamieson, G., & Gruzelier, J. (2005). Hypnosis decouples cognitive control from conflict monitoring processes of the frontal lobe. *NeuroImage, 27,* 969–978.

Ersland, L., Rosen, G., Lundervold, A., Smievoll, A. I., Tillung, T., Sundberg, H., & Hugdahl, K. (1996). Phantom limb imaginary finger tapping causes primary motor cortex activation: An fMRI study. *NeuroReport, 8,* 207–210.

Faymonville, M. E., Laureys, S., Degueldre, C., DelFiore, G., Luxen, A., Franck, G., et al. (2000). Neural mechanisms of antinociceptive effects of hypnosis. *Anesthesiology, 92,* 1257–67.

Fellows, B. J., & Richardson, J. (1993). Relaxed and alert hypnosis: An experiential comparison. *Contemporary Hypnosis, 10*, 49–54.

Gandhi, B., & Oakley, D. A. (2005). Does "hypnosis" by any other name smell as sweet? The efficacy of "hypnotic" induction depends on the label "hypnosis." *Consciousness and Cognition, 14*, 304–315.

Graffin, N. F., Ray, W. J., & Lundy, R. (1995). EEG concomitants of hypnosis and hypnotic susceptibility. *Journal of Abnormal Psychology, 104*, 123–131.

Green, J. P., Barabasz, A. R., Barrett, D., & Montgomery, G. (2005). Forging ahead: The 2003 APA Division 30 definition of hypnosis. *International Journal of Clinical and Experimental Hypnosis, 53*, 259– 264.

Grond, M., Pawlik, G., Walter, H., Lesch, O. M., & Heiss, W. D. (1995). Hypnotic catalepsy-induced changes of regional cerebral glucose metabolism. *Psychiatry Research, 61*, 173–179.

Gruzelier, J. H. (1998). A working model of the neurophysiology of hypnosis: A review of the evidence. *Contemporary Hypnosis, 15*, 3–21.

Gusnard, D. A., & Raichle, M. E. (2001). Searching for a baseline: Functional imaging and the resting human brain. *Nature Reviews Neuroscience, 2*, 685–694.

Guye, M., Parker, G. J., Symms, M., Boulby, P., Wheeler-Kingshott, C. A., Salek-Haddadi, A., et al. (2003). Combined functional MRI and tractography to demonstrate the connectivity of the human primary motor cortex in vivo. *Neuroimage, 19*, 1349–1360.

Halligan, P. W., Athwal, B. S., Oakley, D. A., & Frackowiak, R. S. J. (2000, March 18). Imaging hypnotic paralysis: Implications for conversion hysteria. *The Lancet, 355*, 986–987.

Hilgard, E. R. (1977). *Divided consciousness: Multiple controls in human thought and action.* New York: Wiley.

Hofbauer, R. K., Rainville, P., Duncan, G. H., & Bushnell, M. C. (2001). Cortical representation of the sensory dimension of pain. *Journal of Neurophysiology, 86*, 402–411.

Horton, J. E., & Crawford, H. J. (2004). Neurophysiological and genetic determinants of high hypnotizability. In M. Heap, R. J. Brown, & D. A. Oakley (Eds.), *The highly hypnotizable person: Theoretical, experimental, and clinical issues* (pp. 133–151). London: Routledge.

Hull, C. L. (1933). *Hypnosis and suggestibility: An experimental approach.* New York: Appleton-Century-Crofts.

Hull. C. J., & Huse, B. (1930). Comparative suggestibility in the trance and waking states. *American Journal of Psychology, 52*, 279–286.

Jamieson, G. A., & Sheehan, P. W. (2004). An empirical test of Woody and Bowers's dissociated control theory of hypnosis. *International Journal of Clinical and Experimental Hypnosis, 52*, 232–249.

Jamieson, G. A., & Woody, E. (2007). Dissociated control as a paradigm for cognitive neuroscience research and theorizing in hypnosis. In G. A. Jamieson (Ed.),

Hypnosis and conscious states: The cognitive neuroscience perspective (pp. 111–129). Oxford, England: Oxford University Press.

Jasiukaitis, P., Nouriani, B., Hugdahl, K., & Spiegel, D. (1997). Relateralising hypnosis: Or, have we been barking up the wrong hemisphere? *International Journal of Clinical and Experimental Hypnosis, 45,* 159–177.

Jasiukaitis, P., Nouriani, B., & Spiegel, D. (1996). Left hemisphere superiority for event-related potential effects of hypnotic obstruction. *Neuropsychologia, 34,* 661–668.

Kaiser, J., Barker, R., Haenschel, C., Baldeweg, T., & Gruzelier, J. H. (1997). Hypnosis and event-related potential correlates of error processing in a Stroop-type paradigm: A test of the frontal hypothesis. *International Journal of Psychophysiology, 27,* 215–222.

Kallio, S., & Revonsuo, A. (2003). Hypnotic phenomena and altered states of consciousness: A multilevel framework of description and explanation. *Contemporary Hypnosis, 20,* 111–164.

Kihlstrom, J. F. (2003). The fox, the hedgehog, and hypnosis. *International Journal of Clinical and Experimental Hypnosis, 51,* 166–189.

Killeen, P. R., & Nash, M. R. (2003). The four causes of hypnosis. *International Journal of Clinical and Experimental Hypnosis, 51,* 195–231.

Kirsch, I., & Lynn, S. J. (1995). The altered state of hypnosis: Changes in the theoretical landscape. *American Psychologist, 50,* 846–858.

Kosslyn, S. M., Thompson, W. L., Constantini-Ferrando, M. F., Alpert, N. M., & Spiegel, D. (2000). Hypnotic visual illusion alters color processing in the brain. *American Journal of Psychiatry, 157,* 1279–1284.

LaBerge, S., & Zimbardo, P. G. (1999). Event-related potential correlates of suggested hypnotic amnesia. *Sleep and Hypnosis, 1,* 122–128.

Lynn, S. J., Kirsch, I., Knox, J., Fassler, O., & Lilienfeld, S. O. (2007). Hypnosis and neuroscience: Implications for the altered state debate. In G. A. Jamieson (Ed.), *Hypnosis and conscious states: The cognitive neuroscience perspective* (pp. 145–165). Oxford, England: Oxford University Press.

Maquet, P., Faymonville, M. E., Degueldre, C., Delfiore, G., Franck, G., Luxen, A., & Lamy, M. (1999). Functional neuroanatomy of hypnotic state. *Biological Psychiatry, 45,* 327–333.

Marshall, J. C., Halligan, P. W., Fink, G. R., Wade, D. T., & Frackowiak, R. S. J. (1997). The functional anatomy of a hysterical paralysis. *Cognition, 64,* B1–B8.

Naish, P. (2007). Time distortion and the nature of hypnosis and consciousness. In G. A. Jamieson (Ed.), *Hypnosis and conscious states: The cognitive neuroscience perspective* (pp. 271–292). Oxford, England: Oxford University Press.

Nordby, H., Hugdahl, K., Jasiukaitis, P., & Spiegel, D. (1999). Effects of hypnotizability on performance of a Stroop task and event-related potentials. *Perceptual and Motor Skills, 88,* 819–830.

Oakley, D. A. (1999). Hypnosis and conversion hysteria: A unifying model. *Cognitive Neuropsychiatry, 4,* 243–265.

Oakley, D. A., (2001). Hypnosis and suggestion in the treatment of hysteria. In P. W. Halligan, C. Bass, & J. C. Marshall (Eds.), Contemporary approaches to the study of hysteria: Clinical and theoretical perspectives (pp. 312–329). Oxford, England: Oxford University Press.

Oakley, D. A. (2006). Hypnosis as a tool in research: Experimental psychopathology. *Contemporary Hypnosis, 23*, 3–14.

Oakley, D. A. (2008). Hypnosis, trance, and suggestion: Evidence from neuroimaging. In M. R. Nash & A. J. Barnier (Eds.), *The Oxford handbook of hypnosis* (pp.365–392). Oxford, England: Oxford University Press.

Oakley, D. A., Deeley, Q., & Halligan, P. W. (2007). Hypnotic depth and response to suggestion under standardized conditions and during fMRI scanning. *International Journal of Clinical and Experimental Hypnosis, 55*, 32–58.

Oakley, D. A., Gracey-Whitman, L., & Halligan, P. W. (2002). Hypnotic imagery as a treatment for phantom limb pain: Two case reports and a review. *Clinical Rehabilitation, 16*, 368–377.

Oakley, D. A., & Halligan, P. W. (2009). Hypnotic suggestion and cognitive neuroscience. *Trends in Cognitive Sciences, 13*, 264–270.

Oakley, D. A., Ward, N. S., Halligan, P. W., & Frackowiak, R. S. J. (2003). Differential brain activations for malingered and subjectively "real" paralysis. In P. W. Halligan, C. Bass, & D. A. Oakley (Eds.), *Malingering and illness deception* (pp. 267–284). Oxford, England: Oxford University Press.

Orne, M. T. (1959). The nature of hypnosis: Artifact and essence. *Journal of Social and Abnormal Psychology, 58*, 277–299.

Ott, U. (2007). States of absorption: In search of neurobiological foundations. In G. A. Jamieson (Ed.), *Hypnosis and conscious states: The cognitive neuroscience perspective* (pp. 257–270). Oxford, England: Oxford University Press.

Pekala, R. J., & Kumar, V. K. (2007). An empirical–phenomenological approach to quantifying consciousness and states of consciousness: With particular reference to understanding the nature of hypnosis. In G. A. Jamieson (Ed.), *Hypnosis and conscious states: The cognitive neuroscience perspective* (pp. 167–194). Oxford, England: Oxford University Press.

Polczyk, R., & Pasek, T. (2006). Types of suggestibility: Relationship among compliance, indirect, and direct suggestibility. *International Journal of Clinical and Experimental Hypnosis, 54*, 392–415.

Raij, T. T., Numminen, J., Narvanen, S., Hiltunen, J., & Hari, R. (2005). Brain correlates of subjective reality of physically and psychologically induced pain. *Proceedings of the National Academy of Sciences, 102*, 2147–2151.

Rainville, P., Duncan, G. H., Price, D. D., Carrier B., & Bushnell, M. C. (1997, August 15). Pain affect encoded in human anterior cingulate but not somatosensory cortex. *Science, 277*, 968–971.

Rainville, P., Hofbauer, R. K., Bushnell, M. C., Duncan, G. H., & Price, D. D. (2002). Hypnosis modulates activity in brain structures involved in the regulation of consciousness. *Journal of Cognitive Neuroscience, 14*, 887–901.

Rainville, P., Hofbauer, R. K., Paus, T., Duncan, G. H., Bushnell, M. C., & Price, D. D. (1999). Cerebral mechanisms of hypnotic induction and suggestion. *Journal of Cognitive Neuroscience, 11*, 110–125.

Rainville, P., & Price, D. D. (2003). Hypnosis phenomenology and the neurobiology of consciousness. *International Journal of Clinical and Experimental Hypnosis, 51*, 105–129.

Ramachandran, V. S., & Hirstein, W. (1998). The perception of phantom limbs. *Brain, 121*, 1603–1630.

Ray, W. J. (1997). EEG concomitants of hypnotic susceptibility. *International Journal of Clinical and Experimental Hypnosis, 45*, 301–333.

Ray, W. J., & De Pascalis, V. (2003). Temporal aspects of hypnotic processes. *International Journal of Clinical and Experimental Hypnosis, 51*, 147–165.

Ray, W. J., & Oathes, D. (2003). Brain imaging techniques. *International Journal of Clinical and Experimental Hypnosis, 51*, 97–104.

Ray, W. J., & Tucker, D. M. (2003). Evolutionary approaches to understanding the hypnotic experience. *International Journal of Clinical and Experimental Hypnosis, 51*, 256–281.

Raz, A. (2005). Attention and hypnosis: Neural substrates and genetic associations of two converging processes. *International Journal of Clinical and Experimental Hypnosis, 53*, 237–258.

Raz, A., Fan, J., & Posner, M. I. (2005). Hypnotic suggestion reduces conflict in the human brain. *Proceedings of the National Academy of Sciences of the United States of America, 102*, 9978–9983.

Raz, A., Kirsch, I., Pollard, J., & Nitkin-Kaner. Y. (2006). Suggestion reduces the Stroop effect. *Psychological Science, 17*, 91–95.

Raz, A., & Shapiro, T. (2002). Hypnosis and neuroscience: A cross talk between clinical and cognitive research. *Archives of General Psychiatry, 59*, 85–90.

Reyher, J. (1962). A paradigm for determining the clinical relevance of hypnotically induced psychopathology. *Psychological Bulletin, 59*, 344–352.

Rhue, J. W., Lynn, S. J., & Kirsch, I. (1993). *Handbook of clinical hypnosis*. Washington, DC: American Psychological Association.

Rosen, G., Willoch, F., Bartenstein, P., Berner, N., & Rosjo, S. (2001). Neurophysiological processes underlying the phantom limb pain experience and the use of hypnosis in its clinical management: An intensive examination of two patients. *International Journal of Clinical and Experimental Hypnosis, 49*, 38–55.

Sabourin, M. E., Cutcomb, S. D., Crawford, H. J., & Pribram, K. (1990). EEG correlates of hypnotic susceptibility and hypnotic trance: Spectral analysis and coherence. *International Journal of Psychophysiology, 10*, 125–142.

Schumaker, J. F. (1991). *Human suggestibility: Advances in theory, research, and application*. New York: Routledge.

Sheehan, P. W., Donovan, P. B., & MacLeod, C. M. (1988). Strategy manipulation and the Stroop effect in hypnosis. *Journal of Abnormal Psychology, 97*, 455–460.

Shor, R. E., & Orne, E. C. (1962). *Harvard Group Scale of Hypnotic Susceptibility: Form A*. Palo Alto, CA: Consulting Psychologists Press.

Simos, P. G., Papanicolaou, A. C., Breier, J. I., Fletcher, J. M., Wheless, J. W., Maggio, et al. (2000). Insights into brain function and neural plasticity using magnetic source imaging. *Journal of Clinical Neurophysiology, 17,* 143–162.

Spiegel, D. (2003). Negative and positive visual hypnotic hallucinations: Attending inside and out. *International Journal of Clinical and Experimental Hypnosis, 51,* 130–146.

Spiegel, D., & Barabasz, A. (1988). Effects of hypnotic instructions on P300 evoked potential amplitudes: Research and clinical implications. *American Journal of Clinical Hypnosis, 31,* 11–17.

Spiegel, D., Cutcomb, S., Ren, C., & Pribram, K. (1985). Hypnotic hallucination alters evoked potentials. *Journal of Abnormal Psychology, 94,* 249–255.

Stroop, J. R. (1935). Studies of interference in serial verbal reactions. *Journal of Experimental Psychology, 18,* 643–661.

Szechtman, H., Woody, E., Bowers, K. S., & Nahmias, C. (1998). Where the imaginal appears real: A positron emission tomography study of auditory hallucinations. *Proceedings of the National Academy of Sciences, 95,* 1956–1960.

Wagstaff, G. (2000). Can hypnosis cause madness? *Contemporary Hypnosis, 17,* 97–111.

Walters, V. J., & Oakley, D. A. (2003). Does hypnosis make in vitro, in vivo? Hypnosis as a possible virtual reality context in cognitive behavioral therapy for an environmental phobia. *Clinical Case Studies, 2,* 295–305.

Ward, N. S., Oakley, D. A., Frackowiak, R. S. J., & Halligan, P. W. (2003). Differential brain activations during intentionally simulated and subjectively experienced paralysis. *Cognitive Neuropsychiatry, 8,* 295–312.

Wark, D. M. (2006). Alert hypnosis: A review and case report. *American Journal of Clinical Hypnosis, 48,* 293–303.

Weitzenhoffer, A. (2000). *The practice of hypnotism.* New York: Wiley.

Weitzenhoffer, A., & Hilgard, E. R. (1962). The Stanford Hypnotic Susceptibility Scale: Form C. Palo Alto, CA: Consulting Psychologists Press.

Williams, J. D., & Gruzelier, J. H. (2001). Differentiation of hypnosis and relaxation by analysis of narrow band theta and alpha frequencies. *International Journal of Clinical and Experimental Hypnosis, 49,* 185–206.

Willoch, F., Rosen, G., Tolle, T.R., Oye, I., Wester, H. J., Berner, N., et al. (2000). Phantom limb in the human brain: Unraveling neural circuitries of phantom limb sensations using Positron Emission Tomography. *Annals of Neurology, 48,* 842–849.

Woody, E. Z., & Szechtman, H. (2003). How can brain activity and hypnosis inform each other? *International Journal of Clinical and Experimental Hypnosis, 51,* 232–255.

II
THEORIES OF HYPNOSIS

5

PSYCHOANALYTIC AND PSYCHODYNAMIC MODELS OF HYPNOANALYSIS

MARLENE R. EISEN

There is a strong historical precedent for the use of hypnosis as a therapeutic modality. Freud studied with two early hypnosis practitioners, Charcot and Breuer, and used this art in his practice. In discussing the idealization of the object (i.e., the image of the significant person in the mind of the individual), Freud (1905/1953b) was impressed by hypnotized subjects' credulous submissiveness to the hypnotist. Comparing hypnosis with being in love, Freud pointed out that just as the loved object often stands in the place of the idealized aspect of the self, the essence of hypnosis resides in an unconscious fixation of the subject's libido to the hypnotist as an ego ideal. Schilder and Kauders (1927/1956) agreed with Freud that hypnosis and suggestion have an erotic root. Submission to authority has an erotic–masochistic component. Subjects project their desires for magical powers onto the hypnotist and, subsequently, by the process of identification, attain those powers that they would not otherwise be able to ascribe to themselves.

Ferenczi (1965) proposed that the hypnotic relationship represents a reactivation of the Oedipus complex, with the subject standing in a child–parent

---

All clinical material has been disguised to protect patient confidentiality.

relationship with the hypnotist. He differentiated between maternal (i.e., based on love) and paternal (i.e., based on fear) forms of hypnosis. In contemporary terms, maternal hypnosis would be defined as *nondirective hypnosis*, whereas paternal hypnosis would be defined as *directive hypnosis*.

These concepts are important insofar as the patient's various perceptions of the therapist (e.g., maternal or paternal figure, ego ideal, magician, healer) represent manifestations of the cornerstone of psychoanalytic therapy: *transference*. In psychoanalysis, transference is thought to be a basically regressive phenomenon in which the patient's feelings, attitudes, and expectations, which were once directed at significant people in his or her past, are projected or "transferred" onto the therapist. Transference is considered to be a fundamental tool for helping the patient (Brown & Fromm, 1986). It is in the interpretation of the meaning of the transferential relationship with the patient that conflicts are resolved and personality integration ultimately occurs. Later in this chapter I discuss transference in greater depth and present research that supports the claim that hypnosis potentiates transference phenomena.

PRIMARY AND SECONDARY PROCESS THOUGHT

Freud (1900/1953a) identified two distinct modes of mental functioning: *primary process functioning*, typical of early childhood thinking; and *secondary process functioning*, a more mature, cognitively based mode of thinking. The main format of primary process thinking is preverbal—imagery that is highly mobile, fluid, and undifferentiated. In this mode, anything is possible, even the impossible. Logical thinking and critical, analytical abilities are dramatically reduced, if evident at all, and several ideas may be condensed into a single image. Dreams and hypnosis share this primitive, regressive mode of thinking (see Nash, 1991): the "stuff that dreams are made of." By contrast, secondary process thinking is logical and sequential. It functions by way of language rather than images, and it is reality oriented, guided by the critical and analytical functions of the ego. Although primary process thinking precedes secondary process thinking in the developmental sequence, it does not disappear with age. Instead, it takes other forms, including imagery and the illogical characteristics of playful activities, jokes, and dreams that persist through adulthood. Furthermore, according to Brown and Fromm (1986), the full range of mental experience, from strictly reality-oriented cognition to the more fluid and undifferentiated primary process thought, continues to interact in adulthood. Various states of consciousness can be described as existing on a continuum from primary to secondary process as one moves from fantasy to reality; from nocturnal dreams to full wakefulness; and from unfocused, free-floating attention to focused attention.

Even in adulthood, play and creativity (i.e., mind play) use regression in the service of the ego, a rich reservoir that hypnosis taps for healing purposes. It was Hartmann (1936/1958) who first referred to *adaptive regression*. This concept was derived from his belief that the ego and id were relatively autonomous, a hypothesis that established the theoretical base for ego psychological psychotherapy. Kris (1934/1952) termed the same process *regression in the service of the ego* and described how the creative artist experiences a more or less intentional return to, or resumption of, irrational, archaic modes of imagination, thought, and sensibility. Fenichel (1945) described how adaptive regression enables the hypnotist to take over the function of the patient's superego and even parts of the ego, thus allowing for regression within a safe milieu.

Nash (1987) suggested that this form of regression common to hypnosis is topological rather than temporal (i.e., patients do not exhibit truly childlike behavior during hypnosis) and is related to alternative modes of mature thought rather than to immature thought patterns. According to Loewald (1981),

> regression in service of the ego is not simply a means for increased ability to make the irrational rational, for extending the range of rationality. It frees the ego from the excessive domination of rationality and increases the dimensions and range, not of rationality, but of the ego as an organization encompassing the totality of human experience, including the irrational. (p. 40)

ACTIVITY, PASSIVITY, AND RECEPTIVITY LEVELS OF EGO FUNCTION

The psychoanalytic theory of ego activity and passivity was introduced by Rapaport (1953/1967) and Hart (1961) and extended by Fromm (1972). The concept of *ego receptivity* was developed by Deikman (1971) and was discussed in the context of hypnosis by Fromm and Shor (1979). The ego is active or autonomous when the individual can make an *ego-syntonic choice* (i.e., a choice that is consciously or implicitly consistent with the individual's goals and objectives). It is passive when the person is overwhelmed by instinctual drives or demands from the environment or superego. Ego activity and passivity are related to coping. The ego may cope in a masterful or defensive mode. In hypnotherapy, ego activity may be represented by resistance or by the patient's countertherapeutic self-suggestions taking precedence over the therapist's suggestions (Fromm & Shor, 1979). Ego passivity manifests itself when the patient feels overwhelmed by the therapist or by the perceived demand characteristics of the therapeutic situation. When this occurs, the results are usually ego-dystonic and associated with subjective discomfort.

In ego receptivity, critical judgments, a strict adherence to the demands of reality, and active, goal-oriented thinking are minimal. Receptive in this manner, patients experience a free-flowing stream of consciousness characterized by the emergence of unconscious and preconscious material. In hypnotherapy the patient becomes more receptive both to the therapist's suggestions and to a clearer awareness of the internal flow of images and thoughts. This mode in which experience is organized around taking in and letting things happen can be contrasted with the ego-active mode in which the individual makes things happen and actively manipulates the environment.

A fourth mode of ego function, often reported in certain forms of meditation, is ego inactivity. The individual reports experiencing nothing and coming away from the experience refreshed and relaxed. Meares (1960), working in Australia with patients who were severely ill, found that a nonverbal induction of a deep state of calm had a remarkably curative effect on many patients. He used such nonverbal techniques as humming and gently stroking the hand or arm. These techniques are not unlike the drumming and chanting often used in Shamanic healing. Of course, more research needs to be done in the area of defining and differentiating between the different levels of ego function in hypnotic and nonhypnotic situations.

TRANCE DEPTH AS A DIMENSION OF THERAPY

The hypnotic experience can be characterized by the capacity to sustain a state of attentive, receptive, intensely focused concentration with diminished peripheral awareness. In this chapter I refer to this state as *trance*, which fluctuates on a continuum between focal and peripheral awareness (H. Spiegel & Spiegel, 1978). The degree to which peripheral awareness, or general reality orientation, fades in relation to focused attention determines trance depth.

Although there is no direct correlation between the depth of trance and the degree of primary process thought, in general, it has been found that the deeper the altered state of consciousness, the more likely one is to experience vivid, often free-floating attention; diminished critical thought; and increased ego receptivity (Fromm & Kahn, 1990). Under these circumstances, cognition is less likely to be reality-oriented and more likely to be idiosyncratic or influenced by suggestions from a strong environmental stimulus (i.e., the therapist).

For the most part, the patient's depth of trance is not a crucial issue in hypnotherapy. A light or moderate trance is sufficient to achieve the major goals of psychodynamic hypnotherapy: uncovering, reframing, and reintegrating repressed or disowned aspects of the personality. If the trance is not deep, the patient is more likely to be able to interact verbally with the therapist. Many patients who go into deep trance states have difficulty with verbal communications, and the therapist may need to resort to ideomotor signaling. This is not an insurmountable problem, but if the patient can carry on a dialogue with either the therapist or other ego states within the self (i.e., the "inner child"), the work of therapy proceeds much more satisfactorily.

The traditional psychoanalytic goals of uncovering drives and defenses, working through affects, and achieving new levels of personality integration can be effectively realized by way of psychodynamic hypnotherapy or hypnoanalysis. The characteristics of hypnosis discussed in this section—the preponderance of primary process thinking stimulated by regression in the service of the ego and the patient's receptivity to the emerging mental representations of neurotic defenses and areas of conflict—facilitate achieving these goals quickly and effectively. Hypnosis enhances the process of uncovering dynamically relevant material by stimulating increased awareness of symbolic processes, memories, and affective states (Nash, 1987). Hypnosis can also provide opportunities for cognitive and perceptual changes that lead to new opportunities for insight and conflict resolution (Frankel, 1976). In the next section I discuss the use of hypnosis as a tool in the clinical setting and how its distinctive qualities facilitate and enrich the therapeutic experience.

DOUBLE CONSCIOUSNESS: THE PARTICIPATING AND OBSERVING EGO

E. R. Hilgard (1977), Fromm and Shor (1979), and others have distinguished between two levels of ego function common to the hypnotic experience: (a) the *participating ego*, which relinquishes the critical function (i.e., reality testing) to the control of the hypnotist or to self-directives in self-hypnosis; and (b) the *observing ego*, which maintains the critical function and monitors the level of involvement of the participating ego. Nash (1991) referred to this phenomenon as an *experienced separation* between intent to comply and awareness of that intent.

Hypnotized subjects are not automatons, and they clearly demonstrate will and volition in refusing to comply with ego-dystonic suggestions (Lynn, Rhue, & Weekes, 1990). It is this capacity of the observing ego or *hidden observer* (i.e., the volitional aspect) that makes the hypnotic experience feel safe enough to allow the ego to move into a more regressed state. It is also the hidden observer that is able to interpret the symbolic representations of imagery and dreams because of its access to information dissociated from or split off from conscious experience (E. R. Hilgard, 1973, 1974).

In their research on hypnotic dreams, with or without the evocation of hidden observer as interpreter, Pinnell, Lynn, and Pinnell (1998) found that the effect of the suggestion requesting the engagement of the hidden observer results in less primary process material. Without that suggestion, the hidden observer still functions, but the participating ego has more freedom to engage in primary process activity. One might posit that the hidden observer, when called on, stands on the bridge between the dreamer and the thinker, between ego-receptive and ego-active functions. They also found that the dream reports of individuals who are hypnotized contained more primary process than dream reports of nonhypnotized simulating participants, thus reinforcing the efficacy of hypnosis in enhancing primary process.

HOMEOSTASIS: ADAPTIVE SYNCHRONY

The human being constantly strives for a state of *adaptive synchrony*, or homeostasis in time and space. According to Restak (1979), the brain has the primary responsibility for maintaining itself and the body; it succeeds in this task largely through an automatic set of regulating mechanisms that serve to maintain body integrity. Restak referred to this process as a *feedback loop*. This feedback loop process can be viewed from a psychodynamic perspective. In wakeful states of consciousness, the ego is cognizant of messages from both the id and the environment, which it processes, evaluates, and responds to on the basis of relevance, urgency, or both. During waking moments, the senses are busy gathering volumes of information from the environment, whereas physical and emotional states are pervasive and inescapable. The mind selects environmental features that are the most salient (i.e., most likely to reduce physical and emotional tension levels and attain balance or homeostasis).

When environmental information is restricted, as in the trance state, mental or physical inner processes take precedence. The perception of the environment is restructured through internal, primary process functioning. Becoming involved in a TV show, a book, music, deep breathing, or any activity in which the focus of attention is so intense that elements of the environment fade or are gated out of awareness alters customary cognitive processing.

Neuroscience now documents the activity of *mirror neurons*, a function of the brain that develops empathic understanding by matching the brain patterns of others with whom one is interacting (Rossi, 2007; Rossi & Rossi, 2006). This phenomenon seems to validate a hypothesis that understanding the behavior of others involves translating actions we observe into the neural language of our own actions. This discovery may explain why children of traumatized adults (i.e., Holocaust survivors) develop emotional patterns that mirror those of the actual victims of the trauma. This *observation/execution matching system*, which provides a necessary connection from "doing" to "communicating" as the link between actor and observer, appears to provide a neural mirroring system that could be an essential mechanism for the sensitive, highly focused empathy between therapist and subject in hypnosis.

From the perspective of therapeutic hypnosis, the experience of empathy and understanding "other minds" would appear to be the essence of what has been termed *rapport*, a necessary correlate of therapeutic hypnosis. Further exploration of the function of mirror neurons promises to provide a neuroscientific explanation of the psychological impact of hypnotherapy (Rossi & Rossi, 2006).

Fenichel (1945) declared that hypnosis represents a nostalgic reversion to the phase of life when "passive–receptive" mastery represented the primary means of coping with the world. Security was achieved by participating in or encompassing a greater unit, the all-powerful parent. The hypnotist comes to represent the powerful parent who both guides and protects and who promises, or is believed to promise, surcease from pain or displeasure. It often becomes apparent that the patient's greatest satisfaction derives from the giving over of the troubled aspects of self to the powerful, well-controlled adult in a permissive setting.

Hypnosis satisfies that universal infantile core in each person that longs for wholesale abdication of his or her usual powers and responsibilities (Gill & Brenman, 1959). In my experience, "good hypnotic subjects" may present with intense unconscious needs to be both passive and aggressively demanding, much like the infant. In everyday life these people relentlessly defend against such feelings, both through denial and reaction formation, to such an extent that the manifest personality is frequently that of a self-sufficient "high achiever."

TRANCE AND AFFECT

Clinical experience suggests that during hypnosis, intense absorption and involvement leads to much greater affect intensity, particularly in participants who are highly hypnotizable. Changes in the nature and quality of affect, such as outbursts of weeping and intense expressions of rage, anxiety, fear, and despair, are not uncommon. Encouraging the subject to "sit with" the intense affect and accept it, perhaps asking the self, "What is this?" in an effort to understand the meaning of the particular emotion in the moment, can be used in the therapeutic engagement. In a culture that negates intense emotional responses, the knowledge that one can express such heightened emotional expression without serious consequences, may in itself have a healing effect. It is as if the trance state itself represents a generalized amplification of affect (Brown & Fromm, 1986). A dramatic aspect of the subject's affective response is the abruptness with which it can be turned off when trance is terminated.

In his study of empathy and absorption as correlates of hypnosis, Wickramasekera (2007) found that empathy appears positively related to absorption, which is a characteristic of high hypnotizability. He also found that some individuals engage in behavior he calls *repressive coping*. These individuals avoid attending to environmental stimuli or affective responses that are perceived as emotionally threatening.

THE "ILLOGIC" OF TRANCE LOGIC

Because the ego releases the critical function in hypnotic trance and regresses to more primary thought processes, individuals can visualize anger in concrete form and speak to it or act on it without regard for the irrationality of the act. For example, they can simultaneously visualize the angry self sitting in one place and the contented self in another place, representing different affective states. Individuals in a trance state may find nothing unusual about visualizing someone sitting beside them and also standing across the room. This phenomenon has been referred to as *trance logic* (Orne, 1959).

NURTURING IMAGES: THE INNER CHILD

A powerful image used to reinforce self-nurturing is the adult caring for his or her inner child. Typically, the patient spontaneously evokes in the trance the image of himself or herself as a sad, lonely little child. The therapist can suggest that the adult patient provide the child with the kind of parenting the child needs and desires. Patients often use this image to their advantage in self-hypnosis, becoming self-nurturing, giving the inner child loving, accepting messages (Eisen & Fromm, 1983). Nurtured until it becomes more content, the child ego state can then experience joy and liberate creativity. Of course, the caring and accepting therapist serves as a model for such patient behavior.

THE USE OF DREAMS

Using dreams in hypnoanalysis provides valuable insights. When a patient brings in dream material, the hypnotherapist can suggest that the patient reexperience the dream in trance, this time with a clear understanding of the meaning of the images. Dreams may also be induced in the heterohypnotic hour. The focus can be on a particular conflict or issue raised in therapy. The patient may be encouraged to redream the dream once or several times with different, perhaps more effective, resolutions. A posthypnotic suggestion that the patient will have dreams that foster understanding and problem resolution and that these dreams will be readily recalled and comprehended can stimulate a spate of dreaming, as can recording dreams in a journal.

DEFENSES AND RESISTANCES

Interpretation of defenses and resistances should be handled carefully, gently, and respectfully. Defenses should not be attacked prematurely but need to be acknowledged and understood in the context of their unique and personal meaning. Resistance also serves an adaptive function that must be understood and respected. A common form of resistance in hypnoanalysis is refusal to go into a trance. Rather than interpreting this maneuver as a resistance, the therapist would do well to note the issues being worked with at the time and find different or safer ways of approaching the subject or simply defer exploring the particular topic to a more appropriate time. Resistance can also be manifested when a patient's communications in relation to a particular issue are ambiguous. Interpreting this communication style as resistance can, on occasion, be helpful and move the therapy forward. Finally, there are occasions when acknowledging the resistance will be sufficient to overcome it.

TRANSFERENCE

Transference is a term that indicates the patient's distorted perceptions, feelings, or behaviors toward the therapist, who comes to represent a significant figure from childhood such as a parent or sibling. When there is a positive transference, the therapist is loved and idealized. However, when the transference is negative, the therapist is hated or feared. Hypnosis intensifies transference, bringing conflicts and repressed affects associated with internal representations into focus more rapidly and intensely.

Most frequently, three types of neurotic transferences are encountered. Infantile dependency transferences are the most common in hypnotherapy, especially at the beginning of treatment when the patient comes to be taken care of and wants the therapist to solve all of the problems for him or her. Like the small child, the patient hopes that the therapist is omniscient, possessing the healing power of the perfect parent. Often, significant others and referring professionals share this unrealistic fantasy or wish. Not infrequently, magical thinking accompanies this positive transference. For example, one patient may say, "I carry your voice and the image of your couch, and I feel the healing power."

Transferences can also take the form of seduction or competition. A patient who falsely accuses the therapist of attempting to seduce him or her may actually be acting out an old fantasy of wishing to be seduced by the opposite-sex parent. A patient's attempt to outdo or to compete with the therapist, rooted in early sibling rivalry, may be expressed by statements such as, "I get much better imagery in self-hypnosis," or by regaling the therapist with stories of personal successes while finding fault with the current therapy or therapist (Brown & Fromm, 1986).

Using such transferential feelings may be more effective than interpreting them. For instance, patients who attempt to outshine the therapist can be praised for their excellent abilities. It can be demonstrated that outdoing is not destroying and that such special abilities allow for greater success in using trance states. There are also specific transference reactions related to idiosyncratic experiences. For example, a patient whose analyst had committed suicide wanted to use trance work but feared it would increase her dependence on the current therapist, reenacting her great loss when the analyst on whom she had become so dependent abandoned her. The former analyst had assured her that he would not die after having made a previous attempt. Therefore, even if her current therapist said she was not planning to kill herself it would do little to relieve the patient's distress. Instead, her fears of dependency were acknowledged, and the ways in which this therapist was different from the former one were consistently pointed out.

EGO STATES: RELEVANCE IN TREATMENT

Watkins and Watkins (1981) modified and expanded the ego-state theories of Federn (1952) and Weiss (1952), who described a continuum of permeability and flexibility of ego-state boundaries within each individual. Healthy ego states with fluid boundaries occur in everyday life as people move from one situational context or role to another (e.g., student, daughter, date). As ego-state boundaries become more rigid and impermeable, they become increasingly maladaptive until, at the opposite end of the continuum, there are dissociative states, manifesting in some cases as multiple personality disorders. Lemke (2005) posited the "far left" of the ego-state continuum, where internal conflicts create barriers to fully realizing one's adaptive functions. These barriers act to contain the psyche in a single rigidly held ego state (e.g., workaholic, martyr mom). Hypnosis in the context of ego state therapy can help the patient reconnect the more imaginal parts of the self with the rigidly cognitive self, thus creating a framework for a more balanced life.

When significant figures are internalized or acknowledged in the form of consistent, ongoing mental representations, they are originally recognized as *not self* or as *other*. In object relations theory, they are referred to as *objects*. Eventually, the individual may identify so strongly with this internalized other that it begins to feel like part of the self and ultimately becomes part of the self.

The concepts of object and self ego states have important implications for understanding hypnosis and for dealing with transferences (Watkins & Watkins, 1990). Hypnosis can be used to manipulate the patient's perceptions of ego states. For example, during hypnosis, suggestions can be given for the "frightened child" ego state to be protected by the "competent adult" ego state. In dealing with transference, it is important to understand that it may not be the "whole patient" who has projected the abusing parental figure onto the therapist but a particular ego state that has done so, which represents a relatively vulnerable fragment of the whole.

Ginandes (2006) uses ego state therapy with the medically ill. She suggested that symptoms of medical illness often speak through vivid embedded metaphors that contain complex unconscious meanings. Therapeutic attunement to these multi-layered illness-associated issues can be instrumental in both psychological and physiological healing. In working with ego states, it is important not to cast out those that appear to be flawed. They are, after all, still part of the self, often internalizations of significant others. Rather, these "shadow selves" need to be acknowledged and integrated (Watkins & Watkins, 1979).

PERSONALITY DISORDERS

People diagnosed with narcissistic personality disorder respond strongly to therapists' failures of empathy. Patients diagnosed as mildly narcissistic may express anger or disappointment to the therapist during the therapy hour. By contrast, those diagnosed as highly narcissistic react with rage and disillusionment by missing appointments, making suicide threats or gestures, or making midnight phone calls to the therapist. In such instances, the hypnoanalyst must actively play the role of the good parent, fulfilling the hitherto unmet needs of the patient for admiration and unconditional positive regard.

People diagnosed with borderline personality disorder are unable to form stable self- and object transferences. Instead, the transference is characterized by boundary diffusion and splitting, panic states, and transient loss of self- and object representations (Adler, 1985). Many therapists hesitate to use hypnosis with such patients, fearing an exacerbation of boundary diffusion, destabilizing an already fragile sense of self. Baker (1983, 1990) has written extensively and has carefully explicated a way of successfully using hypnosis with this population. To counter these tendencies, the therapist must provide a *holding environment* (Winnicott, 1975). The environment must be safe, all nurturing, and all accepting, with clear boundaries delineated. Distinctions must be made between reality and fantasy as a step toward integration. First, however, it may be necessary for the therapist to join the patient in a fantasy world, together exploring the meaning of the patient's inner life. The therapist becomes an internalized good object by being all-giving within the context of firm limits. It is in the relationship with the therapist that the patient begins to build an integrated sense of self.

In working with patients diagnosed with borderline personality disorder, the value of hypnosis rests with the power of imagery to provide as-if situations or imaginative scenarios, in which the patient can try out different ways of being and relating to others. Much like the sociodramatic play of young children, hypnosis can be used by borderline patients to regress to an early stage of life when psychological development was truncated and to begin to build a new, healthier personality structure.

COUNTERTRANSFERENCE

When an attitude or behavior on the patient's part calls forth feelings in the therapist that are not appropriate to the therapeutic relationship, this is referred to as *countertransference*. Patients diagnosed with borderline personality disorder are particularly likely to evoke intense feelings because of their insatiable demands on the therapist's time and attention. Traumatized patients' stories of their horrific past may provoke countertransference feelings, whereas patients' problems that trigger unresolved issues from the therapist's past might also engender countertransference reactions.

It is important for the therapist to recognize countertransference issues so that they do not contaminate the therapeutic alliance. When therapists recognize that they may be acting out feelings on the basis of countertransference (e.g., forgetting appointments with a particular patient, being late, using up time on superficial issues to avoid the hypnotic work), it is a good idea to seek consultation. If the relationship with the patient is resilient enough, direct discussion may prove to be the most beneficial.

CLINICAL APPLICATIONS

Hypnotic techniques particularly suited to hypnoanalysis include age regression for tracing early developmental stages of personality organization, for identifying life themes, and for recovery of repressed memories and affects. Metaphors, automatic writing or drawing, and guided and spontaneous imagery can all be used to access emotional states and personal myths and to resolve emotional traumata. Hypnosis can be used to stimulate dissociation of the observing ego from the participating ego (Fromm & Shor, 1979), to integrate dissociated ego states (Watkins & Watkins, 1979), and to differentiate the body self from the mind self to facilitate healing (Eisen, 1990). Some practitioners, particularly those involved in forensic work, have questioned the validity of repressed memory. I believe recalled memories are of great psychological relevance because they represent the patient's present efforts to create a consistent narrative of self. Their historical veracity is not at issue in the therapeutic context.

The purpose of hypnoanalysis is to help the patient achieve insight, conflict resolution, and mastery (Fromm, 1992). Whereas symbolic fantasy or imagery can help uncover repressed material, reality testing, fantasy, or imagery rehearsal techniques can help integrate new insights into novel behavior patterns. Working with a supportive therapist who promotes insight, the patient can safely practice different coping strategies and visualize the successful implementation of one or another. Regressing into the inner world of fantasy and practicing more successful adaptations allows the patient to return to a state of greater active consciousness feeling stronger and more competent.

Some tools of hypnotherapy—in particular, imagery and primary process thought—give patients a creative way to use their inner potential for problem solving and growth. Both fantastic imagery and reality-based imagery can be used in treatment to access the inner world of the mind. Often, the ritual of trance (the "excuse" of the altered state) facilitates the patient's adaptive regression.

In hypnoanalysis, the ego ideal can be used to help the patient to identify with the healthier, stronger parts of the self. The therapist can suggest the presence of a strong, positive figure that has achieved what the patient wants to achieve and with whom the patient can have a dialogue. This can be done by having the patient imagine a split screen or a couch with the "self" at one end and the "ideal self" at the other end. As they interact, the two selves can come closer together and finally meld into one. The therapist can then suggest that the patient look out at the world through the eyes of the ideal, or competent, self.

The therapist can suggest that a *spirit guide* or *inner healer* lives in the quiet, calm center of the mind and knows all that the patient needs to know about himself or herself and all that can be known about human experience. For patients with cancer, this inner spirit is a healer. For others, it becomes a creative force to unblock higher functioning or a good mother from a previous life who can provide warmth and nurturing. Each patient finds the image needed to promote healing. This power within the self, like the ego ideal, can be an excellent source of mastery and fuels a sense of personal power. It mitigates the helpless feeling engendered by the vulnerability of serious illness.

CLINICAL MATERIAL

The following cases are made up of a collage of bits and pieces from years of clinical notes. They have been selected to elucidate the various ways hypnosis is used by patients to further the healing process. I have always been impressed by the creative metaphors people derive in trance as they struggle with their personal demons. Before embarking on the hypnotic process, I generally use Speigel's eye-roll technique to ascertain level of hypnotizability (Speigel & Speigel, 1978). Over the years, I have used a number of different induction techniques, both ideomotor and visualization. I have found that an induction technique that includes deep breathing, progressive relaxation, and visualization is effective with most patients. Finding a safe, quiet inner space, then connecting with a wise inner voice, sets the stage for whatever follows. I assure my patient, because I believe it is true, that the mind will go where it needs to go to do what it needs to do.

A number of hypnotic techniques have been described, and various issues germane to hypnotherapy have been discussed in this chapter. Case material provides another dimension to illuminate and understand the concepts presented in the previous discussion of therapeutic modalities.

Healing Images: The Mask

My discussion indicates that hypnosis can promote primary process thinking that can be used to advantage in hypnoanalysis. Certain images have a historical precedent, a mythic power to evoke intense affective states. One such image is the *mask*. I begin with two cases in which the mask became a healing metaphor.

The first case is that of a patient diagnosed with narcissistic personality disorder who feared self-exploration but also sought it out with great intensity (Eisen & Fromm, 1983). He had created a "living myth" for himself consisting of a perfect family, a loving wife, two beautiful, accomplished children, and a successful career. In truth, he avoided all sexual contact with his wife, his daughter was showing signs of becoming anorexic at age 11, the son was withdrawn and depressed at age 5, and the patient was having difficulties with his job. He came into hypnotherapy because of persistent severe headaches and insisted that this was his only problem.

In a trance, this patient felt compelled to create strong images of power. He envisioned himself as an armored knight on a great horse and used this image in hypnotherapy and also in self-hypnotic episodes at home. As he became more comfortable with his capacity for self-soothing through hypnosis and his headaches abated, he was given the suggestion that perhaps he was wearing a mask that he could remove when he was ready. It took some months before he could risk removing the mask, which had eventually expanded to cover his whole body. What he found behind the mask was not an empty shell, as he had feared, but a humanly flawed yet acceptable self, with some ambivalence about his sexual orientation.

The second patient was the healthier of twin girls who felt that she had been "punished" by her parents because of her crippled sister. She came into therapy to deal with profuse sweating under her arms that was a constant source of embarrassment. She was always fearful that she would not perform well enough to please her parents, her teachers, and her employers. Once she learned to use self-hypnosis to control her tension and sweating, she was able to use her vivid imagination to work on more dynamic issues. In imagery she found herself trapped behind a mask-like gate. Sitting on a stool, she manipulated strings that allowed the mask to maintain adult-like features. Behind her on a hill, a castle full of treasure beckoned. Once she could accept her "childlike" need to engage in spontaneous activities without feeling she would be punished, she was able to drop the strings, destroying the mask of adulthood (i.e., the false self), and to let her whole being respond to the "treasures" life offered. Note that she not only hid behind the mask of adulthood but also distanced herself from it. As a gate, it not only protected her but also kept the world out. When she could acknowledge the child within (i.e., her dependency needs), she could become her true adult self.

Ego States: The Inner Child and the Nurturing Adult

Hypnosis not only provides ample opportunities to use adaptive regression and primary process thinking to advantage, it also provides a context for using metaphors relevant to altering the relation between and among the patient's ego states and promoting personal integration. For instance, the adult who nurtures the child self, or inner child, is a powerful metaphor. It gives the patient permission to acknowledge the needy, dependent part of the self.

A patient who needed to give up smoking for health reasons but found herself "sneaking" cigarettes whenever she could was enraged with herself. A tough professional woman who lived alone, she began questioning her mental stability when she experienced a childlike glee each time she "got away with" another quick puff. When she was given the suggestion that her adult self begin a dialogue with her child self, she found that the little girl within felt unacknowledged. "She," the child, needed to have some fun in this woman's demanding, responsible life. Smoking became the "child's" outlet. When this woman began actively acknowledging this "little kid" (e.g., "My friends think I'm nuts, but my nephews love it!") and finding other ways to "play," it became relatively easy for her to decrease and finally give up the cigarettes.

Hypnotic Dreams

When dreams are reexperienced in trance, the results can be therapeutically powerful. A devoutly religious cancer patient dreamed of a surgical amphitheater with many patients lying on tables. An audience sat in a surrounding chamber behind windows. Three hooded figures stood silently at the door. Calm pervaded the scene. He realized that all the patients were, in fact, himself. The hooded figures (i.e., his brother-in-law, a priest, the surgeon) and the patient himself embodied the cornerstones of his life (i.e., family, church, and his own responsibility), along with the professional healer. He "knew" that with this structure firmly in place the surgery would be successful. There was no place for death in his vision, although he was aware that death lurked just beyond. His initial fear of looking under the hoods was that one of them would be death itself.

A male victim of paternal incest had a recurrent dream that he lived in a strange, scary house that his father had built. He wandered through that house trying to "find his way," seeking help from his father who remained hidden. Several months into therapy, he dreamed that he was in a house that he was building himself. It was not finished yet, but it felt safe and was brightly lit. His wife and friends were helping him with the construction. I suggested that, under hypnosis, he redream his dream while his hidden observer understood its true meaning. He saw this as a metaphor for working on himself, with help from others. He realized that the old dream represented his hopeless efforts as an adult to connect with his abusive, abandoning father and to find a safe home or haven. His new dream symbolized his efforts to construct a healthier self in a safer world with the help of people he could trust and depend on.

Defenses and Resistances

Interpretation of defenses and resistances is an important aspect of hypnoanalysis. Interpretation should be handled carefully, gently, and respectfully. Defenses should not be broken down prematurely. A patient diagnosed with global amnesia (Eisen, 1989) had seen two psychiatrists prior to her current therapy. Both had focused on reviving memories, as her mother had demanded. Terrified of what this had felt like, she entered therapy with fear and trepidation. It was clear that she was using enormous energy to maintain the "not knowing" because her ego was too fragile to "know" the "unknowable."

First, my patient and I worked with images to build ego strength. The consistent message was, "You will begin to know what you need to know when you are ready to know." With this fragile patient each step brought new resistances. As her memories began to emerge, she fled periodically into not knowing, fearful that she would be deluged with a flood of nightmare images. Providing her with the image of a large book on a pedestal with a lock on it, and pictures as well as words, allowed her to titrate her awareness at her own pace. She could unlock the book, glance briefly at a picture, or focus on reading a page of words. It took more than a year for memories to return with any historical validity, by which time she was ready to let down her defensive walls and return to the world. An interesting aftermath of this case is that this woman, healthy now and living a fully functional life, went back to school and became a librarian. The image of a book, her own personal history, brought her back to life, and she now finds great satisfaction in encouraging others to read.

I noted earlier that a common form of resistance in hypnoanalysis is refusal to go into a trance. This is the most typical of patients who want to explore past trauma but have some ambivalence about reliving painful and hitherto repressed experiences. An incest victim, terrified of what would be revealed in the trance, avoided the hypnosis she had originally requested by talking excessively from the moment she entered the office. It was suggested that she allow herself to just relax at home and let her left hand (not her writing hand) write freely, perhaps a short story, poem, or thoughts. She appeared at the following session with her writing: a frightening story of incest and cult abuse. Horrified by what had surfaced, she was now willing to work with trance states. Her argument was, "At least in trance I know what's coming, and I am not alone!" This patient often uses trance states to activate her creativity and then writes poems and stories that reflect her affective states. She has joined a computer poetry group and shares her poems with others whom she will never meet in person yet who are supportive and encouraging. Through this long-distance sharing, she is learning to trust people again.

Narcissistic and Borderline Personality Disorders

Patients diagnosed with narcissistic personality disorder find creative ways to respond to what they perceive as failure of empathy on the part of the therapist. A young woman began therapy because she felt a sense of isolation even though she was seemingly well-accepted in the academic program she was pursuing. She identified herself as the adult child of alcoholic parents. She was the only girl in a large Irish Catholic family and was the family caretaker. She kept a journal beautifully detailed in calligraphy. In it she recorded her anger and disappointment as well as her idealizations in pictures, prose, and poetry, which she shared regularly with her therapist.

Initially, the primary theme was idealization of the therapist. With the inevitable failures of empathy came anger and despair. As therapy progressed her responses became more benign. Recognizing her transference issues she wrote of the therapist, "She reminded me of my mother today, sitting there looking smug and self-righteous . . . but of course she isn't my mother." Eventually, this young woman was able to separate herself from her family and develop a loving relationship with a mentoring older woman. She has found success and satisfaction in her work and is growing more comfortable with a broader range of social relationships.

A woman diagnosed with a borderline personality disorder had difficulty recognizing when her feelings were "real" and when they were "made-up." She had been hospitalized several times in the past and was in an outpatient program at a local hospital when she began therapy. She had had numerous job positions, including actress, waitress, computer analyst, and boutique salesperson. She did each job well initially and then became obsessively immersed in the work. She was unable to leave at night when the job was over, but she was also unable to get herself together to arrive at work at the appropriate time. Eventually, she lost each job. She was also totally obsessed about the workings of her body and harbored a pervasive feeling that others were trying to control her, notably her mother or anyone she worked for.

One of the first tasks was to give her a sense of her autonomy in the therapeutic alliance. Because she felt that only her physical sensations were real, therapy started with that awareness, using ideomotor actions. She was free to ask for exactly what she needed in the experience of hypnosis, which she did before the trance was induced. Some days she wanted to breathe and stretch, and other days she wanted a hand on her forehead or her solar plexus applying light, rhythmic pressure. Eventually, she asked for more complex body work in the trance, asking for the therapist to pull her arms up or press down on her shoulders, during which violent feelings of anger, fear, and grief emerged in deeply regressed form. She kicked and pounded and screamed blood-curdling screams, rolling up in a fetal position.

She dissociated these feeling states to a little girl aged 5. When this little girl state became more firmly established, she began taking over the therapy sessions. She and the therapist together developed outrageous stories of attack rabbits and protective armor while the patient was in the trance, with humor occasionally replacing the negative feelings. The "little girl" and the "adult" sometimes competed for the therapist's attention, often in the form of demands for more. The patient, whose financial resources were extremely limited, began to complain about having to pay for her sessions, claiming that if the therapist really cared for her this would not be an issue. The therapist firmly maintained boundaries and insisted on regular but much reduced payments.

Slowly, this previously semifunctional patient became more adept at relationships. She has been able to live independently for about a year and a half and has not had to be hospitalized since therapy began. She is aware of her limitations but is also learning to capitalize on her strengths. She is now working for her mother, using her computer skills to organize her mother's business, working on her own time schedule, and because her mother recently became ill, assuming caretaking functions she never thought herself capable of.

She has come to recognize and differentiate the real and the unreal. Fearing both the loss of self in the other and abandonment by the much-needed other, this woman has learned that she can control the level of intimacy in a relationship without losing herself or the other (i.e., the therapist). She can become angry without being abandoned or destructive and be her damaged child self without relinquishing her fragile adult self. Doing this through hypnosis also gives her a feeling for her power to use her mind and control her world in a self-guided way.

The Healer Within

For certain patients, getting in touch with an internal spirit guide, or healer within, constitutes a powerful symbol. A bright, creative artist— a weaver—was going through chemotherapy for breast cancer. Determined not to experience debilitating side effects, she needed a way to take control and therefore chose hypnosis. An excellent, highly motivated subject, she quickly got in touch with her inner spirit guide. The original suggestion by the therapist was that there may be a wise inner spirit who lives in the quiet place in the center of her mind. Her spirit guide was an elderly Indian woman, a healer and a weaver, who not only helped her remain symptom-free during the full course of chemotherapy but also imparted ancient weaving skills. The patient's skills improved greatly, collectors now enthusiastically seek her work, and she feels healed in body and in spirit.

Transference

Positive transference can be an important ally in the healing process, which sometimes takes an unexpected form. The fact that the patient views the therapist as the good parent with magical abilities may be a logical extension of the fact that hypnosis (and psychotherapy) has an aura of mystery surrounding it.

One woman consulted me in the midst of a long analysis for the amelioration of a specific symptom. Psychiatrists frequently call me to help patients with specific issues who are deemed likely to respond well to hypnosis. It soon became clear that the patient was using her male analyst and me as surrogate parents to work through unresolved issues. On occasion, she would attempt to manipulate the feelings of one therapist against the other, watching carefully for a response. After 18 months of hypnotherapy, during which time the problem for which she sought hypnotherapy was alleviated, she and I agreed that our work together was completed. She spent several weeks working through termination. In the end, she reported that she could say goodbye to both her mother (who had died several years before) and me and move on. Her mother had never given her permission to leave, as I had, but our parting made it possible for her to see herself as an adult separate from her mother. In her rich trance fantasies, she was always surrounded by three protective figures: her analyst, me, and her husband, in that order. Eventually, her husband took over the protecting role in her fantasies, and the therapists faded into the background. A favorable outcome of therapy was a closer, more spontaneous relationship with her husband and the final termination of her 20-year analysis.

These cases exemplify some of the seminal issues dealt with in psychodynamic hypnotherapy. One can see the broad diversity in the type of patient, in the form the therapy takes, and in the kind of therapeutic relationship established. The one common theme is the ultimate goal: autonomy for the patient, the sense that healing comes from within so that when therapy is terminated, the individual leaves with a strong belief in the power of the internal healer, the spirit of the self.

RESEARCH AND APPRAISAL

Psychoanalysis and psychodynamic therapy are rich clinical traditions. In recent years, research inspired by these traditions has made valuable contributions to understanding psychoanalytic and ego psychology constructs as they pertain to the hypnotic situation. Psychoanalytic and psychodynamic theorists (e.g., Fromm, 1992; Gill & Brenman, 1959; Nash, 1991, 1992) are in agreement that "regression in service of the ego" is a central psychotherapeutic mechanism that is intimately related to manifestations of primary process thinking in hypnotic and nonhypnotic contexts. One interesting question is, What is the nature of the regression that occurs in hypnosis?

On the basis of a literature review of more than 100 studies, Nash (1987) concluded that individuals who are hypnotized neither truly function in a childlike manner nor literally relive childhood experiences in response to suggestions for age regression. Instead of a literal regression, what occurs is a topographic regression that has the following characteristics: an increase in primary process material, the experience of nonvolition, unusual body sensations, more spontaneous and intense emotion, and the tendency to displace core attributes of important others onto the hypnotist and to be receptive to inner and outer experience. These hypnotically stimulated features of topographic regression constitute a useful framework of psychoanalytically derived hypotheses. Memories, though not necessarily veridical, are reworked in conjunction with long-term goals and expectations, revealing the individuals' fundamental views of themselves and their world (Singer & Salovey, 1993).

There is a great deal of support for the idea that during hypnosis, there is an increased availability of primary process thinking. Research indicates that fantasy, imagery, and imaginative involvement are modestly correlated with hypnotizability (see J. R. Hilgard, 1970; Kirsch & Council, 1992; Lynn & Rhue, 1988; Roche & McConkey, 1990), although the relationship may be partly moderated by expectations and situational influences (see Kirsch & Council). However, several studies (Hammer, Walker, & Diment, 1978; Wiseman & Reyher, 1973) have suggested that increased primary process mentation cannot be fully accounted for in terms of compliance with role demands.

Consistent with the idea that primary process thought is a frequent accompaniment of certain altered states of consciousness, Fromm and Kahn's (1990) research showed that imagery is a prominent characteristic of self-hypnosis as well as therapy-guided hypnosis. This research also indicated that the more spontaneous, self-actualized, and open to internal impulses the subject is, the more likely he or she is to have a rich, satisfying hypnotic experience. A particularly fascinating aspect of this study was an exploration of journals kept by self-hypnosis participants, which dramatized the impact of personality characteristics on the nature of the self-hypnotic experience for each individual. Additional studies are needed to determine whether the changes in cognitive processing during hypnosis and self-hypnosis are attributable to specific or unique characteristics of hypnosis rather than to general concomitants of hypnotic suggestions for eye closure and relaxation, for example.

Research comparing hypnotic and nonhypnotic control groups is important in evaluating several other psychoanalytic hypotheses. Consistent with Fromm's (1992) view of ego receptivity, a great deal of research (see Lynn et al., 1990) supports the hypothesis that many individuals who are hypnotized relinquish a consciously directed, task-oriented mode of ego functioning during hypnosis. Instead, they respond to the tacit demands of the hypnotic situation and experience suggestion-related movements, for example, as having an effortless, automatic, and involuntary quality.

Although hypnotized subjects often report that their responses are involuntary occurrences rather than goal-directed actions, many nonhypnotized subjects who receive passively worded suggestions with imagery that encourages them to attribute their responses to an external agency (e.g., "Your hand will rise higher and higher, lift right off the resting surface as the balloons that are attached to that wrist of yours lift it higher and higher") also report that their responses are involuntary (for a review, see Lynn & Sivec, 1992). This implies that the suggestions that individuals receive, along with their interpretation of the suggestions that are administered, play an important role in how they come to experience hypnosis. Of course, this by no means disqualifies the psychoanalytic hypothesis; it simply suggests that a variety of stimulus conditions and situational factors may be involved in instigating primary process thinking and automatized experiences associated with the topographic regression hypothesized by psychoanalytic theorists. Wilson (1990) discussed the "construction of a cohesive narrative" in his work with Holocaust survivors and their family members. He wrote of cultivating a narrative competence through successive regressions, creating a historic framework for containing, explaining and understanding hitherto unbearable life experiences.

Research (see Brentar & Lynn, 1989, for a review; Crawford, Hilgard, & Macdonald, 1982) is generally supportive of the psychoanalytic hypothesis that hypnosis results in shifts in body experience from the baseline of body awareness during mundane task-oriented activities and cognitive processes. However, several experimental studies (Brentar, Lynn, Carlson, Kurzhals, & Green, 1992; Kirsch, Mobayed, Council, & Kenny, 1990) have shown that hypnotized subjects' subjective experiences, including bodily experiences, cannot be reliably distinguished those of from nonhypnotized subjects who are relaxed, asked to imagine suggested activities, or invited to focus on body parts that parallel the focus of hypnotic suggestions.

Although hypnotized subjects report a wide variety of altered body and perceptual experiences (Brentar & Lynn, 1989; Gill & Brenman, 1959), the evidence is mixed regarding the ability of hypnosis to enhance affect. Whereas several studies (Nash, Johnson, & Tipton, 1979; Nash, Lynn, Stanley, Frauman, & Rhue, 1985) have shown that individuals who are age-regressed have greater access to intense emotions than do those in a simulating control group, other studies have shown that simulating subjects can mimic the nature (Bryant & McConkey, 1989) and intensity (Mare, Lynn, Kvaal, Segal, & Sivec, 1994) of hypnotized subjects' emotions. Additional studies with subtle measures conducive to eliciting affect will be necessary to delineate the conditions in which hypnosis may enhance the expression of affect.

One of the cornerstones of psychoanalytic thinking is that transference is a fundamental psychotherapeutic process. Research (for a summary, see Sheehan, 1991) supports the hypothesis that certain hypnotized subjects evidence an especially motivated involvement with the hypnotist and a cognitive commitment to the task of responding to hypnotic suggestions. This research also indicates that hypnotized subjects' investment in the hypnotist and the hypnotic relationship cannot be duplicated by nonhypnotized simulating and task-motivated subjects instructed to do their best to respond to suggested events.

Recent developments in this area of inquiry include the study of the intricate and sometimes subtle nature of the interaction between hypnotist and subject (see Amundson & Nuttgens, 2008; Banyai, 1991; Norcross, 2002) and the development of reliable and valid instruments (Nash & Spinler, 1989; Spiegel, 2008; Sutcher, 2008) to measure transference and archaic involvement with the hypnotist. Shor (1979) defined *archaic involvement* as "the extent to which there occurred a temporary displacement or 'transference' onto the hypnotist, of core personality emotive attitudes . . . most typically in regard to parents" (p. 133). This research promises to advance understanding of the nature of hypnotic rapport, transference, and subjects' motivations to respond to hypnotic suggestions.

In addition to the experimental tradition, the use of psychodynamic hypnotherapy is a rich source of data, providing a strong base for increased understanding of this mode of therapy in relation to a wide variety of cases. Baker (1981) and Brown (1985) have written extensively on the use of hypnosis with patients who were severely disturbed. Adler (1981, 1985), among others, discussed borderline and narcissistic personalities and their responses to hypnotherapeutic intervention. A large number of clinicians have described their work with veterans diagnosed with posttraumatic stress disorders (e.g., Kingsbury, 1988; Peebles, 1989; D. Spiegel, 1981, 1984), and there also is a growing body of clinical literature on hypnotherapy with victims of sexual abuse and those with multiple personality disorders (Bliss, 1986; Kluft, 1984). Ideally, clinical research will supplement more rigorous laboratory investigations of psychoanalytic and ego psychology constructs to enrich the understanding of relevant constructs, treatment mechanisms, and the effectiveness of hypnoanalytic psychotherapy relative to alternative therapeutic approaches.

CONCLUSION

I have touched on a number of key concepts related to hypnosis as a therapeutic tool. As the literature review indicates, there is empirical support for a number of constructs pivotal to psychodynamic and psychoanalytic therapy, including hypnoanalysis. I have viewed hypnosis as an altered state of consciousness, during which the subject experiences his or her physical, cognitive, emotional self in a dissociated manner. The body sense changes, parts of the body appear to function as separate entities, sensory experiences become a function of inner processes rather than external stimuli, and movement or lack of it seems to be under a different control system. As we learn more about ego-state therapy, we may be able to conceptualize these differentiated bodily experiences as a consequence of differing ego states, which may be addressed in hypnotherapy.

Cognitively, there is a clear split between the experiencing and the observing ego. This means that at one level, the critical function is set aside and the subject can accept mutually exclusive possibilities as natural (i.e., trance logic), which is a function of the participating ego, while on another level, the observing ego maintains its integrity and monitors the proceedings from a steadfast reality orientation. This would explain the results of the Pinnell et al.

(1998) study, which found that when the hidden observer is evoked in hypnotic-dream therapy, there is a decrease in primary process material. Emotionally, the subject is capable of strong responses that can be evoked or terminated at will and do not necessarily seem connected to ongoing, logical thought processes.

I have also conceptualized hypnosis as a regression in the service of the ego, during which the subject may revert to a more intuitive, imaginative, free-flowing mode of functioning (primary process), allowing for archaic involvement with the hypnotist and with elements of the self. In pathological regression, the ego is helplessly inundated with a sense of uncontrollable feelings and unmet needs. However, in regression in the service of the ego, it initiates, lends itself to, and uses regressive mental activity as a healing process.

The experience of involvement with the therapeutic process over time and the eventual conscious understanding and integration, which is called *working through*, potentiates structural change in intensive psychoanalytic treatment. Hypnosis can help to direct the experience, contain and modulate the process, and facilitate internal representation and integration in a direct and efficient manner not usually possible in more traditional psychotherapy (Baker, 1990).

Finally, hypnosis can be viewed as a ritual that provides a framework for working through grief and mourning, unresolved relationship conflicts, and developmental discontinuities. Many patients use the special therapeutic relationship hypnotherapy provides to engage in magical thinking and experience strong emotional abreactions they could not allow themselves in more cognitively or intellectually oriented therapy settings. It is not only the regressive nature of hypnosis but also the implied "magic" connected historically to hypnosis that gives it this special power.

The hypnotherapist needs to remain cognizant of the demand characteristics of this interaction and to respect the patient's dual need for a safely dependent relationship and autonomy. The patient must be allowed to create the therapeutic agenda and not bow to the agenda of the therapist. Psychodynamic hypnotherapy provides a technique for uncovering repressed material, reworking the meaning of that material into the fabric of one's present life, and reintegrating one's history with a contemporary sense of self. The therapist serves as a benign guide on this journey through the shadows. Hypnoanalysis adds a new dimension to psychoanalysis because of its unique and special tools: imagery, primary process, age regression, hyperamnesia, dissociation, and automatic writing. The hypnoanalyst attempts to help patients achieve new levels of mastery as they sort out and come to terms with conflicts, fears, painful memories, and destructive habits. Patients can acquire more mature levels of object constancy and more benign, growth-promoting object representations that help in the development of more integrated, healthier self-representations.

As researchers explore the dynamics of hypnoanalysis, they also learn more about the primary and secondary process operations, the various ego states, the function and process of memory, and the way human beings use mental "playfulness" to achieve more joyful, mature, fully functioning levels of self.

REFERENCES

Adler, G. (1981). The borderline-narcissistic personality disorder continuum. *American Journal of Psychiatry, 138*, 46–50.

Adler, G. (1985). *Borderline psychopathology and its treatment.* Northvale, NJ: Jason Aronson.

Amundson, J. K., & Nuttgens, S. A. (2008). Strategic eclecticism in hypnotherapy. *American Journal of Clinical Hypnosis, 50*, 233–245.

Baker, E. L. (1981). A hypnotherapeutic approach to enhance object relatedness in psychotic patients. *International Journal of Clinical and Experimental Hypnosis, 124*, 136–147.

Baker, E. L. (1983). The use of hypnotic dreaming in treatment of the borderline patient. *International Journal of Clinical and Experimental Hypnosis, 31*, 19–27.

Baker, E. L. (1990). Hypnoanalysis for structural pathology: Impairments of self-representation and capacity for object involvement. In M. Fass & D. Brown (Eds.), *Creative mastery in hypnosis and hypnoanalysis* (pp. 255–262). Hillsdale, NJ: Erlbaum.

Banyai, E. (1991). Towards a social–psychobiological model of hypnosis. In S. J. Lynn & J. W. Rhue (Eds.), *Theories of hypnosis: Current models and perspectives* (pp. 564–600). New York: Guilford Press.

Bliss, E. L. (1986). *Multiple personality, allied disorders, and hypnosis.* New York: Oxford University Press.

Brentar, J. P., & Lynn, S. J. (1989). Negative effects and hypnosis: A critical examination. *British Journal of Experimental and Clinical Hypnosis, 6*, 75–84.

Brentar, J. P., Lynn, S. J., Carlson, B., Kurzhals, R., & Green, J. P. (1992, August). *The Posthypnotic Experiences Scale: Reliability and validity studies.* Paper presented at the 100th Annual Convention of the American Psychological Association, Washington, DC.

Brown, D. P. (1985). Hypnosis as an adjunct to the psychotherapy of the severely disturbed patient: An affective development approach. *International Journal of Clinical and Experimental Hypnosis, 33*, 281–301.

Brown, D. P., & Fromm, E. (1986). *Hypnotherapy and hypnoanalysis.* Hillsdale, NJ: Erlbaum.

Bryant, R. A., & McConkey, K. M. (1989). Hypnotic blindness: A behavioral and experiential analysis. *Journal of Abnormal Psychology, 98*, 71–77.

Crawford, H. J., Hilgard, J. R., & Macdonald, H. (1982). Transient experiences following hypnotic testing and special termination procedures. *International Journal of Clinical and Experimental Hypnosis, 30,* 117–126.

Deikman, A. J. (1971). Bimodal consciousness. *Archives of General Psychiatry, 25,* 481–489.

Eisen, M. (1989). Return of the repressed: Hypnoanalysis of a case of total amnesia.? *International Journal of Clinical and Experimental Hypnosis, 37,* 107–119.

Eisen, M. (1990). From the magical wish to the belief in the self. In M. L. Fass & D. Brown (Eds.), *Creative mastery in hypnosis and hypnoanalysis* (pp. 147–157). Hillsdale, NJ: Erlbaum.

Eisen, M. R., & Fromm, E. (1983). The clinical uses of self-hypnosis in hypnotherapy: Tapping the functions of imagery and adaptive regression. *International Journal of Clinical and Experimental Hypnosis, 31,* 243–255.

Federn, R. (1952). *Ego psychology and the psychoses.* New York: Basic Books.

Fenichel, O. (1945). *The psychoanalytic theory of the neuroses.* New York: Norton.

Ferenczi, S. (1965). Comments on hypnosis. In R. Shor & M. T. Orne (Eds.), *The nature of hypnosis: Selected basic readings* (pp. 177–182). New York: Holt, Rinehart & Winston.

Frankel, E. H. (1976). *Hypnosis: Trance as a coping mechanism.* New York: Plenum Press.

Freud, S. (1953a). The interpretation of dreams. In J. Strachey (Ed. & Trans.), *The standard edition of the complete psychological works of Sigmund Freud.* London: Hogarth Press. (Original work published 1900)

Freud, S. (1953b). Three essays on the theory of sexuality. In J. Strachey (Ed. & Trans.), *The standard edition of the complete psychological works of Sigmund Freud* (Vol. 7, pp. 125–245). London: Hogarth Press. (Original work published 1905)

Fromm, E. (1972). Ego activity and ego passivity in hypnosis. *International Journal of Clinical and Experimental Hypnosis, 18,* 79–88.

Fromm, E. (1992). An ego–psychological theory of hypnosis. In E. Fromm & M. R. Nash (Eds.), *Contemporary hypnosis research.* New York: Guilford Press.

Fromm, E., & Kahn, S. (1990). *Self-hypnosis: The Chicago paradigm.* New York: Guilford Press.

Fromm, E., & Shor, R. E. (1979). *Hypnosis: Developments in research and new perspectives* (2nd ed.). Chicago: Aldine Publishing.

Gill, M. M., & Brenman, M. (1959). *Hypnosis and related states.* Madison, CT: International Universities Press.

Ginandes, C. (2006). Players on the inner stage: Using ego state therapy with the medically ill. *International Journal of Clinical and Experimental Hypnosis, 54,* 113–129.

Hammer, A. G., Walker, W., & Diment, A. D. (1978). A nonsuggested effect of trance induction. In E. H. Frankel & H. S. Zamansky (Eds.), *Hypnosis at its bicentennial: Selected papers* (pp. 91–100). New York: Plenum Press.

Hart, H. H. (1961). A review of the psychoanalytic literature on passivity. *Psychiatric Quarterly, 35*, 331–352.

Hartmann, H. (1958). *Ego psychology and the problem of adaptation* (D. Rapaport, Trans.). Madison, CT: International Universities Press. (Original work published 1936)

Hilgard, E. R. (1973). A neodissociation interpretation of pain reduction in hypnosis. *Psychological Review, 80*, 396–411.

Hilgard, E. R. (1974). Toward a neodissociation theory: Multiple cognitive controls in human functioning. *Perspectives in Biology and Medicine, 17*, 301–316.

Hilgard, E. R. (1977). *Divided consciousness: Multiple controls in human thought and action.* New York: Wiley.

Hilgard, J. R. (1970). *Personality and hypnosis: A study of imaginative involvement.* Chicago: University of Chicago Press.

Kingsbury, S. J. (1988). Hypnosis in the treatment of posttraumatic stress disorder: An isomorphic intervention. *American Journal of Clinical Hypnosis, 31*, 81–90.

Kirsch, I., & Council, J. R. (1992). Situational and personality correlates of hypnotic responsiveness. In E. Fromm & M. R. Nash (Eds.), *Contemporary hypnosis research.* New York: Guilford Press.

Kirsch, I., Mobayed, C. P., Council, J. R., & Kenny, D. A. (1990, August). State of the state debate: Can experts detect hypnosis? In R. St. Jean (Chair), *Social and cognitive aspects of hypnosis: Papers honoring W. C. Coe.* Symposium conducted at the 98th Annual Convention of the American Psychological Association, Boston.

Kluft, R. P. (1984). Treatment of multiple personality disorder. *Psychiatric Clinics of North America, 7*, 9–29.

Kris, E. (1952). *Psychoanalytic explorations in art.* Madison, CT: International Universities Press. (Original work published 1934)

Lemke, W. (2005). Utilizing hypnosis and ego state therapy to facilitate healthy adaptive differentiation in the treatment of sexual disorders. *American Journal of Clinical Hypnosis, 47*, 179–189.

Loewald, H. W. (1981). Regression: Some general considerations. *Psychoanalytic Quarterly, 50*, 22–43.

Lynn, S. J., & Rhue, J. W. (1988). Fantasy proneness: Hypnosis, developmental antecedents, and psychopathology. *American Psychologist, 43*, 35–44.

Lynn, S. J., Rhue, J. W., & Weekes, J. R. (1990). Hypnotic responsiveness: A social cognitive analysis. *Psychological Review, 97*, 169–184.

Lynn, S. J., & Sivec, H. (1992). The hypnotizable subject as creative problem-solving agent. In E. Fromm & M. R. Nash (Eds.), *Contemporary hypnosis research* (pp. 292–333). New York: Guilford Press.

Mare, C., Lynn, S. J., Kvaal, S., Segal, D. & Sivec, H. (1994). The dream hidden observer: Primary process and demand characteristics. *Journal of Abnormal Psychology, 103*, 316–327.

Meares, A. (1960). *A system of medical hypnosis*. Philadelphia: W. B. Saunders.

Nash, M. R. (1987). What, if anything, is regressed about hypnotic age regression? A review of the empirical literature. *Psychological Bulletin, 102,* 42–52.

Nash, M. R. (1991). Hypnosis as a special case of psychological regression. In S. J. Lynn & J. W. Rhue (Eds.), *Theories of hypnosis: Current models and perspectives* (pp. 171–194). New York: Guilford Press.

Nash, M. R. (1992). Hypnosis, psychopathology, and psychological regression. In E. Fromm & M. R. Nash (Eds.), *Contemporary hypnosis research* (pp. 149–169). New York: Guilford Press.

Nash, M. R., Johnson, L. S., & Tipton, R. D. (1979). Hypnotic age regression and the occurrence of transitional object relationships. *Journal of Abnormal Psychology, 88,* 547–555.

Nash, M. R., Lynn, S. J., Stanley, S. M., Frauman, D., & Rhue, J. W. (1985). Hypnotic age regression and the importance of assessing interpersonally relevant affect. *International Journal of Clinical and Experimental Hypnosis, 33,* 224–235.

Nash, M. R., & Spinler, D. (1989). Hypnosis and transference: A measure of archaic involvement with the hypnotist. *International Journal of Clinical and Experimental Hypnosis, 37,* 129–144.

Norcross, J. C. (Ed.). (2002). *Psychotherapy relationships that work: Therapist contributions and responsiveness to patients*. Oxford, England: Oxford University Press.

Orne, M. (1959). The nature of hypnosis: Artifact and essence. *Journal of Abnormal and Social Psychology, 58,* 277–299.

Peebles, M. J. (1989). Through a glass darkly: The psychoanalytic use of hypnosis with posttraumatic stress disorder. *International Journal of Clinical and Experimental Hypnosis, 37,* 192–206.

Pinnell, C., Lynn, S., & Pinnell, J. (1998). A primary process, hypnotic dreams, and the hidden observer: Hypnosis versus alert imagining. *International Journal of Clinical and Experimental Hypnosis, 46,* 351–362.

Rapaport, D. (1967). Metaphysical considerations concerning activity and passivity. In M. M. Gill (Ed.), *The collected papers of David Rapaport* (pp. 530–568). New York: Basic Books. (Original work published 1953)

Restak, R. M. (1979). *The brain: The last frontier*. New York: Doubleday.

Roche, S. M., & McConkey, K. M. (1990). Absorption: Nature, assessment, and correlates. *Journal of Personality and Social Psychology, 59,* 91–101.

Rossi, E. (2007). The breakout heuristic: The new neuroscience of mirror neurons. Phoenix, AZ: MHE Press.

Rossi, E., & Rossi, M. (2006). The neuroscience of observing consciousness and mirror neurons in therapeutic hypnosis. *American Journal of Clinical Hypnosis, 48,* 263–279.

Schilder, P. F., & Kauders, O. (1956). Hypnosis. (G. Corvin, Trans.). In P. F. Schilder (Ed.), *The nature of hypnosis* (pp. 43–184). Madison, CT: International

Universities Press. (Reprinted from *Nervous and Mental Disease Monographs, 46*, S. Rosenberg, Trans, 1927)

Sheehan, P. W. (1991). Hypnosis, context and commitment. In S. J. Lynn & J. W. Rhue (Eds.), *Hypnosis: Current models and perspectives* (pp. 520–541). New York: Guilford Press.

Shor, R. E. (1979). A phenomenological method for the measurement of variables important to an understanding of the nature of hypnosis. In E. Fromm & R. E. Shor (Eds.), *Hypnosis: Developments in research and new perspectives* (2nd ed., pp. 105–135). Chicago: Aldine.

Singer, J., & Salovey, P. (1993). *The remembered self: Emotional and memory in personality*. New York: Free Press.

Spiegel, D. (1981). Vietnam grief work using hypnosis. *American Journal of Clinical Hypnosis, 24*, 33–40.

Spiegel, D. (1984). Multiple personality as a posttraumatic stress disorder. *Psychiatric Clinics of North America, 7*, 101–110.

Spiegel, H. (2008). Commentary. *American Journal of Clinical Hypnosis, 51*, 149–151.

Spiegel, H., & Spiegel, D. (1978). *Trance and treatment: Clinical uses of hypnosis*. New York: Basic Books.

Sutcher, H. (2008). Hypnosis, hypnotizability, and treatment. *American Journal of Clinical Hypnosis, 51*, 57–68.

Watkins, J. G., & Watkins, H. (1979). The theory and practice of ego state therapy. In H. Grayson (Ed.), *Short term approaches to psychotherapy* (pp. 176–220). New York: National Institute for the Psychotherapies and Human Sciences Press.

Watkins, J. G., & Watkins, H. H. (1981). Ego-state therapy. In R. J. Corsini (Ed.), *Handbook of innovative therapies* (pp. 252–270). New York: Wiley.

Watkins, J. G., & Watkins, H. H. (1990). Ego-state transferences in the hypnoanalytic treatment of dissociative reactions. In M. Fass & D. Brown (Eds.), *Creative mastery in hypnosis and hypnoanalysis* (pp. 255–261). Hillsdale, NJ: Erlbaum.

Weiss, E. (Ed.). (1952). *Ego psychology and the psychoses*. New York: Basic Books.

Wickramasekera, I. (2007). Empathic absorption and incongruence. *American Journal of Clinical Hypnosis, 50*, 59–69.

Wilson, A. (1990). On silence and the holocaust: A contribution to clinical theory. In M. Fass & D. Brown (Eds.), *Creative mastery in hypnosis and hypnoanalysis*. Hillsdale, NJ: Erlbaum.

Winnicott, D. W. (1975). *Through pediatrics to psychoanalysis*. New York: Basic Books.

Wiseman, R. J., & Reyher, J. (1973). Hypnotically induced dreams using the Rorschach inkblots as stimuli: A test of Freud's theory of dreams. *Journal of Personality and Social Psychology, 27*, 329–336.

6

DISSOCIATION IN HYPNOSIS: THEORETICAL FRAMEWORKS AND PSYCHOTHERAPEUTIC IMPLICATIONS

PAMELA SADLER AND ERIK WOODY

Largely because of the seminal influence of Hilgard (1977), the concept of *dissociation* has become strongly linked with the domain of hypnosis. Unfortunately, however, dissociation is a complex and elusive construct, and various clinicians and researchers tend to use the term, often quite loosely, to refer to very different ideas about hypnosis. Partly because of this, when clinicians or researchers refer to dissociation in describing a hypnotic phenomenon or in attempting to explain it, their intended meaning is often unclear. For instance, is the word being used descriptively to denote a certain kind of event, and if so, what are the defining features of such an event? Or is the word being used to allude to an underlying mechanism, and if so, what are the essential properties of this putative mechanism?

In this chapter, we examine a set of hypothetical underlying mechanisms of dissociation that provide the basis for several intriguing theories about how hypnosis works. We briefly trace how these proposed mechanisms developed in hypnosis research over the last 100 years. We show that there are actually multiple competing dissociation theories of hypnosis, one stream of which

---

Clinical material has been disguised to protect patient confidentiality.

focuses on alterations of conscious experience and the other on alterations of cognitive control. Finally, we outline some clinical implications of these ideas and present a case example to illustrate some of these implications.

A BRIEF HISTORY OF DISSOCIATION THEORIES OF HYPNOSIS

Interest in the concept of dissociation has waxed and waned over the decades, with much activity in some periods of time and virtually none in others. To begin, we go back to the turn of the 20th century.

Janet's Concept of Dissociation

Janet (1901, 1907) originated the concept of *désagrégation* [dissociation] to explain hypnosis and hysterical disorders, both of which he interpreted as suggestive phenomena. He hypothesized that a particular cluster of mental contents can become split off, or disassociated, from the rest of a person's mental processes. Such ideas thereby become isolated from both awareness and voluntary control. This separation allows those ideas to be activated, outside of awareness, through suggestion.

Janet (1925) proposed that dissociation could often be partial rather than complete, such that the awareness and voluntary control linked with the dissociated content are only reduced somewhat but not eliminated. Nonetheless, subsequent research on Janet's concept of dissociation in hypnosis was designed to test a much stronger interpretation of it, which implied autonomous simultaneous mental processes. Some researchers (Hull, 1933; Rosenberg, 1959; White & Shevach, 1942) inferred that if Janet was correct, then in hypnosis people ought to be able to do two mental tasks at the same time without these tasks interfering with each other as they usually would. Results of the research did not seem to confirm this prediction, and, therefore, interest in Janet's ideas declined.

Hilgard's Neodissociation Theory

Reviving interest in Janet's work, Hilgard (1977) adopted Janet's concept of dissociation as "the splitting off of certain mental processes from the main body of consciousness with various degrees of autonomy" (Hilgard, 1992, p. 69). Hilgard proposed that in hypnosis the mechanism of an *amnesia-like barrier* could block some mental activity from the conscious access it would otherwise have. In addition, he discovered that with appropriate suggestions, a *hidden observer* could be elicited that was able to report the mental activity that was otherwise blocked from awareness in hypnosis. From this finding, he made the bold conjecture that in hypnosis amnesia-like barriers can divide consciousness into parallel, coexisting channels (which, however, can interfere with each other to some extent). These ideas—the amnesia-like barrier and the hidden observer—basically elaborated Janet's theme that hypnosis crucially involves reversible restrictions of awareness.

However, Hilgard (1977, 1991, 1992) also developed other ideas, less indebted to Janet, about the mechanisms that may underlie hypnosis. In particular, he proposed a model of hierarchical levels of cognitive control mechanisms, and he hypothesized that hypnosis alters how this control system operates. At the lower level of the model are numerous coexisting control subsystems, and at the higher level is an executive system that ordinarily governs the activity of the lower subsystems. Hilgard hypothesized that hypnosis changes the function of the executive system and, hence, the way in which behavior is controlled.

One important function of the executive system is planning and initiating new behavior. Hilgard (1979) argued that hypnosis weakens this function, such that in hypnosis a person "does not independently undertake new lines of thought or action" (p. 50). Another important function of the executive system is to monitor activity in the subsystems. Accordingly, Hilgard argued that hypnosis reduces this monitoring, such that in hypnosis people become less aware of some of their mental operations, such as the role of volition in their hypnotic responses. A further important function of the executive system is the use of monitoring to provide corrective feedback for the supervision of control. Hilgard suggested that the loss of this corrective feedback in hypnosis could explain why people may confuse their own imaginings with external reality, as in hypnotic hallucinations.

Although Hilgard attempted to combine this hierarchical-control model of hypnosis with his Janet-inspired ideas about amnesic barriers and the hidden observer, the awkward sutures from the attempt often show in his writings. For example, this unwieldy integration led him to propose multiple, inconsistent explanations for the same hypnotic phenomenon, as we examine next.

Bowers's Reformulation of Neodissociation Theory

Strongly influenced by Hilgard, Bowers was one of the most vigorous proponents of neodissociation theory (e.g., Bowers & Davidson, 1991). However, he eventually became critical of some aspects of the theory. In particular, he pointed out that amnesic barriers were an implausible mechanism for most hypnotic behaviors (Bowers, 1990, 1992b) because spontaneous amnesia is a far more rare response than the hypnotic behaviors that Hilgard claimed it might explain. In addition, Bowers noted that Hilgard's proposed barriers are arbitrarily selective in an uncomfortably ad hoc way. For example, with regard to hypnotic analgesia, "the pain and cognitive effort to reduce it is hidden behind an amnesic barrier, but not the original suggestions for analgesia, nor the goal-directed fantasies that typically accompany the reductions in pain" (Bowers, 1992b, pp. 261–262).

More important, Bowers (1990, 1992b) pointed out that the amnesic barrier and Hilgard's hierarchical-control model pose mutually inconsistent explanations of the core experience of involuntariness in hypnotic behavior. On one hand, Hilgard (1977) proposed that if hypnosis creates amnesic barriers, a hypnotic response might be enacted voluntarily and effortfully, as it would under other circumstances, but in hypnosis this self-agency could be walled off from awareness by such an amnesic barrier. Hence, the person's experience of the response as involuntary and effortless would be illusory, a hypnosis-evoked reduction in self-awareness and not a result of a genuine change in the underlying control of behavior. On the other hand, Hilgard alternatively proposed that if hypnosis alters the hierarchical control of behavior, then a hypnotic suggestion may relatively directly activate a subsystem of control, bypassing much of the executive initiative and effort that would govern such a behavior under other circumstances. Hence, the person's experience of the response as involuntary and effortless would be a result of a real change in the underlying control of behavior and not simply an illusory effect of reduced self-awareness.

In summary, the two branches of neodissociation theory make opposite predictions: There is high versus low executive cognitive effort in hypnosis, and the experience of involuntariness is illusory versus accurate. To resolve this inconsistency, Bowers (1990, 1992b) proposed that neodissociation theory should be split into two distinct subtheories: one involving *dissociated experience* and another involving *dissociated control*.

A dissociated experience explanation of hypnosis focuses on the alteration of how people experience their behavior: In hypnosis, the effort and volition that may be involved in enacting suggestions can become dissociated from awareness, such that "the control being exercised is not consciously experienced" (Bowers, 1990, p. 164). According to this account, executive effort in successfully enacting suggestions is actually relatively high but inaccurately experienced as low: "The hypnotized subject remains for the most part unaware that a good deal of effort may have been exercised in order to produce the suggested state of affairs" (Bowers, 1990, p. 162).

In contrast, a dissociated control explanation of hypnosis focuses on the alteration of how behavior is controlled: In hypnosis, lower subsystems of control can become relatively dissociated from oversight by the higher, executive level of control, largely bypassing its processes of volition and effortful control. According to this account, executive effort in successfully enacting suggestions is actually relatively low and thus correctly experienced as such (Bowers & Davidson, 1991).

Although Bowers (1990) initially viewed dissociated experience and dissociated control as complementary phenomena in hypnosis, he later became much more skeptical of dissociated experience and proposed that dissociated control is the principal dissociative mechanism underlying hypnosis (Woody & Bowers, 1994). In addition to the previously mentioned problem of spontaneous amnesic barriers being an improbable mechanism for most hypnotic behaviors, Bowers (e.g., Bowers & Davidson, 1991) viewed the dissociated experience account as somewhat difficult to discriminate from Spanos's (1986) social–cognitive theory of hypnosis. This theory similarly proposes that in hypnosis people maintain ordinary volitional control over their behavior, but, consistent with situational cues, simply misinterpret their responses as involuntary. Bowers (1992b) eventually advocated a position on dissociation in hypnosis that is remarkably far from Janet's: "Dissociation is not intrinsically a matter of keeping things out of consciousness—whether by amnesia, or any other means" (p. 267). In summary, Bowers believed that hypnosis alters the control of behavior, rather than distorting the self-perception of this control.

Woody and Sadler's Proposal to Reintegrate Dissociation Theories

In an important critique of dissociation theories of hypnosis, Kirsch and Lynn (1998) pointed to the inconsistencies between the different versions, such as dissociated experience and dissociated control. Thus, as is also evident in the foregoing brief review, there seemed to be no reasonably consistent, integrated view about dissociation in hypnosis. In addition, Kirsch and Lynn directed strong criticism at the problematic special mechanisms of the amnesic barrier and the hidden observer, which were assigned such a central role in Hilgard's (1977) highly influential work.

In response to Kirsch and Lynn's (1998) critique, we (Woody & Sadler, 1998) outlined a framework in which the various theoretical positions concerning dissociation in hypnosis may be viewed as closely related and reasonably consistent with one another. In addition, we argued that these positions could be reformulated without reference to the admittedly elusive, metaphorical constructs of the amnesic barrier and the hidden observer. Instead, we proposed that dissociation theories of hypnosis might be anchored in dual-systems models of action, as proposed by various cognitive neuroscientists (e.g., Goldberg, 1987; Lhermitte, 1986; Mesulam, 1986; Norman & Shallice, 1986; Perner, 2003). In these models, two complementary systems are responsible for the initiation and control of action: a higher, centralized executive system, which principally handles volitional, effortfully controlled acts; and a lower, diverse system, which mainly handles more stimulus-driven, routine acts. The close parallel of such dual-systems models with Hilgard's hierarchical-control ideas about hypnosis is practically self-evident. In addition, this perspective has the considerable potential of opening up hypnosis research to a thriving domain of research in cognitive neuroscience rather than stranding it on the shoals of special-purpose, ad hoc constructs such as the amnesic barrier and the hidden observer. In the next section, we provide an updated and expanded version of this reintegration of dissociation theories.

AN INTEGRATIVE PERSPECTIVE ON DISSOCIATION THEORIES OF HYPNOSIS

Figure 6.1 provides a diagrammatic representation of our *integrative model* (Woody & Sadler, 2008). Although this model, as it is described here, is mainly conceptual, the possible neural bases for it are covered in detail elsewhere (Jamieson & Woody, 2007; Woody & Sadler, 2008; Woody & Szechtman, 2007).

The model depicts two levels of control of action. The higher, executive level consists of *executive control* and *executive monitoring*, whereas the lower level consists of diverse *subsystems of control*. In accordance with dual-systems models of action (e.g., Norman & Shallice, 1986), it is the subsystems of control that

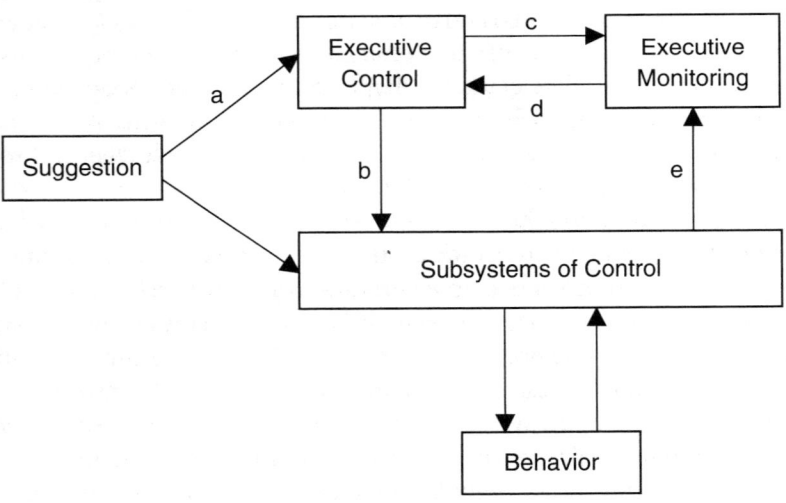

Figure 6.1. An integrative model of dissociation theories of hypnosis. A theory of *dissociated experience* involves the weakening of path *c,* and possibly of path *e.* A theory of *dissociated control* involves the weakening of path *b,* and possibly of path *a.* A theory of *second-order dissociated control* involves the weakening of path *d.* From *Oxford Handbook of Hypnosis* (p. 90), edited by M. R. Nash and A. J. Barnier, 2008, Oxford, England: Oxford University Press. Copyright 2008 by Oxford University Press. Reprinted with permission.

are hypothesized to be directly involved in the selection and tracking of behavior. The executive system provides a second level of control, associated with the sense of volition, which can modulate and monitor the subsystems of control to fine-tune their function. The model posits a major feedback loop by which executive oversight of action occurs. This loop runs from executive control, to subsystems of control, to executive monitoring, and back to executive control. Within the loop, the model posits another important feedback loop, between executive control and executive monitoring. It provides reciprocal connections by which information about intentions and goals passes from executive control to executive monitoring, and, in turn, information about ongoing activity in the subsystems of control passes from executive monitoring to executive control. Dissociation theories of hypnosis may be conceptualized as involving changes in the function of these feedback loops. In Figure 6.1, the lower-case letters along the arrows label functional connections, the weakening of which, according to different dissociation theories, may be hypothesized to yield characteristically hypnotic responses.

First, the *theory of dissociated experience* can be interpreted as crucially involving the weakening of the path labeled *c*, the functional connection from executive control to executive monitoring. Accordingly, when behavior is initiated and modulated in a voluntary fashion by executive control, this information would not be fully passed to the executive monitor and, therefore, not represented well in awareness. The theory of dissociated experience may also imply a weakening of the path labeled *e*, from subsystems of control to the executive monitor. In both cases, the executive monitor would be cut off, or dissociated, from information about the self-mediated nature of ongoing behavior. Hence, in response to hypnotic suggestions, highly responsive individuals could deliberately initiate and modulate their behavior without accurately monitoring this volition. As a result, they would have the illusion that the behavior occurred extravolitionally.

Second, the *theory of dissociated control* can be interpreted as crucially involving the weakening of the path labeled *b*, the functional connection from executive control to the subsystems of control. Accordingly, hypnotic suggestions could bypass the influence of executive control and more directly activate lower subsystems of control. The theory of dissociated control may also imply a weakening of the path labeled *a*, from the suggestion to executive control. In both cases, executive control would be relatively cut off, or dissociated, from the activation of behavior, and, thus, processes of volition and effortful control would be minimized. Hence, in response to hypnotic suggestions, highly responsive individuals could enact behavior without the usual executive initiative and effort. As a result, they would have the correct impression that the suggested behavior occurred with less volition and effort than is typical in ordinary circumstances.

Third, a further important variant of dissociated control not previously addressed by us (Woody & Sadler, 1998) can be readily integrated into this overarching model. This variant, which can usefully be termed the *theory of second-order dissociated control* (Woody & Sadler, 2008), crucially involves the path labeled *d*, from executive monitoring to executive control. As mentioned earlier, Hilgard (1992) posited that, ordinarily, actions initiated by executive control are tracked by the executive monitor to provide information for ongoing adjustments to the executive control process, and he proposed that hypnosis might block this correction process. This idea is at the core of a revision of dissociated control theory recently proposed by Jamieson and colleagues (Egner, Jamieson, & Gruzelier, 2005; Jamieson & Sheehan, 2004; Jamieson & Woody, 2007). They advanced the idea that, in hypnosis, monitoring feedback becomes functionally dissociated from executive control, as represented in our integrative model by the weakening of path *d*. Accordingly, in hypnosis, the executive control process would not be corrected and fine-tuned by the executive monitor in the usual way. Thus, monitor-detected inconsistencies that would ordinarily evoke changes in control in other circumstances would have relatively little impact on the executive control process in hypnosis. This type of dissociation would involve weakening in the control of control, a second-order level of cognitive control normally grounded on executive monitoring.

The integrative model, as shown in Figure 6.1, indicates both how the three types of dissociation theory may be distinguished from one another and also how they fit together conceptually. The three theories represent alternative hypotheses about the mechanisms underlying hypnosis; however, the model indicates that these hypotheses are potentially compatible rather than mutually exclusive. Although in future research one of these dissociative mechanisms may prevail over the others, it is alternatively possible that hypnosis may involve some kind of flexible mixture of multiple processes, depending on the individual's characteristics and the type of suggestions (Woody & McConkey, 2003).

In the next sections, we offer more detail about how hypnotic responses may be conceptualized from each of the three perspectives. For clarity, we discuss pure versions of each of the three theoretical positions, presuming the absence of the types of effects hypothesized by the alternative dissociation theories.

Dissociated Experience Theory

According to *dissociated experience theory*, in hypnosis, people enact suggestions voluntarily, with the same degree of executive control as in nonhypnotic circumstances; however, because they do not self-monitor their volition accurately, they have the illusory impression that their responses are involuntary (Kihlstrom, 1992; Shor, 1979). Hypnotic responses, therefore, are essentially delusions of control, in which people mistakenly attribute self-generated thoughts and actions to causes outside the self. Similarly, the failure to accurately monitor the self-generation of thoughts and images could lead to experiences incorrectly attributed to extravolitional origins, such as positive hallucinations and confabulations of memory. Likewise, the failure to accurately self-monitor the voluntary inhibition of thoughts and images could lead to experiences such as negative hallucinations and amnesia.

A critical aspect of self-monitoring may be a felt or emotive component. Two types of monitoring appear to be of particular relevance to hypnosis: the sense of volition, whether or not an action is attributable to one's own intentions; and the sense of reality, whether or not an experience is attributable to the external environment (Woody, Barnier, & McConkey, 2005). It has been argued that both of these discriminations are fundamentally emotive rather than cognitive (James, 1890; Proust, 2003).

Woody and Szechtman (2000) hypothesized that hypnosis may exert its effects by altering these underlying, felt experiences, which they labeled with the broader term *feelings of knowing*. Various psychopathological conditions—including delusional misidentification syndromes, derealization and depersonalization, and obsessive–compulsive disorder (Szechtman & Woody, 2004)—indicate that such felt components are highly potent. For example, in Capgras syndrome, patients recognize that acquaintances possess all their usual objective characteristics, such as face and tone of voice, yet the patients insist that the others are imposters. This misperception is caused by the absence of the covert emotional "glow" normally experienced in the presence of familiar others (Ellis & Young, 1990). Similarly, consistent with dissociated experience theory, hypnosis may temporarily alter such covert, affective components and thereby powerfully change people's perceptions of the accompanying experiences.

Dissociated Control Theory

According to *dissociated control theory*, in hypnosis, people's behavior is governed less by higher, executive control and more by unmodulated lower subsystems of control, compared with nonhypnotic circumstances (Woody & Bowers, 1994). Given a reduced role for executive control, responses in hypnosis should be more contextually dependent and stimulus-driven than usual, and less readily redirected in a deliberate, effortful way. Thus, the characteristic hypnotic experiences of involuntariness and effortlessness would accurately reflect a genuine change in the hierarchy of control.

In addition to the core hypnotic experiences of involuntariness and effortlessness, dissociated control theory explains other hypnotic phenomena quite differently from dissociated experience theory. To illustrate, consider a motor challenge suggestion in which an initially suggested state of affairs, arm rigidity, is followed by the explicit instruction to try to overcome it by bending one's arm. In carrying out the instruction to try, the individual must exert will, which represents a bid for the executive system to modulate lower subsystems of control (Norman & Shallice, 1986). However, according to dissociated control theory, this executive control is weakened in hypnosis, and therefore the individual should have the experience that effortful control is less effective than it is in normal circumstances. Because exerting will does not counteract stimulus-driven behavior as well as it usually does, the arm is hard to bend.

Dissociated control theory also provides an intriguing explanation of hypnotic alterations of memory. For this purpose, Woody and Bowers (1994) applied a model of the executive control of memory, proposed by Norman and Bobrow (1979) and Shallice (1988). These researchers argued that the executive system (which they termed the *supervisory system*) offers a higher-order level of control over memory, just as it does for action. Confronted with a nonroutine problem that cannot be handled readily by lower-level retrieval subsystems, the executive system formulates preliminary descriptions of what the relevant records would be like if indeed they existed and then compares candidate records with these descriptions to verify their relevance.

Accordingly, if hypnosis weakens executive functioning, it should differentially interfere with memory tasks that require such description and verification phases. The description phase seems particularly relevant to hypnotic suggestions for amnesia: Hypnosis should interfere with access to memories when they require the formulation of preliminary descriptions, as in free recall, but not when they are externally cued, as in cued recall and recognition. The laboratory evidence on hypnotic amnesia is generally consistent with these implications (Barnier, Bryant, & Briscoe, 2001; Evans, 1979: Kihlstrom, 1980; Kihlstrom & Shor, 1978; McConkey & Sheehan, 1981; McConkey, Sheehan, & Cross, 1980; Spanos, Radtke, & Dubreuil, 1982). The verification phase seems particularly relevant to the problem of suggestions that may lead to confabulation: Hypnosis should interfere with verification, leading to irrelevant associations and incorrect confidence that they match the searched-for material. The laboratory evidence on hypnotic distortion of memory is consistent with these implications (Dywan & Bowers, 1983; Laurence & Perry, 1983; Orne, Whitehouse, Dinges, & Orne, 1988).

Woody and Bowers (1994) also advanced a dissociated-control explanation for hypnotic analgesia. Pain typically captures attention in a peremptory fashion (McCaul & Malott, 1984), such that awareness of pain repeatedly interrupts any ongoing deliberative activity in the executive system (Norman & Shallice, 1986). Woody and Bowers hypothesized that hypnotic suggestions for analgesia may lower the sensitivity of the executive system to these pain-based interruptions, such that pain, in effect, no longer draws attention to itself. Presumably, the executive monitor would normally generate such interruptions; thus, this explanation seems to imply a dissociation of executive control from executive monitoring, as in second-order dissociated control theory.

Second-Order Dissociated Control Theory

Rather than focusing on the dissociation of lower subsystems of control from executive control, as in the original version of dissociated control theory (Woody & Bowers, 1994), *second-order dissociated control theory* focuses on the dissociation of executive control from executive monitoring (Egner, Jamieson, & Gruzelier, 2005; Jamieson & Sheehan, 2004; Jamieson & Woody, 2007). According to a pure version of this account, hypnosis does not affect the modulation of subsystems of control by executive control (i.e., a first level of executive control); however, it weakens the feedback from executive monitoring to executive control (i.e., a second level of cognitive control). The normal role of such feedback is to provide information about how well control is working, which allows ongoing adjustments in control to make it more flexible and responsive to changing task demands (Cohen, Aston-Jones, & Gilzenrat, 2004). Thus, in hypnosis, after initiating behavior at the first level of executive control, the individual is relatively incapable of flexibly adjusting this control on the basis of executive monitoring.

Second-order dissociated control theory provides a further explanation for the phenomenon of hypnotic involuntariness. Discussing the dual-control model of action, Perner (2003) hypothesized that "intentional action is defined by the match between what the lower level produces and what the higher level stipulates should be done" (p. 239; see also Haggard, 2003). Thus, if hypnosis weakens the fine-tuning of executive control by executive monitoring, the mismatches that result should be experienced as nonvolitional.

In summary, whereas the original dissociated control theory implies that the initiation of executive control is the issue, the second-order theory implies instead that it is the ongoing adjustment of executive control that is the issue. To illustrate the second-order theory, consider our example of the motor challenge suggestion. Proprioceptive information, such as the lack of changes that should be associated with trying to bend one's arm, may indicate that the control program requires updating. However, in hypnosis, the executive monitor fails to pass this information to executive control, and therefore the control strategy and concomitant suggested state of affairs remain unchanged.

Another intriguing distinction between the original and the second-order dissociated control theories concerns the capacity to generate novel responses in hypnosis. Generally, an important role of the executive system is to aid the production of novelty when circumstances require it (Norman & Shallice, 1986). In a pure version of second-order dissociated control theory, the first level of cognitive control—the governing of subsystems of control by executive control—is unaffected, allowing greater novelty in hypnotic responses than the original dissociated control theory, in which this level of control is weakened (Bowers, 1992a). Indeed, the second-order theory implies strong persistence of novelty. In particular, after setting up unusual cognitive control strategies, individuals who are high hypnotizable should be able to sustain them in a quasi-perseverative way, whereas those who are low hypnotizable would have such attempts overturned by conflict monitoring (Jamieson & Sheehan, 2004; Raz, Fan, & Posner, 2005; Woody & Farvolden, 1998).

Individuals who are high hypnotizable may differ in the degree to which they generate novelty. In a detailed comparison of two hypnotic virtuosos, McConkey, Glisky, and Kihlstrom (1989) found that for one of them, the suggested effects just happened passively by themselves, whereas the other person actively produced a variety of rather complex cognitive strategies in responding to the suggestions. A passive style of hypnotic response seems to fit the original formulation of dissociated control better, whereas a cognitively active style seems to fit the second-order dissociated control theory better.

CLINICAL APPLICATIONS

Before sketching out some possible clinical implications of the foregoing ideas, we want to raise a few caveats. First, we make no attempt to cover applications of hypnosis to a wide range of psychopathologies and other problems, because these applications are specifically covered in detail elsewhere, particularly in many other chapters of this volume. Instead, we focus on some issues common to various applications of hypnosis. These issues derive from the conceptualization of hypnosis as a way of altering the nature of awareness, as in dissociated experience, and as a way of altering the nature of control, as in dissociated control.

Second, we emphasize that the foregoing theoretical framework is somewhat provisional and incomplete. As such, it cannot explain all possibly effective applications of hypnosis. Dissociation theories of hypnosis can enrich clinicians' conceptualizations of how hypnosis works but do not tell them what is impossible.

Third, we need to address the issue of individual differences. Modern dissociation theories of hypnosis, from Hilgard's (1965, 1977) work onward, were devised, to a large extent, to explain the differences in hypnotic behavior between people who score high in hypnotic responsiveness on standardized hypnosis scales versus those who score low. Thus, it is possible that these theories best explain the response to hypnosis of people who are high hypnotizable, whereas they may be less applicable to people with low to moderate hypnotic susceptibility.

Indeed, Bowers (1984) posited that treatment effects should be regarded as genuinely hypnotic if and only if they correlate with hypnotic susceptibility, as assessed with standardized scales. Although hypnosis can lead to improvement in clients of relatively low hypnotic susceptibility, Bowers argued that such improvement is attributable to placebo effects and other nonhypnotic processes at work in the therapeutic situation rather than to hypnotic suggestion per se.

Accordingly, along with many other hypnosis researchers, we strongly recommend that clinicians use standardized hypnosis scales in their hypnotherapeutic work. Information from standardized scales is necessary so that clinicians can verify, over an aggregate of cases, that the treatment effects involved are actually hypnotic. Without this information, hypnotherapy seems wide open to the criticism that it may be an assortment of nonspecific effects masquerading under an exotic label. (For a further discussion of these issues, see Woody & Barnier, 2008.)

Implications of Dissociated Experience

A major implication of the concept of dissociated experience is that hypnosis may be useful for effecting therapeutic changes in awareness. For example, an important, classic use of hypnosis to alter awareness is hypnotic analgesia. However, from the theoretical vantage point, the crucial issue concerns the underlying process by which hypnotic analgesia is achieved. According to the dissociated experience account, individuals who are high hypnotizable and who experience analgesia in response to hypnotic suggestions are voluntarily using the same kinds of effortful cognitive strategies to reduce pain that they would use outside of hypnosis; the difference is that in hypnosis they become less aware of their own volition and effort. As Bowers (1990) pointed out, the dissociated experience view of hypnosis appears to restrict hypnotizability and hypnotherapy to a rather minor role:

> The only conceivable advantage of high hypnotizability would thus be a very limited one: Patients high in hypnotic ability would be more able than their low-hypnotizable counterparts to dissociate from consciousness any special effort or motivation involved in achieving treatment success. (p. 166)

Unlike Bowers, some other clinicians have been reasonably comfortable with the idea that hypnosis mainly affects clients' experience of therapy, leaving the underlying mechanisms of therapeutic change mostly unaffected. For example, Kirsch (1993) made the following memorable comment:

> For the cognitive–behavioral therapist, *hypnosis* is merely a new label for what is already being practiced. However, it is a label that can potentiate treatment for many clients. Unlike a rose, a therapy by a different name may not be experienced as the same. (p. 168)

Although dissociated experience theory implies that hypnosis is more than a new label, its treatment implications appear to be similar: The impression of effortlessness that clients who are high hypnotizable have in hypnosis may enhance how engaging and motivating the treatment is, even though this impression is illusory.

However, there is another, far bolder, rationale for the clinical application of hypnosis that stems from dissociated experience theory. Janet (1901, 1907) proposed that hypnosis and dissociative disorders closely parallel each other and, in fact, share the same underlying mechanisms, including a crucial underlying restriction of awareness. Similarly, there is currently a fairly widespread belief among clinicians that dissociative clinical phenomena, such as fugue states and depersonalization, represent "the spontaneous mobilization of hypnotic experience" (Spiegel, 1990, p. 127). That is, dissociative disorders may have an important autosuggestive core, such that these clients have spontaneously walled off certain material from consciousness using the same underlying, awareness-altering mechanisms that are at work in hypnosis (Allen, 1995).

The apparent clinical implication of this point of view is that hypnosis has special relevance for the treatment of dissociative disorders. Because hypnosis may be conceptualized as engaging the underlying mechanisms that played a role in causing the disorder, it allows the therapist a unique window to manipulate and redirect these underlying processes for therapeutic aims. For example, Smith (1995) commented that,

> Hypnosis is increasingly thought of as a 'controlled dissociation' and dissociation as a form of 'self-hypnosis' . . . . What was originally evoked in the individual by traumatic experiences can be beneficially influenced in treatment by controlled hypnotic interventions. (p. 66)

Similarly, Horevitz (1993) characterized hypnosis as an "indispensable tool" (p. 416) in the treatment of multiple personality disorder (or dissociative identity disorder).

We see reasons for some caution about this line of reasoning. First, clinicians use the term *dissociation* rather loosely to describe diverse phenomena, many of which may possibly have little to do with hypnosis and hypnotizability (Frankel, 1994). For example, attempts to measure real-life dissociative tendencies, such as with the Dissociative Experiences Scale (Bernstein & Putnam, 1986), tend to yield negligible relations to hypnotizability (e.g., Faith & Ray, 1994; Kirsch & Council, 1992). Second, the research on whether dissociative disorders are related to hypnotizability presents a mixed picture at best. Although some relatively early reports indicated a strong relation (e.g., Bliss, 1984), subsequent research has found only a quite modest relation (e.g., Moene, Spinhoven, Hoogduin, & van Dyck, 2003; Roelofs, Hoogduin, Keijsers, Naring, Moene, & Sandijck, 2002) or results suggesting no relation at all (e.g., Nash, Hulsey, Sexton, Harralson, & Lambert, 1993).

For these reasons, we believe it is unwarranted for clinicians to make any blanket assumption that dissociative psychopathology implies a role for hypnotizability and underlying hypnotic-like processes. Instead, we argue that the hypothesis of such a connection requires careful case-by-case evaluation, one part of which should include the administration of a standardized hypnosis scale. In our opinion, individuals who are relatively unresponsive to a formal hypnosis scale are unlikely to have autosuggestion as a core component of their difficulties.

We also raise a final reservation about a dissociated experience conceptualization of the hypnotic treatment of dissociative disorders. If we conceptualize both dissociative disorders and hypnosis as involving restrictions of awareness (e.g., Kihlstrom, 1994), the hypnotherapist seems to be put in the strange position of fighting fire with fire. In other words, why would a technique that restricts awareness be a good way to treat disorders having to do with a restriction of awareness?

Recent research linking hypnosis with dissociative disorders, conducted by Oakley and colleagues (Halligan, Athwal, Oakley, & Frackowiak, 2000; Oakley, 1999; Ward, Oakley, Frackowiak, & Halligan, 2003) and by Roelofs and colleagues (Hagenaars, Roelofs, Hoogduin, & van Minnen, 2006; Roelofs, Hoogduin, & Keijsers, 2002; Roelofs, Hoogduin, Keijsers, Naring, et al., 2002), strongly favors the dissociated control account rather than the dissociated experience account. For example, in conversion disorder, it is not simply a change in awareness that is implicated, but a change in the hierarchy of control. Roelofs Hoogduin, and Keijsers (2002) noted that "in conversion paralysis and hypnotic paralysis the linkage between higher-level and lower-level information processing is impaired, resulting in disturbances that predominantly affect the intentional motor functions" (p. 52). Thus, dissociated control may provide a more useful conceptualization.

Implications of Dissociated Control

As stated earlier, the concept of dissociated control is that hypnosis modifies underlying control processes, or the manner in which behavior is executed. The main clinical implication of this idea is that hypnotherapy should be useful for changing how clients control their behavior and for helping them to develop new ways of control. More specifically, according to the dissociated control account, hypnotic suggestions tend to bypass the intentional level of control and invoke control mechanisms that involve low cognitive effort. For example, according to this theory, hypnotic suggestions for analgesia given to individuals who are high hypnotizable elicit a type of pain control that is different from nonhypnotic control and involves much less effort. In contrast, according to the dissociated experience account, individuals achieving hypnotic analgesia are actually working hard in the same ways as they would control pain in nonhypnotic circumstances but are not aware of this effort.

The critical distinction, therefore, concerns how much effortful cognitive control is being expended in hypnotic responding. In a series of laboratory studies, Bowers and his colleagues provided important evidence that hypnotic phenomena do not depend on effortful control or other deliberate cognitive strategies. Miller and Bowers (1993) demonstrated that, in contrast to a cognitive–behavioral stress-inoculation procedure, hypnotic analgesia did not impair concurrent performance on a cognitively demanding task. This result indicated both that hypnotic analgesia uses negligible cognitive effort and that it taps mechanisms that are different from the effortful cognitive strategies of cognitive–behavioral therapy. Hargadon, Bowers, and Woody (1995) showed that the effectiveness of hypnotic analgesia in individuals who are high hypnotizable was not enhanced at all by deliberate cognitive strategies, such as engaging in counter-pain imagery. This study convincingly indicated that such deliberate cognitive strategies, which often spontaneously accompany suggestions for analgesia, actually have no role in producing the analgesia, which takes place through other, relatively effortless mechanisms. In a further study of hypnotic analgesia, Eastwood, Gaskowski, and Bowers (1998) verified that it requires low attentional resources or cognitive load, unlike stress inoculation.

Similarly, another series of laboratory studies by Bowers and his colleagues showed that hypnotic amnesia does not depend on any of a variety of proposed effortful cognitive strategies (Bowers & Davidson, 1991; Davidson & Bowers, 1991). Indeed, Bowers and Woody (1996; see also King & Council, 1998) showed that intentional efforts to suppress thoughts had the opposite effect from hypnotic suggestions for amnesia, increasing the rate of spontaneous occurrence of such thoughts. In addition, studies of other types of hypnotic suggestions likewise supported the hypothesis that the control mechanisms involved in hypnotic responding actually involve low cognitive effort (e.g., Ruehle & Zamansky, 1997; Sadler & Woody, 2006). Such studies require that researchers devise ways of measuring cognitive effort that avoid self-report because both dissociated experience and social cognitive theories posit that self-report is an inaccurate indicator of actual effort.

The clinical implications of the foregoing body of research are quite important, because they indicate that hypnosis may offer clients genuinely new ways of controlling behavior. There are some major potential advantages of the shift toward low-effort control that hypnosis facilitates. First, compared with more effortful strategies, hypnotic control may free up cognitive resources for other purposes. For example, deliberate cognitive strategies for controlling pain exert a considerable drain on the individual's cognitive resources (Farthing, Venturino, & Brown, 1984) and are subject to disruption by fatigue and distraction (McCaul & Malott, 1984). When such strategies are being used, there may be relatively little cognitive capacity available for other tasks (Miller & Bowers, 1993). According to dissociated control theory, hypnosis offers individuals who are high hypnotizable a way to control pain with lower cognitive costs, such that these clients not only obtain relief from pain but also retain more of the cognitive resources needed to engage in other desired activities. A related hypothesis advanced by Bowers (1992b) is that, compared with strategic efforts to reduce pain, analgesia through hypnotic suggestion should be less vulnerable to disruption by fatigue and distraction.

Second, intentional, effortful control can become maladaptive, and hypnosis offers important therapeutic opportunities to shift clients to alternative kinds of control that may be more effective. Deliberate, effortful control is relatively slow and limited in capacity, and in many types of behavior—for example, sports and music performance—it can readily become counterproductive, interfering with skilled performance (Norman & Shallice, 1986). Furthermore, when such control proves inadequate, people may respond by exerting even greater effort, which can propel them into a vicious circle in which increasing effort produces a worsening of control rather than the intended improvement. Wegner (1994) showed that trying too hard to exert control ironically impoverishes control and leads to persistent unwanted thoughts, emotions, and behaviors. Wegner argued that the solution is often to relinquish effortful control; however, intentionally reducing overcontrol can be difficult because it involves the paradox of exerting yet more effort.

Accordingly, Woody and Bowers (1994) proposed that an important practical use of hypnosis is to provide "a therapeutic opportunity to relinquish some kinds of control in order to further others" (p. 74). With hypnosis, the bypassing of executive initiative and effort may help overturn maladaptive intentional control. In addition, by temporarily assuming some planning and control functions, the hypnotherapist may help elicit new patterns of control, eventually replacing old ones that might otherwise be difficult for clients to relinquish. Bowers and Woody (1996) pointed out that Ericksonian uses of hypnosis, such as paradoxical manipulations of intention (e.g., Haley, 1967), might be viewed in this way.

A Case Study

The following case illustrates some of the foregoing points, particularly the use of a standardized hypnosis scale in therapy and the broad relevance of dissociated control in the conceptualization of hypnotherapy. The client, a woman in her 70s, was referred for persistent breathing difficulties (i.e., dypsnea). These difficulties, which had begun 5 years earlier and eventually began occurring several times per day, consisted of episodes of fairly severe shortness of breath due to the sudden inability to move air through the throat, which interfered with her physical activity and speaking. A series of diagnostic workups showed that the problem stemmed from the tendency of the client's vocal chords to close spontaneously during inhalation and exhalation (i.e., paradoxical vocal fold motion), but these workups were unable to determine whether the problem was principally organic or psychological in origin. A series of treatments, including voice therapy, massage therapy, and biofeedback, had provided only limited improvement. Subsequently, diagnostic impressions had shifted toward conceptualizing the breathing problem as related to anxiety, culminating in inpatient treatment of 2 months' duration, in which the client was given the diagnosis of generalized anxiety disorder. At this time, she was told her breathing difficulties were psychological in origin, connected psychologically to an emotionally abusive upbringing and the stress of a previous period of financial difficulties. However, treatment on the basis of this conceptualization did not lead to any improvement of the breathing problems. The client was also put on several psychoactive medications to treat the presumed anxious basis of her breathing problems and also depressive tendencies.

At the first session in our clinic, the breathing difficulties were abundantly evident: jerky inhalation and exhalation with sudden arrest of air flow, gasping for air, and interrupted, labored speech in a hoarse, low-pitched voice. Although the client said that her breathing problems were the result of anxiety, she could not explain what she meant by the word *anxiety* and could not report any thoughts or feelings consistent with this term. For example, when asked whether she experienced distressing thoughts in association with her breathing problems, she said, "Not really; I just wish I could breathe properly and get on with my life." However, these comments were somewhat difficult to evaluate because she appeared to be a somewhat limited informant, often unable to remember details of her condition and past treatments.

At the beginning of the therapy, when some of the foregoing medical history was not yet available, the client had two expectations. First, she anticipated further exploration of earlier hardships in her life, presumably to bring to awareness and resolve unconscious motivations underlying the problem. The therapist, under the supervision of the second author (Woody), declined to pursue this avenue. Second, the client wanted help to relax better and hence lower her anxiety level. Given the plausibility that anxiety might be a factor that exacerbated the breathing difficulties, the therapist began treatment by using progressive muscle relaxation.

The first such session revealed a striking phenomenon. The early part of the progressive muscle relaxation protocol included instructions for steady, deep breathing. These immediately produced extremely disrupted breathing, full of gasping and choking. Subsequently, with instructions to focus on relaxing muscle groups, the client's breathing returned rapidly to a closer approximation of normal. In the next session, the therapist was readily able to replicate this phenomenon: Whenever the client was asked to voluntarily regulate her breathing, her difficulties worsened dramatically; in contrast, whenever her attention was drawn away from her breathing, the problem relented quite quickly. The client's medical history became available at this time, revealing that other professionals had in the past sometimes noted improvement of the breathing problem with distraction.

Continued progressive muscle relaxation practice, now with the breathing instructions removed, led to reduction in the client's breathing problems both in sessions and, more important, at home. However, it was not the anxiety-reducing effect of this intervention that seemed important; indeed, it became clear that the client had simply adopted the word *anxiety* as a quasi-technical term to denote her breathing difficulties. Instead, the relaxation appeared to work because it shifted the client's attention away from her breathing and her deliberate attempts to fix it. Thus, our case conceptualization was as follows: (a) the client's voluntary regulation of breathing was dysfunctional, whereas her automatic regulation of breathing was reasonably normal; and (b) her expectation or noticing of incipient breathing problems led to a vicious circle in which deliberate attempts to regulate breathing rapidly and paradoxically produced the problem.

This control-based conceptualization suggested the possible treatment relevance of hypnosis. In particular, the dissociated control account of hypnosis posits the minimization of higher-level, voluntary control of behavior—the level that functioned paradoxically for this client—and the relatively direct activation of alternative, lower levels of control. Hypnosis offered not only more variety in distraction-based coping strategies but also some novel treatment possibilities based on suggestion.

In preparation for the therapeutic use of hypnosis, the therapist administered a standardized hypnosis scale, the Harvard Group Scale of Hypnotic Susceptibility, Form A (HGSHS:A; Shor & Orne, 1962). For this case, this scale had the advantage of a comparatively extensive sampling of motor suggestions, of both the direct motor type (e.g., hand lowering) and the motor challenge type (e.g., trying to bend an arm after the suggestion it has become stiff). The therapist explained that the rationale for administering the scale was twofold: to give the client some practice with hypnosis before applying it therapeutically and to get some information about what kinds of interventions might work best for her.

After the scale was administered, the client and therapist scored the client's responses. The client's pattern of response was clear: She tended readily to pass the direct motor suggestions, but passed none of the motor challenge suggestions or the hallucination suggestion, which are more indicative of the capacity for dissociative processes (Woody & Sadler, 1998). Inquiry into her subjective experience revealed relatively little sense of involuntariness but a state of strong motivation consistent with what Barber (1999) termed a *positive set*.

These results have some useful implications. First, in our opinion, the client's modest level of hypnotic suggestibility is not consistent with a conceptualization of the problem as autosuggestive in origin ("the spontaneous mobilization of hypnotic experience," in Spiegel's [1990] terms, p. 127). However, as our control-based conceptualization of the problem indicates, hypnosis could potentially be useful nonetheless because of its relevance for modifying the control of behavior. Second, the client's modest level of suggestibility indicated that relatively straightforward suggestions of limited difficulty were more likely to be helpful. In addition, it was reasonable to expect that the extent of her response to therapeutic suggestions would likely be relatively modest.

At the next session, the therapist used a hypnotic induction consisting of suggestions for relaxation, but without any preliminary muscle tensing, and deepening (similar to the induction of the HGSHS:A). To encourage a passive style of attention to breathing, the following passage was included:

> If at any time you find yourself noticing your breath, see how beautifully it works *all by itself*. *Just observe* how your breath can work all by itself, and *just leave it alone*. Then let your attention move back to the rest of your body, to release any tension. . . . Your body will effortlessly take care of breathing, as you search elsewhere, for any last bits of tension in any of your muscles.

There were also the following kinds of suggestions:

> Your breath knows what to do *all by itself*. You don't need to help it. Your body knows what to do, to breathe free and easy, free, free, and easy. Your body is wise; it knows what to do all by itself. *Just let it do what it does naturally*. You don't need to tell it anything—it already knows what to do.

And later, the following:

> Your throat knows what to do to relax. Feel it opening up gently and relax-
> ing. It is opening up, allowing the breath to travel smoothly without any
> effort. Feel the ease with which you are breathing. The breath is warm and
> soothing. It is creating a sensation of warmth from your lungs to your throat
> and to your nose. It is free to wander back and forth, in and out.

The client's breathing, which had been rather poor early in this session, improved markedly during the induction and became almost completely silent. Similar to the progressive muscle relaxation earlier, the hypnotic induction was recorded for the client's use at home. The therapist encouraged the client to use either tape several times per day, as she saw fit.

At later sessions, the client noted that she preferred to use the hypnosis because her mind wandered less during the sessions and the hypnosis seemed more effective in eliciting feelings of calm. She reported that she used the hyp-nosis tape every morning and evening, which tended to be times when the breathing problems were worse, as well as periodically throughout the day. The therapist introduced a variant of the hypnotic induction by including imagery of a favorite, peaceful place. The client also continued to use the progressive relaxation tape occasionally, for variety.

With improved breathing, the client was able to expand her range of phys-ical activities. For example, she started doing housework (e.g., doing laundry, making beds, mopping floors) again, which she had previously avoided because of her breathing difficulties. However, she complained that she thought she could no longer walk for more than 5 or 10 minutes before her breathing diffi-culties would force her to stop. To further assess this difficulty, the therapist took the client on a walk outside for part of a session. The client was able to walk and simultaneously hold a conversation for more than 20 minutes without any undue difficulty. The therapist instructed the client to take walks at home while listening to a hypnosis tape on a portable tape player, which was effective.

Both the client's breathing in sessions (e.g., during discussion before any hypnosis) and her reports of physical activity at home improved considerably. However, an additional issue to address was the client's unrealistic expectation that hypnosis should completely eliminate all her breathing difficulties. (To some extent, this expectation stemmed from the client being told previously that her problems were purely psychogenic.) Instead, the therapist described hypnosis as a coping tool to help make better use of the client's automatic breathing, which was quite good, and to circumvent her deliberate regulation of breathing, which was dysfunctional.

Despite the low likelihood of the client's problem being dissociative in origin and the client's modest level of hypnotic suggestibility, this case illus-trates the practical use of a dissociated control perspective on hypnosis.

CONCLUSION

The use of the construct of dissociation to explain hypnosis has a history stretching back more than a century. Recent developments in dissociation theories have proposed a specific set of underlying mechanisms. These include alterations in self-monitoring, affecting conscious experience, and alterations in the initiation and ongoing adjustment of cognitive control. Although future research may selectively favor one of these hypothesized mechanisms, it is also possible that hypnosis involves a fluid plurality of dissociative mechanisms, as Hilgard (1992, 1994) suggested.

Dissociation theories imply that hypnosis should be clinically beneficial for altering unpleasant or unwanted aspects of conscious experience and for altering maladaptive mechanisms of control. Because these theories focus on abilities for which there are strong individual differences, they also imply that assessment of clients with standardized hypnosis scales provides important information for tailoring interventions. Finally, dissociation theories provide a useful and informative perspective for the application of hypnosis in clinical therapy, even in the treatment of people with modest hypnotic responsiveness, as our case study illustrated.

REFERENCES

Allen, J. G. (1995). Dissociative processes: Theoretical underpinnings of a working model for clinician and patient. In J. G. Allen & W. H. Smith (Eds.), *Diagnosis and treatment of dissociative disorders* (pp. 1–23). Northvale, NJ: Jason Aronson.

Barber, T. X. (1999). A comprehensive three-dimensional theory of hypnosis. In I. Kirsch, A. Capafons, E. Cardeña-Buelna, & S. Amigó (Eds.), *Clinical hypnosis and self-regulation: Cognitive–behavioural perspectives* (pp. 21–48). Washington, DC: American Psychological Association.

Barnier, A. J., Bryant, R. A., & Briscoe, S. (2001). Posthypnotic amnesia for material learned before or during hypnosis: Explicit and implicit memory effects. *International Journal of Clinical and Experimental Hypnosis, 49,* 286–304.

Bernstein, E. M., & Putnam, F. W. (1986). Development, reliability, and validity of a dissociation scale. *Journal of Nervous and Mental Disease, 174,* 727–735.

Bliss, E. L. (1984). Hysteria and hypnosis. *Journal of Nervous and Mental Disease, 172,* 203–206.

Bowers, K. S. (1984). Hypnosis. In N. S. Endler & J. M. Hunt (Eds.), *Personality and behavior disorders* (2nd ed., Vol. 1, pp. 439–475). New York: Wiley.

Bowers, K. S. (1990). Unconscious influences and hypnosis. In J. L. Singer (Ed.), *Repression and dissociation: Implications for personality theory, psychopathology, and health* (pp. 143–179). Chicago: University of Chicago Press.

Bowers, K. S. (1992a). Dissociated control and the limits of hypnotic responsiveness. *Consciousness and Cognition, 1*, 32–39.

Bowers, K. S. (1992b). Imagination and dissociation in hypnotic responding. *International Journal of Clinical and Experimental Hypnosis, 40*, 253–275.

Bowers, K. S., & Davidson, T. M. (1991). A neodissociative critique of Spanos's social–psychological model of hypnosis. In S. J. Lynn & J. W. Rhue (Eds.), *Theories of hypnosis: Current models and perspectives* (pp. 105–143). New York: Guilford Press.

Bowers, K. S., & Woody, E. Z. (1996). Hypnotic amnesia and the paradox of intentional forgetting. *Journal of Abnormal Psychology, 105*, 381–390.

Cohen, J. D., Aston-Jones, G., & Gilzenrat, M. S. (2004). A systems-level perspective on attention and cognitive control: Guided activation, adaptive gating, conflict monitoring, and exploitation versus exploration. In M. I. Posner (Ed.), *Cognitive neuroscience of attention* (pp. 71–90). New York: Guilford Press.

Davidson, T. M., & Bowers, K. S. (1991). Selective hypnotic amnesia: Is it a successful attempt to forget or an unsuccessful attempt to remember? *Journal of Abnormal Psychology, 100*, 133–143.

Dywan, J., & Bowers, K. S. (1983, October 14). The use of hypnosis to enhance recall. *Science, 222*, 184–185.

Eastwood, J. D., Gaskowski, P., & Bowers, K. S. (1998). The folly of effort: Ironic effects in the mental control of pain. *International Journal of Clinical and Experimental Hypnosis, 46*, 77–91.

Egner, T., Jamieson, G., & Gruzelier, J. (2005). Hypnosis decouples cognitive control from conflict monitoring processes of the frontal lobe. *NeuroImage, 27*, 969–978.

Ellis, H. D., & Young, A. W. (1990). Accounting for delusional misidentifications. *British Journal of Psychiatry, 157*, 239–248.

Evans, F. J. (1979). Contextual forgetting: Posthypnotic source amnesia. *Journal of Abnormal Psychology, 88*, 556–563.

Faith, M., & Ray, W. (1994). Hypnotizability and dissociation in a college age population: Orthogonal individual differences. *Personality and Individual Differences, 17*, 211–216.

Farthing, G. W., Venturino, M., & Brown, S. W. (1984). Suggestion and distraction in the control of pain: Test of two hypotheses. *Journal of Abnormal Psychology, 93*, 266–276.

Frankel, F. H. (1994). Dissociation in hysteria and hypnosis: A concept aggrandized. In S. J. Lynn & J. W. Rhue (Eds.), *Dissociation: Clinical and theoretical perspectives* (pp. 80–93). New York: Guilford Press.

Goldberg, G. (1987). From intent to action: Evolution and function of the premotor systems of the frontal lobe. In E. Perecman (Ed.), *The frontal lobes revisited* (pp. 273–306). New York: IRBN Press.

Hagenaars, M. A., Roelofs, K., Hoogduin, K., & van Minnen, A. (2006). Motor and sensory dissociative phenomena associated with induced catalepsy. *International Journal of Clinical and Experimental Hypnosis, 54*, 234–244.

Haggard, P. (2003). Conscious awareness of intention and action. In J. Roessler and N. Eilan (ed.), *Agency and self-awareness: Issues in philosophy and psychology* (pp. 111–127). Oxford, England: Oxford University Press.

Halligan, P. W., Athwal, B. S., Oakley, D. A., & Frackowiak, R. S. J. (2000, March 18). Imaging hypnotic paralysis: Implications for conversion hysteria. *The Lancet, 355*, 986–987.

Hargadon, R., Bowers, K. S., & Woody, E. Z. (1995). Does counter-pain imagery mediate hypnotic analgesia? *Journal of Abnormal Psychology, 104*, 508–516.

Haley, J. (1967). *Advanced techniques of hypnosis and therapy: Selected papers of Milton H. Erickson, M. D.* New York: Grune & Stratton.

Hilgard, E. R. (1965). *Hypnotic susceptibility.* New York: Harcourt, Brace & World.

Hilgard, E. R. (1977). *Divided consciousness: Multiple controls in human thought and action.* New York: Wiley.

Hilgard, E. R. (1979). Divided consciousness in hypnosis: The implications of the hidden observer. In E. Fromm & R. E. Shor (Eds.), *Hypnosis: Developments in research and new perspectives* (2nd ed., pp. 45–79). Hawthorne, NY: Aldine.

Hilgard, E. R. (1991). A neodissociation interpretation of hypnosis. In S. J. Lynn & J. W. Rhue (Eds.), *Theories of hypnosis: Current models and perspectives* (pp. 83–104). New York: Guilford Press.

Hilgard, E. R. (1992). Dissociation and theories of hypnosis. In E. Fromm & M. R. Nash (Eds.), *Contemporary perspectives in hypnosis research* (pp. 69–101). New York: Guilford Press.

Hilgard, E. R. (1994). Neodissociation theory. In S. J. Lynn & J. W. Rhue (Eds.), *Dissociation: Clinical and theoretical perspectives* (pp. 32–51). New York: Guilford Press.

Horevitz, R. (1993). Hypnosis in the treatment of multiple personality disorder. In J. W. Rhue, S. J. Lynn, & I. Kirsch (Eds.), *Handbook of clinical hypnosis* (pp. 395–424). Washington, DC: American Psychological Association.

Hull, C. L. (1933). *Hypnosis and suggestibility: An experimental approach.* New York: Appleton-Century-Crofts.

James, W. (1890). *The principles of psychology.* New York: Holt.

Jamieson, G. A., & Sheehan, P. W. (2004). An empirical test of Woody and Bowers's dissociated-control theory of hypnosis. *International Journal of Clinical and Experimental Hypnosis, 52*, 232–249.

Jamieson, G. A., & Woody, E. Z. (2007). Dissociated control as a paradigm for cognitive-neuroscience research and theorising in hypnosis. In G. A. Jamieson (Ed.), *Hypnosis and conscious states: The cognitive-neuroscience perspective* (pp. 111–129). Oxford, England: Oxford University Press.

Janet, P. (1901). *The mental state of hystericals*. New York: Putnam.

Janet, P. (1907). *The major symptoms of hysteria*. New York: Macmillan.

Janet, P. (1925). *Psychological healing: A historical and clinical study*. New York: Macmillan.

Kihlstrom, J. F. (1980). Posthypnotic amnesia for recently learned material: Interactions with "episodic" and "semantic" memory. *Cognitive Psychology, 12,* 227–251.

Kihlstrom, J. F. (1992). Hypnosis: A sesquicentennial essay. *International Journal of Clinical and Experimental Hypnosis, 50,* 301–314.

Kihlstrom, J. F. (1994). One hundred years of hysteria. In S. J. Lynn & J. W. Rhue (Eds.), *Dissociation: Clinical and theoretical perspectives* (pp. 365–394). New York: Guilford Press.

Kihlstrom, J. F., & Shor, R. E. (1978). Recall and recognition during posthypnotic amnesia. *International Journal of Clinical and Experimental Hypnosis, 26,* 330–349.

King, B. J., & Council, J. R. (1998). Intentionality during hypnosis: An ironic process analysis. *International Journal of Clinical and Experimental Hypnosis, 45,* 295–312.

Kirsch, I. (1993). Cognitive–behavioral hypnotherapy. In J. W. Rhue, S. J. Lynn, & I. Kirsch (Eds.), *Handbook of clinical hypnosis* (pp. 151–171). Washington, DC: American Psychological Association.

Kirsch, I., & Council, J. R. (1992). Situational and personality correlates of hypnotic responsiveness. In E. Fromm & M. R. Nash (Eds.), *Contemporary Perspectives in Hypnosis Research* (pp. 267–291). New York: Guilford Press.

Kirsch, I., & Lynn, S. J. (1998). Dissociation theories of hypnosis. *Psychological Bulletin, 123,* 100–115.

Laurence, J.-R., & Perry, C. (1983, November 4). Hypnotically created memory among highly hypnotizable subjects. *Science, 222,* 523–524.

Lhermitte, F. (1986). Human autonomy and the frontal lobes. Part II: Patient behavior in complex and social situations: The "environmental dependency syndrome." *Annals of Neurology, 19,* 335–343.

McCaul, K. D., & Malott, J. M. (1984). Distraction and coping with pain. *Psychological Bulletin, 95,* 516–533.

McConkey, K. M., Glisky, M. L., & Kihlstrom, J. F. (1989). Individual differences among hypnotic virtuosos: A case comparison. *Australian Journal of Clinical and Experimental Hypnosis, 17,* 131–140.

McConkey, K. M., & Sheehan, P. W. (1981). The impact of videotape playback of hypnotic events on hypnotic amnesia. *Journal of Abnormal Psychology, 90,* 46–54.

McConkey, K. M., Sheehan, P. W., & Cross, D. G. (1980). Posthypnotic amnesia: Seeing is not remembering. *British Journal of Social and Clinical Psychology, 19,* 99–107.

Moene, F. C., Spinhoven, P., Hoogduin, K. A. L., & van Dyck, R. (2003). A randomized controlled clinical trial of a hypnosis-based treatment for patients with conversion disorder, motor type. *International Journal of Clinical and Experimental Hypnosis, 51*, 29–50.

Mesulam, M.-M. (1986). Frontal cortex and behavior. *Annals of Neurology, 19*, 320–325.

Miller, M. E., & Bowers, K. S. (1993). Hypnotic analgesia: Dissociated experience or dissociated control? *Journal of Abnormal Psychology, 102*, 29–38.

Nash, M. R., Hulsey, T. L., Sexton, M. C., Harralson, T. L., & Lambert, W. (1993). Long-term sequelae of childhood sexual abuse: Perceived family environment, psychopathology, and dissociation. *Journal of Consulting and Clinical Psychology, 61*, 276–283.

Norman, D. A., & Bobrow, D. G. (1979). Descriptions: An intermediate stage in memory retrieval. *Cognitive Psychology, 11*, 107–123.

Norman, D. A., & Shallice, T. (1986). Attention to action: Willed and automatic control of behavior. In R. J. Davidson, G. E. Schwartz, & D. Shapiro (Eds.), *Consciousness and self-regulation* (Vol. 4, pp. 1–18). New York: Plenum Press.

Oakley, D. A. (1999). Hypnosis and conversion hysteria: A unifying model. *Cognitive Neuropsychiatry, 4*, 243–265.

Orne, M. T., Whitehouse, W. G., Dinges, D. F., & Orne, E. C. (1988). Reconstructing memory through hypnosis: Forensic and clinical implications. In H. M. Pettinati (Ed.), *Hypnosis and memory* (pp. 21–63). New York: Guilford Press.

Perner, J. (2003). Dual control and the causal theory of action: The case of non-intentional action. In J. Roessler & N. Eilan (Eds.), *Agency and self-awareness: Issues in philosophy and psychology* (pp. 218–243). Oxford, England: Oxford University Press.

Proust, J. (2003). Perceiving intentions. In J. Roessler & N. Eilan (Eds.), *Agency and self-awareness: Issues in philosophy and psychology* (pp. 296–320). Oxford, England: Oxford University Press.

Raz, A., Fan, J., & Posner, M. I. (2005). Hypnotic suggestion reduces conflict in the human brain. *Proceedings of the National Academy of Sciences USA, 102*, 9978–9983.

Roelofs, K., Hoogduin, C. A. L., & Keijsers, G. P. J. (2002). Motor imagery during hypnotic arm paralysis in high- and low-hypnotizable subjects. *International Journal of Clinical and Experimental Hypnosis, 50*, 51–66.

Roelofs, K., Hoogduin, C. A. L., Keijsers, G. P. J., Naring, G. W. B., Moene, F. C., & Sandijck, P. (2002). Hypnotic susceptibility in patients with conversion disorder. *Journal of Abnormal Psychology, 111*, 390–395.

Rosenberg, M. J. (1959). A disconfirmation of the descriptions of hypnosis as a dissociative state. *International Journal of Clinical and Experimental Hypnosis, 7*, 187–204.

Ruehle, B. L., & Zamansky, H. S. (1997). The experience of effortlessness in hypnosis: Perceived or real? *International Journal of Clinical and Experimental Hypnosis, 45*, 144–157.

Sadler, P., & Woody, E. (2006). Does the more vivid imagery of high hypnotizables depend on greater cognitive effort? A test of dissociation and social–cognitive theories of hypnosis. *International Journal of Clinical and Experimental Hypnosis, 54*, 372–391.

Shallice, T. (1988). *From neuropsychology to mental structure.* Cambridge, England: Cambridge University Press.

Shor, R. E. (1979). The fundamental problem in hypnosis research as viewed from historic perspectives. In E. Fromm & R. E. Shor (Eds.), *Hypnosis: Developments in research and new perspectives* (2nd ed., pp. 15–41). Chicago: Aldine.

Shor, R. E., & Orne, E. C. (1962). *Harvard Group Scale of Hypnotic Susceptibility, Form A.* Palo Alto, CA: Consulting Psychologists Press.

Smith, W. H. (1995). Incorporating hypnosis into the psychotherapy of patients with multiple personality disorder. In J. G. Allen & W. H. Smith (Eds.), *Diagnosis and treatment of dissociative disorders* (pp. 65–75). Northvale, NJ: Jason Aronson.

Spanos, N. P. (1986). Hypnotic behavior: A social–psychological interpretation of amnesia, analgesia, and "trance logic." *Behavioral and Brain Sciences, 9*, 449–467.

Spanos, N. P., Radtke, H. L., & Dubreuil, D. L. (1982). Episodic and semantic memory in posthypnotic amnesia: A reevaluation. *Journal of Personality and Social Psychology, 43*, 565–573.

Spiegel, D. (1990). Hypnosis, dissociation, and trauma: Hidden and overt observers. In J. L. Singer (Ed.), *Repression and dissociation: Implications for personality theory, psychopathology, and health* (pp. 121–142). Chicago: University of Chicago Press.

Szechtman, H., & Woody, E. (2004). Obsessive–compulsive disorder as a disturbance of security motivation. *Psychological Review, 111*, 111–127.

Ward, N. S., Oakley, D. A., Frackowiak, R. S., & Halligan, P. W. (2003). Differential brain activations during intentionally simulated and subjectively experienced paralysis. *Cognitive Neuropsychiatry, 8*, 295–312.

Wegner, D. M. (1994). Ironic processes of mental control. *Psychological Review, 101*, 34–52.

White, R. W., & Shevach, B. J. (1942). Hypnosis and the concept of dissociation. *Journal of Abnormal and Social Psychology, 37*, 309–328.

Woody, E. Z., & Barnier, A.J. (2008). Hypnosis scales for the 21st century: What do we need and how should we use them? In M. R. Nash & A. J. Barnier (Eds.), *Oxford handbook of hypnosis* (pp. 255–281). Oxford, England: Oxford University Press.

Woody, E. Z., Barnier, A. J., & McConkey, K. M. (2005). Multiple hypnotizabilities: Differentiating the building blocks of hypnotic performance. *Psychological Assessment, 17*, 200–211.

Woody, E. Z., & Bowers, K. S. (1994). A frontal assault on dissociated control. In S. J. Lynn & J. W. Rhue (Eds.), *Dissociation: Clinical and theoretical perspectives* (pp. 52–79). New York: Guilford Press.

Woody, E., & Farvolden, P. (1998). Dissociation in hypnosis and frontal executive function. *American Journal of Clinical Hypnosis, 40,* 206–215.

Woody, E. Z., & McConkey, K. M. (2003). What we don't know about the brain and hypnosis, but need to: A view from the Buckhorn Inn. *International Journal of Clinical and Experimental Hypnosis, 51,* 309–338.

Woody, E., & Sadler, P. (1998). On reintegrating dissociated theories: Comment on Kirsch and Lynn (1998). *Psychological Bulletin, 123,* 192–197.

Woody, E., & Sadler, P. (2008). Dissociation theories of hypnosis. In M. R. Nash & A. J. Barnier (Eds.), *Oxford handbook of hypnosis* (pp. 81–110). Oxford, England: Oxford University Press.

Woody, E., & Szechtman, H. (2000). Hypnotic hallucinations: Toward a biology of epistemology. *Contemporary Hypnosis, 17,* 4–14.

Woody, E., & Szechtman, H. (2007). Emotion, motivation, and hypnosis. In G. A. Jamieson (Ed.), *Hypnosis and conscious states: The cognitive-neuroscience perspective* (pp. 241–244). Oxford, England: Oxford University Press.

7

THE COGNITIVE–BEHAVIORAL MODEL OF HYPNOTHERAPY

GRAHAM F. WAGSTAFF, DANIEL DAVID, IRVING KIRSCH, AND STEVEN JAY LYNN

Cognitive–behavioral therapy (CBT) is a set of theories and treatment procedures developed by cognitive therapists and behavior therapists beginning in the 1950s. Many of these procedures were derived from experimental psychology, and their use is based on a conception of psychological problems as learned maladaptive responses sustained by dysfunctional cognitions. More precisely, according to the cognitive perspective, people experience various activating events (A), about which they have functional, rational, adaptive, healthy beliefs and/or dysfunctional, irrational, maladaptive, unhealthy beliefs and cognitions (B). Functional beliefs lead to adaptive, healthy consequences (C), whereas dysfunctional beliefs lead to maladaptive, unhealthy consequences. These consequences can be affective, cognitive, behavioral, and/or physiological. Thus, CBT views most complex human responses as cognitively penetrable (David, Opre, & Miclea, 2004). *Cognitive penetrability* means that (a) human responses are an effect of cognitive processing (i.e., cognitions), be it conscious or unconscious, and (b) a change in cognitions by various procedures (e.g., cognitive–behavioral interventions) will induce a change in the expressed response.

All clinical material has been disguised to protect patient confidentiality.

In this chapter, we discuss the integration of hypnotherapy (i.e., hypnotic inductions and suggestions) with CBT, or what is called *cognitive–behavioral hypnotherapy*, to increase the effectiveness of cognitive–behavioral interventions. Our chapter begins with a review of the development of CBT, and an examination of the cognitive–behavioral interpretation of hypnosis through the work of several important theorists. We then provide an overview of clinical applications of the use of hypnosis with CBT, and present several vignettes of case material as illustrations. Finally, we examine recent research on the efficacy and implications of using cognitive–behavioral hypnotherapy.

THE DEVELOPMENT OF COGNITIVE–BEHAVIORAL THERAPY

The development of behavior therapy in the 1950s and 1960s (Eysenck, 1960; Wolpe, 1958) represented a radical departure in the conceptualization and treatment of behavioral and emotional problems. Instead of viewing presenting problems as symptoms of underlying disorders, behavior therapists saw them as maladaptive learned responses that were to be the direct targets of therapeutic interventions. Assuming that operant and classical conditioning were the mechanisms by which learning occurred, early behavior therapists developed treatments in which conditioning procedures were used to teach clients more adaptive responses.

The term *cognitive therapy* is generally used to designate the treatment techniques described by Aaron Beck (1976) and his colleagues (Beck, Rush, Shaw, & Emery, 1979). However, the *rational emotive therapy* developed by Albert Ellis (1962) should be recognized as the first contemporary cognitive therapy. According to cognitive therapists, emotional problems are not caused by the stimulus events themselves, but rather by the ways in which those events are interpreted. Emotional disturbance is seen as a consequence of unwarranted assumptions and illogical thinking. The strategy of cognitive therapy is to alleviate emotional distress by teaching clients to interpret events in a more rational and adaptive manner.

Although initially distinct schools of therapy, a number of developments have brought about a convergence between cognitive and behavior therapies. First, Bandura (1969) presented an influential overview of behavior therapy that stressed the role of cognitive factors in human learning. Two years later, Arnold Lazarus (1971), who a decade earlier had been one of the pioneers of behavior therapy, added Ellis's *cognitive restructuring* to the broad spectrum of techniques used by behavior therapists. Conversely, virtually all of the methods of behavior therapy have been incorporated into cognitive therapy (Beck et al., 1979; Ellis & Grieger, 1977). In 1974, Donald Meichenbaum presented *cognitive behavior modification*, a formal integration of cognitive and behavioral psychotherapy. In the 1990s, Albert Ellis (1995)changed the name of rational emotive therapy (previously called *rational therapy*) to *rational emotive behavior therapy* to better reflect this integration between cognitive and behavioral approaches. Finally, though once regarded as behavioral mechanisms, classical and operant conditioning are now more widely viewed as cognitive processes that change behavior through their effects on cognitions (Bolles, 1972; Kirsch, Lynn, Vigorito, & Miller, 2004; Rescorla, 1988, 1991).

With this much convergence, the distinction between cognitive therapy and behavior therapy is no longer useful, and the appellation *cognitive–behavior therapy* is the most accurate characterization of these treatment procedures. Indeed, the label *behavior therapy* has always been somewhat problematic, given that some of the earliest and most widely studied "behavioral" procedures were based on the use of imagery (Wolpe, 1958).

THE COGNITIVE–BEHAVIORAL VIEW OF HYPNOSIS: FUNDAMENTALS

Within the cognitive–behavioral model of hypnotherapy, the role of hypnotic inductions is also construed from cognitive–behavioral perspective. The cognitive–behavioral view of hypnosis embraces what has variously been termed the *social psychological*, and more recently, *sociocognitive* approach to hypnosis, which emphasizes the importance of social and cognitive processes in producing, guiding, and interpreting hypnotic behaviors (Lynn & Rhue, 1991; Spanos, 1982, 1986; Wagstaff, 1986, 2004).

Traditionally, hypnosis has been portrayed as a special sleeplike state in which people are more suggestible than they are in the normal waking state and behave in ways that differ fundamentally from normal everyday behavior. In contrast, cognitive–behavior theorists have challenged the hypothesis that hypnotic phenomena are due to an altered state of consciousness; that is, they doubt that the concept of a hypnotic "trance" is useful in explaining changes in behavior and experience that accompany hypnosis (Barber, 1969; Kirsch, 1990; Lynn, Rhue, & Weekes, 1990; Sarbin & Coe, 1972; Spanos & Chaves, 1989; Wagstaff, 1981). In their view, hypnotic phenomena are best explained by the same variables that account for nonhypnotic behavior. This rejection of the altered state construct is based on the following data:

1. No specific physiological markers of the hypothesized hypnotic states have been found (Lynn, Kirsch, Knox, & Lilienfeld, 2006; see also chap. 4, this volume).

2. All of the phenomena produced by suggestion following a hypnotic induction can also be produced without a hypnotic induction (Braffman & Kirsch, 1999). Furthermore, the increases in suggestibility that are produced by hypnotic inductions are small and can often be duplicated or even surpassed by a variety of other procedures, including placebo pills (Barber & Glass, 1961) and imagination training (Katz, 1979; Vickery, Kirsch, Council, & Sirkin, 1985).

3. Rather than describing their experience as an altered state, most hypnotized subjects describe hypnosis as a "normal state of consciousness that simply involves the focusing of attention [and] thinking along with and imagining the suggestions given by the hypnotist" (McConkey, 1986, p. 314). These descriptions of the hypnotic experience are especially common among highly responsive subjects.

4. Descriptions of the state of consciousness produced by typical hypnotic inductions appear to be indistinguishable from those produced by progressive relaxation training (Kirsch, Mobayed, Council, & Kenny, 1992).

Because hypnosis has traditionally been defined as an altered state, the nonstate position could be seen as challenging the concept of hypnosis. As a result, the cognitive–behavioral approach to hypnosis has sometimes been misinterpreted as a denial of the reality or importance of hypnotic phenomena (e.g., Kihlstrom, 1997). The cognitive–behavioral view of hypnosis, however, rejects the position that all hypnotic phenomena are faked or unimportant. Indeed, although some have argued that hypnotic subjects may be capable of faking certain responses (e.g., Orne, 1959, 1962; Spanos, 1992; Wagstaff, 1981, 1991), cognitive–behavioral theorists have conducted a variety of studies demonstrating that hypnotic responses are not merely sham enactments (e.g., Kirsch, Silva, Carone, Johnston, & Simon, 1989; Perugini et al., 1998).

It can also be emphasized that although cognitive–behavioral theorists reject the definition of hypnosis as an altered state of consciousness, they do not deny that hypnosis can exist as a meaningful construct. For example, from a cognitive–behavioral perspective, the concept of hypnosis can be defined operationally as a *belief* or *suggestion* that there exists a hypnotic condition with certain definable characteristics; these characteristics may vary, depending on the context, but typically include, for example, the experience of involuntariness and increased responsiveness to suggestions. In addition, hypnosis can be defined as any *procedure*, or ritual in which participants are invited to respond to this kind of belief or suggestion (i.e., any procedure explicitly or implicitly defined or labeled as a hypnotic induction procedure) and any situation involving such a procedure (Wagstaff, 1998, 2004).

Moreover, although cognitive–behavioral theorists emphasize the point that most hypnotized subjects describe hypnosis as a normal state of focusing of attention and thinking along with and imagining the suggestions, such theorists do not deny that some subjects may experience altered states when undergoing inductions and performing hypnotic suggestions; rather, they question the usefulness of postulating a special hypnotic altered state to account for hypnotic behavior and experience. For example, for some people, relaxation and meditation procedures may result in experiences that could be construed as "an altered state" (Benson & Klipper, 1976). Hence, if a person undergoes relaxation procedures within the context of hypnosis, he or she could experience an altered state. But this is not to say that this relaxed state is uniquely responsible for the phenomena associated with hypnosis. It is critical, for instance, that in the absence of the label *hypnosis*, relaxation procedures are ineffective in raising baseline responses to suggestions (Brown, Antonova, Langley, & Oakely, 2001).

Development of the Cognitive–Behavioral View of Hypnosis

The beginnings of hypnosis have often been linked to the techniques of *mesmerism*, as practiced by Franz Anton Mesmer and his followers in the late 18th and early 19th centuries. But even in these early days, the idea that the phenomena under scrutiny were attributable to some kind of special process had its critics. For example, the Franklin Report of 1785 concluded that all of the effects attributed to mesmerism were the result of "imagination" (Mackay, 1869). And, in 1819, the Portuguese priest and healer, Abbé José Custodio di Faria, argued that the therapeutic cures claimed by mesmerists were the result of "suggestion"; indeed, Faria frequently used suggestions in his treatments, noting, "a glass of water swallowed with the notion that it is *eau-de-vie* completely intoxicates" (Wagstaff, 1981, p.4). In the sense that these critics attempted to explain mesmeric phenomena in terms of everyday processes, without necessarily denouncing them as fraudulent, they could be considered early pioneers of the cognitive–behavioral approach to hypnosis. However, according to Spanos and Chaves (1989), the modern precursor to the cognitive–behavioral view of hypnosis was Robert White (1941).

Although White actually argued that hypnosis involved an altered state of consciousness, he also viewed hypnotic behavior in terms of an interaction between subjects' implicit expectations concerning what was to happen to them and their active attempts to present themselves in a manner appropriate to their interpretation of what the hypnotist expected of them. Thus, to White, hypnotic behavior should be viewed as a social interaction in which hypnotized subjects are active, cognizing agents, using their previous knowledge, and information conveyed to them by the hypnotist, to present themselves as hypnotized, as they understand the term. White's ideas had considerable influence on the views of those such as Martin Orne (1959, 1962, 1970) who, although adhering to the traditional notion of a hypnotic state, nevertheless stressed the influence of social factors on hypnotic responding, in particular, the influence of contextual influences or what he termed the *demand characteristics* of the situation.

However, it was Theodore Sarbin who pioneered the idea of abandoning the notion of hypnosis as a special state altogether by viewing hypnotic behaviors as entirely continuous with concepts and processes found in everyday behavior (see, e.g., Sarbin, 1950; Sarbin & Coe, 1972). Sarbin construed hypnosis to be an active, goal-directed role-enactment in which the subject and the hypnotist are enacting roles appropriate to their conceptions of a developing script. From Sarbin's perspective, therefore, hypnotic responses are not automatic "happenings" but purposeful activities. Moreover, hypnotic behaviors appear to be unusual not because they have unusual causes but because the hypnotic role calls for unusual behavioral enactments.

Sarbin also pioneered research from a nonstate perspective into individual differences in hypnotizability. One of the most significant features of state accounts of hypnosis has been the idea that susceptibility to this state is a relatively fixed and unmodifiable trait; from this point of view, a core feature of subjects who are highly hypnotizable is an aptitude to enter the hypnotic state or trance (e.g., Bowers, 1976). However, Sarbin, working closely with William Coe, rejected this position. Instead, Coe and Sarbin (1966) argued that individual differences in hypnotic responding are dependent on variables such as role congruence and role expectation; that is, they depend on appropriate attitudes toward and expectancies concerning the performance of the hypnotic role (see chap. 13, this volume). They also argued that certain role aptitudes, such as a propensity to become engrossed in and to enact imaginings, are advantageous in enacting the hypnotic role.

At the time, however, Sarbin's role theory approach met with considerable resistance from those who continued to maintain the traditional position that there is something special about hypnosis that enables hypnotized participants to transcend their waking capacities. It was this belief in the special status of hypnosis that motivated the research program of Theodore X. Barber (1969). Barber proposed that all hypnotic phenomena could be explained in terms of concepts and processes drawn from general psychology without postulating the intervention of a special altered state of consciousness. Indeed, Barber argued that the notion that hypnosis involves a special hypnotic state or trance was often used circularly; the concept was used to explain the unusual nature of hypnotic behaviors, but also, the unusual nature of hypnotic behaviors was assumed to be evidence of a special state.

Barber also identified a number of key methodological issues in the way hypnosis experiments and clinical studies were conducted. He pointed out that hypnotic procedures typically include a number of instructions that may have physiological, behavioral, and experiential consequences independently of any assumption about the existence of a hypnotic state. For example, there are often fairly definable patterns of physiological and experiential responses related to fairly mundane activities such as relaxation and sitting quietly, which may be involved in hypnosis procedures. Imaginative suggestions, in the absence of hypnosis, can also have profound behavioral and experiential consequences. Consequently, to test whether it is necessary to invoke some kind of extra trance component to explain hypnotic phenomena, Barber argued that it is important to ensure that nonhypnotic control groups are appropriately instructed regarding these activities. Barber argued that an appropriate control group for hypnosis studies is not, for example, one, commonly used, in which subjects act as their own "waking" controls; that is, in the same or within subjects design. A variety of evidence indicates that individuals who are highly hypnotizable may strategically "hold back" or fail to respond optimally in the "waking" situation so that their performance in the hypnosis condition will look "special" (e.g., Barber, 1969; Wagstaff, 1981).

Of fundamental interest to Barber was the repeated finding, both in his own studies and in the literature, that hypnotic induction procedures tend to increase responsiveness to test suggestions (e.g., arm levitation, body immobility, amnesia). In his research program, therefore, he tried to account for the increases in suggestibility that accompany hypnotic induction procedures without postulating the intervention of a special state. Barber proposed that, because of expectancies and the contextual demands placed on them, subjects given hypnotic induction procedures, particularly if they are classified as high hypnotizable, are more motivated to carry out suggestions and instructions than individuals acting as controls. Also, they have higher expectations that they will respond positively to, or pass, suggestions given to them. Hence, any differences in responsiveness to suggestions between participants in hypnotic and control conditions are likely to due to increased motivation and positive expectancies rather than the effects of an altered state. Consequently, Barber argued that, in most cases, the most appropriate design to assess the effects of hypnosis per se is one in which participants given suggestions or instructions with hypnosis are compared with a motivated independent group of participants who otherwise share similar psychological characteristics and are given the same kinds of imaginative suggestions or instructions as the hypnosis group but without an induction ritual. Arguably, Barber's arguments in this respect are as relevant to research into hypnosis and hypnotherapy today as they were when his seminal work *Hypnosis: A Scientific Approach* was published in 1969.

Because most of Barber's research concentrated on the importance of motivation and expectancies in accounting for hypnotic behaviors, he tended to use simple experimental designs that compared participants receiving hypnotic inductions with those who were given instructions aimed to motivate them and raise their expectations regarding their abilities to respond successfully to suggestions (i.e., task-motivational instructions). On the basis of his own studies and a review of the relevant literature, Barber concluded that suitably motivated nonhypnotized groups can equal hypnotic groups on a variety of performance measures, including test suggestions, feats of strength and endurance, age regression, pain tolerance, and harmful acts. Barber also argued that participants' descriptions of the experience of being hypnotized do not provide evidence of some unique process; indeed, they can be accounted for by factors such as relaxation, eye closure, suggestions for drowsiness and sleep, and the effects of imaginative suggestions (Barber, Spanos, & Chaves, 1974).

Those working with Sarbin and Barber, in particular, Nicholas Spanos, John Chaves, and William Coe, then further developed and refined these ideas, stressing the social psychological nature of hypnotic responding and the importance of context, attitudes, expectancies, and imaginative involvement in guiding and interpreting the behavior of the hypnotic subject. One of the most highly influential and, in terms of research output, certainly the most prolific, of these researchers was Nicholas Spanos (1986, 1991). Spanos researched a wide spectrum of hypnotic phenomena. He argued that hypnotic responding is essentially a strategic role enactment that can be facilitated by the construction of goal-directed imaginings. One issue that particularly interested him was the paradox of how a sentient, goal-directed, hypnotic subject could remain in control of his or her behaviors while apparently experiencing many of them as involuntary. Spanos maintained that hypnotic subjects often become highly involved in conveying the impression that they have lost behavioral control because this impression is required in the hypnotic context; hence, they try to convince not only the hypnotist but also themselves that their behaviors are involuntary, and they sometimes succeed in this. However, they do not actually lose control of their behaviors. To illustrate the latter point, Spanos and his coworkers showed that even highly hypnotizable subjects would readily counter hypnotic suggestions if they were led to believe that maintaining (i.e., rather than losing) voluntary control is a sign of deep hypnosis (Spanos, Cobb, & Gorassini, 1985).

Spanos's work in this respect was a precursor to modern cognitive–behavioral views on hypnotic voluntariness, which were based on models of working memory and attention. According to this latter perspective, much everyday behavior is routinized and scripted to be carried out fairly automatically without continual monitoring from an executive cognitive process; a good example would be driving a car on a familiar route to work. Consequently, all that is needed for a hypnotizable subject to respond to suggestions is to intend to enact the hypnotic role. Having established this intention, the subject is then in a position to essentially relinquish the executive control of his or her actions to the hypnotist in the same way that a driver might hand over control of directing the car he or she is driving to a navigator; as a result, hypnotic responses may be experienced as relatively involuntary or automatic. However, in doing this, the hypnotized subject does not actually lose control of his or her behavior anymore than a driver loses control of his or her behavior while being directed by a navigator (see, e.g., Kirsch & Lynn, 1999).

Among his wide range of achievements, Spanos also made a significant contribution to our understanding of the modification of hypnotizability. Spanos (1986) showed how, by changing negative and unrealistic expectations about the nature of hypnosis and instructing participants in appropriate ways of responding to and interpreting hypnotic suggestions, many participants, who previously appeared to be relatively unresponsive to hypnotic suggestions, can be taught to be responsive. For example, for some clients to learn to be responsive to hypnotic suggestions, it is necessary to show them how hypnotic responding requires their active involvement; that is, a good hypnotic subject does not just wait passively for something to happen. Spanos and other researchers demonstrated that hypnotizability could be modified substantially (see chap. 13, this volume). By the same token, some clients may fail to respond because they fear that a person who is hypnotized loses control of his or her behavior and is at the mercy of the hypnotist. Consequently, if they are to respond successfully to suggestions, it is important to dispel such misconceptions.

Spanos also made a substantial contribution to our understanding of the effects of hypnosis on the perception of pain. The groundwork for Spanos's approach to hypnotic analgesia was laid in his early collaborations with Theodore Barber and John Chaves. Barber, Spanos, and Chaves argued that accounts of painless surgery with hypnosis were explicable in a variety of ways without postulating the intervention of a special altered state of consciousness; for example, they noted that procedures for hypnotic analgesia typically involve a variety of nonspecific pain coping strategies that are potent pain relievers; these include suggestions for pain relief (e.g., numbness, coldness), relaxation and distraction, and preoperative preparation to alleviate fear and anxiety (Barber, Spanos, & Chaves, 1974; Spanos & Chaves, 1989). In a series of detailed and conceptually ingenious laboratory experiments, Spanos and his colleagues claimed to demonstrate that it is not necessary to postulate special hypnotic processes to explain reports of hypnotic analgesia;

rather, reports of hypnotic analgesia represent a mixture of real effects moderated by attitudes, expectancies, interpretational sets and pain coping strategies, and response bias effects that arise as participants in studies of hypnotic analgesia attempt to play the roles expected of them (Spanos, 1991; Spanos & Chaves, 1989).

Significantly, the work of those such as Barber, Spanos and Chaves (1974), had implications far beyond the understanding that all hypnotic phenomena are potentially explicable in terms of everyday psychological processes. The fact that certain clinical phenomena, such as the experience and reporting of pain, could be profoundly influenced by such apparently mundane factors as attitudes, motivation, expectancies, and imaginative suggestions, was important in itself and clearly had implications for therapeutic interventions, regardless of any association with hypnosis. However, their research also suggested that the contexts and rituals associated specifically with hypnosis might be particularly effective in harnessing and promoting these factors for some individuals. As Barber (1969) demonstrated on many occasions, for some, hypnotic induction procedures can be effective in enhancing responsiveness to a variety of suggestions and instructions through raising motivation and positive expectancies for success. Indeed, he showed that even simply labeling a procedure as hypnosis can increase responsiveness to suggestions and instructions.

Irving Kirsch has taken a similar stance, contending that, like placebos, hypnosis produces therapeutic effects by changing the client's expectancies. Kirsch's research has shown that a wide variety of hypnotic responses covary with people's beliefs and expectancies about their occurrence (Kirsch, 1990). In fact, expectancy, along with waking suggestibility, is one of the few stable correlates of hypnotic suggestibility (Kirsch & Lynn, 1995). But unlike placebos, hypnosis does not require deception in order to be effective. Rather than avoid expectancy effects, Kirsch has made the compelling argument that clinicians should maximize them by way of techniques such as hypnosis, which many people expect will be effective in conquering vexing habits and in ameliorating emotional suffering. Honestly informing clients about what researchers have learned about the nature of expectancy may reduce resistance and increase responsiveness to hypnotic interventions.

Steven Jay Lynn (1994) suggested that research originating from a sociocognitive perspective implies that taking the following steps may optimize responses to hypnotherapy: (a) develop a positive rapport and therapeutic alliance with the client that promotes the free-flowing quality of hypnotic experience; (b) understand the client's motives and agenda in relation to experiencing hypnosis; (c) identify the personal connotations that hypnosis has for each client; (d) assess the individual's stream of awareness and internal dialogue during hypnosis; (e) modify suggestions and hypnotic communications so as to minimize resistance and increase a sense of perceived control; (f) encourage clients to adopt lenient or liberal criteria for passing suggestions (e.g., "You don't have to imagine what I suggest 'as real as real,' even a faint image is fine."); and (g) encourage absorbed involvement in suggestions, the use of imagination, and attention to subtle alterations in experiences and responses.

In short, cognitive–behavioral theorists do not deny that for some clients, hypnotic inductions may have highly beneficial therapeutic effects. Indeed, they actively promote this view and set the stage for the development and applications of cognitive–behavioral hypnotherapy.

Cognitive–Behavioral Hypnotherapy

The use of hypnosis in CBT is actually as old as behavior therapy itself. Wolpe and Lazarus (1966), for example, reported using hypnotic inductions instead of progressive relaxation with about one third of their systematic desensitization clients. From a cognitive–behavioral perspective, the main aim of adding a ritual or label to therapeutic procedures that convey to the client that hypnosis is involved is to provide a context in which the effects of cognitive–behavioral interventions can be potentiated for some clients (Barber, 1985; Kirsch, 1999; Kirsch, Montgomery, & Sapirstein, 1995). However, there are other advantages of adding hypnotic inductions to therapeutic procedures. For instance, they can provide a disinhibiting context, allowing clients to exhibit responses that they do not realize they are capable of making; also, hypnosis can disinhibit therapists by providing a context for therapeutic behaviors that might seem inappropriate in other settings (Barber, 1985). For example, the hypnotic context permits the therapist to repeat statements over and over again, thereby enhancing their forcefulness and salience. Outside of the hypnotic context, this style of communication would seem strange and inappropriate. Nevertheless, though potentially beneficial to those with positive attitudes and expectancies toward hypnosis, the addition of hypnosis to cognitive–behavior therapies may not be beneficial for all. In fact, it is likely to degrade the effects of treatment among clients who view hypnosis with fear or derision.

CLINICAL APPLICATIONS

Cognitive–behavioral interventions are best known as treatments of phobic anxiety and depression. However, there are also CBTs for personality disorders, autism, stuttering, enuresis, encopresis, Tourette's disorder, marital distress, hypertension, asthma, obsessive–compulsive disorders, sexual dysfunctions and deviations, pain, addictions, obesity, and various other problems and disorders. The rest of this chapter focuses on the cognitive–behavioral procedures that are common to these various applications.

Relaxation

Relaxation training is a component of many cognitive–behavioral treatments. Frequently, it is taught as a coping skill with which anxiety and stress can be countered. It may be paired with stressful imagery, as in systematic desensitization, or clients may be instructed to generate relaxation as a way of reducing anxiety and tension when it is encountered in daily life. Relaxation training is often used in treating phobias, hypertension, cardiac arrhythmias, asthma, chronic diarrhea, irritable bowel syndrome, pain, headaches, epilepsy, and insomnia.

The traditional method of teaching relaxation is to instruct clients to alternately tense and relax various groups of muscles, until the whole body is relaxed (Jacobson, 1929). However, many therapists omit the instructions for muscle tension and instead maintain a consistent focus on relaxation. In either case, the requests to relax particular muscle groups are interspersed with suggestions for general relaxation, such as, "[You feel] deeply relaxed . . . more and more relaxed . . . all the tension is draining from your body."

The striking similarity between relaxation training and typical hypnotic inductions is easily recognized. In fact, all that is needed to transform relaxation training into a hypnotic induction is the addition of the word *hypnosis*. Thus, whenever relaxation training seems indicated in treatment, a hypnotic induction can be used in its place. Similarly, relaxation exercises at home can be replaced by training in self-hypnosis, the essential difference being the label itself.

The use of the relaxation response in real-life settings can be encouraged by a posthypnotic suggestion to the effect that one will become better and better at producing relaxation at will. For example, the client can be told the following:

> Whenever you find yourself experiencing stress or anxiety, you can relax the tension away. All you need do is take a deep breath, think the word "relax" as you exhale, and let the tension drain from your body. As you practice self-hypnosis, you will find this easier and easier to do, and you may be surprised at how easy it becomes to just let yourself relax.

Imagery

In CBT, relaxation is often paired with guided imagery of stressful encounters with the aim of enabling the client to experience the stressor with reduced anxiety. In traditional systematic desensitization, client and therapist work together to construct a hierarchy of anxiety-related scenes. Clients are then instructed to relax and to begin imagining the least anxiety-provoking scene from their hierarchies. When anxiety is experienced, they are instructed to discontinue the imagined stressful encounter. Brief relaxation instructions are given until relaxation is regained, at which point the anxiety imagery is resumed. Once the image can be tolerated without eliciting anxiety, the next scene on the hierarchy is imagined. Desensitization is a robust treatment in that it retains its effectiveness over a remarkably wide range of variations in procedure (Kirsch, 1990). For example, rather than discontinuing stress-related imagery when anxiety is experienced, clients can be instructed to stay with the imagined scene while breathing slowly, relaxing away their anxiety and imagining themselves applying these coping strategies in the anxiety-provoking situation. Another variation in procedure is to condense or even eliminate the hierarchy entirely so that the client begins by imagining a relatively stressful scene. Imagery can also be used without relaxation. This is particularly useful in practicing assertive interpersonal behavior, which might be inhibited by relaxation. Here too, imagery can be preceded by a hypnotic induction; however, in this case, an *alert induction* (e.g., see chap. 11) might be better than the more traditional relaxation induction. Instead of suggesting relaxation, the therapist induces hypnosis with suggestions for increased energy and focused attention using phrases similar to the following: "With each breath you take, you can feel yourself becoming more and more alive and vital. Feel the energy flow through your body . . . through your feet . . . your legs . . . your thighs."

Behavioral Generation and Behavioral Practice

In most applications, practice in imagination is followed by real life practice. In the treatment of phobias, this is termed *exposure*. Phobic clients are instructed to enter the feared situation while making use of the coping strategies they have learned during hypnosis sessions. Those with panic disorders practice slow, shallow breathing to counteract the tendency to hyperventilate. For clients who are depressed, the aim of behavioral practice may be to (a) increase activity levels, (b) provide pleasurable experiences that have the potential of changing affect and of convincing clients that pleasure is possible, and/or (c) provide experiences of mastery and success that can enhance self-esteem and generalized self-efficacy.

Specific environments activate some beliefs and cognitions (i.e., those congruent with the environment and/or our specific tasks) whereas they inhibit and/or deactivate other beliefs (i.e., those incongruent with the environment and/or our specific tasks). Activated knowledge, in turn, generates behaviors. By means of a hypnotic induction, whether performed by a therapist or the client him- or herself, it is possible to reduce the constraints of the environment on human cognitions and thus deactivate most of our cognitions. Under these conditions, people experience an expanded *operational readiness* (see David, 1999). Moreover, specific suggestions can create diverse mental environments (e.g., to imagine being in a social situation) that can, in turn, activate related cognitions (e.g., how to speak in public) and support desired behaviors (e.g., speaking). Thus, hypnosis is a good tool to create and manipulate operational readiness and impact the behaviors clinicians want to generate in a clinical setting.

Successive Approximation

The reinforcement of successive approximations of a desired response is termed *shaping*. It is through shaping that animal performers are taught the complex behaviors they display in movies and public exhibitions, and it is through shaping that autistic children have been taught to speak (Lovaas, 1969).

The principle of graduated practice is a ubiquitous aspect of cognitive–behavioral treatments. It can be seen, for example, in the hierarchy of anxiety-provoking scenes that is constructed during systematic desensitization. Similarly, behavioral exposure to anxiety situations typically involves progressively longer exposures to increasingly difficult situations. Clients who are depressed may initially be asked only for modest increases in behavior; it is wise to choose initial mastery exercises that are easy enough so that success is virtually guaranteed. The usefulness of successive approximation in hypnosis is implicitly recognized in the structure of hypnosis scales, which tend to begin with relatively easy suggestions and progress to more difficult items.

Cognitive Restructuring

The object of cognitive restructuring is to identify and modify the dysfunctional cognitions that may contribute to emotional and behavioral disorders. The nature of these cognitions varies from disorder to disorder and person to person. People diagnosed with panic disorders, for example, often believe that their attacks are due to a fatal physical condition (e.g., cardiac arrest) or that they are in danger of "going crazy." Depressed individuals may hold negative beliefs about themselves, their world, and the future, a set of beliefs that Beck (1976) termed a *negative cognitive triad*.

Cognitive restructuring typically consists of three phases (David, Macavei, Szentagotai, & McMahon, 2005): (a) the identification of dysfunctional beliefs and/or cognitions; (b) modification of dysfunctional cognitions; and (c) the assimilation of functional cognitions in our cognitive architecture. Dysfunctional beliefs may be maintained against disconfirming evidence because of distortions in logical processing of information. These distortions include attending to confirmatory information and ignoring disconfirmatory information (i.e., selective abstraction), drawing arbitrary inferences in the absence of supportive data, overgeneralizing, magnifying the significance of some events and minimizing the significance of others, personalizing external events without any factual basis for making such a connection, and thinking in dichotomous black and white terms (Beck et al., 1979; Lazarus, 1971).

When dysfunctional thoughts or beliefs are identified, they are evaluated through Socratic questioning. Clients are urged to treat them as hypotheses rather than facts. These hypotheses are then tested by mutual examination of available data. If the data are insufficient for a conclusion to be drawn, behavioral homework may be assigned as a means of testing the validity of old beliefs and potential alternatives. When the client reaches the conclusion that a particular thought or belief is invalid, it is replaced by a more adaptive alternative that is to be integrated into the client's belief system.

It is at this point that hypnosis and self-hypnosis can be particularly useful. New adaptive beliefs that the client has accepted as valid are given as hypnotic suggestions to facilitate their full incorporation into the client's cognitive structure. Without hypnosis, some clients may feel foolish or silly, intentionally repeating sentences to themselves, despite the fact that the content of those sentences is accepted as valid and important and that this repetition, in fact, increases the activation value of cognitions, helping them to be integrated into personal belief-systems and control desired behaviors. The purpose of hypnosis in this process is to provide a special context in which clients can feel comfortable practicing their new cognitions. Montgomery, David, DiLorenzo, and Schnur (2007) found that the impact of dysfunctional beliefs on various human responses is often mediated by response expectancies (i.e., expectancies for nonvolitional outcomes; for details, see Kirsch, 1990). As hypnosis is one of the most powerful techniques used to change response expectancies (Kirsch, 1999), its basic role in cognitive restructuring can be exploited to good advantage.

Hypnosis in Cognitive–Behavioral Therapy: Conclusions

One of the premises of the cognitive–behavioral perspective is that whatever can be done with hypnosis can also be done without it. This is one implication of the hypothesis that hypnosis is not a special state or condition. Conversely, anything that can be done without hypnosis might also be done in a hypnotic context. Given these premises, how is one to decide whether to augment an intervention by establishing a hypnotic context?

Some clients come to therapy requesting hypnosis or are referred for hypnotic treatment by another therapist. The latter occurs with increasing frequency as a therapist gains a reputation as a hypnotherapist. These clients almost invariably hold positive attitudes and expectations about hypnosis, and this makes them good candidates for hypnotic interventions. The danger in these cases is that the client's expectations may be too positive. They may think of hypnosis as a powerful procedure that will do the work for them, so that little effort on their part is required. This, of course, is a set-up for failure, and hypnotic treatment should not be started without first educating the client about the real nature of hypnosis.

Although some clients come to a therapist requesting hypnosis, most come asking for help because of a particular set of problems they are facing, and they look to the therapist to suggest the treatment procedures that will be used. One way that therapists sometimes evaluate the suitability of clients for hypnotic treatment is to assess their hypnotic suggestibility. However, treatment outcome is not always correlated with hypnotic suggestibility (Wadden & Anderton, 1982), and even when it is, the correlation is quite modest. Baker and Kirsch (1993), for example, reported a correlation of .25 between suggestibility and hypnotic analgesia. Many clients who are only moderately hypnotizable may benefit from the use of a hypnotic induction. This tends to be the case for clients who have positive attitudes toward hypnosis and for whom the use of hypnosis makes therapy more credible.

CASE MATERIAL

To illustrate some of these issues, the following case material is presented, taken from the experience of actual clients. Obviously, before including hypnosis as part of a therapeutic intervention it is necessary to decide whether or not hypnosis will be suitable with a particular client.

Deciding Whether to Use Hypnosis

Rather than assessing suggestibility, an excellent way of determining whether to use hypnosis is to ask the client. This is illustrated in the following excerpt. The client had presented with a fear of flying and had disclosed, during the assessment interview, that she also experienced a fear of heights and tunnels. Intentional hyperventilation produced sensations similar to those she experienced in these situations, leading to the supposition that stress-cued hyperventilation may have been contributing to feelings of panic she experienced. The choice of procedures was presented to her as follows:

Therapist: There are two procedures that we can use to help you with your fear. One of these is hypnosis. We would use hypnosis here in the office, and I would also teach to you use self-hypnosis at home. A second possibility is to use a desensitization procedure that involves relaxation training and imagery. In either case, once you achieve some initial fear reduction, either through hypnosis or through the relaxation and imagery exercises, I'll ask you to begin practicing these skills in real-life settings, probably beginning with heights, because airplane trips are rather expensive. Do you have any initial reactions about whether to use hypnosis or muscle relaxation as a method of coping with your fears?

Client: Well, I'd want to use whatever works best. Does one work better than the other?

Therapist: Hypnosis and the imagery/relaxation procedures seem to be about equally effective. But some people find hypnosis more helpful, whereas others benefit more from relaxation training. What it really depends on is how comfortable you are with one method or the other. Because you know yourself much better than I do, you're probably the best judge of which method would work better for you. What do you think?

Client: I don't really know. But, I have a pretty strong will, so I don't think I would be able to be hypnotized. I want to do whatever will work best.

Therapist: Well, based on what you've told me, my sense is that relaxation training may be the best way to begin.

This client's comments indicated that she held some fairly common misconceptions about hypnosis and that these led her to have negative expectations about her hypnotic ability. An alternative response might have been to educate her about the nature of hypnosis in an effort to change her attitude. There are a number of reasons for thinking that accepting the client's judgment was a better tactic. First, regardless of the therapist's educational efforts, the client might still hold the suspicion that responding to hypnosis was an indication of a weak will. Second, the actual procedures that would be used once the choice was made are virtually identical. Third, research indicates that allowing clients to choose between therapeutic alternatives enhances treatment outcome (Devine & Fernald, 1973; Kanfer & Grimm, 1978; Lazarus, 1973).

Hypnosis can also be turned to when problems are encountered in the use of nonhypnotic procedures. For example, some people respond to relaxation training with a paradoxical anxiety reaction. The switch to hypnosis in such a case is illustrated in the following vignette. After a few minutes of relaxation instructions, a 17-year-old client suddenly sat upright with eyes wide open.

> Client: This is stupid. I can't do it. It just makes me feel more uptight and nervous.
>
> Therapist: What happened?
>
> Client: I don't know. I tried to relax. But the more I tried, the more antsy I got. I just can't do it.
>
> Therapist: Okay, it's clear that the relaxation exercise is not working for you. Perhaps we should try something else. I wonder what you think about hypnosis. It might be an alternative that we could try.
>
> Client: [with evident excitement] Do you do hypnosis?
>
> Therapist: Yes, I sometimes use it in therapy. You seem pretty interested in the idea. I wonder what you know about hypnosis or what ideas you have about it.

After discussing the nature of hypnosis from a cognitive–behavioral perspective, a muscle-relaxation, eye-closure induction was begun. In the hypnotic context, the client responded to relaxation suggestions with relaxation instead of discomfort.

Finally, hypnosis can be useful in working with clients who are unreflective and tend to give quick, "I don't know" answers to questions, rather than working on finding an answer. With these clients, the following suggestion is often helpful:

> We all have hidden wisdom of which we are unaware, parts of us that know more than we think we know. In a moment, I'm going to ask you a question. But I don't want you to answer it right away. Instead, I want you to repeat the question to that hidden, wise part of yourself that knows more than you know. And when you've asked the question, I'd like you to wait. Just wait quietly until you become aware of an answer.

From a psychodynamic perspective, instructions of this sort may be seen as a way of accessing unconscious material. Neodissociation theorists (e.g., Hilgard, 1986) might view it as a means of accessing dissociated cognitive structures. From a cognitive–behavioral perspective, however, it is a method of interrupting a habitual response, slowing the client down, and encouraging reflective thought.

Hypnotic Skill Training

Hypnotherapists often devote considerable effort to sharpening their skills at administering hypnotic inductions. Workshops are given in which indirect

inductions, double inductions, special deepening techniques, and other procedures of this sort are taught. In contrast to the amount of attention devoted to
teaching and learning these procedures, relatively little effort has been
expended in evaluating their efficacy. The studies that have been done to investigate these procedures indicate that they are not particularly effective (Lynn,
Neufeld, & Matyi, 1987; Mathews, Kirsch, & Mosher, 1985).

Instead of devoting energy to fancy inductions, cognitive–behavioral
therapists emphasize adequate preparation of clients for hypnosis. This consists of explaining the cognitive–behavioral view of hypnosis and demonstrating how hypnotic experiences can be produced even without a hypnotic
induction. The following is a condensed example of a cognitive–behavioral
approach to hypnotic skill training:

> Many people think of hypnosis as a mysterious altered state of conscious-
> ness, in which the person goes into a trance and loses control over his or
> her behavior. Hypnosis really isn't like that at all. Most people describe
> hypnosis as just a normal state of focused attention. When you are hyp-
> notized, you remain awake and in full control of your behavior, and after
> hypnosis, you can remember everything that happened while you were
> hypnotized.
>
> Hypnosis isn't something that I do to you. Instead, it's something that
> you do yourself. In fact, it's sometimes said that all hypnosis is really self-
> hypnosis. My job isn't to hypnotize you; it's to show you how to hypnotize
> yourself.
>
> The purpose of using hypnosis is to make it easier for you to experi-
> ence suggestions. When I suggest something to you, either in or out of
> hypnosis, my suggestion doesn't make the experience happen. You have
> to decide whether you want to accept the suggestion, and if you do, it's
> you who makes the suggestion happen. If you don't like a suggestion I
> make, you can ignore it, just as you can outside of hypnosis. Or you can
> change it into a suggestion that you would like to experience. But if you
> want to experience the suggestion, hypnosis may make it easier for you
> to do so.
>
> Let me give you an example of what I mean. [*The therapist holds up a
> pendulum.*] Now, when I show you this pendulum, it probably makes you
> think of those old movies in which the hypnotist says, "Watch the
> watch! Watch the watch!" Well, I'm not going to use this to hypnotize
> you. What I want to do with it is show you how you can experience
> hypnotic suggestions without hypnosis. Let me show you what I mean. If
> I hold the pendulum between my thumb and forefinger, and if I concen-
> trate on the pendulum moving in a particular direction, let's say clock-
> wise, just by imagining it moving, I can get it to move that way. [*The
> pendulum begins to move.*] As I concentrate on it, it begins to move in
> wider and wider circles, and I can get it to change direction, to back and
> forth, let's say, just by imagining it. [*The pendulum changes direction.*] It

happens pretty quickly for me, because I've done this a lot. For a lot of people, it happens more slowly. But most people can do it, if they try.

Now, I could easily just swing the pendulum intentionally, but that would be meaningless. Or I could focus my attention on keeping my hand still, and then the pendulum probably wouldn't move at all. But I don't do any of those things. Instead, I ignore my hand and focus all my attention on the pendulum and on the way I want it to move. And a funny thing happens. It seems like the pendulum is moving all by itself, as if the thought went right from my head to the pendulum, bypassing my hand and arm altogether. Now that couldn't really be happening. Somehow, my imagination is causing my hand to move, and those movements are being amplified by the pendulum. But I'm not aware of moving my hand at all. It feels as if the pendulum is moving all by itself. Why don't you try it? [*The therapist hands the pendulum to the client.*]

In what direction would you like the pendulum to move? [*Client answers "clockwise."*] All right, now just concentrate on the pendulum. But stay awake. I don't want you to be hypnotized yet. Just picture the pendulum moving in a clockwise direction . . . round and round . . . round and round [. . . *The pendulum begins to move.*] . . . making wider and wider circles . . . wider and wider. Why not make it change directions now? How about making it move sideways? Back and forth . . . back and forth.

Okay! Now here's what I'd like you to notice. First of all, you weren't hypnotized, were you? You weren't in some kind of trance. Second, I didn't make the suggestion happen. You did! You could have ignored what I said. You could have made it move in any direction you wanted to, right? That's just what hypnosis is like. In hypnosis, I make a suggestion, and you decide whether you want to experience it. And if you do, you have to make it happen. You have to concentrate on the suggestion and imagine along with it. If I ask you to hold out your arm and to imagine it becoming heavy, and if you want to experience that, then you have to imagine something that would make your arm feel very heavy, and you have to imagine the feeling of heaviness. If you concentrate on it, you can probably generate a feeling of heaviness and make it feel like your arm is being dragged down all by itself. But I can't make your arm feel heavy or move down. That's something that you have to do.

Most clients feel quite comfortable with this description and demonstration. They often express amazement when the pendulum starts to move, smiling and exclaiming, "This is weird!" Their fears about giving up control are assuaged. They have learned that taking an active role as a hypnotic subject will make it easier for them to respond to suggestion. More important, they have learned that they must take an active role as client, rather than wait passively for the therapist to "cure" them.

Hypnosis and Cognitive Restructuring

When a dysfunctional interpretation, thought, or belief has been evaluated, and the client has accepted the conclusion that it is illogical or unwarranted, it is replaced by an alternative, more adaptive cognition. However, old thought patterns might not disappear automatically once their fallacy has been demonstrated. Clients often report thinking dysfunctional thoughts that they know to be erroneous; they report knowing one thing in their heads but feeling another in their hearts. Clients prone to panic attacks, for instance, might know intellectually that their attacks are not dangerous. But the irrational thought that it is the beginning of a heart attack may occur nevertheless, and it may occur with enough conviction to generate panic. We refer to this as a *head–heart split* (David et al., 2005). With cognitive restructuring, we can increase the activation of functional cognitions and their assimilation into clients' belief-systems while we facilitate novel adaptive responses and inhibit habitual dysfunctional cognitions. In this way, we can reduce the head–heart split.

Repetition

Hypnosis and self-hypnosis are useful techniques for helping the head convince the heart of what the head knows to be true. Hypnosis is particularly useful in this process because it allows the therapist to speak in ways that would be inappropriate in other contexts. It is normal, during hypnosis, for the therapist to speak slowly and forcefully, put more emphasis than usual on particular words or phrases, and to repeat the same idea many times. The following is an example of a repetitive message that is designed to increase activation of functional cognitions and that sounds normal in a hypnotic context, even when spoken in a slow, deliberate, and emphatic manner:

> Even though the thought sometimes occurs that feelings of anxiety might be the beginning of a heart attack, you know that they are not. They are a normal response to stress . . . a normal response . . . and they are not dangerous. And when the thought that they may be dangerous occurs, you can think, "I know . . . that this is only my anxiety. . . . It cannot hurt me. . . . It cannot hurt me. . . . All I need to do is slow my breathing and relax. . . . Breathe slowly and relax . . . slowly and relax." Whenever you feel anxious, you can tell yourself that you know that it is only anxiety and that it cannot hurt you, and you will know that you are safe. You will remember to relax your muscles and to breathe slowly . . . relax and breathe slowly. And even if a scary thought occurs, you will know that it is just a thought and that it isn't true. Anxiety may be scary, but it can't hurt you. It isn't a heart attack, and you're not going crazy. It's not a heart attack, and you're not going crazy. And as you practice these new thoughts during your self-hypnosis sessions at home, the old thoughts will

come less and less often . . . less and less often . . . and you'll know in your heart that they aren't true.

It is important to remember that suggestions such as these are given only after maladaptive thoughts have been evaluated and the client has concluded intellectually that they are wrong. This is not the way to convince the client of the truth of alternative beliefs; it is a way to help the client become more confident of his or her changed beliefs so that the old thoughts lose their force and new thoughts surface more automatically.

Global Restructuring Technique

Mental contamination is defined as the phenomenon whereby a client experiences an unwanted cognition, emotion, or behavior because of mental processing that is unconscious or uncontrollable (Wilson & Brekke, 1994). Mental contamination is involved in the process of cognitive restructuring (David et al., 2005). Thus, (a) there is a point in cognitive restructuring when clients recognize that their past cognitions are false and/or dysfunctional; then (b) clients agree to assimilate new functional beliefs; however, (c) although clients have assimilated new functional beliefs, they respond emotionally and behaviorally according to past dysfunctional beliefs; typically (d) clients are not aware of this process, or if aware, they cannot control it (see the "head–heart" split, discussed earlier).

To control this mental contamination and to favor the assimilation of the new adaptive beliefs, David et al. (2005) designed and tested in a single-case series the *global restructuring technique*. This technique is based on the *global intentional forgetting paradigm*. In global intentional forgetting, individuals learn new information and then they are told to forget this information (F-cued) because it is false and/or irrelevant and will not be further tested. Then they are given a second set of information to learn and remember (R-cued). However, during the memory test, they are asked to remember both sets of information. Research showed (David et al., 2005; Johnsson, 1994) that subjects create separate representations for F-cued and R-cued information and then inhibit the retrieval of F-cued information. In clinical settings, this procedure was adapted for use during hypnosis and/or waking imagery, as in the following series of steps (see David et al., 2005):

1. Clients are told to imagine a blackboard on which both new functional and past dysfunctional beliefs are written.
2. Clients are instructed to forget everything written on the blackboard (e.g., to experience hypnotic amnesia), namely, both functional and dysfunctional cognitions (F-cued), thus aiming to inhibit the mental representation of both functional and dysfunctional cognitions.

3. Clients are instructed to visualize and repeat only the functional beliefs (R-cued) on the blackboard; thus, clients create a new mental representation containing only the functional cognitions, segregated from the past one containing both functional and dysfunctional cognitions.

The results in single-case series studies (David et al., 2005) showed that global restructuring technique can be implemented in clinical settings and that it contributes to positive outcome in cognitive restructuring, as compared with standard cognitive restructuring.

Converting adaptive cognitions into hypnotic and self-hypnotic suggestions is also useful as a means of countering rationalization. Smokers trying to quit the habit, for example, often relapse because they rationalize that they can have one cigarette without becoming addicted again. This is reinforced when they do not feel especially strong cravings following that one cigarette. But these lapses then occur with greater and greater frequency, until the person concludes that he or she has become a smoker again. The likelihood of relapse may be decreased by frequent forceful repetition of the following self-suggestion: "This is a rationalization! It is how I fooled myself into failing in the past. If I give in now, it will only be harder to resist the next time I'm tempted. This time I won't give in." The client is instructed to use this suggestion during self-hypnotic practice at home and also whenever a temptation to smoke is experienced. Once again, it is important that the client has accepted the validity of this conclusion before it is assigned for use as a self-hypnotic suggestion.

RESEARCH AND APPRAISAL

More than any other treatment, CBT is closely linked to empirical research. Many of the treatment techniques were derived from experimental research, and their efficacy has been tested in an exceptionally large number of therapy outcome studies. Similarly, the cognitive–behavioral approach to hypnosis is backed by an extensive body of research (e.g., Spanos & Chaves, 1989).

Kirsch, Montgomery, and Sapirstein (1995) located 18 published studies in which the effects of a cognitive–behavioral treatment were compared with the effects of the same treatment supplemented by hypnosis. In all but two of these studies, sufficient data were reported to calculate effect sizes. We analyzed these data by treating the groups receiving nonhypnotic treatment as control groups and those receiving hypnotic treatment as experimental groups. The difference between hypnotic and nonhypnotic treatment was statistically significant with a mean effect size of 0.87 standard deviations. An effect size of this magnitude indicates that the average client receiving cognitive–behavioral hypnotherapy is better off at the end of it than more than 80% of clients who receive the same treatment in a nonhypnotic context.

More recent studies have reinforced these meta-analytic findings. Alladin and Alibhai (2007) determined that clients who received hypnosis in addition to CBT for depression scored as much as 8% greater reductions over and above the standard CBT group on measures of anxiety, depression, and hopelessness. Bryant, Moulds, Nixon, Mastrodomenico, Felmingham, and Hopwood (2006) found that hypnosis plus CBT was better than standard CBT and supportive counseling for reexperiencing symptoms in acute stress disorder, but CBT and CBT plus hypnosis were comparable at 6 months and 3-year follow-ups, and they were both better than supportive counseling at all three assessments. The authors of the study suggested that the initial benefits of adding hypnosis to CBT might be retained if hypnosis were used in ways other than just imaginal exposure. In a third study, Schoenberger, Kirsch, Gearan, Montgomery, and Pastyrnak (1997) showed that cognitive–behavioral hypnotherapy was superior to standard CBT in treating subjective and behavioral symptoms of anxiety when people with public speaking anxiety gave an impromptu speech.

Despite the promise of hypnosis as an adjunctive method in cognitive–behavioral interventions, hypnosis is not for everyone. Some people are frightened by the loss of control that they mistakenly associate with hypnosis. Others think that hypnotizability is an indication of a weakness in will or that hypnotizable people are gullible. Such attitudes tend to result in poor responsiveness to hypnotic suggestions (Spanos, Brett, Menary, & Cross, 1987). It is also significant that a variety of evidence suggests that subjects who respond poorly to hypnotic suggestions are more likely to be deliberately uncooperative in situations defined as hypnosis (Jones & Flynn, 1989). For clients with negative attitudes toward hypnosis, therefore, the hypnotic context is likely to diminish rather than enhance the effectiveness of treatment. Consequently, a modest overall effect is the most that would be expected when participants are assigned to conditions randomly.

For these reasons, the size of the effect in the Kirsch et al. (1995) study is surprising. It is about the same magnitude as the effect size for psychotherapy in general compared with no treatment at all (Smith et al., 1980). An effect of this magnitude might be expected if clients were selected for inclusion in studies only if they preferred hypnotherapy. However, this does not seem to be the case in most of the studies we found (for a notable exception, see Lazarus, 1973). Perhaps the settings in which some of these studies were conducted attracted individuals who were particularly interested in hypnotherapy. Alternatively, it is possible that hypnosis is currently viewed in a sufficiently positive light as to generate these results among a representative selection of clients. In any case, these data and the more recent studies we cited indicate that the question of whether hypnosis enhances treatment effects deserves far more attention among cognitive–behavioral researchers than it has been given to date.

CONCLUSION

Cognitive–behavioral hypnotherapy is the addition of hypnosis to the treatment procedures currently used by cognitive–behavioral therapists. These procedures have demonstrated effectiveness for a wide variety of dysfunctions, and meta-analyses indicate that they are significantly more effective than other psychotherapeutic methods. Though relatively sparse, research on the addition of hypnosis to these procedures indicates that the hypnotic context can enhance the efficacy of cognitive–behavioral therapy, especially for clients who are positively disposed to hypnosis.

Because hypnotic inductions and suggestions are similar to standard cognitive–behavioral procedures, a competent cognitive–behavioral therapist needs little additional training to incorporate hypnosis into treatment. In fact, cognitive–behavioral relaxation and imagery procedures can be thought of as hypnotic inductions and suggestions without the *hypnosis* label. Thus, for the cognitive behavior therapist, *hypnosis* is a merely a new label for what is already being practiced. But it is a label that can potentiate treatment for many clients. Unlike a rose, a therapy by a different name might not be experienced as the same.

REFERENCES

Alladin, A., & Alibhai, A. (2007). Cognitive hypnotherapy for depression: An empirical investigation. *International Journal of Clinical and Experimental Hypnosis*, 55, 147–166.

Baker, S. L., & Kirsch, I. (1993). Hypnotic and placebo analgesia: Order effects and the placebo label. *Contemporary Hypnosis*, 10, 117–126.

Bandura, A. (1969). *Principles of behavior modification*. New York: Holt, Rinehart and Winston.

Barber, T. X. (1969). *Hypnosis: A scientific approach*. New York: Van Nostrand Reinhold.

Barber, T. X. (1985). Hypnosuggestive procedures as catalysts for psychotherapies. In S. J. Lynn & J. P. Garske (Eds.), *Contemporary psychotherapies: Models and methods* (pp. 333–375). Columbus, OH: Merrill.

Barber, T. X., & Glass, L. B. (1962). Significant factors in hypnotic behavior. *Journal of Abnormal and Social Psychology, 64*, 222–228.

Barber, T. X., Spanos, N. P., & Chaves, J. F. (1974). *Hypnosis, imagination, and human potentialities*. New York: Pergamon Press.

Beck, A. T. (1976). *Cognitive therapy and the emotional disorders*. New York: International Universities Press.

Beck, A. T., Rush, A. J., Shaw, B. F., & Emery, G. (1979). *Cognitive therapy of depression*. New York: Guilford Press.

Benson, H., & Klipper, M. Z. (1976). *The relaxation response*. London: Collins.

Bolles, R. C. (1972). Reinforcement, expectancy, and learning. *Psychological Review, 79*, 394–409.

Bowers, K. S. (1976). *Hypnosis for the seriously curious*, Monterey, C A: Brooks/Cole.

Braffman, W., & Kirsch, I. (1999). Imaginative suggestibility and hypnotizability: An empirical analysis. *Journal of Personality and Social Psychology, 77*, 578–587.

Brown, R. J., Antonova, E., Langley, A., & Oakley, D. A. (2001). The effects of absorption and reduced critical thought on suggestibility in a hypnotic context. *Contemporary Hypnosis, 18*, 62–72.

Bryant, R. A., Moulds, M. L., Nixon, R. D., Mastrodomenico, J., Felmingham, K., & Hopwood, S. (2006). Hypnotherapy and cognitive behavior therapy of acute stress disorder: A 3-year follow-up. *Behavioral and Research Therapy, 44*, 1331–1335.

Coe, W. C., & Sarbin, T. R. (1966). An experimental demonstration of hypnosis as role enactment. *Journal of Abnormal Psychology, 71*, 400–416.

David, D. (1998). Hypnosis and operational readiness theory. *Studia Universitatis, 1–2*, 91–111.

David, D., Macavei, A., Szentagotai, A., & McMahon, J. (2005). Cognitive restructuring and mental contamination: An empirical re-conceptualisation. *Journal of Rational–Emotive & Cognitive–Behavior Therapy, 23*, 21–55.

David, D., Opre, A., & Miclea, M. (2004). The information processing approach to the human mind: Basic and beyond. *Journal of Clinical Psychology, 60*, 353–368.

Devine, D. A., & Fernald, P. S. (1973). Outcome effects of receiving a preferred, randomly assigned or nonpreferred therapy. *Journal of Consulting and Clinical Psychology, 41*, 104–107.

Ellis, A. (1962). *Reason and emotion in psychotherapy*. Secaucus, NJ: Lyle Stuart.

Ellis, A. (1995). *Better, deeper, and more enduring brief therapy: The rational emotive behavior therapy approach*. New York: Brummer/Mazel.

Ellis, A., & Grieger, R. (Eds.). (1977). *Handbook of rational–emotive therapy*. New York: Springer.

Eysenck, H. J. (Ed.). (1960). *Behavior therapy and the neuroses*. New York: Pergamon Press.

Hilgard, E. R. (1986). *Divided consciousness: Multiple controls in human thought and action* (Rev. ed.). New York: Wiley.

Jacobson, E. (1929). *Progressive relaxation*. Chicago: University of Chicago Press.

Johnsson, H. M. (1994). Processes of successful intentional forgetting. *Psychological Bulletin, 116*, 274–292.

Jones, W. J., & Flynn, D. M. (1989). Methodological and theoretical considerations in the study of "hypnotic" effects in perception. In N. P. Spanos & J. F. Chaves (Eds.), *Hypnosis: The cognitive–behavioral perspective* (pp. 149–174). Buffalo, NY: Prometheus Books.

Kanfer, F. H., & Grimm, L. G. (1978). Freedom of choice and behavioral change. *Journal of Consulting and Clinical Psychology, 46*, 873–878.

Katz, N. (1979). Comparative efficacy of behavioral training, training plus relaxation, and a sleep/trance induction in increasing hypnotic susceptibility. *Journal of Consulting and Clinical Psychology, 47*, 119–127.

Kihlstrom, J. F. (1997). Convergence in understanding hypnosis? Perhaps, but not so fast. *International Journal of Clinical and Experimental Hypnosis, 45*, 324–332.

Kirsch, I. (1990). *Changing expectations: A key to effective psychotherapy*. Pacific Grove, CA: Brooks/Cole.

Kirsch, I. (1999). Clinical hypnosis as a nondeceptive placebo. In I. Kirsch, A. Capafons, E. Cardeña-Buela, & S. Amigó (Eds.), *Clinical hypnosis and self-regulation* (pp. 211–225). Washington, DC: American Psychological Association.

Kirsch, I., & Lynn, S. J. (1995). Altered state of hypnosis: Changes in the theoretical landscape. *American Psychologist, 50*, 846–858.

Kirsch, I., & Lynn, S. J. (1999). Hypnotic involuntariness and the automaticity of everyday life. In I. Kirsch, A. Capafons, E. Cardeña-Buelna, & S. Amigó (Eds.), *Clinical hypnosis and self-regulation: Cognitive–behavioral perspectives* (pp. 49–72). Washington, DC: American Psychological Association.

Kirsch, I., Lynn, S. J., Vigorito, M., & Miller, R. R. (2004). The role of cognition in classical and operant conditioning. *Journal of Clinical Psychology, 60*, 369–392.

Kirsch, I., Mobayed, C. P., Council, J. R., & Kenny, D. A. (1992). Expert judgments of hypnosis from subjective state reports. *Journal of Abnormal Psychology, 101*, 657–662.

Kirsch, I., Montgomery, G., & Sapirstein, G. (1995). Hypnosis as an adjunct to cognitive behavioral psychotherapy: A meta-analysis. *Journal of Consulting and Clinical Psychology, 63*, 214–220.

Kirsch, I., Silva, C. E., Carone, J. E., Johnston, J. D., & Simon, B. (1989). The surreptitious observation design: An experimental paradigm for distinguishing artifact from essence in hypnosis. *Journal of Abnormal Psychology, 98*, 132–136.

Lazarus, A. A. (1971). *Behavior therapy and beyond*. New York: McGraw-Hill.

Lazarus, A. A. (1973). "Hypnosis" as a facilitator in behavior therapy. *International Journal of Clinical and Experimental Hypnosis, 21*, 25–31.

Lovaas, O. I. (1969). *Behavior modification: Teaching language to psychotic children* [Motion picture]. New York: Appleton-Century-Crofts.

Lynn, S. J. (1994). The interface of hypnosis research and clinical practice. *American Journal of Clinical Hypnosis, 37*, 81–83.

Lynn, S. J., Kirsch, I., Knox, J., & Lilienfeld, S. (2006). Hypnosis and neuroscience: Implications for the altered state debate. In G. Jamieson (Ed.), *Hypnosis and conscious states: The cognitive–neuroscience perspective*. New York: Oxford University Press.

Lynn, S. J., Neufeld, V., & Matyi, C. L. (1987). Inductions versus suggestions: Effects of direct and indirect wording on hypnotic responding and experience. *Journal of Abnormal Psychology, 96*, 76–79.

Lynn, S. J., & Rhue, J. W. (1991). An integrative model of hypnosis. In S. J. Lynn, & J. W. Rhue (Eds.), *Theories of hypnosis: Current models and perspectives* (pp. 397–438). New York: Guilford Press.

Lynn, S. J., Rhue, J., & Weekes, J. R. (l990). Hypnotic involuntariness: A social cognitive analysis. *Psychological Review, 97*, 169–184.

Mathews, W. J., Kirsch, I., & Mosher, D. (1985). The "double" hypnotic induction: An initial empirical test. *Journal of Abnormal Psychology, 94*, 92–95.

McConkey, K. M. (1986). Opinions about hypnosis and self-hypnosis before and after hypnotic testing. *International Journal of Clinical and Experimental Hypnosis, 34*, 311–319.

Mackay, C. (1869). *Memoirs of extraordinary popular delusions and the madness of crowds*. London: Routledge.

Meichenbaum, D. (1974). *Cognitive behavior modification*. Morristown, NJ: General Learning Press.

Montgomery, G. M., David, D., DiLorenzo, T. A., & Schnur, J. B. (2007). Response expectancies and irrational beliefs predict exam-related distress. *Journal of Rational–Emotive & Cognitive–Behavior Therapy, 25*, 17–32.

Orne, M. T. (1959). The nature of hypnosis: Artifact and essence. *Journal of Abnormal Psychology, 58*, 277–299.

Orne, M. T. (1962). On the social psychology of the psychological experiment: With particular reference to demand characteristics and their implications. *American Psychologist, 17*, 776–783.

Orne, M. T. (1970). Hypnosis, motivation, and the ecological validity of the psychological experiment. In W. J. Arnold & M. M. Page (Eds.), *Nebraska Symposium on Motivation*, 187–265. Lincoln, NB: Nebraska Press.

Perugini, E. M., Kirsch, I., Allen, S. T., Coldwell, E., Meredith, J., Montgomery, G. H., & Sheehan, J. (1998). Surreptitious observation of responses to hypnotically suggested hallucinations: A test of the compliance hypothesis. *International Journal of Clinical and Experimental Hypnosis, 46*, 191–203.

Rescorla, R. A. (1988). Pavlovian conditioning: It's not what you think it is. *American Psychologist, 43*, 151–160.

Rescorla, A. (1991). Associative relations in instrumental learning: The eighteenth Bartlett Memorial Lecture. *Quarterly Journal of Experimental Psychology, 43B*, 1–23.

Sarbin, T. R. (1950). Contributions to role theory: 1. Hypnotic behavior. *Psychological Review, 57,* 255–270.

Sarbin, T. R., & Coe, W. C. (1972). *Hypnosis: A social psychological analysis of influence communication.* New York: Holt, Rinehart & Winston.

Schoenberger, N. E., Kirsch, I., Gearan, P., Montgomery, G., & Pastyrnask, S. L. (1997). Hypnotic enhancement of cognitive behavioral treatment for public speaking anxiety. *Behavior Therapy, 28,* 127–140.

Smith, M. L., Glass, G. V., & Miller, T. I. (1980). *The benefits of psychotherapy.* Baltimore, MD: John Hopkins University Press.

Spanos, N. P. (1982). A social psychological approach to hypnotic behavior. In G. Weary & H. L. Mirels (Eds.), *Integrations of clinical and social psychology* (pp. 231–271). Oxford, England: Oxford University Press.

Spanos, N. P. (1986). Hypnotic behavior: A social psychological interpretation of amnesia, analgesia, and 'trance logic.' *The Behavioral and Brain Sciences, 9,* 449–502.

Spanos, N. P. (1991). A sociocognitive approach to hypnosis. In S. J. Lynn & J. W. Rhue (Eds.), *Theories of hypnosis: Current models and perspectives* (pp. 324–363). New York: Guilford Press.

Spanos, N. P. (1992). Compliance and reinterpretation in hypnotic responding, *Contemporary Hypnosis, 9,* 7–14.

Spanos, N. P., Brett, P. J., Menary, E. P., & Cross, W. P. (1987). A measure of attitudes toward hypnosis: Relationships with absorption and hypnotic susceptibility. *American Journal of Clinical Hypnosis, 30,* 139–150.

Spanos, N. P., & Chaves J. F. (Eds.). (1989). *Hypnosis: The cognitive–behavioral perspective.* Buffalo, NY: Prometheus Books.

Spanos, N. P., Cobb, P. C., & Gorassini, D. R. (1985). Failing to resist test suggestions: A strategy for self-presenting as deeply hypnotized. *Psychiatry, 48,* 282–292.

Vickery, A. R., Kirsch, I., Council, J. R., & Sirkin, M. I. (1985). Cognitive skill and traditional trance hypnotic inductions: A within-subject comparison. *Journal of Consulting and Clinical Psychology, 53,* 131–133.

Wadden T. A., & Anderton, C. H. (1982). The clinical use of hypnosis. *Psychological Bulletin, 91,* 215–243.

Wagstaff, G. F. (1981). *Hypnosis compliance and belief.* New York: St Martin's Press.

Wagstaff, G. F. (1986). Hypnosis as compliance and belief: A sociocognitive view. In P. L. N. Naish (Ed.), *What is hypnosis?* (pp. 59–84). Philadelphia: Open University Press.

Wagstaff, G. F. (1991). Compliance, belief, and semantics in hypnosis: A nonstate sociocognitive perspective. In S. J. Lynn & J. W. Rhue (Eds.), *Theories of hypnosis* (pp. 362–396). New York: Guilford Press.

Wagstaff, G. F. (1998). The semantics and physiology of hypnosis as an altered state: Towards a definition of hypnosis. *Contemporary Hypnosis, 15,* 149–165.

Wagstaff, G. F. (2004). High hypnotizability in a sociocognitive framework. In M. Heap, D. Oakley, & R. Brown (Eds.), *The highly hypnotisable person* (pp. 85–114). London: Brunner-Routledge.

White, R. W. (1941). A preface to a theory of hypnotism. *Journal of Abnormal Psychology, 36,* 477–505.

Wilson, T. T., & Brekke, N. (1994). Mental contamination and mental correction: Unwanted influences on judgments and evaluations. *Psychological Bulletin, 116,* 117–142.

Wolpe, J. (1958). *Psychotherapy by reciprocal inhibition.* Stanford, CA: Stanford University Press.

Wolpe, J., & Lazarus, A. A. (1966). *Behavior therapy techniques.* Oxford, England: Pergamon Press.

8

AN ERICKSONIAN MODEL OF CLINICAL HYPNOSIS

STEPHEN R. LANKTON AND WILLIAM J. MATTHEWS

Milton Erickson (1901–1980) was generally acknowledged to be the world's leading practitioner of medical hypnosis. He had a life-long dedication to exploring hypnotic phenomena and published more than 100 articles on a variety of subjects related to his interest during his professional life. Erickson was an innovator in his approach to therapeutic change in that he often used hypnosis to help bring about change in his clients. He thought of therapy as a way of helping people to extend beyond their self-perceived limits. Although such a perspective seems reasonable to therapists today, this notion was at odds with traditional psychiatry during much of Erickson's professional life. Before presenting an Ericksonian approach to hypnosis followed by a case example, we discuss the philosophical underpinnings of Erickson's work, which can provide an important context in which to understand his interventions.

In this chapter, we first examine the philosophical basis of Erickson's technique and approach to hypnosis. Next, we discuss clinical applications of the approach through an extended case example and through a discussion of the various ways in which Erickson has been interpreted in clinical settings. Finally,

---

All clinical material has been disguised to protect patient confidentiality.

we examine recent research into the efficacy and implications of Ericksonian hypnotherapy.

RATIONALE, PHILOSOPHY, AND APPROACH

According to Rossi (Erickson & Rossi, 1980a), the limitations of most schools of psychotherapy arise from three general assumptions:

1. Therapy based on observable behavior and related to the present and future circumstances of the client is often viewed as superficial and lacking depth compared with therapies that seek to restructure clients' understanding of the distant past,
2. The same approach to therapy (e.g., classical analysis, gestalt therapy, transactional analysis, nondirective therapy) is appropriate for all clients in all circumstances. This assumption denies the context of the problem, the unique learning, experiences, and resources of clients, and the type of symptoms presented.
3. Effective therapy occurs through an interpretation and explanation of a client's inner life in accordance with the assumptions of the given theory. Change, from this perspective, occurs mainly through insight by a client into his or her behavior.

Rossi (Erickson & Rossi, 1980a), in his introduction to Erickson's approach, indicated that the elaborate and involved theoretical interpretations of human behavior, in conjunction with rigid therapeutic procedures, have made the process of psychotherapy longer and more expensive than it needs to be, making it unavailable to many people. Most therapies require, at least indirectly, that clients adapt to the therapist's worldview even when it may not be in their best interests to do so. From early in his life, Erickson began to challenge traditional notions and expectations, and the limitations they placed on him, and this attitude was also reflected in his approach to therapy.

Focusing on history to the exclusion of the client's daily life contradicts basic experience. Events in daily life can have a profound influence in the development of character or personality. These events can occur completely out of the immediate situation and dramatically affect the client's present and future. As Rossi (Erickson & Rossi, 1980a) correctly pointed out, these events do not need to be considered extensions of earlier unresolved infantile traumata to be understood.

Although people have memories, perceptions, and feelings regarding their past, current realities impinge on them and affect their daily and future interactions in the world. Preoccupation with the past and a disregard of present and future needs unnecessarily prolong and complicate the process of therapy.

Certainly one hallmark of an Ericksonian approach is an emphasis on current interpersonal relationships and their influence on the development and resolution of problems. Although an individual might have developed a symptomatic behavior in the distant past, the Ericksonian view focuses on how the problem is maintained in the present. Thus, in this approach, the unique interpersonal interactions in the client's daily life are more important than relying on the application of a rigid theory and set of techniques. Ericksonian therapy is based on identifying client strengths and increasing the possibility of new learning and experiences that can be used in resolving a given problem in the client's present life. In addition, this work focuses on orienting a given solution toward future developmental changes.

Ericksonian Approaches to Hypnosis

Hypnosis means sleep in Greek, and many practitioners of clinical hypnosis at one time or another have probably used the expressions "going to sleep" or "waking up" when doing hypnosis. However, the act of sleeping seems to have little connection to the process of hypnosis. As Araoz (1982) indicated, hypnosis is a construct that can mean a special state of mental functioning, the technique to create that state, the experience of oneself in that special state of mental functioning, or all of these.

Many in the scientific community view hypnosis as a particular state of consciousness (Bowers, 1966; M. Gill & Brenman, 1959; Hilgard, 1966; Orne, 1959) that can be experienced only by those with the personality trait of *hypnotizability* (Hilgard, 1965, 1975; Hilgard, Weitzenhoffer, Landes, & Moore, 1961). Hypnotizability as a trait has often been measured by classical scales of hypnotizability (Shor & Orne, 1962; Weitzenhoffer & Hilgard, 1959, 1962). The trance state is assumed to exist because of the behaviors manifested by hypnotized people. Because these behaviors do not usually occur in the normal waking state, it is assumed that inducing hypnotizable people puts them in this special state of mental functioning. This model is an approach common to most psychological research (i.e., the influence of the independent variable, *hypnotic induction*, on the dependent variable, *hypnotic behaviors*; Araoz, 1982). The approach of using the independent variable of hypnotic induction on the dependent variable of hypnotic behaviors is common to most psychological research (Araoz, 1982).

Ericksonian approaches to hypnosis emphasize the intervening variables of the inner processes of the individual. It is these mediational variables of both the conscious and unconscious mind (i.e., that which is outside of conscious awareness) that allow the individual to experience hypnosis. In the traditional approach, it is accepted that hypnosis will not occur with uncooperative individuals. Embedded in this position is the notion that hypnosis can occur when the person allows it to occur. The notions of trait and hypnotizability (i.e., constructs viewed as being in the individual) become significantly less relevant when the hypnotist/client context is considered. The essence of the Ericksonian approach is creating a context that will allow hypnosis to occur.

Hallmarks of the Ericksonian Approach

Rossi (Erickson & Rossi, 1980a) among others (S. Lankton, 2004; S. Lankton & Lankton, 1983, 1986; Matthews, 1985a, 1985b; O'Hanlon, 1987; Zeig, 1980, 1982), has identified four basic principles of Erickson's work. Rossi (Erickson & Rossi, 1980a) has indicated that these principles represent a paradigmatic shift to an entirely different way of using hypnosis in therapy. These principles are as follows:

1. The unconscious need not be made conscious. Unconscious processes can be facilitated such that they can remain outside of conscious awareness and be used for problem solving. For Erickson, the unconscious was considered to be a complex set of associations that covered a broad range of human experience. It is the unconscious patterns of the individual that regulate, control, and guide the moment-to-moment conduct of an individual. These patterns are resources that can be used in clinical hypnosis to create different perceptions, experiences, and behaviors by the individual. For Erickson, the unconscious was a repository of positive resources and skills that could be used for positive therapeutic change. This conscious/unconscious splitting or differentiation provides for the possibility of multiple levels of communication between the hypnotherapist and client. S. Lankton and Lankton (1983) stated that everything done by, to, or for the body at an unconscious level is done either for maintaining health, prohibiting it, or promoting it (p. 9). Thus, it is at the unconscious level that stories, double binds, and paradoxes are directed. Rossi (Erickson & Rossi, 1979) observed that "if we translate the terms 'conscious' and 'unconscious' into 'dominant' and 'nondominant' hemispheres, we may have the neuropsychological basis for describing a new hypnotherapeutic approach" (p. 247).

2. Mental mechanisms and personality characteristics need not be analyzed for the client. They can be used as processes for facilitating therapeutic goals. One of Erickson's major contributions to the process of clinical hypnosis specifically, and to therapy in general, is the notion of utilizing the client's ongoing behavior,

perceptions, and attitudes for therapeutic change. Clients are not asked to conform to the therapist's mode of interaction; rather, their behavior is accepted and used in the treatment process. Haley (1967) cited a dramatic example of use in the client who could not stop pacing in Erickson's office. Rather than trying to force the man to sit in the chair and relax in order to begin (which might have resulted in an escalation of wills between Erickson and the client and perhaps a termination of therapy), Erickson asked the individual if he were willing to cooperate by continuing to pace the floor. The man replied that he must continue to pace the floor to remain in the office.

In accepting this behavior, Erickson then made fairly direct and simple suggestions that coincided with the man's pacing. Over a period of time, suggestions of relaxation and the desire to eventually sit in a particular chair were embedded in Erickson's offerings. Erickson offered suggestions in such a manner that anything the client did was construed as a positive response. Over a period of time, the client was able to sit in the chair and develop a therapeutic trance. Thus, behaviors that might have been viewed as antithetical to therapeutic success were considered to be a part of the process of therapy and were used to increase the expectation for a positive therapeutic outcome by both therapist and client.

3. Suggestions need not be direct. Indirect suggestion permits (a) the subject's individuality, previous life experience, and unique potentials to become manifest; (b) the classical psychodynamics of learning with processes such as association, contiguity, similarity, and contrast to be involved on a more or less unconscious level so that (c) the client's conscious limitations and criticism can be bypassed and therefore increase therapeutic effectiveness (Erickson & Rossi, 1980b, p. 455).

Direct suggestion occurs when the hypnotherapist makes a clear, direct request for a certain response. With *indirect suggestion,* the relation between the hypnotherapist's request and the client's response is less clear. For example, using direct suggestion in trance induction, the therapist may say to the client, "Close your eyes and become more and more relaxed." In using a more indirect approach, the same suggestion could be, "As you develop a level of comfort necessary for your own learning, perhaps you will notice your eyes closing, closing partway, or remaining as they are, as you go deeper into trance." Here, the client is given a wide range of options in developing a trance state that is unique to him or her.

Erickson's early approach reflected an authoritative manner characteristic of "one-up" or the dominant interpersonal style common to the medical profession at the time. He created that impression with frank nonverbal and verbal communication such as in the following statement: "I can *put you* [italics added] in any level of trance" (Haley, 1967, p. 64). However, in the latter part of his life, he used indirection more heavily. He observed that indirection allowed him to show respect for clients by not directly challenging them to do what their conscious minds, for whatever reason, might not wish to do. Indirection is the basis for the therapeutic use of metaphors, stories, paradox, binds, and so forth, because they allow clients to create meanings that are relevant for them and to explore their potential to facilitate new responses. Rather than telling a patient what to do, Erickson stated that he "offered" ideas and suggestions (Erickson & Rossi, 1981, pp. 1–2). Surprisingly, he even added, "I don't like this matter of telling a patient *I want you* [italics added] to get tired and sleepy" (p. 4). In other words, with regard to his use of suggestion, there is clear evidence that he evolved his practice to a point by the late 1970s where he had all but abandoned his earlier techniques of direct suggestion, redundancy, and authoritarianism during induction and replaced these with forms of indirection and permissive suggestions.

4. Hypnotic suggestion is not a process of programming the client with the therapist's point of view but an interactive process for creating new meanings, attitudes, or beliefs that can lead to different perceptions, feelings, and behaviors. Erickson (Erickson & Rossi, 1980a) was clear that in all of his years of clinical experience he never found any validity to claims of miraculous healing by any unusual power arising out of hypnosis. He simply maintained that people have more potential and resources than they realize. The value of hypnosis lies in its ability to evoke and use the client's vast storehouse of hidden potential. The evocation and use of the client's potential is a process unique to the individual that seems less likely to occur with a purely direct, rigid, or programmed approach.

Length of Typical Treatment

At the beginning of his career, Erickson worked in a psychiatric hospital. Patients receiving care in such facilities were often considered long-term patients. Even after Erickson began his private practice, he was willing to engage in therapeutic journeys with his clients that might have lasted several years. Published descriptions of his therapy show that during the early 1950s, cases treated by Erickson took several months or years. Although Erickson often made himself available to clients for an indefinite period of time, while practicing in Phoenix, his published cases gradually illustrate that the duration of his treatment became shorter For instance, the 1973 case of the 8-year-old "stomper" took just 2 hours (Haley, 1973). Various cases of his "shock" technique conducted in 1973 entailed 1- to 2-hour-long sessions (Erickson & Rossi, 1980a, p. 447). Overall, the movement to brief therapy is evident in his work as it progressed and became prominent in his later practice.

Use of Metaphor

Erickson's first published account of using a story in therapy was published with reluctance in 1944 and pertained to a case he conducted in 1935. He titled it "The Method Employed to Formulate a Complex Story for the Induction of the Experimental Neurosis" (Erickson, 1980d, pp. 336–355). He understood at that point that a complex story that paralleled a client's problem could actually heighten discomfort and bring the neurosis closer to the surface where it could be better recognized, understood, and treated. Some 2 decades after the first use of metaphor, in 1954, Erickson was regularly using many "fabricated case histories" of fleeting symptomatology (Erickson, 1980e, p. 152). The purpose of telling a metaphor, or any intervention other that reasoning with a client, is to shift and enrich perception, cognition, and imagination and to retrieve needed experience. Erickson reported finding that these outcomes were best achieved when the metaphors paralleled the clients experience or were relevant to the listener; this was sometimes even achieved by melding the case stories of different clients.

Yet another 2 decades later, in 1973, Erickson provided several examples of case stories for making a therapeutic point (Haley, 1973). Finally, in 1979, Erickson assigned the term *metaphor* to represent a special class of interventions (Erickson & Rossi, 1979). As mentioned earlier, this corresponds to his movement from direct and authoritarian therapy to indirect and permissive therapy.

Erickson took a traditional analytic view of neurosis and various symptoms during his earliest years as a psychiatrist and at least up to the mid 1950s. He stated that the development of neurotic symptoms "constitutes behavior of a defensive, protective character" (Erickson, 1980e, p. 149). Such a statement could not be more psychoanalytic. However, he continued to evolve his clinical understanding such that his view in the mid 1960s had become interactional. Perhaps this was a result of his collaboration with Jay Haley, Gregory Bateson, John Weakland and the Palo Alto Communication Project, and the general rise in interactional therapies sparked by the work of Kurt Lewin, Eric Berne, and others. In any case, Erickson wrote in 1966, "Mental disease is the breaking down of communication between people" (Erickson, 1980b, p. 75). Once again, we find that by the end of his career he had moved even further from the original psychoanalytic and adopted the communication or systems theory of disease. He stated, "Symptoms are forms of communication," and added that they are "signs or cues of developmental problems that are in the process of becoming conscious" (Erickson & Rossi, 1979, p. 143). His evolution of thought about problems or symptoms became less and less oriented toward a pathological model until, in the end, they could be seen as communications that signaled a client's desired direction of growth. Erickson took such signals to be a request for change, and even unconscious contracts for therapeutic engagement.

Erickson stated as early as 1948 that a patient's cure was not the result of a response to suggestion but rather was from the reassociation of experiences. Erickson wrote, "It is this experience of reassociating and reorganizing [the patient's] own experiential life that eventuates in a cure" (Erickson, 1980c, p. 38). We find this theme repeated time and again in the later years of his career (Erickson & Rossi, 1979; 1980b, p. 464; 1981).

Therapeutic Trance

Within the Ericksonian framework, hypnotic trance provides a time when the client's conscious limitations are at least partially suspended so that the individual can be receptive to alternative associations and ways of mental functioning that are supportive of problem solving. Rossi (Erickson & Rossi, 1979) conceptualized the dynamics of trance into a five-stage process. Stage 1 is the fixation of attention, in which the client's beliefs and behaviors focus on inner realities. Stage 2 uses distraction, surprise, shock, metaphor, and confusion. This disrupts the client's typical conscious functioning and thus appends the client's typical frames of reference and belief systems with ideas not previously present. This then creates the possibility for Stage 3, an unconscious search for new meanings or experiences that may lead to problem resolution. This unconscious search leads to, and overlaps with, Stage 4, an unconscious process that is the activation of personal associations and mechanisms whereby a reorganization of one's experience can take place. Finally, Stage 5 is the hypnotic behavior in which the individual often reports or exhibits a behavior as seemingly being independent of his or her typical conscious control. The so-called *Eureka!* experience is a naturalistic example of an unconscious search and process that often occurs without formal trance induction. Hand levitation as the result of hypnotic induction is a more typical example of an unconscious search and process leading to a behavior that the client often reports as spontaneous.

In the section that follows we present a conceptual model of assessment and intervention in conjunction with a case study. One should note that there is no definitive Ericksonian method or approach. The following material was developed from Erickson's work on the basis of the interpretation of C. Lankton and Lankton (1989); S. Lankton and Lankton (1983, 1986); S. Lankton, Lankton, and Matthews (1991); Matthews (1985a, 1985b), and Matthews and Dardeck (1985).

CLINICAL MATERIAL

The following case material is from a treatment demonstration conducted by Stephen Lankton (1989) in December 1988. The actual client is referred to as "Linda," and the only modifications made to the transcript are those that conceal her identity, employment, and geographical location. Linda had a history of physical and sexual abuse in her home. She was unmarried and living alone at the time of the therapy. Her presenting complaint was that she avoided others because of self-imposed criticisms and thoughts that she was not acceptable to others. Linda specifically requested therapy to help her accept compliments. The partial transcript of portions of the treatment (conducted by Lankton) is followed by commentaries (by Matthews).[1]

> *Lankton:* Would you be willing to tell us your age?

A simple question, but in asking it, Lankton implied that Linda had control of the information she decided to share and what she had the right to withhold. Linda then explained that she engaged in a lot of negative and self-deprecating thoughts that she wanted to stop.

> *Lankton:* I would like to change it, if it were me. I'm not quite sure what your motivation is for changing it. Why do you want to? Woody Allen does fine with it.
>
> *Linda:* It is really unhelpful for me!
>
> *Lankton:* But what is your motivation for getting rid of this self-effacement? How do you imagine your life would be improved somehow if you did?
>
> *Linda:* I wouldn't be, um, I would be able to be less afraid about being in groups and more able to receive credit when people try to give it to me. I would be able to teach easier without it being traumatic. I mean those are the things that I am doing.

---

[1]The dialogue is from "Motivating action with hypnotherapy for a client with a history of early family violence," by S. Lankton, 1989, *Ericksonian Monographs*, 6, pp. 43–56. Copyright 1989 by The Milton H. Erickson Foundation (http://www.erickson-foundation.org). Adapted with permission.

In this exchange, Lankton sought to determine (a) the context and logic of this behavior in her life, (b) what behaviors would indicate positive identifiable change, and (c) what the cost of change would be. Perhaps in changing the self-effacing behavior, Linda would be unhappier if, for example, by being more self-assured, Linda were challenging a family rule of communication or some notion of how one is supposed to act in interpersonal relationships.

> *Lankton:* We remember the past for the ways we are doing this stuff, or we credit the past for the ways we are doing it. What do you blame or credit for how come you are self-effacing? In some ways I reckon it's a real strength that helped: kept you somehow from getting more punishment that you expect you might have gotten. And by keeping yourself self-critical, you've anticipated punishment and maybe removed some of the actual punishment that you would have gotten; so in a way it's been real handy, and it's sort of survival strength. But why did you do it in the first place?

Lankton offered the possibility of reframing a perceived limitation (self-effacing behavior) as a strength. In doing so, the meaning of this behavior for Linda could have dramatically changed. Linda responded to Lankton's last question with uncertainty as to why she learned this behavior. Lankton reiterated that, given the unpleasantness of her home life, rather than being self-critical, she could have said to herself, "I survived another day!" (which is also an indirect suggestion for future positive self-talk). Following this suggestion, Lankton introduced the idea of hypnosis.

> *Lankton:* We might/could talk for 2 hours and really get something accomplished that would be useful just by talking. I wonder what we could accomplish that would be useful in trance. That's what I would like to attempt to do. And I know you will seek further help and so on afterward to the extent you need it, and you are capable of doing that.

This brief introduction is a good example of the use of indirect suggestion. Lankton said much could be accomplished in just talking, but his wondering about what would be accomplished in trance is an indirect suggestion to Linda to experience trance to find out. He also reminded her that she could seek additional therapy after this demonstration if it was in her best interest.

> *Lankton:* You go into trance in your own way, of course, and in your own time into the depth that is appropriate for you. And although you may have your eyes open in trance, you may begin by closing them. Sooner or later, the sense of concentrating your attention and becoming comfortable, by letting your conscious mind focus "in" on certain thoughts that are least distressing for you so that your unconscious can have some

freedom to play with other thoughts, entertain other ideas, investigate experiences. You can lean back in the chair, all right? Or is that a problem? [*Linda leans back in the chair.*]

In this interaction, Lankton offered Linda a range of ideas and opportunities that would be valuable to her in developing her own trance experience. He suggested that although she could experience a trance with her eyes open, she could begin by closing them. The implication was that, with her eyes open or closed, she could experience a trance that would be useful for her. In his next offering to Linda, Lankton suggested that, although her conscious mind had the specific task of focusing on relaxing thoughts, her unconscious mind could begin to investigate new possibilities that, by definition, would be outside of her conscious awareness. He created with Linda the possibility for new ideas and associations to occur, although her conscious mind might have had doubts and concerns.

> Lankton: One of the things that I sometimes ask people to do in trance is to dissociate their experience in trance from everything else—to never have the generalization of the successful experience in the trance—not to anticipate having it, not to worry about having it. Just let the experience be all by itself, like standing on the observation deck of the Eiffel Tower. Thinking about all that history, and you're not part of it.

Linda's presenting issue was self-effacing behavior in which she examined her ongoing experience and criticized herself for not doing "better," regardless of what she was doing. To circumvent her critical conscious mind, Lankton suggested that this trance experience need not be generalizable. Instead, she could learn to dissociate from her experience and perhaps develop a different understanding. He then offered her a number of anecdotes of how one dissociates. Lankton suggested the importance of Linda learning to dissociate from her experience to develop a different perspective and then told a story demonstrating a natural, everyday dissociative experience he had. Although one cannot assume that Linda had exactly the same sort of experience Lankton described, we can assume that Linda derived some meaning related to comfort, relaxation, and dissociation. Her nonverbal behavior was consistent with a relaxed state. At the end of the story, Lankton stated that his role in the trance experience with Linda was to help stimulate conscious and unconscious thinking in ways that could be useful to her. Following the story, Lankton gave Linda feedback about her physical state that enhanced the trance experience (e.g., her cheek muscles were relaxed, rapid eye movement had decreased, swallow reflex had slowed, breathing was deeper and slower).

Lankton reiterated that this trance experience could be valuable in itself and did not have to be generalizable to her daily life. He then told another story about a woman with whom he worked who had chronic back pain that was significantly diminished in their trance work. Lankton suggested that the woman make sure that the pain came back after the trance and that this experience need not influence her daily life in any way unless she wanted it to. Lankton continued with the value of metaphor.

> *Lankton:* There's another problem in telling metaphors to people in trance, and that is: Who will the person identify with? I think it would be perfectly legitimate for you to identify with everybody I talk about in the metaphor. I might talk about my daughter and my conduct with my daughter. After all, you can't really understand the situation that occurs to people in the metaphor unless you have projected into it. I don't know if you have ever thought of holding yourself as a little girl. Everyone sooner or later has the idea. Maybe your conscious mind has had the experience a little bit and allowed your unconscious mind to flirt with the idea.

Lankton was then ready to help Linda recreate or invent some pleasant childhood experiences but, prior to doing so, he directly suggested to Linda the importance of identifying with all of the characters in his metaphors, specifically, having the feelings and experiences of a little girl. Lankton was fully aware that Linda's childhood experiences were not predominantly positive, so he told her that she could identify with his daughter and her experiences. This created the likelihood that she would have the positive experiences that Lankton soon detailed.

Lankton proceeded with a series of stories describing the tender relationship he had with his daughter and that his daughter had with her mother. In these stories he detailed the tender physical and emotional connection with his daughter. The intention was to have Linda identify with and have those tender feelings as she projected herself into the story Lankton told. To enhance this learning for Linda, Lankton offered a description of the physical feelings his daughter had during these tender interactions. However, rather than refer to his daughter by name or as "she," as one would typically do when speaking with a third person (i.e., Linda), he repeatedly used the pronoun "you," which may have confused Linda with regard to about whom he was talking (i.e., his daughter or Linda); this thereby became a suggestion for Linda to identify with the positive feelings being discussed.

> *Lankton:* And I wonder how it makes a child feel—where you'd feel it on your face. What would happen with regard to your heart rate, your breathing rate, your feelings of your musculature, your sense of self? You learn it; it becomes a part of

you. You bring it with you the next time you walk into the living room.

Lankton sought to have Linda's physiological experience in trance coincide with her psychological state, thus enhancing the positive connection between the two. He then continued with the importance of having feelings of mastery in one's life. He offered a series of anecdotes of how children achieve mastery by pretending.

> *Lankton:* And there is no harm in pretending; it is very good rehearsal to make space somewhere inside for that new feeling to develop.

In the midst of the anecdotes of how children pretend, Lankton offered a statement about the value and importance of pretending. Lankton then became more direct with Linda and suggested how she could use the experience she had in trance.

> *Lankton:* Then you can think about my daughter and you can have those experiences. What is memory anyway except imagination? So go into trance to a depth necessary to allow you to have the imagination of the memory. Feeling that degree of safety and comfort with the agreement that if you have it now, it's disconnected from everything. It's a trial period. It has no meaning. There is no threat it will generalize into the rest of your life. Just like an ant digging a little bitty tunnel down into the sand and making a great big hole in which he can live, or a little rabbit that makes a little burrow, down a little thin hole up to the earth. But inside the burrow who knows what the rabbit is doing? Maybe just storing jars of honey before Pooh Bear comes to visit.

Lankton, with references such as those to Pooh Bear, directed Linda to have a memory and imagine having feelings like his daughter had but without worrying about having to generalize those feelings to her everyday life. He probed for associations to a deeper sense of hope and childhood dreams. Like the rabbit in the burrow, one cannot know what positive experiences she has stored in her unconscious for use at a later time.

> *Lankton:* And let the feeling of safety be something that you feel more now than you ever felt before. Know what it's like for your little finger to feel it, for your ankle [to feel it]. Feel the skin temperatures change with it. And know that your conscious mind needn't even remember it but that you have made an agreement that you are going to the depth of the trance necessary to have the experience now more than you have ever had it. Let it radiate to the tips of your fingers. Let it radiate out your

fingers and toes. Ooze safety, security, belonging, in a way you most imagined that my daughter probably does. And then I want you to keep it constant for the next 5 minutes with the agreement that if there is any difficulty for you having that experience, you can be fully assured that you won't have it again after the trance is over. It's just a little experiment. Now memorize it and hold on to it. Does it feel good? [*Linda slightly nods her head and smiles.*]

Lankton continued to emphasize that this experience for Linda should be considered only as an experiment with no lasting effects; she had the control to make such a decision. In response to his question about whether the experience she was having felt good, she answered affirmatively. He then asked her to open her eyes while having these positive feelings and know that she was able to open her eyes while holding onto these feelings. Linda was able to do so. He then asked her to look at the group (i.e., the audience) while holding onto the positive feelings, and Linda was able to do this. To further stabilize her desirable state of consciousness, he checked whether she was able to project her current emotional state onto the audience and verified that she believed the audience to be accepting of her. After establishing that Linda could have her eyes open and look at the audience while holding onto these feelings, Lankton asked her to try to have self-effacing thoughts while she was holding onto the positive feelings. He exhorted her to try to have negative memories from her childhood while maintaining these positive feelings and images and looking at the audience. Lankton commented to the audience, and indirectly to Linda, that this is a form of reciprocal inhibition that floods a person's negative experience with positive feelings rather than the reverse.

> Lankton: Sometimes I work with people and I mention that they will do an experience in trance and they'll gain an idea that they just won't be able to shake when the trance is over. Something will seize their mind as a useful concept or an idea and it will stay with them.

Lankton offered, indirectly, the possibility that Linda may have wanted to keep the positive experience without challenging her with a direct posthypnotic suggestion that she would continue to have the experience. Thus, there was no chance of Linda failing, regardless of what she did. At this point, Lankton continued his challenge to Linda to try to have negative memories of experiences in the past that proved she was wrong and should be self-effacing.

> Lankton: So I would like you to try really hard to feel bad while you are holding this feeling and looking at the group that you become

aware that you failed at feeling bad. And maybe criticize yourself for that. [*Linda laughs.*]

To help reduce her performance anxiety, Lankton used a paradox with Linda
to challenge her to feel bad and, when she failed at this task, to criticize herself for failing at failing. Prescribing the symptom creates the possibility of
new meaning for the symptom (e.g., taking conscious control of what was
thought to be involuntary). While in the trance, Lankton asked Linda how
this experience worked. She was clear that this experience (i.e., to look at
others without thinking they are criticizing her) was new to her. She indicated that she felt relaxed and comfortable with this new learning. Lankton
then asked Linda, who continued in the trance, to close her eyes and appreciate what she had just done. He explicitly reminded her of her accomplishment and the fact that this experience could have many different meanings
for her. To illustrate his point metaphorically, he then told Linda a series of
short anecdotes about his own learning experiences as a child in which he
learned significant things, such as riding a bike and swimming, almost as if by
accident. He reminded her that there are many things that one does by accident that have important connections to the rest of one's life. This interaction was a direct attempt to strengthen the significant experience that Linda
had just had while in the trance and to create the possibility that she would
take the experience with her into her everyday life. Lankton then began a
5-minute metaphoric story about a fictitious youth who lived "before the age
of technology."

> Lankton: And he had lived kind of in isolation with a wall around him
> for a long time, in a city with a wall around it. It seemed per-
> fectly reasonable. It was all he knew. He had very few posses-
> sions, and he carried them with him most of the time: a key
> [that] didn't open any lock; a feather that he pretended was
> an eagle feather, which actually just came from a seagull that
> had gotten lost in the desert; a whistle that he hardly ever
> used because when he blew it, it didn't make any sound; and
> a crystal.
>
>   In the story, the young man then left his town to explore
> the desert, only to return to find that his beloved town was
> gone. Not knowing what to do, he went to see the region's
> magistrate, who listened to his story. The Magistrate said,
> "Well, it's always different in each case. And this one of
> course, is unique. But one thing that is certain to me is that
> sometimes it's a matter of trust and sometimes it's a matter of
> wit, and sometimes it's a matter of courage and sometimes it's
> a matter of the heart. And the tests that you have will be a
> test of your heart."

Clearly, the intention here was for Linda to identify with the protagonist of the story and to follow his quest with the parallels in her own life. Lankton took his protagonist through a series of trials for which he needed courage, heart, trust, and wit to overcome. In each of the trials, the protagonist used one of his possessions (i.e., the key, feather, whistle, crystal) to solve his dilemma. In doing so, however, he lost each possession. For instance, he found himself locked in a cage for which he used his key to free himself, but the key became lodged in the lock. In each trial, a different emotion and character trait were emphasized. However, the protagonist thought he was a failure and was certain that the magistrate would think the same. However, in the end, the magistrate reviewed each of the trials that the protagonist had to overcome.

> Lankton: The Magistrate congratulated him on a job well done. He passed the test. . . . The Magistrate said, "You have a heart filled with truth and you saw it. And you could have thought that the beast was evil and malicious, but to you it was humorous, and your heart passed the test of being a light heart. And you saw that the cage had come undone, and you could have thought that it was evil and malicious, but you decided it was an accident and proved you have the capricious and forgiving heart. And when the animals threatened you, you could have tried to be brave and pretend, but you have the trusting heart and you asked for help. . . . Go back to where you came from now, and you will find, I think, free of delusion, that the home you look for is there."

Remembering that the overall contract was to reduce her debilitating self-criticism, the story offered Linda a way to draw conclusions for herself about herself. A story of this structure invites the listener to reevaluate isolated experiences previously thought to be failures in light of a larger context of one's growth and life accomplishments. This act of maturing is one of the natural ways in which people learn to forgive themselves and perhaps others. Lankton then offered the idea of amnesia for what they had done in this session and reminded her that she did not need to change anything if she chose not to. Again, he attempted to relieve any pressure on Linda to have immediate success with this experience. He then returned to his initial story about the client with back pain. He reported that her pain had gone.

> Lankton: You can use those unconscious accidental experiences that occur to you, in your own unconscious way, at your own speed, and let your unconscious discover just how or if you'll use what you've done here today.

Within 4 months after this initial therapy session, Linda reported being surprised to find that she sought out and engaged in more social contact, including allowing others to touch her for the first time. It is interesting that the social contact increased even while Linda was receiving a great deal of criticism from a coworker who was in disagreement or in competition with her. She stated that she was more aware of incidents in her past and that she was not self-critical as a result of this increased awareness. She subsequently engaged in additional therapy to resolve important aspects of her past that she had refused to share with others before this session.

In this session, Lankton emphasized three different areas that focused on Linda's major presenting issues: (a) the method of dealing with social avoidance and posttraumatic stress in which a secure reality was created and Linda was given the opportunity to experience others as noncritical; (b) the repeated paradoxical restraint from change, to reduce Linda's anxiety and inhibit her self-critical faculties from undermining the potential of change; and (c) the emphasis in the final metaphor on reevaluating her life as that of a person with a "good heart." The implication in this metaphor was that perhaps Linda might begin to reevaluate her life and to appreciate her qualities and strengths.

These three aspects of Linda's treatment emphasize key elements of an Ericksonian approach, which are (a) a focus on the present and future with an opportunity to reexperience previously negative stimuli from a different perspective, (b) the therapeutic use of reframing in which any response the client makes can be considered to be positive and a part of the therapeutic process, and (c) the challenging and shifting of negative attitudes about the self that have created limitations in the client's worldview and subsequent experience.

RESEARCH AND APPRAISAL

Most of the Ericksonian interventions reported in the literature are either clinical case studies or anecdotes and not systematic investigations of clinical claims. Although clinical case studies are both fascinating and informative to practitioners, this method has well-known weaknesses in terms of making causal connections between treatment and outcome. The following is a brief overview of some of the research on Ericksonian techniques and principles.

Bandler and Grinder (1975) used two separate hypnotists speaking simultaneously to the participant and hypothesized that this induction procedure would be particularly effective. Matthews, Kirsch, and Mosher (1985), in comparing a standard induction (Stanford Hypnotic Susceptibility Scale, Form C; Weitzenhoffer & Hilgard, 1963) with a double hypnotic induction, found no significant differences between the two inductions in terms of depth of trance (i.e., as measured by behavioral responses to suggestion). In addition, they reported that the double hypnotic induction might have actually decreased hypnotic responsiveness.

An important element of the Ericksonian approach, both in the induction of trance and in treatment intervention is the use of indirect suggestion (Erickson & Rossi, 1979, 1980; Haley, 1973; S. Lankton & C. Lankton, 1983; Matthews, 1985b). *Indirect suggestions* are defined as suggestions that have a degree of ambiguity and allow for increased latitude in responding on the participant's part. By contrast, *direct suggestions* are clear requests for a particular response by the hypnotist to the participant. Alman and Carney (1980), using audiotaped inductions of direct and indirect suggestions, compared male and female participants on their responsiveness to posthypnotic suggestions. They reported that indirect suggestions were more successful in producing posthypnotic behavior than were direct suggestions.

McConkey (1984) used direct and indirect suggestions with real and simulating hypnotic subjects. He found that although all of the simulating subjects recognized the expectation for a positive hallucination, half of the real subjects responded to the indirect suggestions and half did not. Floda (2003) found no statistically significant relationships or differences between the level of adolescent oppositional behavior and responsiveness to direct or indirect suggestion.

Van Gorp, Meyer, and Dunbar (1985), in comparing direct and indirect suggestions for analgesia in the reduction of experimentally induced pain, found direct suggestion to be more effective as measured by verbal self-reports and autonomic ability scores. Stone and Lundy (1985) investigated the effectiveness of indirect and direct suggestions in eliciting body movements following suggestions. They reported that indirect suggestions were more effective than direct suggestions in eliciting the target behaviors. Rovelli (1997) found that subjects listening to indirect suggestion were more likely to think that therapists had a personal involvement and as a result they showed more curiosity and willingness to explore than subjects who heard direct suggestions.

A major misunderstanding exists in this debate between direct and indirect suggestion. Direct suggestion is aimed at creating a particular change; indirect suggestion is not. Indirect suggestion is aimed at creating an environment in the therapy session that can essentially create a permissive atmosphere for clients to project relevant meaning and motivation into the words spoken by the therapist. In other words, indirect suggestion does not "make" or "cause" a particular change that is defined by the operator but rather allows the subjects to reveal their own personal experience at which the operator "hinted." As a result, the operator is not expecting a specific and predetermined outcome, but is rather cocreating the outcomes that emerge from the ongoing interaction with the subject. It should be clear to the reader that typical research comparing direct and indirect suggestion is quite problematic in the Ericksonian paradigm (Fourie, 1997).

There have been few research reports on the use of therapeutic metaphor. Mosher and Matthews (1985) investigated the claim by S. Lankton and Lankton (1983) that series of metaphors embedded within one another will create a natural structure for amnesia for material presented in the middle of the metaphoric material. A *multiple embedded metaphor* is created when an initial metaphor is left unfinished and another metaphor is begun and is thus embedded in the first. This metaphor is a tangent that can itself be interrupted by still another metaphor embedded within it. The third metaphor is completed before returning to the unfinished second metaphor, which is then completed before then returning to the original metaphor and completing it. The authors compared treatment groups who received multiply embedded stories with indirect suggestion for amnesia with control groups who received multiple embedded metaphors without indirect suggestions for amnesia. They found support for the structural effect of embedding metaphors on amnesia, but they also reported that indirect suggestion did not enhance the effect of amnesia.

Comparing guided imagery with therapeutic metaphor, researchers found that the use of metaphors while conducting hypnotherapy showed a slight advantage over the use of guided imagery therapy in treating patients with pruritus (Scholz & Meise, 2004). This is significant in light of the proposition that the use of metaphor allows clients to select their own unique meaning for the ideas offered from the therapist or operator. It was found that children prefer instructions delivered by metaphor to those delivered by direct literal communication (Heffner, Greco, & Eifert, 2003).

Matthews, Bennett, Bean, and Gallagher (1985) compared subjects' responses on the Stanford Hypnotic Clinical Scale (Morgan & Hilgard, 1978) with subjects' responses on the same scale rewritten to include only indirect suggestions. They found no significant behavioral differences between the two scales. However, they did report that individuals who received the indirect suggestions perceived themselves to be more hypnotized than those who received the Stanford Hypnotic Clinical Scale.

In a follow-up study, Matthews and Mosher (1988) compared direct and indirect hypnotic induction with direct and indirect suggestions. Thus, one quarter of the participants received direct induction followed by direct suggestions, one quarter received indirect induction followed by indirect suggestion, and the remaining half of the participants received a mixed procedure. The results did not support the efficacy of indirect induction and suggestion over direct induction and suggestion. Contrary to expectations, the data also revealed that participants who received indirect induction and suggestions reported feeling more resistant to the hypnotist than did participants who received direct induction and suggestion.

Weekes and Lynn (1990) also compared direct and indirect suggestions for a range of hypnotic behaviors and found no significant behavioral differences; however, they did find that participants who received direct suggestions perceived their hypnotic responses to be more involuntary than did those who received indirect suggestions. Weekes and Lynn also found that participants who received indirect suggestions reported a greater fear of negative appraisal by the experimenter than did participants who received direct suggestions. This latter result may be similar to the earlier finding by Matthews and Mosher (1988) of an increase in resistance to the hypnotist by participants who received indirect suggestions. The research to date appears to be mixed at best in support of indirect suggestion as compared with direct suggestion in producing trance depth and a range of hypnotic and posthypnotic behaviors.

The reader should remember that the tests in this research were done using audiotaped suggestions to standardize the intervention and that it was therefore not possible to tailor the suggestions (whether direct or indirect) and stories to the individual. As a result, the tests do not emphasize the importance Erickson attached to adapting and using the unique responses of the individual. Similarly, and perhaps more important, these tests were not designed in a context that attempted to address the relevant goals of each individual. Therefore, in this regard, the research may not represent an accurate picture of how a clinical client would experience the interventions.

Systematic study of Erickson's ideas in the clinical setting may provide more useful information with regard to process and efficacy than the more limited analogue studies previously mentioned. For example, Bank (1985) reported positive results over a 22-month period when hypnotic suggestions (both direct and indirect) were used for the control of bleeding that occurs in patients following the insertion and removal of the angiographic catheter. During this time period, an ABA design was used out of medical necessity with a particular patient who was given suggestions to stop his bleeding, which he did. The patient was then told that to find out what was bleeding, he had to undo the previous suggestion and start bleeding, which he did. Bank concluded that although a causal connection was not established beyond any possible doubt, he believed that the use of hypnotic suggestion was highly effective in the control of this type of bleeding. Bank's study underscores the importance of a context in which certain suggestions have a significant relevance not often found in the analogue study.

Matthews and Langdell (1989) used S. Lankton and Lankton's (1983) multiple embedded metaphor procedure on three separate occasions over eight treatment sessions with six clients who had a range of presenting issues. The purpose of the study was to simply ask the clients what meaning they made about the treatment they were receiving. The assumption in the use of metaphor was that effectiveness was most likely when clients were amnesic for the metaphoric experience. Clients were shown video presentations of their hypnotic inductions and metaphors and were asked a series of structured questions about their experience. Five of the six clients believed that they were completely aware and nonamnesic for the meaning and purpose of the metaphors at the time of the clinical session. They indicated that although the stories seemed obvious to them, they trusted and liked the therapist and thus chose to go along with the treatment. Each reported thinking about the meaning of the therapeutic stories told to them during the intervening week and how they could act differently with regard to the presenting issue. Each of the five clients reported a positive change in the presenting problem. The sixth client reported almost total amnesia for each of the metaphor sessions. He also indicated his dislike of the treatment process and reported no therapeutic change.

Nugent (1989a) attempted to show a causal connection between symptomatic improvement and Erickson's notion of "unconscious thinking without conscious awareness" (p. 35). In a series of seven independent case studies with a range of presenting problems (e.g., fear of injections, performance anxiety, claustrophobia), he used the same methodological procedure and treatment intervention (i.e., orientation, induction, Ericksonian suggestions for change, getting the client to endorse he or she is in trance). Nugent systematically assessed the following: a pretreatment baseline response, the most recent onset of the problem, and therapeutic change relative to the intervention. In all seven cases, each client reported a clear, sustained positive change with respect to the presenting problem. Although the individual case study has clear methodological limitations, Nugent's use of seven independent cases with a carefully followed treatment protocol makes his conclusion of causality more convincing.

In a related study, Nugent (1989b) used a multiple-baseline design to investigate the effect of two Ericksonian hypnotic interventions. These interventions involved "pseudo-orientation in time" (Erickson & Rossi, 1980a) and the "unconscious thinking without conscious awareness" suggestions (Erickson & Rossi, 1979). The target behaviors were two athletic skills performed by a collegiate athlete and her level of confidence to perform those behaviors adequately. The data indicated that the target behaviors changed as a result of the treatment intervention. Each of the Nugent (1989a, 1989b) studies, like the Matthews and Langdell (1989) study, have methodological weaknesses, but represent a legitimate attempt to systematically investigate the clinical validity of Ericksonian interventions.

With the exception of the aforementioned clinically oriented studies, this research review has focused on Ericksonian techniques and has an important contribution to make to scientific knowledge. However, it is perhaps easier to discuss Erickson's techniques than to discuss the subtle but more important contributions of his overall approach. With an overemphasis on technique, novice therapists have frequently been guilty of applying a technique without an adequate sense of how such techniques develop a natural interaction with clients. The effective application of Ericksonian techniques relies heavily on the principles of use and cooperation that emerge in the clinical context. The same criticism may be applied to researchers who attempt to study a particular technique separate from the therapeutic context.

It is possible for anyone to use the term *Ericksonian* to describe his or her particular orientation. Lacking a precise definition of the term, many studies have been conducted that would not qualify in the present authors' minds as being representative of Erickson's approach. These studies range from simply having a group exposed to self-hypnosis and calling it the "Ericksonian group" (Larkin, 2001) to studies that administered numerous interventions, including what was called "Ericksonian metaphors" among a list that also included the following: self-hypnosis, meditation, guided imagery, music therapy, neurolinguistic programming, breath control, thought distraction, unconditional acceptance, cognitive challenging of the idealized self-image, assertiveness training, inner-child work, and gestalt therapy (Edwards, 1999). In peer-reviewed journals, there are many such manuscripts and research studies that offer anecdotal studies of outcomes and are said to be following the approach of Erickson; we will only mention a few to illustrate the point (S. T. Gill, 2001; Jacobs, 1998; Marcus, 1999).

Matthews (2000) published an opinion that research is scarce on relevant areas of Erickson's work; these included the following: (a) the belief in an altered state of consciousness and the existence of specific markers indicating an altered state, (b) the superiority of indirect suggestion over direct suggestion, and (c) client hypnotizability as a function of the hypnotist's skill. He concluded that the research literature does not provide empirical support for these key assumptions or for the efficacy of Ericksonian methods. Although there can be little argument with this conclusion, a few remarks are required. The efficacy of Erickson's work does not rely on substantiation of hypnosis as a state of consciousness. This issue is merely one of interest and not one of pragmatics. During his career, Erickson used both direct and indirect suggestion; the concern is not which is superior but, rather, which is most appropriate for each particular client.

Finally, the importance of the therapist's skill in using hypnosis is no small concern. Many research articles state that hypnosis "was used" to produce this or that outcome. However, descriptions of the specific interventions, wording, phrasing, and timing of delivery are almost always absent from research studies. The interaction of the individual hypnotist and client is, although understandably elusive, absolutely essential to study the crucial aspects of hypnosis. The ability to measure and specify communication is challenged by the creativity and sensitivity of the work of Milton Erickson. We must begin to direct our research to the moment-to-moment communications with clients and apply the increasingly well-specified categories of intervention that exist for describing hypnosis, such as the interventions carefully exemplified by S. Lankton and Lankton (1983, 1986), C. Lankton and Lankton (1989), and S. Lankton (2004).

An interesting and relevant study by Tamalonis and Mitchell (1997) compared the effect of traditional direct suggestion with that of neo-Ericksonian indirect suggestion on the performance of memory and skin temperature change in hypnosis. Eighty female college students and employees completed the Stanford Hypnotic Susceptibility Scale, Form C (Weitzenhoffer & Hilgard, 1963) and were randomly assigned to four experimental groups: taped traditional hypnosis, taped Ericksonian hypnosis, Ericksonian hypnosis presented by an experimenter, and a control group assigned to a cognitive task. Participants viewed a series of slides and were tested on their memory of details before being subjected to the experimental conditions. Although no differences were found for the physiological variable, visual data recalled were significantly greater in both Ericksonian conditions.

Future research that may have more bearing on Erickson's approach is that which examines the differences between pathological and nonpathological models (i.e., Ericksonian). Researchers may need to look beyond traditional hypnosis research, such as the frequently cited Rosenthal and Jacobson (1968) study in which randomly selected students were described to their teachers as having exceptional intelligence and could be expected to perform better than their peers, which they did. When retested 9 months later, these students continued to outperform their peers simply as a function of teacher expectations (i.e., positive, nonpathological). The work of Kirsch (1985, 1990) on the importance of expectancy and its relation to behavior may capture more of the essence of Erickson's approach, which was to create a context in which expectancy for change will occur. Thus, the gestalt of the therapist's epistemology, beliefs, attitudes, and expectancies create the context in which a given technique may have meaning for clients. Future research must not focus on techniques to the exclusion of the context in which they occur and should consider the inclusion of qualitative designs in addition to quantitative ones.

CONCLUSION

Fisch (1990) stated that perhaps Erickson's greatest contribution to psychotherapy was not his innovative techniques of metaphor and paradox but his ability to "depathologize" people. Instead of considering a client's problematic behavior as indicative of an underlying personality deficit, he viewed people as making the best choice they can in an unfolding life cycle. Family therapist Lynn Hoffman once described Erickson as "a human dialysis machine" (L. Hoffman, personal communication, November 17, 1987). He filtered out people's negative self-perceptions and focused on what clients could do, not what they could not.

Erickson's approach to therapeutic change was to help the client access the resources needed to solve a given problem. If the resources needed were not fully developed, Erickson would create opportunities within and outside of the hypnotic session for the client to develop and use the needed resources for problem resolution. One is reminded of the time when an inpatient at a state hospital kept insisting that he was Jesus Christ. The more the staff confronted the patient on the falseness of his belief, the more insistent he became. Erickson simply said to the man, "I hear you are a carpenter" and then asked him to make some bookcases (Haley, 1973). The process of change had begun.

An Ericksonian approach to clinical hypnosis is solution focused. The therapeutic orientation is to identify what are the concerns of the client, the solutions that have been used to date, and the desired outcome. These questions are considered within a developmental and systemic framework. The essence of this approach is the reassociation of positive resources to the needed situation such that the client has an increased sense of agency in terms of affect, cognition, and/or behavior. The client is always considered within some interpersonal context. The ultimate goal of therapy is to promote more adaptive and satisfying interpersonal relationships.

Erickson developed many techniques to help create the desired therapeutic change. His use of paradox (i.e., asking a resistive or rebellious client to do the opposite of what is desired); symptom prescription (i.e., asking a client to purposely produce and continue a symptom); and metaphor, jokes, and puns—with and without a hypnotic trance—have become legend. Underlying these interventions is the importance of using the client's behavior to promote change. Ericksonian work also emphasizes indirect use of suggestions to bypass conscious resistance and access unconscious resources and associations. Of equal importance is the metaphor of the splitting of the conscious mind, where the presenting problem resides, from the unconscious mind from which the necessary tools and resource experiences can emerge. The Ericksonian approach to problem solving in clinical hypnosis, because of its focus on solution, tends to be brief, with the focus on present and future functioning over various developmental stages.

The research on concepts such as indirect suggestion, metaphor, and Ericksonian approach as causal to therapeutic change is relatively new. The data reviewed in this chapter are mixed in their support for the importance of indirect suggestion and the necessity of amnesia for a given metaphor. However, two studies did reveal preliminary support for the effectiveness of

Ericksonian hypnosis as a clinical intervention (Heffner, Greco, & Eifert, 2003; Scholz & Meise, 2004). More research on this approach and its various claims needs to be conducted and used as part of a feedback loop to inform both clinicians and future research. Although Erickson has become a legendary figure, those who use his clinical principles need to have more than anecdotal evidence to support their belief systems. Researchers, however, need to develop methodologies that accurately reflect the clinical setting.

As has been stated, there is no one Ericksonian approach. The essence of this work is to help the client to develop creative ways of being. The range of behaviors used by therapists in helping clients to achieve this creativity should not be limited by the tyranny of clinical orthodoxy. Each client offers the therapist a unique opportunity to create a positive climate for change. The legacy of Milton Erickson is not to use clever techniques arbitrarily but to stimulate each therapist to act as creatively as possible for the client's benefit.

Erickson's clinical work continues to inspire study, research, and theory building about the nature of hypnosis, interpersonal influence, and how life experience and the mind interact. His professional influence is far reaching. Beyond his clinical expertise, he was instrumental in starting the American Society of Clinical Hypnosis (ASCH) in 1958 and, in the same year, the *American Journal of Clinical Hypnosis*, which he edited for the next decade. ASCH is a large professional society of health care professionals and academics with component organizations throughout the United States. Although ASCH and its membership represent a broader approach to hypnosis, it is clear that many of Erickson's techniques influence a vast portion of its membership. However, in 1980 the Milton H. Erickson Foundation was established to promote the awareness of Erickson's work among professionals by means of education, training, and archival records. The foundation has established more than 130 training institutes throughout the world. Each of these institutes furthers Erickson's influence within its respective locality. Erickson's effect on the fields of hypnosis and psychotherapy is still expanding. With it, the unique approach to hypnosis and unique approach to clients and their problems, developed and promoted by Erickson, continues to evolve.

REFERENCES

Alman, B., & Carney, R. (1980). Consequences of direct and indirect suggestion on success of posthypnotic behavior. *American Journal of Clinical Hypnosis, 23,* 112–118.

Araoz, D. (1982). *Hypnosis and sex therapy.* New York: Brunner/Mazel.

Bandler, R., & Grinder, R. (1975). *Patterns of the hypnotic techniques of Milton H. Erickson, M.D.* Cupertino, CA: Meta Publications.

Bank, W. O. (1985). Hypnotic suggestion for the control of bleeding in the angiography suite. *Ericksonian Monographs, 1*, 76–89.

Edwards, L. A. (1999). Self-hypnosis and psychological interventions for symptoms attributed to Candida and food intolerance. *Australian Journal of Clinical Hypnotherapy and Hypnosis, 20*(1), 1–12.

Erickson, M. (1980a). February man: Facilitating new identity in hypnotherapy. In E. L. Rossi (Ed.), *The collected papers of Milton H. Erickson on hypnosis: Vol. 4. Innovative hypnotherapy* (pp. 525–542). New York: Irvington Publishers.

Erickson, M. (1980b). Hypnosis: It's renaissance as a treatment modality. In E. L. Rossi (Ed.), *The collected papers of Milton H. Erickson on hypnosis: Vol. 4. Innovative hypnotherapy* (pp. 3–75). New York: Irvington Publishers.

Erickson, M. (1980c). Hypnotic psychotherapy. In E. L. Rossi (Ed.), *The collected papers of Milton H. Erickson on hypnosis: Vol. 4. Innovative hypnotherapy* (pp. 35–48). New York: Irvington Publishers.

Erickson, M. (1980d). Method employed to formulate a complex story for the induction of an experimental neurosis in a hypnotic subject. In E. L. Rossi (Ed.), *The collected papers of Milton H. Erickson on hypnosis: Vol. 3. Hypnotic investigation of psychodynamic processes* (pp. 336–355). New York: Irvington Publishers.

Erickson, M. (1980e). Special techniques of brief hypnotherapy. In E. L. Rossi (Ed.), *The collected papers of Milton H. Erickson on hypnosis: Vol. 4. Innovative hypnotherapy* (pp. 149–187). New York: Irvington Publishers.

Erickson, M. H., & Rossi, E. (1979). *Hypnotherapy: An exploratory casebook.* New York: Irvington Publishers.

Erickson, M. H., & Rossi, E. L. (Eds.). (1980a). *The collected papers of Milton H. Erickson on hypnosis: Vol. 1. The nature of hypnosis and suggestion.* New York: Irvington.

Erickson, M., & Rossi, E. (1980b). Indirect forms of suggestion. In E. L. Rossi (Ed.), *The collected papers of Milton H. Erickson on hypnosis: Vol. 1. The nature of hypnosis and suggestion* (pp. 452–477). New York: Irvington.

Erickson, M., & Rossi, E. (1981). *Experiencing hypnosis: Therapeutic approaches to altered state.* New York: Irvington.

Fisch, R. (1990). The broader implications of Milton H. Erickson's work. *Ericksonian Monographs, 7*, 1–6.

Floda, T. L. (2003). Hypnotic responsiveness as mediated by oppositionality level of conduct disordered adolescents in residential treatment. *Dissertation Abstracts International: Section B: The Sciences and Engineering, 63* (7 B), 3471.

Fourie, D. P. (1997). "Indirect" suggestion in hypnosis: Theoretical and experimental issues. *Psychological Reports, 80*, 1255–1266.

Gill, M., & Brenman, M. (1959). *Hypnosis and related states: Psychoanalytic studies in regression.* Madison, CT: International Universities Press.

Gill, S. T. (2001). An Ericksonian hypnosis intervention on psychological distress and immune functioning in HIV 1 seropositive patients. *Dissertation Abstracts International: Section B: The Sciences and Engineering, 61* (10 B), 5612.

Haley, J. (Ed.). (1967). *Advanced techniques of hypnosis and therapy: Selected papers of Milton H. Erickson, M.D.* New York: Grune & Stratton.

Haley, J. (1973). *Uncommon therapy: The psychiatric techniques of Milton H. Erickson, M.D.* New York: Norton.

Heffner, M., Greco, L. A., & Eifert, G. H. (2003). Pretend you are a turtle: Children's responses to metaphorical versus literal relaxation instructions. *Child And Family Behavior Therapy, 25,* 19–33.

Hilgard, E. R. (1965). *Hypnotic susceptibility.* New York: Harcourt, Brace & World.

Hilgard, E. R. (1966). Posthypnotic amnesia: Experiments and theory. *International Journal of Clinical and Experimental Hypnosis, 14,* 104–111.

Hilgard, E. R. (1975). Hypnosis. *Annual Review of Psychology, 26,* 19–44.

Hilgard, E. R., Weitzenhoffer, A., Landes, J., & Moore, R. (1961). The distribution of susceptibility to hypnosis in a student population: A study using the Stanford Hypnotic Susceptibility Scale. *Psychology Monographs, 75,* 1–22.

Kirsch, I. (1985). Response expectancy as a determinant of experience and behavior. *American Psychologist, 40,* 1189–1202.

Kirsch, I. (1990). *Changing expectations: A key to effective psychotherapy.* Pacific Grove, CA: Brooks/Cole.

Larkin, D. M. (2001). Ericksonian hypnotherapeutic approaches in chronic care support groups: A Rogerian exploration of power and self defined health-promoting goals. *Dissertation Abstracts International: Section B: The Sciences and Engineering, 62* (2 B), 781.

Lankton, C., & Lankton, S. (1989). *Tales of enchantment: Goal-oriented metaphors for adults and children in therapy.* New York: Brunner/Mazel.

Lankton, S. (2004). *Assembling Ericksonian therapy: The collected papers of Stephen Lankton.* Phoenix, AZ: Zeig-Tucker & Theisen.

Lankton, S. (1989). Motivating action with hypnotherapy for a client with a history of early family violence. *Ericksonian Monographs, 6,* 43–61.

Lankton, S., & Lankton, C. (1983). *The answer within: A clinical framework of Ericksonian hypnotherapy.* New York: Brunner/Mazel.

Lankton, S., & Lankton, C. (1986). *Enchantment and intervention in family therapy: Training in Ericksonian approaches.* New York: Brunner/Mazel.

Lankton, S., Lankton, C., & Matthews, W. (1991). Ericksonian family therapy. In A. Gurman & D. Kniskern (Eds.), *Handbook of family therapy* (pp. 239–283). New York: Brunner/Mazel.

Marcus, J. D. (1999). An Ericksonian approach to crack cocaine addiction: A single session intervention. *Contemporary Hypnosis, 16,* 95–102.

Matthews, W. (1985a). Ericksonian and Milan therapy: An intersection between circular questioning and therapeutic metaphor. *Journal of Strategic and Systemic Therapy, 3,* 16–26.

Matthews, W. (1985b). A cybernetic model of Ericksonian hypnotherapy: One hand draws the other. *Ericksonian Monographs, 1,* 42–60.

Matthews, W. J. (2000). Ericksonian approaches to hypnosis and therapy: Where are we now? *International Journal of Clinical and Experimental Hypnosis, 48,* 418–426.

Matthews, W., Bennett, H., Bean, W., & Gallagher, M. (1985). Indirect versus direct hypnotic suggestions—An initial investigation: A brief communication. *International Journal of Clinical and Experimental Hypnosis, 33,* 219–223.

Matthews, W., & Dardeck, K. (1985). The use and construction of therapeutic metaphor. *American Mental Health Counselors Association Journal, 7,* 11–24.

Matthews, W., Kirsch, I., & Mosher, D. (1985). Double hypnotic induction: An initial empirical test. *Journal of Abnormal Psychology, 94,* 92–95.

Matthews, W., & Langdell, S. (1989). What do clients think about the metaphors they receive? *American Journal of Clinical Hypnosis, 31,* 242–251.

Matthews, W., & Mosher, D. (1988). Direct and indirect hypnotic suggestion in a laboratory setting. *British Journal of Experimental and Clinical Hypnosis, 5*(2), 63–71.

McConkey, K. (1984). The impact of indirect suggestion. *International Journal of Clinical and Experimental Hypnosis, 32,* 307–314.

Morgan, A., & Hilgard, J. (1978). The Stanford Hypnotic Susceptibility Scale for Adults. *American Journal of Clinical Hypnosis, 21,* 148–169.

Mosher, D., & Matthews, W. (1985, August). *Multiple embedded metaphor and structured amnesia.* Paper presented at the 93rd Annual Convention of the American Psychological Association, San Diego, CA.

Nugent, W. (1989a). Evidence concerning the causal effect of an Ericksonian hypnotic intervention. *Ericksonian Monographs, 5,* 35–55.

Nugent, W. (1989b). A multiple baseline investigation of an Ericksonian hypnotic approach. *Ericksonian Monographs, 5,* 69–85.

O'Hanlon, W. (1987). *Taproots.* New York: Norton.

Orne, M. (1959). The nature of hypnosis: Artifact and essence. *Journal of Abnormal and Social Psychology, 58,* 277–299.

Rosenthal, R., & Jacobson, L. (1968). *Pygmalion in the classroom.* New York: Holt, Rinehart & Winston.

Rovelli, P. M. (1997). Direct versus indirect suggestions: Does the manner of entry into hypnosis make a difference in how a person will experience an altered state when the induction is tailored and shaped to the individual and later explored from a qualitative methodology? *Dissertation Abstracts International: Section B: The Sciences and Engineering, 57* (10 B), 6591.

Scholz, O., & Meise, M.(2004). Metaphor guided hypnotherapy in comparison with guided imagery therapy. *Zeitschrift fur klinische psychologie und psychotherapie: Forschung und praxis, 33,* 209–217.

Shor, R. E., & Orne, E. C. (1962). *The Harvard Group Scale of Hypnotic Susceptibility, Form A*. Palo Alto, CA: Consulting Psychologists Press.

Stone, J. A., & Lundy, R. M. (1985). Behavioral compliance with direct and indirect body movement suggestions. *Journal of Abnormal Psychology, 3*, 256–263.

Tamalonis, A. M., & Mitchell, J. (1997). An empirical comparison of Ericksonian and traditional hypnotic procedures. *Australian Journal of Clinical Hypnotherapy and Hypnosis, 8*(1), 5–16.

Van Gorp, W. O., Meyer, R. O., & Dunbar, K, D. (1985). The efficacy of direct versus indirect hypnotic induction techniques on reduction of experimental pain. *International Journal of Clinical and Experimental Hypnosis, 4*, 319–328.

Weekes, J. R., & Lynn, S. J. (1990). Hypnosis, suggestion type and subjective experience: The order effects hypothesis revisited. *International Journal of Clinical and Experimental Hypnosis, 38*, 95–101.

Weitzenhoffer, A. M., & Hilgard, E. R. (1959). *Stanford Hypnotic Susceptibility Scale, Forms A and B*. Palo Alto, CA: Consulting Psychologists Press.

Weitzenhoffer, A. M., & Hilgard, E. R. (1962). Stanford Hypnotic Susceptibility Scale, Form C. Palo Alto, CA: Consulting Psychologists Press.

Weitzenhoffer, A. M., & Hilgard, E. R. (1963). Stanford Hypnotic Susceptibility Scale, Form C. Palo Alto, CA: Consulting Psychologists Press.

Zeig, J. (Ed.). (1980). *A teaching seminar with Milton H. Erickson*. New York: Brunner/Mazel.

Zeig, J. (Ed.). (1982). Ericksonian approaches to hypnosis and psychotherapy. New York: Brunner/Mazel.

9

A MULTIMODAL FRAMEWORK
AND CLINICAL HYPNOSIS

ARNOLD A. LAZARUS

Initially, the use of hypnosis was quite prominent among behavior therapists. For example, during systematic desensitization procedures, clients were routinely hypnotized as part of the relaxation processes (Wolpe, 1958). Subsequently, relaxation instructions were given without any hypnotic suggestions, but those clients who specifically requested hypnosis would receive trance induction methods (Wolpe & Lazarus, 1966). A clinical test revealed that clients who came to therapy seeking a procedure such as hypnosis but did not receive it, were apt to respond less well than those whose requests were granted (Lazarus, 1973b).

Multimodal therapy (MMT), an outgrowth of behavior therapy, is a heuristic framework that can incorporate hypnotic methods at several strategic junctures (see also chap. 10). Many problems call for active methods of behavioral retraining rather than conversational therapy. I was the first to use the terms *behavior therapy* and *behavior therapist* in a scientific article (Lazarus, 1958), and I championed the virtues of action over insight. However, carefully conducted follow-up inquiries led me to conclude that more durable results would ensue from applying behavioral plus cognitive methods, and by the time my volume *Behavior Therapy and Beyond* appeared (Lazarus, 1971/

All clinical material has been disguised to protect patient confidentiality.

1996), I was advocating a broad but systematic range of effective cognitive–behavioral techniques.

Within a couple of years, the outcomes of several follow-up inquiries pointed to the importance of breadth if treatment gains were to be maintained, and led to the development of the multimodal approach (Lazarus, 1973a). Emphasis was placed on the fact that, at base, we are biological organisms (i.e., neurophysiological, biochemical entities) who *behave* (i.e., act, react), *emote* (i.e., experience affective responses), *sense* (i.e., respond to tactile, olfactory, gustatory, visual, auditory stimuli), *imagine* (i.e., conjure up sights, sounds, and other events in our mind's eye), *think* (i.e., entertain beliefs, opinions, values, attitudes), and *interact* with one another (i.e., enjoy, tolerate, or suffer various interpersonal relationships). The first letter of each of these seven discrete but interactive dimensions or modalities, *Behavior, Affect, Sensation, Imagery, Cognition, Interpersonal, Drugs/biologicals*, form the convenient acronym, BASIC I.D.

The BASIC I.D. or multimodal framework rests on a broad social and cognitive learning theory (e.g., Bandura, 1977, 1986; Rotter, 1954) because its tenets are open to verification or disproof. Instead of postulating putative complexes and unconscious forces, social learning theory posits testable developmental factors (e.g., modeling, observational and enactive learning, the acquisition of expectancies, operant and respondent conditioning, various self-regulatory mechanisms). Although drawing on effective methods from any discipline, the multimodal therapist does not embrace divergent theories but remains consistently within social–cognitive learning theory. The virtues of *technical eclecticism* (Lazarus, 1967, 1992; Lazarus, Beutler, & Norcross, 1992) over the dangers of *theoretical integration* have been emphasized in several publications (e.g., Lazarus, 1989b, 1995, 2005; Lazarus & Beutler, 1993). The major criticism of theoretical integration is that it inevitably tries to blend incompatible notions and only breeds confusion. This is discussed in some detail later in this chapter.

In this chapter, I describe the advantages of adopting a holistic and comprehensive orientation to the assessment and treatment of psychological disorders. Before reviewing the research on multimodal approaches and empirical issues in understanding the role of hypnosis in a comprehensive treatment, I describe how hypnosis can be used within the context of such a multimodal approach, and consider the virtues and pitfalls of technical eclecticism and theoretical integration in psychotherapy.

THE HOLISTIC AND COMPREHENSIVE NATURE OF THE MULTIMODAL ORIENTATION

The polar opposite of the multimodal approach is the Rogerian, or person-centered, orientation, which is entirely conversational and virtually unimodal (see Bozarth, 1991). Although the relationship between therapist and client is highly significant and sometimes "necessary and sufficient," in most instances, the doctor–patient relationship is but the soil that enables the techniques to take root. A good relationship, adequate rapport, and a constructive working alliance are "usually necessary but often insufficient" (Fay & Lazarus, 1993; Lazarus & Lazarus, 1991a).

Many psychotherapeutic approaches are trimodal, addressing affect, cognition, and behavior. The multimodal approach provides clinicians with a comprehensive template. By separating sensations from emotions, distinguishing between images and cognitions, emphasizing both intraindividual and interpersonal behaviors, and underscoring the biological substrate, the multimodal orientation is most far-reaching. By assessing a client's BASIC I.D., one endeavors to "leave no stone unturned."

The elements of a thorough assessment involve the following range of questions:

- *Behavior (B)*. What is this individual doing that is getting in the way of his or her happiness or personal fulfillment (e.g., self-defeating actions, maladaptive behaviors)? What does the client need to increase and decrease? What should he or she stop doing and start doing?

- *Affect (A)*. What emotions (affective reactions) are predominant? Are we dealing with anger, anxiety, depression, or combinations thereof and to what extent (e.g., irritation versus rage; sadness versus profound melancholy)? What appears to generate these negative affects—certain cognitions, images, interpersonal conflicts? And how does the person respond (i.e., behave) when feeling a certain way? It is important to look for interactive processes: What impact do various behaviors have on the person's affect and vice versa? How does this influence each of the other modalities?

- *Sensation (S)*. Are there specific sensory complaints (e.g., tension, chronic pain, tremors)? What feelings, thoughts, and behaviors are connected to these negative sensations? What positive sensations (e.g., visual, auditory, tactile, olfactory, gustatory delights) does the person report? The sensory modality includes the individual as a sensual and sexual being. When called for, the enhancement or cultivation of erotic pleasure is a viable therapeutic goal (Rosen & Leiblum, 1995).

- *Imagery (I)*. What fantasies and images are predominant? What is the person's self-image? Are there specific success or failure images? Are there negative or intrusive images (e.g., flashbacks to unhappy or traumatic experiences)? And how are these images connected to ongoing cognitions, behaviors, affective reactions, and so forth?

- *Cognition (C).* Can we determine the individual's main attitudes, values, beliefs, and opinions? What are this person's predominant "shoulds," "oughts," and "musts"? Are there any definite dysfunctional beliefs or irrational ideas? Can we detect any untoward automatic thoughts that undermine his or her functioning?
- *Interpersonal (I.).* Interpersonally, who are the significant others in this individual's life? What does he or she want, desire, expect, and receive from them, and what does he or she, in turn, give to and do for them? What relationships give him or her particular pleasures and pains?
- *Drugs/biologicals (D.).* Is this person biologically healthy and health conscious? Does he or she have any medical complaints or concerns? What relevant details pertain to diet, weight, sleep, exercise, alcohol and drug use?

The foregoing are some of the main issues that multimodal clinicians deal with while assessing the client's BASIC I.D. A more comprehensive problem identification sequence is derived from asking most clients to complete the Multimodal Life History Inventory (Lazarus & Lazarus, 1991b, 2005). This 15-page questionnaire facilitates treatment when conscientiously filled in by clients as a homework assignment, usually after the initial session. Seriously disturbed (e.g., deluded, deeply depressed, highly agitated) clients are obviously not expected to comply, but most psychiatric outpatients who are reasonably literate find the exercise useful for speeding up routine history taking and readily provide the therapist with a BASIC I.D. analysis.

PLACING THE BASIC I.D. IN PERSPECTIVE

In multimodal assessment, the BASIC I.D. serves as a template to remind us to examine each of the seven modalities and their interactive effects. It implies that people are social beings who move, feel, sense, imagine, and think and that, at base, humans are biochemical–neurophysiological entities. Students and colleagues frequently inquire whether any particular areas are more significant or more heavily weighted than the others. For thoroughness, all seven require careful attention, but perhaps the biological and interpersonal modalities are especially significant.

The biological modality wields a profound influence on all the other modalities. Unpleasant sensory reactions can signal a host of medical illnesses; excessive emotional reactions (e.g., anxiety, depression, rage) may all have biological determinants; faulty thinking, and images of gloom, doom and terror may derive entirely from chemical imbalances; and untoward personal and interpersonal behaviors may stem from many somatic reactions ranging from toxins (e.g., drugs, alcohol) to intracranial lesions. Hence, when any doubts arise about the probable involvement of biological factors, it is imperative to have them fully investigated. A person with no untoward medical or physical problems and who enjoys warm, meaningful and loving relationships is apt to find life personally and interpersonally fulfilling. Hence, the biological modality serves as the base and the interpersonal modality is perhaps the apex. The seven modalities are by no means static or linear but exist in a state of reciprocal transaction.

A patient requesting therapy may point to any of the seven modalities as his or her entry point. For example, "I suffer from anxiety and depression" (affect); "It's my compulsive habits that are getting to me" (behavior); "My wife and I are not getting along" (interpersonal); "I have these tension headaches and pains in my jaw" (sensory); "I can't get the picture of my grandmother's funeral out of my mind, and I often have disturbing dreams" (imagery); "I know I set unrealistic goals for myself and expect too much from others, but I can't seem to help it" (cognitive); and "I'm fine as long as I take lithium, but I need someone to monitor my blood levels" (drugs/biological).

It is more usual, however, for people to enter therapy with explicit problems in two or more modalities; for example, "I have all sorts of aches and pains that my doctor tells me are due to tension. I also worry too much, and I feel frustrated a lot of the time. And I'm very angry with my father." Initially, it is usually advisable to engage the patient by focusing on the issues, modalities, or areas of concern that he or she presents (See Kwee & Lazarus, 1986).

Any good clinician will first address and investigate the presenting issues by saying, for example, "Please tell me more about the aches and pains you are experiencing," "Do you feel tense in any specific areas of your body?" "You mentioned worries and feelings of frustration. Can you please elaborate on them for me?" "What are some of the specific clash points between you and your father?" Any competent therapist would flesh out the details. However, a multimodal therapist goes further. She or he will carefully note the specific modalities across the BASIC I.D. that are being discussed versus omitted or glossed over. The latter (i.e., the areas that are overlooked or neglected) often yield important data when specific elaborations are requested, and when examining a particular issue, the BASIC I.D. will be rapidly traversed. An example derived from an actual client may prove helpful in illustrating how hypnotic interventions can be targeted to in the context of a succinct multimodal assessment.

Therapist: So you worry a good deal about losing your job.

Client: I literally lose sleep over it.

Therapist: When you become so worried and preoccupied about your job, what would you usually be doing at the time?

Client: Just worrying. That's what I'd be doing.

Therapist: I'm asking if you would worry no less or no more when out with friends, watching television, or when eating dinner.

Client: No, I don't think about it when I'm keeping active. It happens mainly when I get into bed and try to go to sleep.

Therapist: And when you are dwelling on it, how do you feel? Do you become depressed? Fearful? Discouraged?

Client: All of the above.

Therapist: And does your body feel tense?

Client: I know I grind my teeth. My dentist calls it bruxism, or something like that.

Therapist: What pictures or images come into your mind when you are dwelling on possibly losing your job?

Client: I see myself as a bum, as a sort of bagman. And I can hear and see my father saying, "I always told you that you were a loser!"

Therapist: A loser who goes straight to the poorhouse! So do you actually tell yourself and believe that if you got fired you'd probably end up in dire poverty, thereby fulfilling your father's prophecy?

Client: Not really, when I think about it rationally.

Therapist: That's good to know. One of the things we need to figure out is how to keep your rational thoughts from being undermined by irrational ones. But tell me, who are the people who might want to fire you and on what basis or grounds would they do it?

Client: It's my boss's son. He's really incompetent, but his daddy owns the company and he's the blue-eyed boy. And so I am supposed to report to him and he gets mad when I go straight to his dad.

Therapist: So perhaps we need to figure out some effective strategies here. But tell me, what do you do if you can't get to sleep and you keep on worrying?

Client: I don't know what to do.

Therapist: I mean, do you ever resort to alcohol or sleeping pills?

Client: If it's really bad, I take .5 mg Xanax that my doctor prescribed for me.

A clinician well versed in hypnotic procedures could readily consider various entry points and hypnotic procedures to aid and abet the treatment goals. This brief inquiry into his job-related worries quickly unearthed focal points for subsequent remediation.

Behavior

Given the fact that the client only appears to dwell on his worries while in bed, when trying to go to sleep, several behavioral interventions suggest themselves: (a) He could be induced to use "prescribed time periods for worrying," wherein he would have preset intervals during which to fuss and brood, and he could also be advised to dwell on his worries only in one particular place; (b) he could be taught to switch on soporific images while in bed and to leave the bedroom if his negative mind-set intruded; hypnotic procedures might well enhance his capacity to switch off his worries and immerse himself in calm and slumberous images and sensations; (c) he could use a mild aversive consequence when dwelling on the issues beyond his prescribed times (e.g., a rubber band snapped on his wrist).

Affect

In concert with the other tactics used, the client's negative affective reactions may be quelled by repeating various statements designed to provide self-assurance (e.g., "I will be able to cope with and survive the loss of my job!"). Self-statements of this kind may be reinforced by self-hypnotic suggestions.

Sensation

The use of general and differential relaxation techniques, labeled hypnosis or not, might be helpful (e.g., teaching the client how to relax his entire body and then how to direct the relaxation specifically to his face and jaws). Moreover, hypnosis can be used to become aware of sensations in the jaw as it tenses and to develop a sense of warmth and comfort in the muscles to counter bruxism.

Imagery

Coping images could be prescribed wherein the client pictured himself surviving the loss of his job without ending up as a "bagman." Hypnosis can play an important role in making images more veridical and powerful.

Cognition

The client's panic-driven thinking could be addressed and in place of his penchant toward catastrophic ideation, he could learn self-calming statements and more rational and realistic ideas. Catastrophic thoughts can be reframed as negative self-suggestions that can be modified or replaced with more adaptive self-suggestions that promote confidence and a sense of well-being. Some self-help books have been of considerable value as an adjunct to therapy (e.g., Lazarus, Lazarus, & Fay, 1993; Lazarus & Lazarus, 1997).

Interpersonal

The client's difficulties with his employer's son could be examined and possible social skills could be taught. Imaginative rehearsal, practiced during hypnosis, can be used to shape and reinforce a variety of interpersonal interactions relevant to work, for example, and is an excellent vehicle for mentally practicing assertion skills.

Drugs/Biology

Instead of resorting to Xanax, the client could be encouraged to apply relaxation methods, positive imagery procedures, and self-hypnotic suggestions.

THE TEMPORAL FACTOR

I have been discussing an anxious patient who tended to obsess about losing his job. To offset his worries, at least eight different procedures were recommended. At talks and workshops on MMT, people often ask the following two questions: (a) Wouldn't this be rather time-consuming? (b) Won't it dehumanize the client by dissecting the whole person into convenient particles? The answer, in a word, is no. Most of the specific recommendations would take only a few minutes to elucidate and they blend into a harmonious whole. Those methods that call for practice and rehearsal also need not cut into the actual time spent with the client. Thus, after spending about 10 to 15 minutes in the consulting room, the necessary relaxation and hypnotic skills can usually be fostered by giving or loaning specially prepared or commercially available relaxation or self-hypnosis training cassettes for home use. And giving, recommending, or loaning specific articles, chapters, or books often expedites cognitive restructuring.

Why bother to work multimodally, why involve the entire BASIC I.D. when feasible? Follow-up studies that I have conducted intermittently since 1973 have consistently suggested that durable outcomes are in direct proportion to the number of modalities deliberately traversed (Lazarus, 1973a). Although there is obviously a point of diminishing returns, it is a multimodal maxim that the more someone learns in therapy, the less likely he or she is to relapse.

FOR WHOM IS THE MULTIMODAL APPROACH
PARTICULARLY SUITED?

The multimodal orientation is not yet another system of psychotherapy to be added to the hundreds already in existence (Karasu, 1986). Rather, it is an approach that takes Paul's (1967) mandate seriously: "What treatment, by whom, is most effective for this individual with that specific problem and under which set of circumstances?" (p. 111). But in addition to techniques of choice, the multimodal clinician also tries to be an authentic chameleon who also asks about relationships of choice (Lazarus, 1993). Decisions regarding different relationship stances or styles include when and how to be directive, supportive, reflective, cold, warm, tepid, gentle, tender, tough, earthy, chummy, casual, informal, or formal.

How does the clinician determine or arrive at specific relationships of choice? He or she does this by carefully observing the client's reactions to various statements, tactics, and strategies. One begins neutrally by offering the usual facilitative conditions—listening attentively, expressing caring and concern, exuding empathy—and noting the client's reactions. If there are clear signs of progress, one offers more of the same; if not, the clinician may take a more active or directive position and note whether this proves effective. Moreover, those who complete the Multimodal Life History Inventory (Lazarus & Lazarus, 1991b) are asked to describe their "expectations regarding therapy" (p. 4), including their views of the personal qualities of the ideal therapist. A client who describes the ideal therapist as "a good listener" will probably respond to a different treatment trajectory from a person who wants "a good teacher and coach." Sometimes, the client's expectancies leap out at one. Thus, when I used the word *ephemeral* with a client who was a philosophy professor, she immediately said, "Ephemeral? Did you say ephemeral? Or did you mean to say abstruse, evanescent, transient, cursory, or illusive? And do you know the difference?" She made it clear that she was uninterested in my advice or opinions but wanted a sounding board, an active listener. This was one of the few cases in which a strictly Rogerian or person-centered approach seemed indicated. MMT practitioners endeavor to provide what the client appears to desire, especially the clinical ambiance from which he or she is most likely to benefit.

Thus, the essence of cost-effective MMT underscores the notion that treatment should be custom-made for the client. Similarly, hypnotic suggestions can be created, modified, and adapted to the client's needs, which come before the therapist's theoretical framework. Instead of placing clients on a Procrustean bed and treating them alike, multimodal therapists look for a broad, but tailor-made, panoply of effective techniques to bring to bear on the problem, a practice in keeping with long-standing tradition within the field of hypnosis (Lynn & Kirsch, 2006). The methods are carefully applied within an appropriate context and delivered in a style or manner that is most likely to have a positive impact.

Flexibility is the major impetus. Thus, as already indicated, if an assessment reveals the need to do little more than listen attentively and reflect the client's feelings, a multimodal therapist will do just that. If the situation calls for a directive stance involving role-playing and other active strategies, that is what will be implemented. In searching for the best match in terms of the therapeutic alliance and the specific treatment trajectory, a multimodal practitioner is quite willing to refer a client to someone else—a colleague who may be a more effective resource. This is in stark contrast to many clinical schools of thought wherein the client will receive what the therapist offers, whether or not that is what is required.

SOME SPECIFIC FEATURES OF MULTIMODAL THERAPY

Methods we call "bridging" and "tracking" are two important diagnostic procedures. These procedures are discussed in the sections that follow.

Bridging

A therapist interested in a client's emotional responses to an event asks, "How did you feel when your parents showered attention on your brother but left you out?" Instead of discussing his feelings, the client responds with defensive and irrelevant intellectualizations: "My parents had strange priorities and even as a kid I used to question their judgment. Their appraisal of my brother's needs was way off; they saw him as deficient whereas he was quite satisfied with himself." Additional probes into the client's feelings only yield similar abstractions. It is often counterproductive to confront the client and point out that he is evading the question and seems reluctant to face his true feelings. In situations of this kind, *bridging* is usually effective. First, the therapist deliberately tunes into the client's preferred modality, in this case the cognitive domain. Thus, the therapist explores the cognitive content by saying, "So you see it as a consequence involving judgments and priorities. Please tell me more." In this way, after perhaps a 5- to 10-minute discourse, the therapist endeavors to branch off into other directions that seem more productive by asking, "Tell me, while we have been discussing these matters, have you noticed any sensations anywhere in your body?" This sudden switch from cognition to sensation may begin to elicit more pertinent information, assuming that, in this instance, sensory inputs are probably less threatening than affective material. The client may refer to some sensations of tension or bodily discomfort, at which point the therapist may ask him to focus on them, often with suggestions commonly used in hypnotic contexts. For example, he or she might say, "Will you please close your eyes and now feel that neck tension. [*Pause.*] Now relax deeply for a few moments, breathe easily and gently, in and out, in and out, just letting yourself feel calm and peaceful." The feelings of tension, their associated images and cognitions may then be examined. One may then venture to bridge into affect by asking, "Beneath the sensations, can you find any strong feelings or emotions? Perhaps they are lurking in the background." At this juncture it is not unusual for clients to give voice to their feelings by saying, for example, "I am in touch with anger and with sadness."

By starting where the client is, a fundamental principle of many hypnotic approaches (Lynn & Kirsch, 2006), and then bridging into a different modality, most clients then seem to be willing to traverse the more emotionally charged areas they had been avoiding. Notably, a hypnotic technique, the *affect bridge*, can be helpful in this context. In this technique, clients imagine that feelings they identify are a bridge they cross to foster a connection with similar or other feelings, cognitions, and behaviors in everyday life or in the past.

Tracking the "Firing Order"

A fairly reliable pattern may be discerned behind the way in which people generate negative affect. Some dwell first on unpleasant sensations (e.g., palpitations, shortness of breath, tremors), followed by aversive images (e.g., pictures of disastrous events) to which they attach negative cognitions (e.g., ideas about catastrophic illness), leading to maladaptive behavior (e.g., withdrawal and avoidance). This S-I-C-B (sensation, imagery, cognition, behavior) firing order may require a different treatment strategy from that used with, say, a C-I-S-B sequence, an I-C-B-S sequence, or yet a different firing order. Clinical findings suggest that it is often best to apply treatment techniques in accordance with a client's specific chain reaction. A rapid way of determining someone's firing order is to use hypnosis to foster an altered state of consciousness—deeply relaxed with eyes closed—contemplating untoward events and then describing his or her reactions.

One of my clients was perplexed that she frequently felt extremely anxious "out of the blue." Here is part of an actual clinical dialogue:

Therapist: Now please think back to those feelings of anxiety that took you by surprise. Take your time, and tell me what you remember.

Client: We had just finished having dinner and I was clearing the table. [*pause*] I remember now. I had some indigestion.

Therapist:	Can you describe the sensations?
Client:	Sort of like heartburn and a kind of a cramp over here [*Points to upper abdomen.*].
Therapist:	Can you focus on the memory of those sensations?
Client:	Yes. I remember them well.
Therapist:	[*after about 30 seconds*] What else comes to mind?
Client:	I started to breath more quickly, and then I said, "Here I go again."
Therapist:	Meaning?
Client:	Meaning, I'm probably going to end up having another migraine.
Therapist:	How did you come to that conclusion?
Client:	Well, I started imagining things.
Therapist:	Such as?
Client:	Such as the time I had dinner at Tom's and had such a migraine that I threw up.
Therapist:	Let me see if I am following you. You started having some digestive discomfort, and then you noticed that you were breathing rapidly.
Client:	And my heart started pounding.
Therapist:	And then you had an image, a picture of the time you were at Tom's and got sick.
Client:	Yeah. That's when I stopped what I was doing and went to lie down.

This brief excerpt reveals a sensation-imagery-behavioral sequence. In this case, a most significant treatment goal was to show the client that she attached extremely negative attributions to negative sensations, which then served as a trigger for anxiety-generating images. Consequently, she was asked to draw up a list of unpleasant sensations, to dwell on them one by one, and to prevent the eruption of catastrophic images with a mantra: "This too shall pass."

Only general overviews are possible in a single chapter, and those readers who want more information about bridging and tracking and the multimodal approach may wish to read Lazarus (1989a, 1997) and my chapters in O'Donohue, Fisher, and Hayes (2003), Corsini and Wedding (2008), and Norcross and Goldfried (2005).

Second-Order BASIC I.D. Assessments

The initial modality profile (BASIC I.D. Chart) translates vague, general, or diffuse problems (e.g., depression, unhappiness, anxiety) into specific, discrete, and interactive difficulties. The modality profile is a list of specific problems across the BASIC I.D. Techniques—preferably those with empirical backing—are selected to counter the various problems. Nevertheless, treatment impasses arise, and when this occurs, a more detailed inquiry into associated behaviors, affective responses, sensory reactions, images, cognitions, interpersonal factors, and possible biological considerations may shed light on the situation. This recursive application of the BASIC I.D. to itself adds depth and detail to the macroscopic overview afforded by the initial modality profile (see Corsini & Wedding, 2008; Lazarus, 1997; Norcross & Goldfried, 2005). Thus, a second-order assessment with a client who was not responding to antidepressants and a combination of cognitive–behavioral procedures revealed a central cognitive schema, "I am not entitled to be happy," that had eluded all other avenues of inquiry. Therapy was then aimed directly at addressing this maladaptive cognition.

CLINICAL APPLICATIONS

Hypnosis occurs within the context of a special hypnotist/participant relationship during which suggestions are given pertaining to cognition, perception, memory, and affect (Kirsch, 1994). My early experiences with hypnosis from 1960 to 1966, mainly in South Africa, focused on numerous induction techniques, methods for "deepening trances," procedures for inducing robust posthypnotic suggestions, the feasibility of self-hypnosis, and matters pertaining to specific processes, from pain control (i.e., anesthesia, analgesia) to amnesia. Wide differences in hypnotic susceptibility seemed to be demonstrated clinically and experimentally. Over time, as I grew both weary and wary of eye-fixation, eye-closure, and hand-levitation techniques, I started scouring the literature for other hypnotic procedures and experimented with some of my own. Subsequently, Milton Erickson's unusual and diverse indirect methods (see chap. 8, this volume) lent impetus to the notion that hypnotic methods need to be tailored to individual clients and call for clinical flexibility.

Many years ago, it occurred to me to conduct a little clinical experiment (Lazarus, 1973b). Clients who explicitly asked for hypnosis were randomly assigned to one of two groups. One group was told that data have shown relaxation methods to be more effective than hypnosis because they produce greater self-reliance rather than dependency on a hypnotist's suggestions. The other group received hypnosis. Induction scripts were prepared for each. However, the only difference between the relaxation versus the hypnosis script was that, in the former, phrases contained the words *hypnosis* and *hypnotic* (e.g., "feel the hypnotic relaxation spreading throughout your body . . . as the hypnotic relaxation takes you into deeper levels of tranquility"), whereas in the pure relaxation script, the words *hypnosis* and *hypnotic* were conspicuously absent.

The outcome showed that, in the main, those individuals who requested hypnosis and were given the hypnosis script obtained better results than those who received relaxation. Subsequently, when those who had derived little or minimal benefit from relaxation were treated by the hypnosis script, significant gains accrued. This outcome indicated to me that people's expectancies must often be honored, and the power of the proper word can be of inestimable value. A meta-analysis performed by Kirsch, Montgomery, and Sapirstein (1995) supported these contentions. Hypnosis, then, is defined largely by the context (e.g., labeling the procedures *hypnosis*) and the expectation of clients that they will experience a hypnotic induction. This permits a wide range of suggestions and interventions to be considered hypnotic in nature.

Clinically speaking, the use of the word *hypnosis* and the application of various hypnotic techniques appear to enhance the impact of imagery methods on susceptible clients. These steps also appear to augment the power of most suggestions. There seems to be a greater veridical effect when suggestible clients picture various scenes under hypnosis. Thus, I routinely inquire about clients' attitudes toward hypnosis. I do not waste time endeavoring to persuade skeptics. Those who say they do not believe in hypnosis or who claim to be nonhypnotizable are treated without hypnosis. Given that virtually everyone is suggestible (to a greater or lesser degree), one may wonder to what extent hypnosis is nevertheless often part of the variance.

Those who express some interest in hypnosis may be open to the direct enhancement effects already mentioned. Given numerous unsuccessful attempts to hypnotize certain clients with standard induction techniques (e.g., eye roll, hand levitation, eye fixation, eye closure), I have developed a different patter:

> Hypnosis has nothing to do with sleep, a loss of consciousness, or with profound amnesia. What we aim to achieve is the greater self-empowerment that an altered state of consciousness can provide. When your eyes are closed, you are in a different state of consciousness than when your eyes are open. You enter a different and receptive realm of awareness. Please test it out. Your eyes are open at present. Notice your state of awareness. Now please close your eyes. The moment your eyes close, you immediately cut down on external stimuli and distractions. You become aware of different inputs. If you were attached to an EEG machine, we would

find different brain waves being emitted when your eyes are open and when they are closed. What differences do you notice when your eyes are open and when they are closed? [A *brief discussion ensues*.] Simply by closing your eyes, it becomes easier to bypass the usual barriers and needless defenses via this different realm of consciousness. Thus, if I say to you that you will begin to feel more self-confident, it's likely to go in one ear and out the other, but in an altered state of consciousness, you can more readily absorb that idea and probably make it so.

Now please close your eyes, settle back comfortably, allow your breath to flow in and out, easily and pleasantly as you enter an altered state of consciousness. You should feel relaxed, and as you imagine yourself entering a more profound level of modified consciousness, your mind becomes more receptive to all healing suggestions. A few simple deep breaths can assist you in attaining a better level of altered consciousness. So with your eyes closed, with your body as relaxed as possible, take in a deep breath and hold it for a few seconds. Now exhale and automatically drift into a deeper level of altered consciousness. Just repeat this once or twice.

Hypnotically susceptible individuals report entering a deep trance even from this brief and straightforward induction. In most cases, I have found it uneconomical and needlessly time-consuming to devote time to more intricate inductions. Having gone through the foregoing patter, the multimodal therapist then uses the required imagery methods (especially coping imagery, various past- and/or future-oriented time-tripping techniques) to challenge faulty cognitions and to offer self-statements that enhance self-assurance and self-worth. What are often referred to as *ego-strengthening* suggestions (e.g., "You can feel your own power," "You can develop a sense of independence") are also often worth pursuing.

One of the major elements of hypnotic imagery rests on an assumption that before one can accomplish something in reality, it is often essential first to be able to perceive or picture oneself doing it in imagery (e.g., Lazarus, 1984; Zilbergeld & Lazarus, 1988). Thus, hypnotic suggestions can play a definite and robust role when working with certain clients to alter significant behaviors; enhance different affective states; augment pleasant sensations while diminishing unpleasant ones; intensify positive and coping imagery; attenuate dysfunctional beliefs and replace them with prudent, insightful and discerning ideas; heighten assertive behavior and develop social skills; and persuade them to picture themselves adhering to health promoting activities: exercising, eating sensibly, avoiding noxious substances, and taking prescribed medication when indicated. It is notable that suggestions can be described to clients as *self-hypnosis* insofar as the clients themselves are ultimately responsible for creating the experiences called for by the suggestions. For some clients, framing hypnosis in this manner can counter prevalent, yet inaccurate, cultural beliefs that hypnosis somehow robs individuals of their volition or sense of control.

My identification of the hypnotic state with the change in consciousness that accompanies eye-closure is particularly relevant from a cognitive–behavioral perspective. It suggests that hypnosis is not a distinct or unique condition or state. Instead, it is a name (with positive connotations for some and negative implications for others) for the state of awareness that occurs when people are relaxed with their eyes closed. The parallels between relaxation and hypnosis are well presented by Palmer (1993), who has written a useful booklet that describes step-by-step relaxation and hypnotic scripts.

Although I favor a simple eye-closure/relaxation induction, any number of inductions of hypnosis can be used with equal success with clients, depending on their expectations about hypnosis and their individual preferences (see Lynn & Kirsch, 2006). The next chapter in this volume (chap. 10) provides an in-depth discussion of how a multimodal approach can be used to create individually tailored inductions. Moreover, it is not necessary that clients actually achieve a state of consciousness dramatically or demonstrably different from waking consciousness. Rather, it is more important that clients become immersed in the therapeutic suggestions that follow the induction, which are crafted to meet their needs and achieve their unique therapy agenda. Finally, formal assessment of hypnotic susceptibility is rarely, if ever, necessary; most clients who respond to a hypnotic induction with eye closure and relaxation can easily experience the sorts of suggestions (e.g., relaxation, imagining specific situations, ego strengthening) commonly used in MMTs.

RESEARCH AND APPRAISAL

Hypnosis is almost always used in combination with other treatments, with the exception of pain relief, in which it is sometimes administered as a stand-alone intervention. As noted in chapter 1, a variety of meta-analytic studies indicate that hypnosis can be a useful adjunct to cognitive–behavioral and other treatments, contributing to their efficacy. Moreover, hypnotic suggestions often target and call for changes in sensations, perceptions, cognitions, and behaviors. Accordingly, hypnosis can rightfully be considered a multimodal approach that can expand the breadth of psychological interventions. Indeed, empirically based knowledge regarding the role that hypnosis can play in a broad-spectrum treatment can contribute to addressing the important question of whether there is evidence that a multimodal approach is superior to more narrow or targeted treatments.

During the 1970s and 1980s, issues pertaining to focused versus combined treatment modalities were addressed in several quarters. It is of interest that for some disorders specialized or highly focused interventions appeared superior to broad-spectrum approaches. For example, in weight-loss programs McReynolds and Paulsen (1976) provided data that favored a specialized stimulus-control procedure over multidimensional treatments. Similarly, Agras, Kazdin, and Wilson (1979) listed several problem areas that may respond better to specialized procedures: some phobias, compulsive disorders, sexual problems, eating disorders, cases of insomnia, tension headaches, and the management of oppositional children.

A strong argument for combined treatments was made by Blake (1965), who showed that alcoholics treated only by aversion therapy were more likely to relapse than their counterparts who had also received relaxation training. Sherman, Mulac, and McCann (1974) reported a synergistic effect of relaxation training and rehearsal feedback. Garson's (1978) controlled study clearly showed the superiority of broad-spectrum treatment in smoking reduction. Telch and Lucas (1994) suggested that a combination of imipramine and exposure is more effective in treating panic disorder with agoraphobia than either exposure treatment or drug treatment alone.

In a carefully controlled outcome study, Williams (1988) compared multimodal assessment and treatment with less integrative approaches in helping children with learning disabilities. Clear results emerged in support of the multimodal procedures. Kwee (1984) conducted a treatment outcome study on 84 hospitalized patients diagnosed with obsessive–compulsive disorders or phobias, 90% of whom had received prior treatment without success and 70% of whom had been diagnosed with their disorders for more than 4 years. Implementing multimodal treatment regimens resulted in substantial recoveries and durable 9-month follow-ups. This has been confirmed and amplified by Kwee and Kwee-Taams (1994). Recently, the vast literature on treatment regimens, be they journal articles or entire volumes, has accentuated MMT, although the authors often label their work *multidimensional, multimethod,* or *multifactorial.*

It should be understood that the multimodal approach is not one that insists on treating everyone across the entire BASIC I.D. As already mentioned, it would seem that some problems respond better to focused interventions. However, when progress falters or when no treatment gains are evident, I recommend a BASIC I.D. assessment as a means of shedding light on otherwise concealed issues that may be amenable to change.

Aside from outcome measures, however, there is research bearing out certain multimodal tenets and procedures. For example, multimodal clinicians often use a 35-item Structural Profile Inventory (SPI) that provides a quantitative rating of the extent to which clients favor specific BASIC I.D. areas. Factor analytic studies gave rise to several versions of the SPI until one with good factorial stability was obtained (see Appendix 4 in Lazarus, 1989a). The instrument measures the extent to which people are action-oriented (behavior), their degree of emotionality (affect), the value they attach to various sensory experiences (sensation), how much time they occupy with fantasy day dreaming and "thinking in pictures" (imagery), how analytical they tend to be (cognition), how important other people are to them (interpersonal) and the extent to which they are healthy and health-conscious (drugs/biology). The instrument's reliability and validity have been borne out by research (Herman, 1992a; Landes, 1991). Herman (1991, 1992b, 1994) has conducted extensive research on the Multimodal Structural Profile Inventory. One of his most important findings is that when clients and therapists have wide differences on the SPI, therapeutic outcomes tend to be adversely affected.

Technical Eclecticism and Theoretical Integration

As more therapists have become aware that no one school can possibly provide all the answers, a willingness to incorporate different methods into their own purview and to combine different procedures has become fairly prominent. Indeed, over the past few decades, there has been a growing awareness among researchers and clinicians that hypnosis can be used to augment the effectiveness of a variety of treatment approaches, including empirically supported interventions (Lynn & Kirsch, 2006). There are several different ways in which methods may be combined. The first is to use several techniques within a given approach (e.g., exposure, response prevention, participant modeling from a behavioral perspective). One may also combine techniques from different disciplines, especially when confronted by a seemingly intractable patient or problem. Yet another way of combining treatments is to use medication in conjunction with psychosocial therapies, including hypnosis. In addition, one may treat certain clients with a combination of individual, family and group therapy or look to other disciplines (e.g., social work in the case of vocational rehabilitation).

There are three principal routes to rapprochement or integration: technical eclecticism, theoretical integration, and common factors (Arkowitz, 1989; Norcross & Goldfried, 2005; Norcross & Newman, 1992). Garfield (1994) concluded that "there is no clear agreement on what really constitutes integration" (p. 130). Yet those who attempt to meld different or even disparate theories (i.e., *theoretical integrationists*) differ significantly from those who remain theoretically consistent but use diverse techniques (i.e., *technical eclectics*). And those who dwell on the common ingredients shared by different therapies (e.g., self-efficacy, enhanced morale, corrective emotional experiences) are apt to ignore crucial differences while emphasizing essential similarities (Lazarus, 1989b, 1995). Wilson (1995) maintained that the common factors approach is likely to be a conceptual dead end.

Many integrationists are fully aware that fundamental incompatibilities render only certain aspects of each orientation capable of consolidation or amalgamation. But in my view, in most instances only phenotypical similarities can be blended. For example, when Wolpe (1958) stated that "anxiety is usually the central constituent of [neurotic] behavior" (p. 32), this may have sounded decidedly Freudian. But on examining Wolpe's definition of the term, its presumed etiology, functions, manifestations, and treatment trajectory, it becomes quite obvious that his views bear no basic similarities to any psychodynamic formulations. In essence, there appear to be no data to support the notion that a blend of different theories has resulted in a more robust therapeutic technique or has led to synergistic practice effects.

It cannot be overstated that the effectiveness of specific techniques may have no bearing on the theories that spawned them. Techniques may, in fact, prove effective for reasons that do not remotely relate to the theoretical ideas that gave birth to them. This is not meant to imply that techniques operate or function in a vacuum. The therapeutic relationship is the soil that enables techniques to take root. Theories are needed to explain or account for various phenomena and to try to make objective sense out of bewildering observations and assertions.

Technical Eclecticism and Experimentally Supported Procedures

The arbitrary nature of theoretical beliefs was brought home to me circa 1964 after treating two patients for several months at the Palo Alto V.A. Hospital while a professional audience from the San Francisco Bay area observed the therapy from behind a one-way mirror. At that juncture I was an ardent behavior therapist who downplayed cognitive processes. Week after week, my colleagues observed me implementing relaxation procedures, systematic desensitization, assertiveness training, various imagery methods, and homework assignments. Discussions with the audience vis-à-vis the rationale for applying or withholding certain procedures followed each session. After 8 to 10 sessions, it was clear that the patients had made significant progress. A heated discussion then ensued as to the reasons behind the constructive changes. The audience consisted of theorists from different persuasions, and each one argued vociferously for the veracity of his or her own theoretical position. Because antithetical convictions were being espoused, it occurred to me that whatever the genuine or accurate underlying processes happened to be, most of the speakers (myself included) were probably in error.

Nobody disagreed that progress had been made, but there was considerable contention as to why these gains had occurred. This was the major impetus behind my development of a technically eclectic outlook (Lazarus, 1967, 1989b, 2005). As London (1964) underscored, we apply techniques, not theories, to our patients, although one's theoretical underpinnings will determine, to a large extent, which techniques are admissible or inadmissible (see Davison & Lazarus, 1994, 1995,). It makes sense to select seemingly effective techniques from any discipline without necessarily subscribing to the theories that begot them. Thus, it is not necessary to draw on a single tenet of Frankl's (1967) existential theories to use his method of "paradoxical intention," and one may freely use the "empty chair technique" without embracing any theories from gestalt therapy or psychodrama (see Lazarus, 1995). In the case of hypnosis, it is not altogether clear why clients benefit from it (e.g., enhanced expectations vs. enhanced imagination or relaxation), yet hypnotically framed suggestions appear to be useful in a variety of treatment contexts (see Schoenberger et al., 1997).

In MMT, the selection and development of specific techniques are not at all capricious. My basic position can be summarized as follows: Eclecticism is warranted only when well-documented treatments of choice do not exist for a particular disorder or when well-established methods are not achieving the desired results. Thus, for the treatment of agoraphobia, with or without panic attacks, there are several well-documented, empirically established, and highly recommended treatment procedures (Barlow, 1996; Carter, Turovsky, & Barlow, 1994). For example, Barlow (1994) stated, "Investigators around the world have demonstrated clearly that exposure *in vivo* is the central ingredient in the behavioral treatment of agoraphobia and that this process is substantially more effective than any number of credible alternative psychotherapeutic procedures" (p. 407).

However, when these procedures, despite proper implementation, fail to achieve the desired results, one may look to less authenticated procedures, attempt alternative interventions, or endeavor to develop new strategies (see Davison & Lazarus, 1995). For example, hypnosis can be used to help clients better tolerate exposure, and there are indications that it can increase the effectiveness of imaginal exposure as well as in vivo exposure (Kirsch & Lynn, 1995; Lynn & Kirsch, 2006). Clinical effectiveness is probably in direct proportion to the range of effective tactics, strategies, and methods that a practitioner has at his or her disposal. Nevertheless, the random importation of techniques from anywhere or everywhere without a sound rationale can only result in syncretistic confusion (see Lazarus, 1989b, 1995). A systematic, prescriptive, technically eclectic orientation is the opposite of a smorgasbord conception of eclecticism in which one selects procedures according to unstated and unreplicable processes (Lazarus & Beutler, 1993; Lazarus, Beutler, & Norcross, 1992).

The vast literature on treatment regimens accentuates multidimensional, multifactorial, and multimethod approaches. Manuals written expressly for treatment application typically prescribe combinations of techniques. For example, in treating panic disorder, Barlow and his associates (e.g., Barlow &

Cerny, 1988; Barlow & Craske, 1989) recommended a combination of several components: relaxation training, respiratory retraining, cognitive restructuring, and exposure to the internal cues that trigger panic. Similarly, the treatments of choice for obsessive–compulsive disorder include exposure to the feared stimuli and response prevention, often in conjunction with pharmacological treatment (e.g., serotonin reuptake blockers). Overall case management for schizophrenia calls for social skills training, vocational rehabilitation, and supported employment, along with antipsychotic medication (Mueser & Glynn, 1995).

The aforementioned treatment combinations make use of no eclectic maneuvers but are all drawn from within the established purview of cognitive–behavioral interventions. There are few, if any, data or controlled studies to support the notion that clinical outcomes are enhanced by adding psychodynamic, gestalt, or any other nonbehavioral techniques or procedures to standard cognitive–behavioral methods. Nevertheless, the potential for clinical enrichment exists. It needs to be emphasized again that arbitrary blends of different techniques are to be decried. Lambert (1992) warned that certain eclectic practices "may even produce therapies that are less efficacious than the single-school approaches from which they are derived" (p. 122). Kazdin (1984) arrived at a similar conclusion and emphasized that "premature integration of specific positions that are not well supported on their own may greatly impede progress" (p. 142). Wilson (1995) provided an incisive critique of psychotherapy integration. He stressed that technique selection can rest on rather capricious, arbitrary, and subjective criteria unless proper guidelines are established.

The cognitive–behavioral literature has documented various treatments of choice for a wide range of afflictions, including maladaptive habits, fears and phobias, stress-related difficulties, sexual dysfunctions, depression, eating disorders, obsessive–compulsive disorders, posttraumatic stress disorders, dementia, psychoactive substance abuse, somatization disorder, personality disorders, psychophysiologic disorders, pain management, and diverse forms of violence. There are relatively few empirically validated treatments outside the area of cognitive–behavior therapy (see Chambless, 1995). Two noteworthy exceptions are interpersonal psychotherapy for depression (Klerman, Weissman, Rounsaville, & Chevron, 1984) and bulimia nervosa (Fairburn, 1993). When approached by patients with any of the aforementioned problem areas, the knowledgeable and ethical therapist will administer the established treatments of choice or refer the patient to someone well versed in the necessary procedures.

Important questions regarding hypnosis remain to be addressed. For example, are hypnotic techniques more effective in enhancing therapeutic work in some modalities (e.g., sensation, imagination) than others (e.g., interpersonal)? When hypnosis addresses multiple modalities, is it more effective than when it addresses a single modality (see chap. 10)? By what mechanism does hypnosis bolster the effectiveness of empirically supported procedures? For example, is it the heightened expectancies for therapeutic change that can accompany hypnosis, or is it solidification of the therapeutic alliance that hypnosis often promotes (Nash & Barnier, 2008)? Answers to these questions, as well as the question of whether controlled outcome studies of multimodal hypnosis will reveal that this approach is effective with different treatment populations, should prove to be of great interest and potential benefit to clinicians of diverse stripes.

CONCLUSION

Hypnotic procedures often use multimodal approaches, targeting different and clinically relevant dimensions of human experience. Hypnosis can be incorporated into a wide range of clinical interventions and enhance the treatment effectiveness of these interventions. As a final word, it has been widely stated that virtually any method that will enhance patient compliance and treatment adherence is worth cultivating. Within the multimodal framework, I see hypnosis as one of the most useful devices for attaining this worthy end.

REFERENCES

Agras, W. S., Kazdin, A. E., & Wilson, G. T. (1979). *Behavior therapy: Toward an applied clinical science*. San Francisco: W.H. Freeman.

Arkowitz, H. (1989). The role of theory in psychotherapy integration. *Journal of Integrative and Eclectic Psychotherapy, 8*, 8–16.

Bandura, A. (1977). *Social learning theory*. Englewood Cliffs, NJ: Prentice Hall.

Bandura, A. (1986). *Social foundations of thought and action: A social–cognitive theory*. Englewood Cliffs, NJ: Prentice Hall.

Barlow, D. H., & Cerny, J. A. (1988). *Psychological treatment of panic*. New York: Guilford Press.

Barlow, D. H., & Craske, M. G. (1989). *Mastery of your anxiety and panic*. Albany, NY: Graywind.

Blake, B. G. (1965). The application of behavior therapy to the treatment of alcoholism. *Behaviour Research and Therapy, 3*, 75–85.

Bozarth, J. D. (1991). Person-centered assessment. *Journal of Counseling & Development, 69*, 458–461.

Carter, M. M., Turovsky, J., & Barlow, D. H. (1994). Interpersonal relationships in panic disorder with agoraphobia: A review of empirical evidence. *Clinical Psychology: Science and Practice, 1*, 25–34.

Chambless, D. (1995). Training in and dissemination of empirically validated psychological treatments: Report and recommendations. *The Clinical Psychologist, 48*, 3–23.

Corsini, R. J., & Wedding, D. (Eds.). (2008). *Current psychotherapies* (8th ed.). Belmont, CA: Brooks/Cole.

Davison, G. C., & Lazarus, A. A. (1994). Clinical innovation and evaluation: Integrating practice with inquiry. *Clinical Psychology: Science and Practice, 1*, 157–168.

Davison, G. C., & Lazarus, A. A. (1995). The dialectics of science and practice. In S. C. Hayes, V. M. Follette, T. Risley, R. D. Dawes, & K. Grady (Eds.), *Scientific standards of psychological practice: Issues and recommendations* (pp. 95–120). Reno, NV: Context Press.

Fairburn, C. G. (1993). *Interpersonal psychotherapy for bulimia nervosa.* Washington, DC: American Psychiatric Association.

Fay, A., & Lazarus, A. A. (1993). On necessity and sufficiency in psychotherapy. *Psychotherapy in Private Practice, 12*, 33–39.

Frankl, V. (1967). *Psychotherapy and existentialism.* New York: Simon & Schuster.

Garfield, S. L. (1994). Eclecticism and integration in psychotherapy: Developments and issues. *Clinical Psychology: Science and Practice, 1*, 123–137.

Garson, E. B. (1978). *The application of positive imagery in the maintenance of smoking reduction following broad-spectrum treatment.* Unpublished doctoral dissertation, Rutgers, The State University of New Jersey.

Herman, S. M. (1991). Client–therapist similarity on the Multimodal Structural Profile Inventory as predictive of psychotherapy outcome. *Psychotherapy Bulletin, 26*, 26–27.

Herman, S. M. (1992a). A demonstration of the validity of the Multimodal Structural Profile Inventory through a correlation with the Vocational Preference Inventory. *Psychotherapy in Private Practice, 11*, 71–80.

Herman, S. M. (1992b). Predicting psychotherapists' treatment theories by Multimodal Structural Profile Inventories: An exploratory study. *Psychotherapy in Private Practice, 11*, 85–100.

Herman, S. M. (1994). The diagnostic utility of the Multimodal Structural Profile Inventory. *Psychotherapy in Private Practice, 13*, 55–62.

Herman, S. M., Cave, S., Kooreman, H. E., Miller, J. M., & Jones, L. L. (1995). Predicting clients' perceptions of their symptomatology by multimodal structural profile inventory responses. *Psychotherapy in Private Practice, 14*, 23–33.

Karasu, T. B. (1986). The specificity versus nonspecificity dilemma: Toward identifying therapeutic change agents. *American Journal of Psychiatry, 143*, 687–695.

Kazdin, A. E. (1984). Integration of psychodynamic and behavioral psychotherapies: Conceptual versus empirical synthesis. In H. Arkowitz & S. B. Messer (Eds.), *Psychoanalytic therapy and behavior therapy: Is integration possible?* (pp. 139–170). New York: Basic Books.

Kirsch, I. (1994). APA definition and description of *hypnosis*. *Contemporary Hypnosis, 11*, 142–144.

Kirsch, I., & Lynn, S. (1995). The altered state of hypnosis: Changes in the theoretical landscape. *American Psychologist, 50*, 846–858.

Kirsch, I., Montgomery G., & Sapirstein, G. (1995). Hypnosis as an adjunct to cognitive–behavioral psychotherapy: A meta-analysis. *Journal of Consulting and Clinical Psychology, 63*, 214–220.

Klerman, G. L., Weissman, M. M., Rounsaville, B. J., & Chevron, E. S. (1984). *Interpersonal psychotherapy of depression*. New York: Basic Books.

Kwee, M. G. T. (1984). *Klinische multimodale gegragtstherapie* [Clinical multimodal behavior therapy]. Lisse, Holland: Swets & Zeitlinger.

Kwee, M. G. T., & Kwee-Taams, M. K. (1994). *Klinische gedragstherapie in Nederland & vlaanderen* [Clinical behavioral therapy in the Netherlands and Flanders]. Delft, Holland: Eubron.

Kwee, M. G. T., & Lazarus, A. A. (1986). Multimodal therapy: The cognitive–behavioural tradition and beyond. In W. Dryden & W. Golden (Eds.), *Cognitive–behavioural approaches to psychotherapy* (pp. 320–355). London: Harper & Row.

Lambert, M. J. (1992). Psychotherapy outcome research: Implications for integrative and eclectic therapists. In J. C. Norcross & M. R. Goldfried (Eds.), *Handbook of psychotherapy integration* (pp. 94–129). New York: Basic Books.

Landes, A. A. (1991). Development of the Structural Profile Inventory. *Psychotherapy in Private Practice, 9*, 123–141.

Lazarus, A. A. (1958). New methods in psychotherapy: A case study. *South African Medical Journal, 32*, 660–664.

Lazarus, A. A. (1967). In support of technical eclecticism. *Psychological Reports, 21*, 415–416.

Lazarus, A. A. (1973a). Multimodal behavior therapy: Treating the BASIC ID. *Journal of Nervous and Mental Disease, 156*, 404–411.

Lazarus, A. A. (1973b). "Hypnosis" as a facilitator in behavior therapy. *The International Journal of Clinical and Experimental Hypnosis, 21*, 25–31.

Lazarus, A. A. (1984). *In the mind's eye*. New York: Guilford Press.

Lazarus, A. A. (1989a). *The practice of multimodal therapy*. Baltimore, MD: Johns Hopkins University Press.

Lazarus, A. A. (1989b). Why I am an eclectic (not an integrationist). *British Journal of Guidance and Counselling, 19*, 248–258.

Lazarus, A. A. (1992). Multimodal therapy: Technical eclecticism with minimal integration. In J. C. Norcross & M. R. Goldfried (Eds.), *Handbook of psychotherapy integration*. (pp. 231–263). New York: Basic Books.

Lazarus, A. A. (1993). Tailoring the therapeutic relationship, or being an authentic chameleon. *Psychotherapy, 30*, 404–407.

Lazarus, A. A. (1995). Different types of eclecticism and integration: Let's be aware of the dangers. *Journal of Psychotherapy Integration, 5*, 27–39.

Lazarus, A. A. (1996). *Behavior therapy and beyond*. Northvale, NJ: Jason Aronson. (Original work published 1971)

Lazarus, A. A. (1997). *Brief but comprehensive psychotherapy: The multimodal way*. New York: Springer.

Lazarus, A. A. (2005). Multimodal therapy. In J. C. Norcross & M. R. Goldfried (Eds.), *Handbook of psychotherapy integration* (pp. 105–120). New York: Oxford University Press.

Lazarus, A. A., & Beutler, L. E. (1993). On technical eclecticism. *Journal of Counseling & Development, 71*, 381–385.

Lazarus, A. A., Beutler, L. E., & Norcross, J. C. (1992). The future of technical eclecticism. *Psychotherapy, 29*, 11–20.

Lazarus, A. A., & Lazarus, C. N. (1991a). Let us not forsake the individual nor ignore the data: A response to Bozarth. *Journal of Counseling & Development, 69*, 463–465.

Lazarus, A. A., & Lazarus, C. N. (1991b). *Multimodal life history inventory*. Champaign, IL: Research Press.

Lazarus, A. A., & Lazarus, C. N. (2005). The multimodal life history inventory. In G. P. Koocher, J. C. Norcross, & S. A. Hill (Eds.), *Psychologists' desk reference* (pp. 26–23). New York: Oxford University Press.

Lazarus, A. A., Lazarus, C. N., & Fay, A. (1993). *Don't believe it for a minute!* San Luis Obispo, CA: Impact Publishers.

London, P. (1964). *The modes and morals of psychotherapy*. New York: Holt, Rinehart & Winston.

Lynn, S. J., & Kirsch, I. (2006). *Essentials of clinical hypnosis*. Washington, DC: American Psychological Association.

McReynolds, W. T., & Paulsen, B. K. (1976). Stimulus control as the behavioral basis of weight loss procedures. In G. J. Williams, S. Martin, & J. Foreyt (Eds.), *Obesity: Behavioral approaches to dietary management* (pp. 78–93). New York: Brunner/Mazel.

Mueser, K. T., & Glynn, S. M. (1995). *Behavioral family therapy for psychiatric disorders*. Needham Heights, MA: Allyn & Bacon.

Nash, M. R., & Barnier, A. (2008). *The Oxford handbook of hypnosis: Theory, research, and practice*. New York: Oxford University Press.

Norcross, J. C., & Goldfried, M. R. (Eds.). (2005). *Handbook of psychotherapy integration*. (2nd ed.). New York: Basic Books.

Norcross, J. C., & Newman, C. F. (1992). Psychotherapy integration: Setting the context. In J. C. Norcross & M. R. Goldfried (Eds.). *Handbook of psychotherapy integration* (pp. 3–45). New York: Basic Books.

O'Donohue, W., Fisher, J. E., & Hayes, S. C. (Eds.). (2003). *Cognitive behavior therapy: Applying empirically supported techniques in your practice*. New York: Wiley.

Palmer, S. (1993). *Multimodal techniques: Relaxation and hypnosis*. London: The Centre for Multimodal Therapy.

Paul, G. L. (1967). Strategy of outcome research in psychotherapy. *Journal of Consulting Psychology, 31*, 109–118.

Rosen, R. C., & Leiblum, S. R. (Eds.). (1995). *Case studies in sex therapy*. New York: Guilford Press.

Rotter, J. B. (1954). *Social learning and clinical psychology*. New Jersey: Prentice-Hall.

Schoenberger, N. E., Kirsch, I., Gearan, P., Montgomery, G., & Pastyrnak, S. L. (1997). Hypnotic enhancement of a cognitive–behavioral treatment for public speaking anxiety. *Behavior Therapy, 28*, 127–140.

Sherman, A. R., Mulac, A., & McCann, M. S. (1974). Synergistic effect of self-relaxation and rehearsal feedback in the treatment of subjective and behavioral dimensions of speech anxiety. *Journal of Consulting and Clinical Psychology, 42*, 819–827.

Telch, M. J., & Lucas, R. A. (1994). Combined pharmacological and psychological treatment of panic disorder: Current status and future directions. In B. E. Wolfe & J. D. Maser (Eds.), *Treatment of panic disorder* (pp. 177–197). Washington, DC: American Psychiatric Press.

Williams, T. A. (1988). *A multimodal approach to assessment and intervention with children with learning disabilities*. Unpublished doctoral dissertation, University of Glasgow, Scotland.

Wilson, G. T. (1995). Empirically validated treatments as a basis for clinical practice: Problems and prospects. In S. C. Hayes, V. M. Follette, T. Risley, R. D. Dawes, & K. Grady (Eds.), *Scientific standards of psychological practice: Issues and recommendations* (pp. 163–196). Reno, NV: Context Press.

Wolpe, J. (1958). *Psychotherapy by reciprocal inhibition*. Stanford, CA: Stanford University Press.

Wolpe, J., & Lazarus, A. A. (1966). *Behavior therapy techniques*. Oxford, England: Pergamon Press.

Zilbergeld, B., & Lazarus, A. A. (1988). *Mind power*. New York: Ivy Books.

III

HYPNOTIC TECHNIQUES

10

HYPNOTIC INDUCTIONS: A PRIMER

DON E. GIBBONS AND STEVEN JAY LYNN

Hypnotic inductions are etched into the public consciousness as a defining feature of hypnosis. Historically, a panoply of inductions have been incorporated into hypnotic procedures. Whether the induction has involved clanging gongs; eye fixation on objects such as a moving watch, as popularized in the media; flashing lights; applying pressure to subjects' heads; suggesting relaxation; or suggesting alertness, all inductions share a common feature: They define as *hypnosis* the interaction between the person administering suggestions and the person receiving suggestions, and, in clinical contexts, they typically precede therapeutic suggestions tailored to the client's needs and goals.

Wagstaff (1998) noted that an induction represents a suggestion for participants to enter a hypnotic state. According to this perspective, an *induction* can be defined as any procedure the therapist presents or labels *hypnosis*, which is intended to increase participants' responsiveness to subsequent suggestions. Practitioners use a broad array of inductions, limited only by their creativity. Successful hypnotic inductions foster positive expectations that participants will be able to experience suggestions for changes in thoughts,

We gratefully acknowledge Lynn Hornyak's many thoughtful and important contributions to this chapter.

feelings, behaviors, sensations, perceptions, and memories. Typical inductions are worded so as to direct attention inward, to reduce vigilance, and to diminish the importance of self-directed action. Lynn, Kirsch, and Hallquist (2008) contended that the focus of some inductions on passive or receptive mental states, such as sleep and relaxation, discourages individuals from adopting an analytical attitude and searching for the causes of behaviors outside the hypnotic context. Even when inductions emphasize alertness, the fact that the hypnotist supplies the directions for action implies that the client need not make active choices or judgments.

Clients can experience an altered state when the induction focuses awareness on concrete images, sensations, and behaviors, which diminishes abstract, logical, and self-referential thinking (Field, 1979). Inductions often include direct suggestions for profound changes in consciousness and physical sensations, so it is not surprising that some people report that they experienced an "altered state" during hypnosis. Still, the majority of people who experience hypnosis describe their experiences more in terms of focused attention than a "trance" state (McConkey, 1986). However people construe their experience of hypnosis, the induction provides a powerful context for personal change, allowing clients to generate experiences and exhibit responses they may not realize they are capable of making.

In this chapter we outline a typical hypnotherapy session, with particular focus on the procedures and methods of several hypnotic induction techniques, such as progressive relaxation, eye fixation, and the "empty bucket" technique. We also make recommendations for using hypnosis with children or other clients who may be resistant to typical inductions. We discuss the later stages of the session, including posthypnotic suggestions, possible aftereffects of induction, and concluding the hypnosis session. We conclude the chapter with a discussion of research on different induction techniques.

PREINDUCTION PROCEDURES: PAVING THE WAY

The first hypnosis session often begins with a *preinduction talk*. Whether clients will experience specific suggestions depends, to a considerable extent, on their motives, expectations, and beliefs, as well as their trust and confidence in the therapist (Lynn, Kirsch, & Rhue, 1996). Accordingly, preliminary discussion with clients concerning the nature of the experiences they are about to undergo is equally important, if not more important, than the induction itself. The therapist's preinduction talk serves as a vehicle to educate clients about the empirical foundations of hypnosis and to counter misconceptions and myths about hypnosis popularized by the media that would interfere with therapy. Accordingly, misconceptions should be identified and addressed before any formal induction is administered or therapeutic suggestions are provided to the client.

If the client has experienced hypnosis on a prior occasion, the therapist may inquire about these experiences, both to determine whether there are any misunderstandings that need to be cleared up and to get an idea of how well the client is likely to respond and which induction procedure might be likely to produce the best results. Another useful means of evaluating clients' misconceptions is to ask whether they have any questions about hypnosis. Questions should be addressed with reference to the now substantial research base on hypnosis and suggestibility (see Lynn & Kirsch, 2006). Therapists should have a "mental checklist" of common myths and misconceptions about hypnosis that they are prepared to address. This will help therapists ensure they do not initiate hypnosis before clients are disabused of culturally prevalent, yet mistaken, beliefs about hypnosis.

What are the most common misconceptions clients entertain? Many people believe that hypnosis is something that is done to them rather than something they experience in their highly personal, unique way. They think that hypnotized people lose control of themselves and can be made to do or say whatever the hypnotist wants. They think that they will feel as if they had taken a powerful drug, and they may fear that they will not be able to come out of a radically altered state that has been imposed on them. Some clients believe that subjects who have been hypnotized are unable to remember what transpired. Less common misconceptions include the idea that only weak-willed people are capable of being hypnotized and that hypnosis can transform people into automatons (see Lynn, Neufeld, & Mare, 1993).

To counter such beliefs, clients may be told, "During hypnosis, you still have your own personality, and you're still you. Research shows that you can easily refuse to respond to any suggestion that you don't want to accept; that's why we call them 'suggestions.'" Clients may need to know that they will not reveal any intimate secrets they do not wish to disclose. To allay fears that they may not "come out of hypnosis," the therapist may tell clients, "Sometimes you might not want a movie to end, because it is so enjoyable, but you still come back to everyday life when the session is over, just like you return to everyday life at the end of a movie." Unless amnesia is deemed a useful part of the therapeutic experience, it may contribute to the development of trust and rapport to inform clients as follows that this is not likely to occur: "You will remain completely conscious and aware of everything that's going on, and you will remember most everything that happened when the session is over. As in everyday life, we may forget a few details, but you won't forget anything that's important."

To counter the widely held misconception that hypnosis is something the therapist "does to" a client to bring about a desired result, it may be helpful to describe the therapist's role as similar to that of a coach or a personal trainer. Other clients prefer an explanation of the therapist's role as akin to an Eastern guru who shows a student how to explore new levels of awareness and how to focus and direct thoughts and experiences to facilitate constructive life changes. To highlight the important role of motivation, the therapist can point out that hypnosis is a process that makes change easier, but the client still has to want to change and be ready to do so.

The prehypnotic talk should also include a brief preview of the induction procedure to identify suggestions the client might find threatening or objectionable and to select desirable imagery to accompany the induction. One client, for example, was told, "I'm going to ask you to visualize yourself sinking down in a soft, pink cloud while I count from 1 to 10." The client replied, "Because I'm a pilot, I can't picture myself sinking down into a cloud. That means rough weather; that's turbulence!" The therapist then used the comforting imagery of relaxing on the beach, and the client responded well.

If clients continue to remain dubious as to whether they will respond successfully, they should be encouraged to try hypnosis anyway. Many people are surprised to discover that they respond to suggestions even though they doubted their ability to do so. The therapist might say something along the following lines: "We all have the ability to use our minds in ways of which we are not usually aware. We may have the ability to wake up at the same time each morning, despite the changes of the seasons; some of us have developed these abilities more than others." It has also proven helpful to point out that the experience of hypnosis is similar to such common experiences as when one becomes so involved in watching a motion picture or a television drama that he or she feels like a part of the action instead of part of the audience: "If you just allow your thoughts to respond freely to the words and images that guide you into these experiences, you'll be able to go wherever your mind can take you."

Research indicates that therapists would do well to define successful responding to suggestions as requiring cooperation and involvement in what is suggested, rather than achieving a trance state (Lynn, Vanderhoff, Shindler, & Stafford, 2002). If participants question whether they have achieved such a state, it may dampen their expectations and conviction that they are responding successfully and diminish their overall responsiveness. Also, many people without prior experience of hypnosis are afraid of the idea of going into a trance and actively resist responding to suggestions (Lynn & Kirsch, 2006). Some clients benefit from demonstrating that they can easily respond to nonhypnotic suggestions, for example, to perceive one's arm growing heavy or to imagine a force attracting or repelling their hands.

Prior to the induction, reasonable care should be taken to avoid the possibility that the session might be interrupted. Clients should be asked to turn off their cell phone if they are carrying one and assume a comfortable position, sitting or reclining, as if preparing to take a nap. Just as the effect of a song is enhanced by the proper volume and rhythm, the therapist may facilitate the effect of an induction by adopting a speaking style consistent with cultural preconceptions of a hypnotic induction. For example, it is often helpful if the therapist uses a slow, measured cadence, with considerable repetition and elaboration, far beyond the point of what would be considered boring in ordinary conversation. As the induction proceeds, careful attention should be paid to the client's breathing, posture, facial expression, facial coloring, and general muscle tone to obtain feedback as to how the suggestions should be worded and paced.

METHODS OF INDUCTION

Sometimes an induction may be read from a script after the prehypnotic talk, when the client is comfortably seated or reclining with eyes closed, prepared for the session to begin. Strict adherence to a script, however, does not provide for much flexibility to contend with individual variations in responsiveness. For example, if the client begins to breathe slowly and deeply, the therapist might say, "You are beginning to breathe slowly and deeply now as you continue to go deeper," returning to this theme occasionally as the induction proceeds. However, if the client begins to appear uncomfortable because of the position in which he or she is sitting, the therapist may state, as if it were part of the induction itself, "You can shift your position if you want to make yourself more comfortable." If the client shows actual signs of distress during the induction, the therapist may smoothly terminate the proceedings by stating that at the count of three the client's eyes will open and he or she will be back in the normal, everyday frame of mind. Many times, the client is able to supply the reason if asked what seemed to be the source of the difficulty. Perhaps, for example, the client may have been reminded of a childhood incident in which he or she almost drowned. Sometimes recognition of the differences between the past and the present situation may be all that is necessary for the induction to proceed. However, if the situation cannot be quickly and easily resolved, and if the client does not feel comfortable in continuing, then the session should, of course, be terminated.

The examples that follow illustrate some of the ways suggestions may be used to reframe information provided by imagery and sensory feedback. This helps to bolster the conviction that client's mental processes are beginning to function differently, which in turn legitimizes behaviors and modes of perception commonly considered hypnotic.

Progressive Relaxation

Induction suggestions are frequently presented serially, and in this way acceptance of earlier suggestions facilitates the acceptance of later ones as a means of compounding the conviction that the client is experiencing hypnosis. For example, in the induction that follows, the therapist begins by talking about relaxation in various parts of the body: "Just think of your arms relaxing and your legs relaxing." Then the therapist comments about the ability to experience relaxation: "You can feel a heavy, relaxed feeling throughout your body." This statement is followed by suggestions that the relaxation is deepening and then that the relaxation is carrying the client deeper and deeper into hypnosis. Finally, the therapist begins to speak as if the client were indeed "in hypnosis," which may or may not be stated explicitly. If the client has affirmed that it would be pleasant to imagine relaxing on the beach, the induction may proceed along the following lines:

> Now, with your eyes closed, imagine that you are sitting or lying on a sandy beach, by the side of the ocean. So just picture the scene, and imagine yourself resting there, on that sandy beach by the side of the ocean. You can hear the sound of gulls in the distance and the gentle waves breaking upon the shore. You can smell the freshness of the pure salt air. Feel the warmth of the sand beneath your blanket and the cool ocean breeze blowing softly across your skin and the warm sun shining down, with the temperature just right to make you relaxed and drowsy. It's so calm and so peaceful there, that all you want to do is just let yourself go and begin to drift into a deep, comfortable, relaxing hypnosis. You can feel yourself relaxing now in that warm sunlight, there by the side of the ocean. You can feel a gentle relaxed feeling coming over your entire body. Just think of your arms relaxing and your legs relaxing and your entire body relaxing all over as the gentle sunlight feels like it's warming you through and through. I'm going to count from 1 to 10, and by the time I get to the count of 10 you will be resting comfortably in a deep, peaceful hypnotic state. So just continue to relax, and listen to my voice, as I begin the count from 1 to 10. One. You can feel that relaxed feeling growing stronger now, as you can feel your entire body relaxing more and more and more. Two. You can feel a heavy, relaxed feeling coming over you. And with each count that heavy, relaxed feeling is going to grow and grow until it causes you to fall into a deep, peaceful state of hypnosis. Three. That heavy, relaxed feeling is growing stronger and stronger with each moment that passes and with each word that I speak. Soon, you will be resting comfortably in a deep, peaceful hypnotic state. Four. You are relaxing very deeply now. Relaxing so very, very deeply that you can just let yourself go and begin to drift down and down, deeper and deeper, into a very deep, relaxing state of hypnosis. Five. Every word that

I speak is carrying you deeper and deeper. Deeper and deeper, down and down, into a deep, relaxing hypnotic state. And by the time I get to the count of ten, you will be deeply hypnotized. Six. Deeper and deeper now. And the deeper you go, the more relaxing and the more enjoyable the experience becomes. So just let yourself go completely now as you continue to drift, down and down, down and down, into a deep, peaceful, relaxing experience of hypnosis. Seven. Deeper yet. Deeper and deeper, down and down. Eight. Going very rapidly into a deep, sound hypnosis now. Into a deep, sound hypnosis. Nine. Very deeply drifting into a deep, sound hypnosis, a deep, sound experience of hypnosis. Ten. Very deeply drifting, in a deep, sound hypnosis and continuing to go deeper and deeper with each passing moment.

At this point, it is usually helpful to use a "deepening" procedure, which is described at the end of this section, to increase the client's involvement with the conviction that he or she is now deeply hypnotized.

Eye Fixation

In this type of induction, clients are asked to stare at an object, such as their thumb or a spot on the wall or the ceiling. If the chosen object is slightly above normal eye level, the naturally occurring eye fatigue that results will facilitate the therapist's suggestions of eye closure. The therapist begins the induction with suggestions such as,

Your eyes are getting heavy and tired now. You can feel your eyes becoming heavy and tired. Any moment now, your eyes will close. They are closing, closing. Now your eyes are completely closed, and you are drifting very rapidly into a deep state of hypnosis.

Naturally, the wording and content of the suggestions, and the time taken to provide them, are guided by the client's responsiveness as the eyes begin to close in response to both suggestions and the naturally occurring fatigue from staring at the fixation object.

Inductions Using Kinesthetic Imagery

The *empty bucket technique* is a procedure that may stand on its own as an induction or may serve as a backup induction if the initial one appears to be ineffective. One client, for example, opened her eyes and sat up before the progressive relaxation induction could be concluded, stating, "I'm just not very good at using imagery," despite the fact that she had previously indicated that she would have no trouble picturing herself relaxing on the beach. "That's all right," the therapist said without pausing, "Just stretch your right arm out in front of you and close your eyes again." When this had been done, the therapist asked her to imagine that she was holding a bucket in her outstretched hand. The therapist then suggested,

> Now I've poured a gallon of water into the bucket, and your arm is beginning to sink down. Your arm is getting heavier and heavier, and soon it will sink down and touch your leg or touch the chair, and you will immediately sink into deep hypnosis.

The client's arm did not move as the therapist continued to suggest that he was pouring more and more water into the bucket and that her arm was getting heavier and heavier and beginning to sink down. Slowly, however, she drew her arm back so that her upper arm was braced against her side and only her forearm was extended. At the same time, the therapist noticed that the pulse in her neck appeared to be quite strong and that her eyelids were fluttering. The therapist then began a series of suggestions leading to eyelid catalepsy, which can be used as a postinduction test of responsiveness:

> Your eyelids are beginning to flutter now, and they are becoming tightly closed together. I'm going to count to three, and at the count of three, your eyelids will be stuck together so tightly that you cannot open them no matter how hard you try. But don't try yet; just listen to my voice as I begin the count from one to three. One. Your eyelids are becoming stuck together now, tighter and tighter. Two. Your eyelids are becoming stuck together, glued together, tighter and tighter, and by the time I get to the count of three, you will not be able to open them no matter how hard you try. And the harder you try to open them, the harder it will be to do so. Three. You can try, but you cannot open your eyes. Try as you might, it's impossible. Now I'm going to count from one to five, and by the count of five you will be much deeper than you are right now.

The therapist then proceeded to count and provide suggestions of deepening the experience of hypnosis (but without using imagery); with this "save," the therapeutic suggestions could begin.

The *arm-levitation procedure* is in many ways the opposite of the induction just described. After the client is comfortably seated with eyes closed in preparation for the induction to begin, the client is asked to imagine a balloon tied to his or her left wrist. The therapist then continues as follows:

> As I continue to speak, the balloon is going to pull on your wrist, more and more, until it causes your wrist to rise from your lap. You can feel it beginning to tug now, tugging more and more. (*as the wrist begins to rise*) Now your wrist is rising up, and your forearm is rising up, and soon your arm will have risen all the way up into the air. (*when this is accomplished*) Now it is pulling your arm higher and higher until your arm will soon be stretched straight out in front of you. And when it is, I will cut the string

and your arm will fall back into your lap. Almost ready. Now I've cut the string and your arm is falling back naturally into your lap, and you experience a much deeper state of hypnosis than you are in right now.

One advantage of this procedure and the preceding one is that they allow the therapist to calibrate suggestions to the client's response. If the wrist is slow to rise, the therapist can proceed more slowly and use more repetition until the client's wrist has completely risen off his or her lap. Thus, the therapist's suggestions move apace with the client's movements.

Lynn, Kirsch, and Rhue (1996) proposed using a *fail-safe induction* that uses a combination of arm-levitation and arm-heaviness suggestions that can be given before a more formal induction of hypnosis, in the context of relaxation or "creative imagination," or as incorporated into an induction. The therapist might say the following:

> You may notice that one of your arms is just a bit lighter than the other, and your other arm is heavier. As we talk, your light arm may become even lighter or your heavy arm may become even heavier. And I wonder just how light your lighter arm will feel and how heavy the other arm will feel. Will your light arm become so light that it lifts up into the air all by itself, or will your heavy arm become so heavy that it stays rooted to the arm of your chair? And I wonder which arm feels lighter. Is it your right arm or your left arm? And where do you feel the lightness most? In your wrist, or in your fingers? In all of your fingers, or especially in one of them? (p. 15)

Overt signs of upward movement in one hand or arm provide a signal to focus on suggestions for arm levitation. Otherwise, these are abandoned and suggestions for arm heaviness and immobility are stressed. This method can prevent perceptions of failure, maintain therapeutic rapport, and provide some indication of the client's level of responsiveness. If the client is not able to generate responses of either arm lightness or heaviness, it may indicate the presence of recalcitrant negative beliefs and attitudes, which may preclude using hypnosis as a treatment modality (Lynn, Kirsch, & Rhue, 1996).

EXPANDING ON INDUCTION METHODS: ALERT AND MULTIMODAL APPROACHES

Hypnotic inductions often include suggestions that call for increased alertness as well as relaxation-based and ideomotor (i.e., movement-oriented) suggestions, as we have described (see chap. 11 for a discussion of waking hypnosis). The goal of many hypnotic suggestions is to enhance and modify experience. The term *hyperempiria* (literally, "enhanced experience") has previously been used to refer to an increase in suggestibility in response to inductions based on suggestions for alertness, mind expansion, and increased sensitivity (Gibbons, 1973, 1974). Alert inductions have been found to be as effective as traditional sleepy/drowsy inductions in facilitating subsequent responsiveness to suggestion (Bányai & Hilgard, 1976; Gibbons, 1975, 1976). Such procedures have been referred to as *alert hypnosis* (Bányai & Hilgard).

Suggestions for enhanced alert experience can be presented in the context of relaxation–sleepy/drowsy suggestions, or clinicians may prefer to use the term *hyperempiria* in place of hypnosis to circumvent misconceptions associated with the popular view of hypnosis as a sleeplike state. It is possible to tell clients something such as, "You might associate hypnosis with suggestions such as, 'You are going into a deep, sound sleep.' But in hyperempiria, you're awake and alert the whole time. It's interesting and enjoyable, and you can get a lot out of it." The therapist can then use a wide variety of inductions while continuing to refer to hyperempiria as an enjoyable and effective alternative; in effect, creating such a perception as a form of self-fulfilling prophecy (Barber, 1985). Given the inherent flexibility of hypnotic interventions, inductions can contain a mix of hyperempiric and relaxation-based or even sleepy/drowsy suggestions.

Induction for Children

The following induction can be presented with suggestions for feeling alert and wide awake (i.e., hyperempiric) or following suggestions that emphasize relaxation. The induction is based on a fairy tale format and was originally written for children. However, it also appeals to some college students and may resonate with the childlike imagination in all of us, which is often the key to responding well to suggestions.

> Just sit back, and close your eyes, and I am going to tell you a magic story. It is a story about a very special place, deep in an enchanted forest, where everything I tell you will come true. Imagine now that we are walking together down a long, winding path, which runs through the middle of a large wood. We are walking along early on a bright spring morning. Birds are singing in the trees, and here and there a flower is poking its head out of the soft, green grass, which grows beside the path. And because this is a magic story, the farther we go along the path, the more real everything around us becomes. Now and then a ray of sunlight makes its way down through the branches of the trees and falls upon the dewdrops in the grass, causing them to sparkle like a million tiny diamonds. The air is fresh and cool, with gentle breezes blowing now and then, causing the trees and the grass and the flowers to move ever so slightly, as if everything in the world were feeling so happy on this bright spring morning, that nothing could keep still for very long. And because this is a magic story, the farther we go along the path, the more real everything becomes. As we continue on our walk, we can begin to be aware of the sound of

rushing water. With each passing second, the sound is becoming clearer and clearer still. And now we are standing beside the bank of a forest stream, which is the source of the sound we have been hearing. The water is flowing past us swift and clear, for it has come tumbling down from a magic spring many miles away in the hills. And because the water from the magic spring is enchanted, anyone who drinks it will be enchanted too. And anyone who is enchanted in this way will be easily able to find that special place, deep in the magic forest, where everything I say will come true. We dip our hands eagerly into the bubbling stream and cup them together, bringing the cool, fresh water up to our lips again and again, until we have drunk all that we want. Now it is time to hurry on our way once more, for the water from the magic spring has made it certain that we will soon find that very special place in the enchanted forest where everything I tell you will come true, and we know now that it cannot be far away. As we continue on our journey, we notice a tiny path leading off to one side, and we decide to go up this path to see where it leads. Before very long, we notice that the woods are beginning to thin out and that we are about to enter a clearing. And as we approach nearer and nearer to the edge of the clearing, we can see that the path we have been following leads right up to a small cottage. This is that very special place I have been telling you about, where everything will come true. For as long as we stay here, in this enchanted cottage in the enchanted forest, even my words will be enchanted, and everything I tell you will happen exactly as I say it will. The door to the cottage is standing slightly open as we hurry up the path, and as soon as we reach the entrance, we hurry on inside in order to lose no more time. We have arrived now at that very special enchanted place in the enchanted forest, which we have traveled so far to reach. And as long as we remain here, in this enchanted cottage, everything I say and everything I describe to you will come true as soon as I have said it. For as long as we remain here in this enchanted place, even my words will be enchanted. (Gibbons, 1979, pp. 39–41)

Multimodal Induction

Hypnotic inductions often focus on and access multiple modalities, just as psychotherapeutic approaches, such as those championed by Arnold Lazarus (see chap. 9, this volume), systematically address multiple experiential modalities. Multimodal suggestion uses suggested changes in Belief systems, Expectations, Sensations and perceptions, Thoughts and images, Motives, and Emotions, and therefore may be referred to by the acronym, BEST ME (Gibbons, 1999, 2001). BEST ME suggestions may be presented in any order and repeated with appropriate variations in content. Each suggestion may contain elements of the others, in which case the label applied to describe the modality refers to the element given the greatest emphasis (Gibbons, 2004).

Multimodal suggestions may be used in an induction procedure in the formulation of therapeutic suggestions and in the conclusion of the hypnotic or hyperempiric session (Gibbons, 2004, 2005). Multimodal suggestions in inductions may be worded so as to emphasize one or more categories (e.g., beliefs, sensations), according to the experiential orientation of each participant. Some clients appear to enjoy the individualized approach afforded by the use of a comprehensive multimodal induction tailored to their experiential style. In the multimodal hyperempiric induction that follows, the suggestions emphasize positive emotion. Differently constructed inductions might emphasize other experiential elements, such as imagery or sensations.

> I am going to show you how to focus and concentrate your mind, in a manner that allows your imagination to immediately translate spoken words into thought, feeling, and experience. [*Belief systems*]
>
> First, picture yourself resting comfortably in a safe, outdoor setting, such as a mountainside besides a gently flowing brook, an isolated beach, or a warm, spring meadow. [*Sensations and physical perceptions*]
>
> Just picture the scene, and imagine yourself resting there, waiting for your journey to begin. You will be completely free to talk to me anytime you want to as we plan and explore together new dimensions of reality and of meaning, which will benefit your life in many different ways. [*Expectations*]
>
> It feels like a perfect day for a journey such as this. Just take a moment to let yourself feel the warm sun shining down, to listen to the song of birds in the distance, and to feel the gentle breeze on your skin. [*Sensations and physical perceptions*]
>
> You feel as if you could not have picked a better time or a more perfect spot for your journey, and you are eager to get started. [*Motives*]
>
> You will always be able to hear and to respond to my voice, and you will return to the time and place from which you left when your session is completed. [*Expectations*] But until then, every detail of the situations to which I guide you will become completely real, and you will soon be able to experience them all just as if you were really there.
>
> Now, as your consciousness begins to expand, you can feel waves of happiness and joy slowly flowing out from the innermost depths of your being, like water from a hundred secret springs. [*Emotions*]
>
> With each passing moment, you can feel your awareness expanding more and more, filling you with wonder and making your imagination soar. [*Sensations and physical perceptions*]
>
> It's a wonderful feeling of release and liberation you are experiencing now in many different ways and on many different levels, as your consciousness is becoming freed for its highest possible functioning. [*Thoughts and images*]
>
> Believe it will happen, expect it to happen, and feel it happening, and you will be able to go wherever your mind can take you. [*Expectations*]

DEEPENING OR HEIGHTENING TECHNIQUES

During, and especially at the conclusion of an induction, it is often useful to provide deepening or, in the case of hyperempiria, heightening suggestions to increase the clients' involvement with the idea that they are experiencing their consciousness in a different manner. If counting is used in a hypnotic induction procedure, for example, deepening can be as simple as continuing the count beyond ten, as the therapist might have initially specified, and providing additional suggestions that by the count of fifteen, the client will "go even deeper."

Additional imagery may also be used, such as going down a staircase as the therapist counts the steps, suggesting that the client will go deeper into hypnosis with each step, or going deeper into hypnosis as each wave rolls onto the shore. Analogous procedures, such as descending on an elevator or escalator or going deeper into hypnosis as an arm becomes heavy and moves downward, may be used to heighten clients' involvement with the suggestion that they are experiencing hypnosis. Alternately, simple instructions for becoming more deeply hypnotized as comfort or calmness spreads or with each breath will generally suffice.

Because the purpose of a deepening or heightening procedure is to further clients' involvement with the suggestion that their mental processes are beginning to function differently, virtually any hypnotic procedure may be used as a deepening procedure, and any of the aforementioned deepening procedures may be used as an induction. Some clients with previous experience in hypnosis may benefit from first going "down" into hypnosis and then "up" into hyperempiria. The following example provided by Lynne Hornyak (personal communication, March 15, 2009) combines breathing and muscle relaxation deepening with safe place imagery, frequently used in hypnotic inductions.

> As your body floats, you can relax more and more, moving deeper and deeper, relaxing deeper with each breath you exhale. If there are any sounds in the background, they can just be there and then gradually fade away as you tune in more and more to the rhythm of your breathing, the small shifts in your muscles that add to your sense of comfort as you drift, comfortably, easily, moving into the territory of your own private experience. [*Breathing focus*]
>
> Eyes relaxed, the muscles of your face softening, smoothing out, jaw comfortably relaxed, shoulders easing, arms limp and loose, chest relaxed, the muscles of your back easing and letting go, abdomen soft and easy, legs loose and comfortable, your mind as relaxed as your body. [*Muscle relaxation*]
>
> Imagine being on a path, a very inviting path, which will lead you to a place of safety and security, a very comfortable, special, safe place. Counting from 1 to 20 you can take steps along that path, feeling more

comfortable, relaxed, and secure with each step you take. [*Intersperse numbers with suggestions for comfort and relaxation.*] 1. Stepping along the path. . . . 2. Feeling more comfortable. . . . 3. Becoming more relaxed with each step. . . . 4. And with each step you take going farther, farther along the path, each step will serve as a cue to relax even more. . . . 5. Looking forward to reaching your special place. . . . 6 . . . 7. Feeling more relaxed. . . . 8. Moving along the path. . . . 9. Easy and comfortable. . . . 10 . . . 11 . . . 12 . . . 13. Becoming more relaxed with each step, closer to reaching your safe, special place. . . . 14. Feeling more and more comfortable. . . . 15 . . . 16 . . . 17. So completely relaxed. . . . 18. Soon to be there. . . . 19 . . . 20. [*Path*]

You've arrived. Take some time to explore your special place. It is safe, secure. It may be a place that you've actually been before or some place that you create right now in your mind. As you look around you, notice the details of your special place, see what's there. Notice the shapes and colors, the sounds, the smells. Or, you may not be seeing any detail; you just know that you are there. Whatever you are experiencing is just fine. And you can notice how you feel just a bit more "there," more absorbed in the comfort of your special place with each breath you take.

SELF-HYPNOSIS

Most hypnosuggestive procedures can be truthfully defined as self-hypnosis (Barber, 1985; Orne & McConkey, 1981; Sanders, 1991). Ultimately, patients are responsible for generating suggestion-relevant imagery, experiences, and behaviors. By teaching patients to orchestrate their experience of hypnosis, it is possible for them to practice implementing hypnotic techniques in many real-life situations and to take credit for the success they achieve. Other advantages of defining procedures as self-hypnosis include bypassing resistances and fears associated with being under the control of another, fear of being unaware or unconscious, fear of revealing secrets, and fear of not coming out of trance (Lynn & Kirsch, 2006).

Self-hypnosis is most frequently taught by first introducing the patient to traditional (i.e., heterohypnotic) techniques and then encouraging the patient to assume increasingly greater responsibility for devising suggestions appropriate to achieving treatment goals (Hammond, 1992; Lynn, Kirsch, & Rhue, 1996). This can be done as follows:

> Remember how you learned to ride a bike? If you were like me, at first you might have wondered whether you could do it. Whether you could experience the pleasure of riding a bike, coasting along, feeling the gentle wind. And after a while, you learned that you could do it. And you were able to just get up on the seat and ride and feel the wind in your hair and

the pleasure of moving along, at your own pace, going in a direction of your choice. And didn't it become easier and easier, so that after a while, you didn't even have to think about staying in control, but you knew that you were in control of where you went and how you got there? And, you know, it's the same thing with hypnosis. You do it; you go in a direction of your own choosing. You decide whether to respond or not, to cooperate or not, to imagine or not, to try to make the suggestion seem real. And it gets easier and easier, just like riding a bike. After we practice with me giving you suggestions at first, you'll realize that all hypnosis is self-hypnosis. You make it happen; you create the experiences for yourself. I can't do it for you. And you, too, can devise helpful suggestions tailored just for you, made just for you, by you. I can help if you like, but you can do it too. After all, you know yourself even better than I know you. But for now, just relax, settle in, and I'll give you some suggestions that you can make seem real, real to you, in your own mind, in your own way, as we discussed when I introduced the idea of hypnosis to you. And after that, after you experience hypnosis for yourself, you can begin to generate suggestions of your own, suggestions that can and will help you to achieve your goals, just for you, your suggestions. Not mine, but yours. And we can work together too to devise suggestions, and these suggestions can be "ours." (Lynn & Kirsch, 2006, p. 61–62)

Within this framework, we encourage clients to write down clear, specific suggestions (e.g., how they would like to think, feel, and act in a given situation and in general) and develop scripts consistent with their goals that can be incorporated into self-hypnosis sessions and their everyday lives. Therapists can include the material on 10- to 20-minute tapes that can be played on a regular or as-needed basis before the client experiences self-hypnosis. After a period of experimenting and discovering what suggestions work best, shorter, more focused and customized tapes can be made, recorded in the client's or the therapist's voice, as the client prefers. In either case, clients should be encouraged to integrate helpful suggestions into their internal dialogue or "self-talk" on a routine basis (Lynn & Kirsch, 2006).

THE EXPERIENTIALLY GIFTED CLIENT

As a general rule, the more responsive a client is to suggestion, the less detail is required for an induction to achieve the necessary threshold of plausibility and the less need there is for deepening or heightening techniques. Some high-responders exhibit behavioral signs of being hypnotized almost immediately during their first induction, as indicated by their observable movements and compliance with suggestions, including breathing, posture, and general body language consistent with what is suggested. Other clients exhibit signs of being hypnotized earlier than would be expected during the course of an induction, after only one or two previous full-length inductions. For clients who quickly and easily experience hypnotic suggestions, it is usually possible to use a shortened induction procedure with satisfactory results.

THE DIFFICULT OR "RESISTANT" CLIENT

Many times an initially "resistant" client may experience success if a so-called *challenge item*, such as eyelid catalepsy, which we described previously, or arm catalepsy, is used, as in the following example. One client, at the conclusion of an induction procedure, remained seated with her eyes closed and spontaneously remarked, "Oh, it isn't going to work." Understanding the client's motivational style the therapist responded in a confident tone, "Oh yes it is, and I'll show you. I'm just going to stretch your right arm out straight in front of you, and you hold it out there by yourself after I have done so." Once the client's arm had been extended, the therapist continued, speaking rapidly and in an authoritative tone:

> I'm going to count from one to three, and at the count of three, your arm will be just as rigid as an iron bar. One. You can feel the muscles in your right arm becoming tighter and tighter now. Your right arm is becoming stiff and rigid. And by the time I get to the count of three, your right arm will be as rigid as an iron bar, and you won't be able to bend it at the elbow no matter how hard you try. Two. It's becoming as rigid as an iron bar now, and by the time I get to the count of three, you won't be able to bend it at the elbow until I touch it, no matter how hard you try. Three. Try, but you cannot do so, and the harder you try to bend your arm, the harder it becomes.

A broad smile crossed the client's face as she remained motionless, her arm outstretched. After waiting for only a second or two, the therapist concluded, "Now, and only now as I touch it, can your arm return to normal and sink down, becoming completely normal again. Now your arm is completely normal once more." Then, with the client convinced of the reality of her hypnotic experience, the therapeutic suggestions could proceed.

Challenge items, in which a person is momentarily willing to feel and act as if he is unable to perform a simple act such as bending his arm or opening his eyes, are no longer routinely used with everyone as a measure of the effectiveness of an induction, except under special circumstances, as in the foregoing example. It is likely that many people who resist these challenge items will nevertheless be highly responsive to suggestions they themselves desire to be effective. If "nothing succeeds like success," it is also true that "nothing fails like failure" (A. K. Schreiber, personal communication, January 14, 2006).

THE NONRESPONSIVE CLIENT

The late Martin T. Orne (1927–2000) commented only partially in jest when he observed that in today's hectic culture, almost everybody could benefit from sitting quietly for a while with their eyes closed listening to the positive suggestions of a therapist. However, not all clients respond successfully to hypnotic suggestions: 15% to 25% of clients will respond minimally to suggestions for a variety of reasons. Some individuals have little imagery ability or harbor fears of being controlled despite efforts to disabuse them of this belief regarding hypnosis. Other individuals are concerned about relinquishing long-standing and familiar, yet counterproductive, symptoms or behaviors. Accordingly, hypnosis may not be a treatment of choice for some people, no matter how much they may desire it or how much benefit they might potentially reap from it. Beginning therapists should not be discouraged, therefore, if they encounter one or two clients who do not respond to their induction procedures. It is generally agreed that no unique talent is required to use hypnosis as a treatment modality. If the therapist has presented the induction suggestions in a sufficiently plausible manner, the result is usually much more the responsibility of the client than it is of the therapist. But for every client who responds poorly, one is statistically certain to find one who responds so well that perseverance in using hypnotic techniques will be amply rewarded.

CONCLUDING THE SESSION

Before ending the initial hypnosis session, it may be useful to prepare the client for subsequent sessions so that the time required for inducing hypnosis can be shortened. Kirsch, Lynn, and Rhue (1993) suggest that this can be accomplished in two ways. First, clients can be given the positive suggestion that hypnosis becomes easier to experience with practice so that each time they experience hypnosis, they will find it easier and easier to become hypnotized, and they will enter hypnosis more and more quickly. For example, the hypnotist might say, "The next time you are hypnotized [or experience hyperempiria], you will be able to go even deeper [or higher] than you did this time."

Second, a posthypnotic suggestion (i.e., a suggestion to have particular experiences or engage in specific behaviors after hypnosis is terminated) can be given, establishing a cue or signal for quickly becoming involved with the experience of hypnosis. For example,

> From now on, it is going to be very easy for you to become hypnotized when you want to. We are going to establish a cue that will allow you to become hypnotized instantly. We can use any word or phrase you like. I wonder if there is a particular word or phrase that can symbolize this experience for you or whether you prefer that I suggest the phrase. [*The client or therapist selects a phrase.*] Okay! From now on, the words "hypnosis now" will be a signal to enter hypnosis. But it will only work when I say those words and when you want to become hypnotized. When you want to enter hypnosis and I say the words "hypnosis now," you will immediately become deeply engrossed in the hypnotic experience. But it won't happen if someone else says those words. If you hear those words in normal conversation, they will have no effect at all. And it won't work if you do not wish to experience hypnosis. But if I say "hypnosis now," and if you are ready to be hypnotized, you will be able to enter hypnosis immediately.

In subsequent sessions, once the client is comfortable and indicates readiness to begin hypnosis, the therapist says "hypnosis now," either alone or embedded in a phrase, such as "You can enter hypnosis now," stressing the cue words so that the signal intent is not missed, with deepening suggestions administered as needed. In some cases, it is necessary to retain an induction, albeit a shorter one, if desired, to promote involvement in hypnosis and heighten the client's expectations regarding the benefits of therapeutic suggestions that follow. Before ending the hypnosis session, it may be helpful to provide suggestions for general well-being and pleasant imagery. This approach is especially useful if emotionally stressful work has been done during the session, but soothing suggestions can be included at other times as well to promote feelings of well-being and enhance the enjoyment of the hypnotic experience.

Ending a hypnosis session is even easier than inducing it. One can terminate hypnosis by simply telling the client to become alert now or that "you can become alert as soon as you are ready." But in most cases, there is no need for termination procedures to be abrupt. Instead, the transition from the communication patterns of hypnosis or hyperempiria to the patterns of everyday life should occur gradually to provide the client with an ongoing sense of assurance and support. Therapists should provide posthypnotic suggestions for the client to be fully alert and to easily be able to resume his or her everyday tasks afterward. The session itself should be described as a highly enjoyable experience with pleasant and cheerful feelings persisting throughout the day and night. The transition should also emphasize the benefits the client can derive from the experience, as in the following example:

> I'm going to count backward from five to one, and by the time I get to the count of one you will be back in an everyday state of awareness, and ready

to resume your daily life. One. Beginning to come back now. Your mind will be clear and alert, and you will be feeling pleased and happy from the experiences you have had. Two. You will benefit from today's experience in many different ways, and on many different levels. Three. Coming back more and more. Four. Today's experience will bring about many desirable changes in your life, some of which you may already know and some of which you may not yet be aware of. Five. Now you can open your eyes anytime you are ready.

Occasionally, therapists find that a client opens his or her eyes before suggestions for termination have concluded. However, this is of little consequence, insofar as therapists can usually weave their concluding comments regarding the expected benefits of hypnosis into the ensuing conversation. At the conclusion of a session, some clients may remark, "I don't think I was hypnotized," or "I don't think it worked on me." To comments such as these, the therapist may truthfully respond, "Because there are so many ways to experience hypnosis, there's no such thing as a 'hypnotized' feeling. But if you fully engage with the suggestions and you're ready for them to work, then you will be able to experience them to the best of your ability."

POSTHYPNOTIC SUGGESTIONS: ANCHORING

Generally speaking, it is often helpful to administer posthypnotic suggestions for relaxation, ego-enhancement, and mastery. With *anchoring* or *cue-related techniques*, clients can often transport what they have learned during hypnosis to everyday situations. More specifically, any feeling state, positive cognition, or behavior pattern developed during hypnosis can be associated with a *cue* or *anchor*, such as touching the thumb and forefinger together, that can be actuated in relevant life situations. For example, if a client learns to relax the musculature around the mouth during hypnosis while imagining giving a speech scheduled for the following week, the client can be given the suggestion to use the thumb–forefinger anchor during the actual speech to facilitate relaxation. This technique is illustrated, with respect to smoking cessation in chapter 24, but the technique of cue-controlled relaxation or anchoring has a wide range of application.

POSTSESSION INQUIRY

A basic induction can provide an initial assessment of a person's responsiveness to suggestions and serve as the cornerstone for the application of additional therapeutic suggestions. Lynn, Kirsch, and Rhue (1996) suggested that at the conclusion of the induction, therapists can ask the following questions to guide subsequent interventions: What did you like about your experience? What was particularly helpful? At what point did you feel most deeply involved? Did anything get in the way? Are there any suggestions that were not helpful? How did the experience compare with what you thought you would experience? What could make the experience even better? Do you have any thoughts about suggestions that might be useful in the future?

POSSIBLE AFTEREFFECTS OF INDUCTION

Novice hypnotists sometimes worry needlessly about not being able to bring a client out of hypnosis. The state of consciousness produced by typical hypnotic inductions is similar to meditative or relaxed states. Asking, "What if my client doesn't come out of hypnosis" is like asking, "What if my client doesn't stop relaxing?" (Kirsch, Lynn, & Rhue, 1993). Still, hypnosis and hyperempiria are typically absorbing experiences. Accordingly, occasionally, a client may not open his or her eyes immediately on conclusion of the induction procedure. This is almost always taken care of by suggesting, "Any second now, you will open your eyes," and by taking advantage of any signs of arousal such as by commenting, "Your eyelids are beginning to flutter now. They're fluttering more and more, and any second now, they will open, any second now. There!" said with emphasis as the client's eyes open.

At the conclusion of the hypnosis session, it is important to ask clients how they are feeling. People sometimes, though uncommonly, report negative experiences, such as headaches and anxiety, after hypnosis. It is of interest that research indicates that people report equally frequent and comparable negative experiences after sitting quietly with their eyes closed or after a college exam (see Lynn, Martin, & Frauman, 1996). Accordingly, such negative experiences are neither specific to hypnosis, nor necessarily "caused" by hypnosis. Nevertheless, negative experiences do require clinical attention. Clinicians can state matter-of-factly, "Any remaining discomfort that you may feel will quickly pass," followed a few moments later with a question regarding the client's well-being to ensure that the client indeed does feel better.

RESEARCH

Clinicians have an opportunity to try different inductions with interested clients to "see what works." However, few, if any, differences have been found among different types of inductions in terms of overt responses to suggestions. For example, Lynn and Kvaal (2009) determined that participants responded comparably to a traditional hypnotic induction, an induction that focused on body awareness and imaginative experiences, and an induction that emphasized positive emotional experiences associated with imagined situations in everyday life. Moreover, complex inductions, such as the double induction, championed by Richard Bandler and John Grinder (1976), in which the voice of two hypnotists each speak into a different ear of the participant, are no more effective than a more traditional, relaxation-based induction (Mathews, Kirsch, & Mosher, 1985). As Kirsch (1991) observed, there is apparently no need for clinicians to learn complex induction methods insofar as research indicates that simple as well as more complex inductions can largely be used interchangeably.

In addition, there is also little reason to believe that: (a) indirect and permissive suggestions (e.g., "You may notice that you begin to experience a sense of lightness in your right hand, or perhaps you first notice it in your left hand.") are superior to traditional, authoritatively worded suggestions (J. Barber, 1991; Erickson, Rossi, & Rossi, 1976; Zeig & Rennick, 1991), and (b) low-suggestible participants are especially likely to benefit from indirect suggestions (see Lynn, Neufeld, & Mare, 1993). However, in cases in which participants express concerns about "losing control" during hypnosis, research suggests that permissive suggestions may be useful insofar as they are associated with increased perceptions of voluntary responding (and equivalent behavioral responsiveness) relative to more authoritatively worded suggestions (Lynn, Neufeld, & Matyi, 1987).

Goal-directed fantasies (GDFs) can be defined as "imagined situations, which, if they were to occur, would be expected to lead to the involuntary occurrence of the motor response called for by the suggestion" (Spanos, Rivers, & Ross, 1977, p. 211). People not infrequently generate GDFs spontaneously in response to hypnotic suggestions. For example, in response to a hand-levitation suggestion, they may imagine that a helium balloon is lifting their hand or a basketball is being inflated under their hand. Research indicates that when suggestions for GDFs are included in hypnotic inductions, they facilitate the perception of hypnotic responses as involuntary or automatic (Lynn & Sivec, 1992). It follows that clinicians interested in enhancing the experience of suggestion-related involuntariness can incorporate GDFs into their hypnotic interventions.

It is interesting that GDFs do not determine how many suggestions a person successfully passes during assessments of hypnotizability (Lynn & Sivec, 1992). One reason why GDFs do not determine suggestibility is that some people who receive imaginative suggestions wait passively for something to "happen" to them. This response set virtually guarantees failure. In contrast, when participants associate imagining with lifting their arm, they are much more likely to succeed. It is important that therapists convey to participants either in the hypnotic induction or in information provided before hypnosis that they must enact imagined responses to some extent rather than passively waiting for them to "happen."

Suggestions can be used to advantage even when the procedures are not defined as hypnosis. Amigó (1998), for example, determined that people can be trained to experience a variety of alterations in perceptions and sensations at will, including the taste of lemon juice. Amigó used this demonstration to suggest to patients "with their brains sensitized" by the ability to produce sensory experiences that they would be better able to accept therapeutic suggestions even with their eyes open and when they were able to move about and interact with the therapist. Capafons (1998) documented that this expectancy and imagery enhancing procedure is effective in treating a wide variety of problems with many clients who are normally not responsive to hypnosis, including those who are skeptical or fearful of hypnosis itself.

As Amigó's (1998) research implied, imaginative abilities can be accessed to produce hypnotic-like phenomena. Perhaps not surprisingly, hypnotic-like experiences can be achieved spontaneously in people with at least a modicum of imaginative abilities. Barabasz (2005), for example, reported a brief episode of temporary but complete amnesia while waiting to receive a set of immunization shots in a physician's office, returning to his normal awareness immediately after the shots had been administered. Similarly, a woman who was employed at New Jersey's maximum security prison, and who had never experienced hypnosis until recently, told one of the authors (Gibbons) that she has long been in the habit of "putting up an energy shield" each day before entering the building. This spontaneous use of her imaginative abilities engendered a feeling of relative safety in a job that entailed working with some of the state's most dangerous long-term inmates. These examples suggest that people may use imaginative abilities to create a wealth of profound and compelling alterations of consciousness in everyday life in both hypnotic and nonhypnotic contexts.

Although hypnotic-like phenomena occasionally occur spontaneously, and formal training may facilitate hypnotic-like responses, generally speaking, the most reliable and clinically useful way to facilitate responses to hypnotic suggestions is by means of an induction procedure. Still, if participants are resistant to the idea of experiencing hypnosis, suggestions can be administered in the absence of a formal hypnotic induction and instead defined as imagery or relaxation. Research suggests that a hypnotic induction, compared with nonhypnotic relaxation or imagery suggestions, generally results in a small yet significant increase in suggestibility on the order of 10% to 20% (see Lynn & Kirsch, 2006). However, a relaxation induction that is not presented as hypnosis produces subjective experiences largely equivalent to a traditional hypnotic induction (Meyer & Lynn, 2005), implying that approaches couched in terms of relaxation or imagery can be substituted for interventions presented to clients as hypnotic in nature. Indeed, the hallmark of a successful hypnotherapist is the ability to flexibly adapt interventions to the needs and goals of the client.

CONCLUSION

Clinicians should be well versed in the basics of hypnotic inductions and recognize that how clients respond to suggestions depends less on the nature and success of a particular induction than on the following variables: (a) clients' prehypnotic attitudes, beliefs, intentions, and expectations about hypnosis; (b) their ability to think, fantasize, and absorb themselves in suggestions; (c) their ability to form a trusting relationship with the hypnotist; (d) their ability to interpret suggestions appropriately and view their responses as successful; (e) their ability to discern task demands and cues; (f) their ongoing interaction with the hypnotist; and (g) the appropriateness of the therapeutic methods and suggestions to treating the presenting problem (Barber, 1985, Lynn, Kirsch, & Rhue, 1996). Accordingly, clinicians should devise inductions and suggestions with these variables in mind and tailor their approach to the unique personal characteristics and agenda of each client they encounter.

REFERENCES

Amigó, S. (1998). Self-regulation therapy: Suggestion without hypnosis. In I. Kirsch, A. Capafons, E. Cardeña-Bulena, & Amigó, S. (Eds.) *Clinical hypnosis and self-regulation: Cognitive–behavioral perspectives* (pp. 311–330). Washington, DC: American Psychological Association

Bandler, R., & Grinder, J. (1976). *The structure of magic: A book about language and therapy.* New York: Science and Behavior Books.

Bányai, E. I., & Hilgard, E. R. (1976). A comparison of active–alert hypnotic induction with traditional relaxation induction. *Journal of Abnormal Psychology, 85,* 218–224.

Barabasz, A. (2005, October). Hypnosis and mind–body interactions. Paper presented at the meeting of the Society for Clinical and Experimental Hypnosis, Charleston, SC.

Barber, J. (1991). The locksmith model: Accessing hypnotic responsiveness. In S. J. Lynn & J. W. Rhue (Eds.), *Theories of hypnosis* (pp. 241–274). New York: Guilford Press.

Barber, T. X. (1985). Hypnosuggestive procedures as catalysts for psychotherapies. In S. J. Lynn & J. P. Garske (Eds.), *Contemporary psychotherapies: Models and methods* (pp. 333–376). Columbus, OH: Charles E. Merrill.

Capafons, A. (1998). Applications of emotional self-regulation therapy. In I. Kirsch, A. Capafons, E. Cardeña-Bulena, & Amigó, S. (Eds.) *Clinical hypnosis and self-regulation: Cognitive–behavioral perspectives* (pp. 331–349). Washington, DC: American Psychological Association.

Erickson, M. H., Rossi, E. L., & Rossi, S. I. (1976). *Hypnotic realities: The induction of clinical hypnosis and forms of indirect suggestion*. New York: Irvington.

Field, P. (1979). Humanistic aspects of communication. In E. Fromm & R. E. Schor (Ed.), *Hypnosis: Developments in research and new perspectives* (2nd ed.; pp. 605–636). Chicago: Aldine.

Gibbons, D. E. (1973, December). *Hyperempiria: A new "altered state of consciousness" induced by suggestion*. Paper presented at the meeting of the Society for Clinical and Experimental Hypnosis, Newport Beach, CA.

Gibbons, D. E. (1974, March). *Hyperempiria: Waking up hypnosis*. Paper presented at the meeting of the Southeastern Psychological Association, Orlando, FL.

Gibbons, D. E. (1975, August). Hypnotic versus hyperempiric induction: An experimental comparison. Paper presented at the meeting of the American Psychological Association, Chicago.

Gibbons, D. E. (1976). Hypnotic versus hyperempiric induction: An experimental comparison. *Perceptual and Motor Skills, 42*, 834.

Gibbons, D. E. (1979). *Applied hypnosis and hyperempiria*. New York: Plenum Press.

Gibbons, D. E. (1999, August). Suggestion as an art form: Alternative paradigm for hypnosis? Paper presented at the meeting of the American Psychological Association, San Francisco.

Gibbons, D. E. (2001). *Experience as an art form: Hypnosis, hyperempiria, and the Best Me Technique*. San Jose, CA: Authors Choice Press.

Gibbons, D. E. (2004). Multimodal suggestion for facilitating meditation and prayer. *Hypnos, 31*(2), 90–92.

Gibbons, D. E. (2005). *Kicking it up a notch: Multimodal hyperempiria*. Paper presented at the meeting of the Society for Clinical and Experimental Hypnosis, Charleston, SC.

Hammond, D. C. (1992). *Manual for self-hypnosis*. Des Plaines, IL: American Society of Clinical Hypnosis.

Kirsch, I. (1991). The social learning theory of hypnosis. In S. J. Lynn & J. W. Rhue (Eds.), *Theories of hypnosis: Current models and perspectives* (pp. 439–466). New York: Guilford Press.

Kirsch, I., Lynn, S. J., & Rhue, J. W. (1993). An introduction to clinical hypnosis. In J. W. Rhue, S. J. Lynn, & I. Kirsch (Eds.), *Handbook of clinical hypnosis* (pp. 3–22). Washington, DC: American Psychological Association.

Lynn, S. J., & Kirsch, I. (2006). *Essentials of clinical hypnosis: An evidence-based approach*. Washington, DC: American Psychological Association.

Lynn, S. J., Kirsch, I., & Hallquist, M. (2008). Social cognitive theories of hypnosis. In M. R. Nash & A. Barnier (Eds.), *The Oxford handbook of hypnosis* (pp. 111–140). New York: Oxford University Press.

Lynn, S. J., Kirsch, I., & Rhue, J. W. (1996). Maximizing treatment gains: Recommendations for the practice of clinical hypnosis. In S. J. Lynn, I. Kirsch, & J. W. Rhue (Eds.), *Casebook of clinical hypnosis* (pp. 395–406). Washington, DC: American Psychological Association.

Lynn, S. J., & Kvaal, S. (2004). *A comparison of three different hypnotic inductions*. Unpublished manuscript, Binghamton University, Binghamton, NY.

Lynn, S. J., Martin, D., & Frauman, D. (1996). Does hypnosis pose special risks for negative effects? *International Journal of Clinical and Experimental Hypnosis, 44*, 7–19.

Lynn, S. J., Neufeld, V., & Mare, C. (1993). Direct versus indirect suggestions: A conceptual and methodological review. *International Journal of Clinical and Experimental Hypnosis, 31*, 124–152.

Lynn, S. J., Neufeld, V. & Matyi, C. L. (1987). Hypnotic inductions versus suggestions: The effects of direct and indirect wording. *Journal of Abnormal Psychology, 96*, 76–80.

Lynn, S. J., & Sivec, H. (1992). The hypnotizable subject as creative problem solving agent. In E. Fromm & M. Nash (Eds.), *Contemporary perspectives in hypnosis research*. New York: Guilford Press.

Lynn, S. J., Vanderhoff, H., Shindler, K., & Stafford, J. (2002). The effects of an induction and defining hypnosis as a "trance" versus cooperation: Hypnotic suggestibility and performance standards. *American Journal of Clinical Hypnosis, 44*, 231–240.

Mathews, W. J., Kirsch, I., & Mosher, D. (1985). The "double" hypnotic induction: An initial empirical test. *Journal of Abnormal Psychology, 94*, 92–95.

McConkey, K. M. (1986). Opinions about hypnosis and self-hypnosis before and after hypnotic testing. *International Journal of Clinical and Experimental Hypnosis, 34*, 311–319.

Meyer, E. C., & Lynn, S. J. (2005). *The determinants of hypnotic and nonhypnotic suggestibility*. Unpublished manuscript, Binghamton University, Binghamton, NY.

Orne, M. T., & McConkey, K. M. (1981). Toward convergent inquiry into self-hypnosis. *International Journal of Clinical and Experimental Hypnosis, 29*, 313–323.

Sanders, S. (1991). *Clinical self-hypnosis: The power of words and images*. New York: Guilford Press.

Spanos, N. P., Rivers, S. M., & Ross, S. (1977). Experienced involuntariness and response to hypnotic suggestions. In W. E. Edmonston, Jr. (Ed.), *Conceptual and investigative approaches to hypnosis and hypnotic phenomena* (Vol. 296, pp. 208–221). New York: New York Academy of Sciences.

Wagstaff, G. (1998). The semantics and physiology of hypnosis as an altered state: Towards a definition of hypnosis. *Contemporary Hypnosis, 15*, 149–165.

Zeig, J., & Rennick, P. J. (1991). Ericksonian hypnotherapy: A communications approach to hypnosis. In S. J. Lynn & J. W. Rhue (Eds.), *Theories of hypnosis* (pp. 275–300). New York: Guilford Press.

11

"WAKING" HYPNOSIS IN CLINICAL PRACTICE

ANTONIO CAPAFONS AND M. ELENA MENDOZA

In 1924, Wells introduced *waking hypnosis* to overcome some of the intrinsic difficulties of the usual hypnotic induction, which incorporates relaxing or sleeplike suggestions. According to Wells, there are a number of advantages to using waking hypnosis:

> First, it is less mysterious in appearance, and the total impression is more desirable. The psychologist who uses hypnosis partly for the purpose of teaching against occultism desires to avoid the appearance of an occult procedure. Second, it usually takes less time. With an individual subject or with a group, one usually begins to get results in two or three minutes, if not in five or ten seconds; while sleeping hypnosis, when first used with a subject usually requires a longer time before results are obtained. Third, it is easier, requiring less effort on the part of the experimenter; and it is easier for the beginner to learn. Fourth, it can be employed on a larger percentage of subjects with success at the start than can the usual methods of sleeping hypnosis. Fifth, if for any reason sleeping hypnosis is desired, one can easily change to the methods of

Our acknowledgements to Gemma Costa, Mª José Milán, Belén Miquel, Ángeles Ludeña, and Ana Isabel Villafañe, psychologists.

producing the sleeping state, with greater chance of success if the first suggestions by the method of waking hypnosis have been successful. (pp. 396–397)

It is now known that traditional hypnosis is not sleep and that hypnotized individuals remain wide awake; hence the quotation marks around the term *waking* in the title of this chapter. However, traditional or "relaxation" hypnosis involves a restriction in attention, passivity, and drowsiness, whereas waking hypnosis may be used while the clients keep their eyes open, continue with their everyday life, and are alert.

Currently, some Ericksonian approaches embrace an approach to hypnosis that does not involve a relaxation-based induction (Matthews, Conti, & Starr, 1998), as do clinicians who work with active–alert hypnosis or similar techniques (Bányai, Zseni, & Túry, 1993; Barabasz & Barabasz, 1996; Gibbons, 1979; Kratochvil, 1970; Wark, 1998). Nevertheless, waking hypnosis is not a widely known technique. One of the reasons for the low visibility of waking hypnosis may be its apparent lack of application to clinical problems. However, waking hypnosis can be a useful alternative to the traditional hypnosis induction. Beyond the reasons Wells noted more than 80 years ago, clients can remain self-hypnotized and give themselves self-suggestions with eyes open while talking, walking, driving, and engaging in other activities. In this way, they can experience therapeutic suggestions in situ (i.e., where the problem occurs or arises; Capafons, 1998b, 1999, 2004a, 2004b). Accordingly, therapists using treatments that include homework assignments, for example, find active–alert hypnosis or waking hypnosis, a useful strategy, as we illustrate later in our discussion. Likewise, according to Wells (1924), clients exhibit a greater degree of self-control during waking hypnosis in contrast with traditional hypnosis due to the fact that their eyes remain open. Furthermore, it has been found that the waking hypnosis induction methods are preferred over the traditional self-hypnosis version of the Hypnosis Induction Profile (Martínez-Tendero, Capafons, Weber, & Cardeña, 2001; Spiegel & Spiegel, 1978), and over a more traditional active–alert procedure (Alarcón, Capafons, Bayot, & Cardeña, 1999; Bányai & Hilgard, 1976).

Clients do not usually request waking hypnosis unless former clients have referred them. However, once they learn to use waking hypnosis, they accept it and report they like and enjoy the "new" hypnosis. Our clinical experience is that clients are surprised when they learn to use waking hypnosis. It is something novel that they did not expect; it strengthens their expectancies for success, bolsters their motivation for subsequent sessions and therapy more generally, and magnifies their sense of general efficacy and self-control. Metaphorically speaking, many clients react as if they can see the light outside a dark tunnel.

In the following sections, the Valencia Model of Waking Hypnosis is explained in detail. Assessment methods, procedures for the change and consolidation of attitudes, and waking hypnosis methods of self and hetero-hypnosis induction are included. Finally, its clinical applications as well as the research carried out on this model are described.

THE VALENCIA MODEL OF WAKING HYPNOSIS: FROM EFFICACY TO EFFICIENCY

To achieve good rapport with clients, we implement three procedures as part of the *Valencia Model of Waking Hypnosis*: a cognitive–behavioral introduction to hypnosis, a clinical assessment of hypnotic suggestibility, and a metaphor for hypnosis. The induction methods used (i.e., *rapid self-hypnosis* and *waking-alert hypnosis*, the latter also known as *alert-hand hypnosis*; Cardeña, Alarcón, Capafons, & Bayot, 1998; see Table 11.1 for more detail regarding our use of these and other terms throughout this chapter) are especially important in the general context in which the introduction, assessment, and metaphor are presented. The final underlying idea is that individuals can activate the suggestive processes typical of hypnosis across a radically different behavioral topography (e.g., appearance, activity, open eyes) than traditional hypnosis (Capafons, 1999).

In the sections that follow, we present a script that can serve as a guide to the use of waking hypnosis. It represents a composite case with characteristics and problems that require the implementation of all steps in the protocol. Nevertheless, this script should be adapted to each individual client, his or her circumstances, and personal characteristics.

TABLE 11.1.
Methods of Induction of Hypnosis and Managing Suggestions

Method	Induction	Relaxation	Suggestions of alertness	Physical activation	Eyes open
Focusing Attention	Yes	Yes	No	No	No
Alert	Yes	Yes	Yes	No	No*
Active-Alert	Yes	No	Yes	Yes	No*
Waking-Alert**	Yes	No	Yes	Yes	Yes
Rapid Self-Hypnosis**	Yes	Yes***	Yes	No	Yes
Waking suggestion	No	No	No	No	Yes

*Sometimes it may be suggested to open the eyes, but they are fixed on something or the gaze is lost.
**These are methods of inducing waking hypnosis. They can be used both to activate and to relax.
***Only in its long version.

A Cognitive–Behavioral Introduction to Hypnosis

We initiate the introduction to hypnosis from a cognitive–behavioral standpoint (Capafons, 2001a; Capafons & Amigó, 1993, Coe, 1980; Kirsch, 1994). In presenting the introduction, it is important that hypnotist convey the following ideas to participants:

1. Responses to suggestions are acts committed by the clients and are therefore not dependent on any "power" of the therapist. The hypnotist merely facilitates the experience of suggested responses.
2. Actions during waking hypnosis are automatic; yet, they are voluntary in the sense that individuals have the ability to initiate or resist suggested responses.
3. What happens during hypnosis depends mainly on a person's ability to use his or her resources, which are activated in a manner similar to how they are activated on an everyday basis.
4. In a related way, hypnosis involves reactions in everyday life that can be activated or deactivated at will at any given moment.
5. From this point of view, hypnosis is a form of self-control, even if less conscious effort is required on behalf of individuals to regulate certain behaviors.
6. To be hypnotized does not require entering into a trance or altered state of consciousness but rather involves preparing the mind to access resources that facilitate perceiving responses in daily life as automatic.

This framework is based on experimental research from a cognitive–behavioral perspective. The fundamental proposition of response set theory (Kirsch & Lynn, 1998; Lynn, 1997; Lynn & Kirsch, 2005) is that the acts committed in hypnosis are voluntary but automatic (Capafons, 2001a; Capafons & Amigó, 1993). According to this theory, responses to hypnotic suggestion are intentional but also automatic insofar as relatively little volitional effort and attentional resources are necessary to enact them. Hypnosis can be thought of as a controlled automatic process in which responses (e.g., amnesia, alterations in perception and sensation) occur that may be inappropriate in other contexts but are completely appropriate in the context of hypnosis for therapeutic and experimental ends. The introduction that we propose is also based on the dramaturgical theory of hypnosis and Sarbin's concept of self-deception (Coe & Sarbin, 1991; Gorassini, 1999) and on the theories of goal-directed and rule-governed behavior as well as on the misattribution theory proposed by Spanos (1996; Spanos & Coe, 1992).

The introductory presentation based on the cognitive–behavioral perspective begins with the therapist providing the client with a pocket watch with a chain or anything that can be used as a pendulum. The therapist explains and serves as a model for the following exercise: With the dominant arm stretched out in front of him or her, the therapist holds the pendulum between the thumb and forefinger. At this moment, the therapist asks the watch to perform circular movements or oscillations. When the therapist has finished the exercise, he or she asks the clients to do it in more or less the following way:

Therapist: Now stretch out your arm and allow the pendulum to come to rest completely still. Very good. Now ask the watch to move in some direction or other, to trace circles or move from left to right or backward and forward. Ask it whatever you wish but do not ask it to defy gravity and move up toward the ceiling. That particular one never works when I try it, and, if it did work, I would probably die of shock. So what have you asked the watch? [*The client answers and the watch moves.*] Ah! Fantastic! I can see you are quite good at this. Why do you think the watch moved?

Client: I don't know. It just moved by itself. It's incredible. Maybe I moved it without realizing it.

Therapist: Yes, its fun isn't it? OK, let's try it again, but this time I want you to watch your hand very closely. [*The watch moves.*] Can you notice anything?

Client: I think I notice very minute movements in my hand. But I'm not doing it on purpose!

Therapist: Exactly! Do you know what this pendulum is?

Client: Well, of course I do, it's a pendulum.

Therapist: OK, I guess that's obvious. But in this case it works as an amplifier, which amplifies the almost unnoticeable movements of your hand at the end of the pendulum, and for that reason you can see the movements. If we were to shorten the chain that suspends the watch [*The therapist holds the pendulum near the watch end of the chain.*], it would hardly move at all regardless of what we ask it to do. [*The therapist demonstrates the idea.*] Well, hypnosis, in a way, is like that. Whenever you hear my voice, or indeed your own voice, suggesting things to you, your brain will send "orders" to the organs involved in the response that you experience, and you will do things in order to experience these responses. Generally, they will be so subtle that you will not even notice them and you will experience them as if they happened by themselves, as if they just happen. OK? But remember, it is always you who triggers the things that happen. It is also you who puts an end to them.

Let's do another exercise. Stretch out your arm and ask the watch to move in a specific direction. [*The watch moves.*] Now, I want you to think that what you are doing is really nonsense, just a stupid game, that you are in fact being ridiculous. Or, just think of something urgent that you have to do at home or at work. [*The watch usually comes to a standstill.*] Can you see what happens? If you don't move your hand, the watch will stop moving. This is what we call interference. The word interference usually has negative connotations: Interference impedes us from watching the television or from using our mobile phone. If someone interferes, then they obstruct us in our attempts to achieve some goal or other. However, in my case, interference is something positive: You have shown me that you are an active person and that you control what occurs in hypnosis at any given moment. If there is anything that you do not like or if you think that anything is inappropriate, you can interfere with it and stop it. When a person is hypnotized he or she does not lose control. The reactions that person experiences are automatic but voluntary, given that you yourself initiated and stopped the response once you thought that it was ridiculous or it stopped interesting you. You asked the watch to move, you did not ask your hand to move the watch; however, your brain understood the instruction and activated the hand movements by itself. Talking itself is a voluntary act, I can stop when I wish [*The therapist stops talking for a few moments.*], but I do not have to search for the words in order to talk, they just jump out without having to think of them. In this way, talking is automatic. If I had to speak to you in a different language which was not so familiar to me, I would have to think about many of my words; that is, it would be something voluntary but not automatic. Hypnosis is like that; you will experience voluntary but automatic responses. Do you understand?

Client: Yes I think so: It's just like walking: voluntary but automatic at the same time, right?

Therapist: Precisely! But let us try another exercise. Stretch out your arm and ask the watch to move, but this time ask it as if your life depended on it, ask it forcefully and demandingly. Ask it now! [*The client does so, but the watch does not move.*] You see, this is another form of interference. If you wish to experience something and you are waiting on it and forcefully demanding that it occur, then it most probably will not happen. It is just like when you try to remember something that is on the tip of your tongue: The more you try to remember it, the blanker your mind goes. Have you ever had anything like that happen to you?

Client: Yes, many times. I think I am getting the hang of what it means to be hypnotized.

Therapist: Excellent! Just a moment ago, I mentioned that for me interference is something positive. Nevertheless, there are interferences that would be inappropriate. Do you know what they are?

Client: No. I don't know what you mean.

Therapist: I mean that if at any moment you feel unhappy or do not agree with any of the suggestions or with any of the things we do to help overcome the problem that has brought you here and you do not communicate this to me but instead keep silent, this would be an inappropriate interference. This would not be positive, because it would imply a break in our communication. If this were to happen, then both you and I would be wasting our time here. Do you understand?

Client: Yes. Yes, I believe so.

Therapist: There is still one more thing that I would like to ask you: If you wished to interfere with the suggestions or the therapy, how do you think you might do it?

Client: Well, I don't know. I don't think I will interfere.

Therapist: Probably not, but try now to imagine what you would do in such a case.

Client: I suppose I would think of something else—perhaps not follow the instructions or not offer any ideas about looking for solutions.

Therapist: I see. I am going to ask a favor of you: If you discover that you are doing one of the things that you have just described, please tell me right away. Otherwise our communication will be broken, you will lose confidence in me, and I will not be able to help you. As I said before, in this case we would both be wasting our time. OK?

Client: All right, I'll give it a try.

Therapist: Good. Now I would like to explain something else. I know that you have understood what to expect from hypnosis, but I would still like for us to agree on one more thing. I assure you that all the time that we spend here talking about this will be time saved in the future if we can overcome all possible misunderstandings. Tell me, have you ever seen a horror movie?

Client: Yes.

Therapist: Do they frighten you? Do you notice anything about yourself?

Client: Yes I get scared. I notice tension, fear.

Therapist: Your heart beats faster perhaps, your hands sweat, and you feel a sense of danger?

Client: Yes, sometimes; even though I like the movie, I look away from the most terrifying scenes.

Therapist: Perfect. Now try to imagine that I am an extraterrestrial and that I am observing you while you watch the movie. Do you think that I could believe it possible that you should be frightened by something that you know is not real but is actually a fantasy, a lie? Don't you think that I should believe that you were not very intelligent?

Client: Well, if you look at it like that [*laughter*], then I guess so.

Therapist: But really it's not like that. The cinema is an art form. You know that there is a director, actors, cameras, a scriptwriter, and so forth, and you know that everything is just a story, right?

Client: Yes, of course [*laughter*].

Therapist: In other words, you voluntarily choose not to think of the fact that it is all a fantasy, and you become involved in the story that is being told. You unconsciously "forget" that behind the scenes there is a whole team of people who have recorded the movie and that all you see are the effects of a few lights reflecting consecutive stills on the screen. All things considered, it is actually a great effort, given that you must "forget" something that is obvious.

Client: Exactly, but it doesn't take much effort, unless of course the movie is really badly made.

Therapist: Precisely. So what happens when you watch an interesting movie is that you experience enriching intense automatic reactions? In spite of the fact that you know everything is false, you let yourself go along with the director's proposals, and thus you experience intense emotions. You may even experience certain behaviors—a sudden start, for example—covering your eyes, crying, and so forth. Is that right?

Client: Yes, generally.

Therapist: Well, hypnosis works in a similar way: Sometimes, I will be the director of the movie, directing the hypnotic suggestions, and at other times, you will be the director—self-hypnosis. I will propose that you experience certain things, which deep down you will know are not true—for example, that you cannot lift your arm or that you forget something. However, if you allow things to happen, just as in the cinema, then they will happen. Sometimes these reactions can be very intense, but they will always be under your control. In fact, what do you or, indeed, what do other people do when they don't want to see certain sequences of a horror movie?

Client: I look away, or I leave my seat. Sometimes, I cover my face with my hands and I look out from between my fingers. Some people actually leave the cinema. Sometimes, I think that it is all a lie, and I distance myself from the plot.

Therapist: That's right. Don't you think that these behaviors are like interferences?

Client: Well, now that you mention it, I guess they are.

Therapist: Going to the cinema is a voluntary act, just like "forgetting" that all is fantasy and paying attention to what happens on screen. The reactions that you experience are automatic, just like the fear, happiness, or pity generated by the images. All of these reactions, however, are under your control. All you have to do is avoid going to the movies or stop paying attention to the director's proposals. You can even get up and leave the theatre. Well, hypnosis is just like a story or a film. What happens in hypnosis is voluntary and automatic at the same time. You may wish not to initiate the processes to experience certain reactions, or you may wish to interfere in it. It depends on you. If you like the proposed script, you can experience enriching intense sensations and reactions that will help you to overcome the problem that you have told me about. If you decide that the story does not interest you, just don't listen to it, but do not forget to tell me. OK?

Client: Yes, OK. I never thought that hypnosis worked that way. I think that now I know why I sometimes get a sense that I do things almost without wanting to but without losing control.

Therapist: Perfect. If you wish, we can begin with a few exercises that will give us information about your current level of responding to hypnotic suggestions.

Client: OK, I am looking forward to experiencing what it is like to be hypnotized.

The introduction that we propose links hypnosis to everyday life, and it corrects the popular yet mistaken beliefs that people susceptible to hypnosis are ignorant, stupid, or mentally ill, that hypnosis can somehow endanger the participant or that it involves an altered state of consciousness in which a person can become trapped (Capafons, 1998b). Moreover, the introduction presents hypnosis as a form of self-control, which mitigates excessive dependence on the therapist and also reduces any fear that the individual might have about losing control. In this way, the information transmitted increases the probability that clients will feel comfortable proceeding with hypnotic suggestibility assessment with little reluctance and with more accurate beliefs and expectancies about hypnosis. Recent research shows that the presentation reduces attrition much more than a presentation that emphasizes achieving a trance when people who express reluctance to experience hypnosis are selected and given the opportunity to be hypnotized (Capafons et al., 2006). These findings converge with the results of a study by Lynn, Vanderhoff, Shindler, and Stafford (2002), although they used a different trance explanation that suggested that an altered state of consciousness was instrumental to responding during hypnosis.

In contrast, studies conducted in Valencia show that when a self-hypnosis induction is offered as an option, there are no differences between a trance and cognitive–behavioral presentation in the ability to change participants' negative attitudes about hypnosis (Capafons et al., 2005). Therefore, the key factor in accounting for the differences in results when self-hypnosis is used is that clients believe that they retain personal control when they self-administer suggestions. As will become apparent, self-hypnosis is an excellent means of facilitating the perception of self-control.

Clinical Assessment of Hypnotic Suggestibility

The assessment of hypnotic suggestibility in applied clinical practice continues to be a controversial issue. Some authors believe that it is useful to include standardized suggestibility scales in the context of a comprehensive assessment of the client (Council, 1998), whereas others argue that suggestibility assessment is of little utility, given that hypnotic suggestibility can be modified (Chaves, 1996) and that the probability that clients will fail one or more test suggestions at the beginning of therapy renders assessment inadvisable (Capafons, 2001a, 2001b; Capafons & Amigó, 1993).

In our practice, the initial assessment is done outside the hypnotic context, as a form of assessing clients' collaboration with, and confidence in, the therapist and the hypnosis procedure itself. After we propose the use of hypnosis to clients, demythologize the possible risks and dangers of hypnosis (Capafons, 1998b), and convey the cognitive–behavioral introduction described previously, we gear our actions both toward confirming that hypnosis is not a threatening procedure and that it is highly likely clients will be able to respond successfully to therapeutic suggestions.

Accordingly, the primary data we obtain pertains to clients' attitudes toward hypnosis and the therapist. This information is vital insofar as attitudes (a) are the most consistent predictor of successful treatment in programs that include hypnosis as an adjunctive method (Schoenberger, 2000) and (b) may be compared with the generalized implementation intentions (Kirsch & Lynn, 1998; Lynn, 1997), which motivate behavioral responses through the intention to do so. As Wagstaff (1998) stated, the improvement of expectancies and attitudes toward hypnosis is probably the key to increasing the effectiveness of hypnosis-based therapies.

The assessment exercises are conducted with no previous hypnotic induction (Capafons, 2001a) because of the high correlation between responses to hypnotic and waking suggestions (i.e., approximately 64% of the variance; Hilgard, 1965; Kirsch, 1997) and because it is important that clients gain familiarity with waking hypnosis at the earliest opportunity. Meanwhile, any failure to respond can be attributed to the lack of training, practice, or a difficulty with the hypnotic induction exercises (Capafons, 2001a; 2004a). The first assessment exercise begins with postural sway, which involves direct and repetitive suggestions along the following lines (Hull, 1933): The clients should have their eyes closed and their feet together, an unbalanced position that, in itself, with no hypnotic intervention or suggestions, produces swaying. If clients begin to gently sway following suggestions to do so, they are not interfering with or blocking a naturally occurring response. If the sway is pronounced, we assume that individuals are collaborating and experiencing the effect of the suggestion. Or in the terms of response expectancy theory, it is apparent that clients possess response expectancies that prepare for the automatic activation of the response (Kirsch, 1999; Kirsch & Lynn, 1998). However, if clients do not sway at all, then it is highly likely that they are actively resisting the natural effects of the suggestion. If this occurs, we can determine why they are resisting and probe regarding whether it is due to their fears, reluctances, skepticism, or other interfering beliefs. In addition, we inform clients that everyone sways slightly unless they block the effects of the suggestions.

In the next exercise, "falling back" (Capafons, 2001a, 2004a; Hilgard, 1965), as the name implies, therapists suggest that clients fall backward. With this exercise, therapists can assess client confidence in them with even greater certainty, because therapists are responsible for catching their clients as they fall. The client is asked to close his or her eyes and try to guess the distance and location of the therapist. It is therefore possible to determine whether therapists are in the right place to hold clients when they fall backward. In fact, the angle of fall should be very small, just enough to permit therapists to test whether clients try to avoid the fall somehow.

If clients avoid falling, we determine the reasons for their lack of confidence. In contrast, if clients allow themselves to fall backward, we conclude that they are reasonably confident and collaborative. If clients also state that they felt unbalanced, then we can assume that they have experienced the subjective reaction suggested. This exercise is carried out in a relaxed atmosphere, using jokes to help establish rapport and to decrease tension and concerns about testing.

Certain clients exhibit a preference: They want or need to use their imaginations to fully experience suggested reactions (T. X. Barber, 1999). Thus, therapists can use metaphor to facilitate a "fall backward" response. In a variant of the standard exercise, therapists ask clients to imagine that the therapist is holding a rather powerful magnet in his or her right hand and that the magnet is being passed around the client's head, which feels attracted to the magnet. The therapist then indicates that the magnet is moving to the left and drawing the client's body with it, then to the right, then forward, then backward (the postural sway movements). Finally, the magnet draws the client so strongly backward that balance cannot be maintained, and he or she falls into the supporting hands of the therapist. If we observe and/or the client reports more elaborate responses on application of the magnet metaphor, we conclude that the client is more likely to respond to imaginative suggestions.

The next exercise involves a trick of sorts (Weitzenhoffer, 1989). We ask clients to roll up their eyes and then instruct them to close their eyelids without lowering their eyes. Clients are then told to attempt to raise their eyelids, without moving their eyes from this position, and informed that they will not be able to do so (challenge exercise). At times, clients find it difficult to roll up their eyes and hold them in position with their eyelids closed. In this case, we ask clients to look at a given point on the ceiling, obliging them to lift their gaze and then to lower their eyelids without moving their eyes from the target point.

If the clients do not open their eyes, we ask how they feel and explain the trick (i.e., it is virtually impossible to raise one's eyelids while maintaining your eyes in this position). If clients open their eyes, they are then asked about any reluctance they experienced, and we assess whether they understood the instructions. If the clients open their eyes because they were afraid, we curtail hypnotic suggestibility assessment and address the possible causes of lack of confidence. If these difficulties are overcome, the exercise is repeated, and we inform clients of the trick. At this point, we make it clear to clients that we will always explain tricks to them and that we will use tricks as a part of the treatment to improve their responsivity to suggestions, thus converting them into prompts for suggested responses.

The final exercise is a motor challenge suggestion (i.e., hand clasping). We introduce the exercise as one involving mental self-control and explain that it involves getting the sense that the hands get stuck together following suggestions that the hands are so tightly stuck together that they cannot be separated. If individuals do not interfere (i.e., by being skeptical or interfering with the reaction), they will feel they cannot separate their hands until they "break" the response and no longer experience the sense that their hands are stuck. If clients fail the challenge (i.e., they simply separate their hands), they are asked whether they felt tension in their fingers or whether they felt as if their hands were stuck together. If they felt tension or as if their hands were "stuck," they are asked why they separated their hands. If clients report that they did so because they feared losing voluntary control, we remind them of the trick, namely, the importance of experiencing the tension without interference. If the clients fail to experience any reaction, the exercise is repeated using imagination techniques (e.g., a strong glue sticking the hands together). If none of these endeavors succeeds, clients are told that they are not in hypnosis and that with some practice they will probably be able to perform the exercise while in hypnosis.

If the clients respond appropriately and do not become startled by their failure to separate their hands, then the mechanism behind the exercise is explained, and they are told that there is a high probability that they will respond well to the therapeutic suggestions that follow, given that they have activated the tension response in their hands and have not interfered with it. In fact, the correlation of these motor exercises of primary suggestibility with hypnotic suggestibility is high (Eysenck, 1989), although the magnitude of the correlation depends on the explanations given to the participants (Gheorghiu, 1989).

We tell clients that, so far, our goal has been to assess what kinds of suggestions are most useful. Moreover, we inform clients who fail passing suggestions that it does not mean that they are not hypnotizable but, rather, that the methods we tried did not prove useful and that we will search for effective methods until we succeed. (This goal of determining whether hypnosis will be a valuable treatment adjunct is shared by J. Barber's, 1991, locksmith method of hypnosis). Finally, we reassure clients that hypnosis will not prolong treatment beyond comparable nonhypnotic interventions.

In summary, the hypnotic suggestibility assessment that we propose is standardized, but yields a great deal of information about the client's attitudes and ability to collaborate with the therapist. Likewise, it allows the therapist to transmit important messages to clients, including the following: (a) Responses to the suggestions depend more on the confidence they have in the therapist and in the benefits of hypnosis than on any trait they possess; (b) responses to suggestions can be learned, and a lack of response to some suggestions should not be considered a failure; and (c) tricks or prompts can be used to allow the activation of the desired responses, with the goal of evoking them with suggestions at a later date. Finally, the therapist emphasizes that hypnosis enhances self-control to instill the idea that nonresponsiveness to hypnosis presents a problem that represents nothing more than learning how to gain more self-control. In short, the therapist strives to convey that there always is a solution to any problem that arises and that clients possess the necessary resources to solve problems that emerge. This approach increases response expectancies and involvement with the treatment, while providing a robust sense of personal control, which predictably should facilitate responses to suggestions (Kirsch & Lynn, 1998; Lynn, Rhue, & Weekes, 1990) as well as a strong rapport and therapeutic alliance.

Rapid Self-Hypnosis

Following the introduction and assessment of confidence, cooperation, and suggestibility, clients are invited to initiate their hypnotic experience or, if clients have been hypnotized previously using other methods, to initiate their experience with a new kind of hypnosis: self-hypnosis. In this way, any residual lack of confidence that the clients experience is tempered by labeling the situation *self-hypnosis*, which reaffirms the idea that hypnosis is a self-control skill (Capafons, 1998a, 1998b, 2001a; Katz, 1978). Self-hypnosis, like other psychological procedures, is a potent way to alter personal reactions, even at a physiological level, as Gruzelier, Levy, Williams, and Henderson (2001) and Egner and Gruzelier (2003) demonstrated. Given these considerations, the Valencia model focuses on (rapid) self-hypnosis (see Lynn, Kirsch, & Rhue, 1996, for a similar recommendation). Defining the procedures as self-hypnosis is also supported by the fact that it is associated with lower dropout rates and that it is a valuable self-control method that emphasizes clients' responsibility for their treatment.

In rapid self-hypnosis, clients are told that they will be shown exercises that together form a method of self-hypnosis, which can be carried out quickly in a disguised fashion, with eyes open. This induction method (described in detail by Capafons, 1998a, 1998b) is closely linked to the hypnotic suggestibility exercises practiced earlier (i.e., falling backward and hand clasping), thereby capitalizing on familiarity and positive expectations that the methods will prove effective.

Rapid self-hypnosis consists of three separate steps: (a) hand clasping, (b) falling backward, and (c) a challenge suggestion (i.e., a confirmation exercise). The client is told that the exercises are designed to activate the brain so that it can work in a rapid and effective manner. As in Kroger and Fezler (1976), the therapist appeals to clients' sensory and emotional recall, informing them that the suggestions will evoke (or reproduce) reactions that are already stored in their brains, in the absence of the original stimuli that accompanied the events. Therefore, the hand clasping, falling backward, and the challenge exercises activate the brain so that it can respond effectively, just as participants were taught in the cognitive–behavioral introduction.

Specifically, rapid self-hypnosis begins by showing clients how to perform the hand clasping exercise: They join hands without interlocking their fingers and take a deep breath and exhale slowly while clasping their hands gently together. Without releasing the pressure on their hands, they take another deep breath and exhale again, this time tensing their hands a little more. Finally, they exhale and clasp hands for a third time, allowing their hands to fall abruptly onto their laps. Subsequently, clients learn to fall backward, beginning by sitting comfortably in chairs and then moving approximately 10 centimeters from the back of the chair and allowing themselves to fall abruptly backward onto it. This exercise promotes a comfortable feeling, as well as a brief and faint sensation of paralysis (useful for relaxation and the next challenge suggestion).

Once clients have practiced both exercises separately, they can combine the two, as follows. First, they find a comfortable position in the chair into which they will later fall backward. Next, they lean forward in the chair and, with their arms outstretched, join their hands and put pressure on them while exhaling three times. Then, they allow themselves to fall abruptly backward, while at the same time letting their hands fall down onto their laps in an abrupt manner. At this point, therapists suggest heaviness and relaxation (already prompted in the previous exercises), as well as a sense of greater activation and an expanding capacity of the mind. Finally, therapists suggest that one hand is very heavy and stuck to the leg so that they can suggest later that the more clients attempt to separate them, the heavier and more stuck the hand will become. In this way, the more the clients try to lift their hand, the more difficult it will be for them. This suggestion is carried out while reminding clients of the content of the cognitive–behavioral introduction: The suggested reaction is fictional; however, it can be experienced as if it were real, thus readdressing Sarbin's role enactment theory (Coe & Sarbin, 1991; Sarbin & Coe, 1972).

In the beginning, clients typically experience these exercises with their eyes closed. With practice, however, they are able to experience them with their eyes open, shortening the prominence of the movements until they are almost unnoticeable, as follows: (a) Clients lean forward in the chair, as if they are paying attention to something; (b) the hands join in a nonobvious way, with arms bent and the elbows resting on whatever surface is available (e.g., a desk, the legs, the armrests of the chair); (c) exhalations and hand clasping are performed in a disguised fashion, adopting an appropriate facial expression according to the situation (e.g., interest, great surprise, concentration); (d) finally, falling backward is concealed, so that it looks as if individuals have simply changed positions in the chair. With eyes open and talking normally, clients "evoke" the heavy sensation in their hands and suggest the challenge exercise to themselves. At this point, clients are told that their brains are now ready to respond to the therapist's suggestion (or, in the subsequent sessions, the clients' suggestions), whatever the nature of the suggestions may be, including suggestions for mental activation, alertness, mind expansion, and openness. In other words, clients shift from being relaxed to feeling activated and energized, thus being able to experience the suggested therapeutic reactions (e.g., to feel indifference toward certain foods, happiness and well-being, analgesia) while they carry out their daily tasks.

With practice, this disguised form of self-hypnosis becomes more abbreviated and better disguised. If clients are capable of reproducing extreme heaviness in their arm, with little practice, they can concentrate on the arm (with the eyes open, without interrupting the flow of activities) and self-suggest that the arm is heavy and immobile, as if the arm were not theirs, in effect experiencing a dissociation of the arm from the body. The clients are now in self-hypnosis, and are ready to implement therapeutic suggestions. In other words, rapid self-hypnosis is reduced to a single instruction of reproducing a sensation. It often goes unnoticed by others because it does not require overt exercises, eye closure, or a relaxed posture. Clients thus gain access to self-hypnosis by fading the relaxation exercises and relinquishing the traditional hypnotic appearance (i.e., eyes closed, relaxed, sleepy). Accordingly, all individuals need to do in everyday life is to activate the dissociation of the arm to set the stage for self-administering therapeutic suggestions. However, if they wish, clients can use the rapid self-hypnosis exercises to achieve quick but intense relaxation.

A Metaphor for Attitudinal Consolidation

Once clients have experienced hypnosis (in this case by self-hypnosis), we provide a metaphor that is designed to help them access personal resources and consolidate the following ideas: (a) hypnosis is not dangerous; (b) successful responding does not imply a lack of effort or perseverance to achieve a change in behavior; and (c) hypnosis is an important tool that can act a catalyst of other treatments, such as cognitive–behavioral interventions. The metaphor also helps to engender a less esoteric and more scientific and natural view of hypnosis, based on ordinary and well-known processes, helping clients to appreciate the commonality between hypnotic and "normal" behaviors.

This metaphor, which was published previously (Capafons, Alarcón, & Hemmings, 1999), will not be repeated in entirety here because of its length. However, it involves clients as the main characters in an adventure story in a jungle. They confront various difficult situations and overcome them with their own effort, creativity, and use of a multipurpose tool. The metaphor is intended to be a didactic aid that allows the clients to consolidate and remember information about hypnosis (Porush, 1987), as well as to activate self-efficacy expectations to facilitate therapeutic outcome (Callow & Benson, 1990).

The Role of Heterohypnosis

As we have indicated, our model of therapeutic intervention using hypnosis is based on creating positive attitudes about hypnosis and using waking suggestion to enhance self-control skills, while adapting the method to clients' particular problems. Accordingly, clients learn exercises that help them acquire self-hypnosis skills they can use under most any circumstances and enable them to become the main agents responsible for their own psychotherapy. To do this, therapists can hypnotize clients with the aim of reinforcing the efficacy of the self-administered suggestions. In the waking hypnosis model, alert or active–alert methods are used (see chap. 10, this volume), which encourage the clients to keep their eyes open, adopt a normal everyday appearance, and even maintain pleasant conversations with the therapist (as is the case in rapid self-hypnosis). Normally, the therapist provides suggestions to the effect that rapid self-hypnosis will facilitate the activation of the clients' resources and that they will react in a subjectively compelling manner, allowing them to modulate, regulate, and produce robust therapeutic changes. Stated another way, rapid self-hypnosis is the axis around which heterohypnosis will turn.

As indicated herein, workers in the field have developed various methods of alert hypnosis (Barabasz & Barabasz, 1996; Vingoe, 1973; Wark, 1998), which sometimes is called *hyperempiria* (Gibbons, 1979; see also chap. 10, this volume). In general, hyperempiric methods include relaxation and eye closure. Bányai and colleagues (Bányai et al., 1993; Bányai & Hilgard, 1976) created probably the most researched and well known of these methods. However, Bányai's approach requires an ergonomic bicycle, or a spacious room in which the clients can walk around and activate themselves, which may be incompatible with clients who have cardiovascular problems or with the preferences of certain clients (Capafons, 1998a). The waking-alert hypnosis or alert-hand heterohypnosis method, designed by the first author (Capafons), may be preferable to other action–alert induction methods insofar as clients are required to perform only a gentle physical exercise (i.e., hand movement) that emphasizes keeping the eyes open, general activation, and even walking while remaining "hypnotized."

To reduce reactions of stress and anxiety (Ludwig & Lyle, 1964), clients first carry out a few brief exercises to familiarize themselves with the reactions that they will later experience (Cardeña et al., 1998). Clients are then asked to move their dominant hands up and down until the movement seems automatic. When clients indicate that this objective has been achieved, the therapist suggests that their hearts pump more blood to keep the hands moving and that their heartbeat and breathing rate will increase. The clinician then suggests that the augmented heartbeat and breathing rate will activate the brain, which will become increasingly alert, along with the muscles of the body. When clients report that they feel alert and activated, the therapist suggests that they stand up and walk around while they remain active, alert, and hypnotized. Suggestions can then be given to confirm that the brain is now receptive, activated, and ready to respond to therapeutic suggestions that reinforce expectancies for positive change and the effectiveness of rapid self-hypnosis. On occasion, clients show a marked interest in receiving suggestions from the therapist. When this occurs, their preference is respected, with the understanding that "control" can be gradually passed back to the client.

CLINICAL APPLICATIONS

Therapists who have learned waking hypnosis and use it in their practice, report that they have successfully applied it as an adjunct to the cognitive–behavioral treatment of anxiety disorders, smoking cessation, depression, pain management, obesity, and so forth. Some of these therapists combine waking hypnosis with traditional hypnosis when clients request relaxation and when it better matches their expectancies regarding hypnosis. Moreover, therapists generally agree that waking hypnosis is a useful addition to their repertoire of techniques and that it institutes a brief, pleasant experience for their clients. Indeed, when the procedures are first introduced, many clients are excited about learning them, insofar as they perceive the method as a straightforward means of controlling their emotions and behaviors. Their interest and motivation is spurred by their perception that the rationale for hypnosis is "rational" and focused meaningfully on addressing concerns in their everyday life. Moreover, because the examples provided to clients are easy to understand, education level generally does not limit the advantages of the method. In addition, once the clients have learned to use waking hypnosis, they have a portable tool, which they can disguise and they can implement in situations where anxiety or other problems occur and when they can benefit most from waking hypnosis.

As mentioned earlier, waking hypnosis makes it easier for clients to carry out therapeutic home assignments. For instance, when clients with phobias need to cope with a feared situation they usually avoid, they can use posthypnotic suggestions and rapid self-hypnosis to reduce anxiety and cope with the situation through self-suggestion. Given that the techniques foster self-control, they can be invaluable in treating habit disorders and in coping with cravings for food, alcohol, and other drugs. It is interesting that therapists with considerable experience in using waking hypnosis often comment that their clients develop creative uses of the procedures they are taught and that benefits generalize to an array of problems beyond the presenting complaint. Success breeds further involvement and success, which transfers to many aspects of the therapy as clients gain increasing control of formerly automatic emotions and responses and general self-efficacy expectations are strengthened, often shortening what could be a much longer therapy. Therapists with backgrounds in a variety of helping professions, including medicine, social work, counseling, and psychology, can incorporate cost-effective waking hypnosis methods into their therapeutic regimens. Finally, therapists remark that clients only rarely reject waking hypnosis, and when this happens, it occurs because clients tend to be closed-minded in terms of accepting procedures other than the traditional hypnosis they expected. Figure 11.1 summarizes this process.

RESEARCH AND APPRAISAL

A great deal of our group's research has been focused on the experimental validation of the Valencia Model of Waking Hypnosis. The assessment instruments for beliefs and attitudes toward hypnosis, the introduction of hypnosis, the two methods of induction, as well as the metaphor we developed have

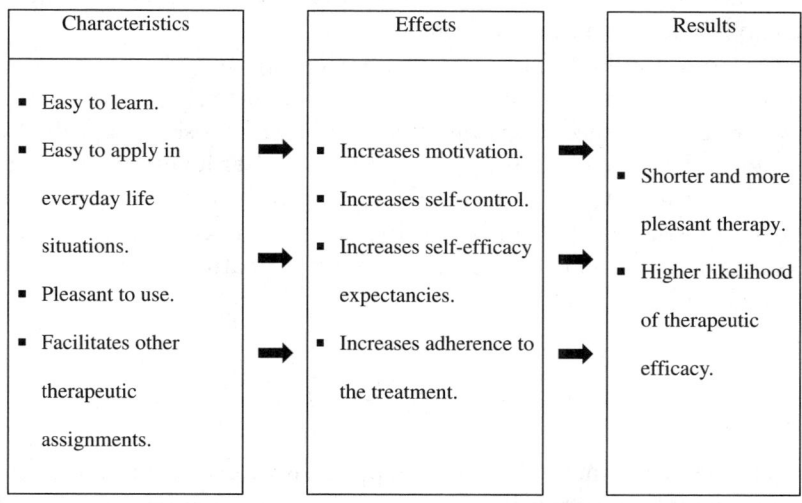

Figure 11.1. Waking hypnosis methods.

garnered empirical support as efficacious methods for their original purposes. However, there is only one published study of its clinical efficacy (Mendoza, 2000), which used a single-case experimental design and provided evidence of the promise of the approach for smoking cessation. In addition, preliminary research (Martínez-Valero et al., 2008) showed that a cognitive–behavioral treatment plus hypnosis and medication is more efficacious than the same treatment without hypnosis, and both are much more efficacious than the treatment using only medication.

Research conducted on the waking-alert method indicates that it produces high levels of responsiveness to test suggestions, that participants rate the experience as pleasant (Cardeña et al., 1998), and that it results in less attrition and greater responsivity than Bányai's method (Alarcón et al., 1999). Research carried out by our group (Martínez-Tendero et al., 2001) showed that rapid self-hypnosis is perceived as pleasant, as well as easy to understand, learn, and use. Moreover, rapid self-hypnosis appears to be just as "powerful" as both other forms of self-hypnosis (Spiegel & Spiegel, 2006) and heterohypnosis with respect to fostering responsiveness to test suggestions. Other research has shown that many people experience the reactions suggested by the method of induction (i.e., relaxation, heaviness, challenge exercise) and also experience the method as pleasant (Reig, Capafons, Bayot, & Bustillo, 2001). In addition, the findings of Reig et al. (2001) indicate that the arm dissociation variant of rapid self-hypnosis is perceived as even more pleasant and that it promotes more responses to the suggestions than the falling backward and hand-clasping variant. In other words, both the long and the short versions of rapid self-hypnosis are well received by participants and, after a few days practice of the exercises described previously, the effectiveness and pleasantness of the technique can be increased by using arm dissociation.

Research conducted by Capafons, Alarcón, and Hemmings (1999) demonstrated that after listening to the metaphor during hypnosis, the majority of volunteers changed their opinions regarding hypnosis, accepting it with greater confidence as a technique to achieve higher levels of self-control. Clearly, controlled trials targeting different problems and components of waking hypnosis, including rapid self-hypnosis, are necessary to expand our understanding of the value and generalizability of treatment gains to a variety of problems in living.

CONCLUSION

We believe the methods of waking hypnosis we described in this chapter have considerable clinical utility. Many participants describe our approach to suggestion management as pleasant, enjoyable, and useful. Waking hypnosis sacrifices none of the efficacy attributed to other forms of hypnotic suggestion management and even surpasses a number of other methods in research support. All of the procedures we have proposed are derived from cognitive–behavioral or sociocognitive conceptions of hypnosis (being, at the same time, permeable enough to incorporate the ideas and methods of other schools that fit with such conceptions) and have been empirically validated. Our waking suggestion approach is not only effective but also efficient (see Seligman's, 1995, 1996, definition) as well as flexible in being adaptable to changing preferences and client needs. At a time when hypnosis is not widely embraced by the general public, we (see Capafons, 2002) are in agreement with Lynn and Fite's (1998) contention that sociocognitive views of hypnosis may gain widespread acceptance as clinicians become better informed of the experimental literature. Without mentioning the words *trance* or *altered state of consciousness*, we have succeeded in creating a context in which both clients and therapist can enjoy creating useful suggestions while their beliefs about hypnosis are in accordance with the information provided by the empirical literature. Paradoxically, the results of scientific investigations validate and confirm well-worn concepts: (a) Waking hypnosis is just as effective and efficient as hypnosis by relaxation, (b) almost everyone can experience hypnosis to some degree or be trained to be hypnotized (see chap. 13, this volume), and (c) hypnotic responses imply that clients can access certain resources that are available in nonhypnotic circumstances. Only time will tell whether Lynn and Fite's prediction that sociocognitive points of view will meet widespread acceptance is correct. Our view is that we can increase the likelihood of this development if clinical psychologists and researchers join to create effective and efficient change methodologies—based on not only sociocognitive principles but also other empirically grounded theories and principles—that can be integrated and translated into viable techniques in an appealing and compelling manner.

REFERENCES

Alarcón, A., Capafons, A., Bayot, A., & Cardeña, E. (1999). Preference between two methods of active–alert hypnosis: Not all techniques are created equal . . . *American Journal of Clinical Hypnosis, 41,* 269–276.

Bányai, E. I., & Hilgard, E. R. (1976). A comparison of active–alert hypnotic induction with traditional relaxation induction. *Journal of Abnormal Psychology, 85,* 218–224.

Bányai, E. I., Zseni, A., & Túry, F. (1993). Active–alert hypnosis in psychotherapy. In J. W. Rhue, S. J. Lynn, & I. Kirsch (Eds.), *Handbook of clinical hypnosis* (pp. 271–290). Washington, DC: American Psychological Association.

Barabasz, A., & Barabasz, M. (1996). Neurotherapy and alert hypnosis in the treatment of attention deficit hyperactivity disorder. In S. J. Lynn, I. Kirsch, & J. W. Rhue (Eds.), *Casebook of clinical hypnosis* (pp. 271–291). Washington, DC: American Psychological Association.

Barber, J. (1991). The locksmith model: Accessing hypnotic responsiveness. In S. J. Lynn & J. W. Rhue (Eds.), *Theories of hypnosis: Current models and perspectives* (pp. 241–274). New York: Guilford Press.

Barber, T. X. (1999). A comprehensive three-dimensional theory of hypnosis. In I. Kirsch, A. Capafons, E. Cardeña, & S. Amigó (Eds.), *Clinical hypnosis and self-regulation: Cognitive–behavioral perspectives* (pp. 21–48). Washington, DC: American Psychological Association.

Callow, G., & Benson, G. (1990). Metaphor technique (story telling) as a treatment option. *Educational and Child Psychology, 7,* 54–60.

Capafons, A. (1998a). Hipnosis clínica: una visión cognitivo–comportamental [Clinical hypnosis: A cognitive–behavioral perspective]. *Papeles del Psicólogo, 69,* 71–88.

Capafons, A. (1998b). Rapid self-hypnosis: A suggestion method for self-control. *Psicothema, 10,* 571–581.

Capafons, A. (1999). La hipnosis despierta setenta y cuatro años después [Waking hypnosis 74 years later]. *Anales de Psicología, 15,* 77–88.

Capafons, A. (2001a). *Hipnosis* [Hypnosis]. Madrid, Spain: Síntesis.

Capafons, A. (2001b). News methods of hypnosis. In T. McIntyre, Â. Costa, & C. Fernandes (Eds.), *Hipnose clínica: Uma abordagem científica* [Clinical hypnosis: A scientific approach] (pp. 121–135). Braga, Portugal: Bial.

Capafons, A. (2002): Dissemination of hypnosis: Don't change the name, change the perspective. *Hypnosis International Monographs, 6,* 225–236.

Capafons, A. (2004a). Clinical applications of "waking" hypnosis from a cognitive–behavioural perspective: From efficacy to efficiency. *Contemporary Hypnosis, 21,* 187–201.

Capafons, A. (2004b). Waking hypnosis for waking people: Why from Valencia? *Contemporary Hypnosis, 21,* 136–145.

Capafons, A., Alarcón, A., & Hemmings, M. (1999). A metaphor for hypnosis. *Australian Journal of Clinical and Experimental Hypnosis, 27,* 158–172.

Capafons, A., & Amigó, S. (1993). *Hipnosis y terapia de auto-regulación (introducción práctica)* [Hypnosis and self-regulation therapy (a practical introduction)]. Madrid: Eudema.

Capafons, A., Cabañas, S., Alarcón, A. Espejo, B., Mendoza, M. E., Chaves, J. F., & Monje, A. (2005). Effects of different types of preparatory information on attitudes toward hypnosis. *Contemporary Hypnosis, 22,* 67–76.

Capafons, A., Selma, M. L., Cabañas, S., Espejo, B., Alarcón, A., Mendoza, M. E., & Natkin, Y. (2006). Change of attitudes toward hypnosis: Effects of cognitive–

behavioral and trance explanations in a setting of heterohypnosis. *Australian Journal of Clinical and Experimental Hypnosis, 34,* 119–134.

Cardeña, E., Alarcón, A., Capafons, A., & Bayot, A. (1998). Effects on suggestibility of a new method of active–alert hypnosis. *International Journal of Clinical and Experimental Hypnosis, 45,* 280–294.

Chaves, J. F. (1996). Hypnotic strategies for somatoform disorders. In S. J. Lynn, I. Kirsch, & J. W. Rhue (Eds.), *Casebook of clinical hypnosis* (pp. 131–151). Washington, DC: American Psychological Association.

Coe, W. C. (1980). Expectations, hypnosis, and suggestions in change. In F. H. Kanfer & A. P. Goldstein (Eds.), *Helping people change* (2nd ed.; 432–469). New York: Pergamon Press.

Coe, W. C., & Sarbin, T. R. (1991). Role theory: Hypnosis from a dramaturgical and narrational perspective. In J. W. Rhue, S. J. Lynn, & I. Kirsch (Eds.), *Handbook of clinical hypnosis* (pp. 303–323). Washington, DC: American Psychological Association.

Council, J. R. (1998). Hypnosis and assessment. *Psychological Hypnosis, 7,* 13–16.

Egner, T., & Gruzelier, J. H. (2003). Ecological validity of neurofeedback: Modulation of slow wave EEG enhances musical performance. *Neuroreport, 14,* 1221–1224.

Eysenck, H. J. (1989). Personality, primary and secondary suggestibility, and hypnosis. In V. A. Gheorghiu, P. Netter, H. J. Eysenck, & R. Rosenthal (Eds.), *Suggestions and suggestibility* (pp. 57–67). Berlin: Springer-Verlag.

Gheorghiu, V. A. (1989). The development of research on suggestibility: Critical considerations. In V. A. Gheorghiu, P. Netter, H. J. Eysenck, & R. Rosenthal (Eds.), *Suggestions and suggestibility* (pp. 3–55). Berlin: Springer-Verlag.

Gibbons, D. G. (1979). *Applied hypnosis and hyperempiria.* New York: Plenum Press.

Gorassini, D. R. (1999). Hypnotic responding: A cognitive–behavioral analysis of self-deception. In I. Kirsch, A. Capafons, E. Cardeña, & S. Amigó (Eds.), *Clinical hypnosis and self-regulation: Cognitive–behavioral perspectives* (pp. 73–103). Washington, DC: American Psychological Association.

Gruzelier, J., Levy, J., Williams, J., & Henderson, D. (2001). Self-hypnosis and exam stress: Comparing immune and relaxation-related imagery for influences on immunity, health, and mood. *Contemporary Hypnosis, 18,* 73–86.

Hilgard, E. R. (1965). *Hypnotic susceptibility.* New York: Harcourt Brace & World.

Hull, C. L. (1933). *Hypnosis and suggestibility: An experimental approach.* New York: Appleton-Century-Crofts.

Katz, N. W. (1978). Hypnotic inductions as training in cognitive self-control. *Cognitive Therapy and Research, 2,* 365–369.

Kirsch, I. (1994). Clinical hypnosis as a nondeceptive placebo: Empirically derived techniques. *American Journal of Clinical Hypnosis, 37,* 95–106.

Kirsch, I. (1997). Suggestibility or hypnosis: What do our scales really measure? *International Journal of Clinical and Experimental Hypnosis, 45,* 212–225.

Kirsch, I. (1999). Hypnosis and placebos: Response expectancy as a mediator of suggestion effects. *Anales de Psicología, 15*, 99–110.

Kirsch, I., & Lynn, S. J. (1998). Social–cognitive alternatives to dissociation theories of hypnotic involuntariness. *Review of General Psychology, 2*, 66–80.

Kratochvil, S. (1970). Sleep hypnosis and waking hypnosis. *International Journal of Clinical and Experimental Hypnosis, 18*, 25–40.

Kroger, W. S., & Fezler, W. D. (1976). *Hypnosis and behavior modification: Imagery conditioning.* Philadelphia: Lippincott Williams & Wilkins.

Lynn, S. J. (1997). Automaticity and hypnosis: A sociocognitive account. *International Journal of Clinical and Experimental Hypnosis, 45*, 239–250.

Lynn, S. J., & Fite, R. (1998). Will the false memory debate increase acceptance of the sociocognitive model of hypnosis? *Contemporary Hypnosis, 15*, 171–174.

Lynn, S. J., & Kirsch, I. (2005). Teorías de hipnosis [Theories of hypnosis]. *Papeles del Psicólogo, 25*, 9–15.

Lynn, S. J., Kirsch, I., & Rhue, J. W. (1996). Maximizing treatment gains: Recommendations for the practice of clinical hypnosis. In S. J. Lynn, I. Kirsch, & J. W. Rhue (Eds.), *Casebook of clinical hypnosis* (pp. 395–406). Washington, DC: American Psychological Association.

Lynn, S. J., Rhue, J. W., & Weekes, J. R. (1990). Hypnotic involuntariness: A social cognitive analysis. *Psychological Review, 97*, 169–184.

Lynn, S. J., Vanderhoff, H., Shindler K., & Stafford J. (2002). Defining hypnosis as a trance vs. cooperation: Hypnotic inductions, suggestibility, and performance standards. *American Journal of Clinical Hypnosis, 44*, 231–240.

Ludwig, A. M., & Lyle, W. H. (1964). Tension induction and the hyperalert trance. *Journal of Abnormal and Social Psychology, 69*, 70–76.

Martínez-Tendero, J., Capafons, A., Weber, V., & Cardeña, E. (2001). Rapid self-hypnosis: A new self-hypnosis method and its comparison with the Hypnosis Induction Profile. *American Journal of Clinical Hypnosis, 44*, 3–11.

Martínez-Valero, C., Castell, A., Capafons, A., Sala J., Espejo, B., & Cardeña, E. (2008). Hypnotic treatment synergizes the psychological treatment of fibromyalgia: A pilot study. *American Journal of Clinical Hypnosis, 50*, 311–321.

Matthews, W. J., Conti, J., & Starr, L. (1998). Ericksonian hypnosis: A review of the empirical data. In W. J. Matthews & J. Edgette (Eds.), *Current thinking and research in brief therapy, solutions, strategies, narratives* (Vol. 2, pp. 239–263). Philadelphia: Taylor & Francis.

Mendoza, M. E. (2000). La hipnosis como adjunto en el tratamiento del hábito de fumar: Estudio de caso [Hypnosis as an adjunct to the treatment for smoking cessation: A case study]. *Psicothema, 12*, 330–338.

Porush, D. (1987). What Homer can teach technical writers: The mnemonic value of poetic devices. *Journal of Technical Writing and Communication, 17*, 129–143.

Reig, I., Capafons, A., Bayot, A., & Bustillo, A. (2001). Suggestion and degree of pleasantness of rapid self-hypnosis and its abbreviated variant. *Australian Journal of Clinical and Experimental Hypnosis, 29*, 152–164.

Sarbin, T. R., & Coe, W. C. (1972). *Hypnosis: A social psychological analysis of influence communication*. New York: Holt, Rinehart & Winston.

Schoenberger, N. E. (2000). Research on hypnosis as an adjunct to cognitive–behavioral psychotherapy. *International Journal of Experimental and Clinical Hypnosis, 48*, 154–169.

Seligman, M. E. (1995). The effectiveness of psychotherapy: The consumer reports study. *American Psychologist, 50*, 965–974.

Seligman, M. E. (1996). Science as an ally of practice. *American Psychologist, 51*, 1072–1079.

Spanos, N. P. (1996). *Multiple identities and false memories*. Washington, DC: American Psychological Association.

Spanos, N. P., & Coe, W. C. (1992). A social–psychological approach to hypnosis. In E. Fromm & M. R. Nash (Eds.), *Contemporary hypnosis research* (pp. 102–130). New York: Guilford Press.

Spiegel, H., & Spiegel, D. (2006). *Trance and treatment: Clinical uses of hypnosis* (2nd ed.). Arlington, VA: American Publishing.

Vingoe, F. J. (1973). Comparison of the Harvard Group Scale of Hypnotic Susceptibility, Form A, and the group alert trance scale in a university population. *International Journal of Clinical and Experimental Hypnosis, 21*, 169–179.

Wagstaff, G. F. (1998). The hypnotic state: Semantics and pragmatics. *Contemporary Hypnosis, 15*, 182–188.

Wark, D. M. (1998). Alert hypnosis: History and applications. In W. J. Matthews & J. Edgette (Eds.), *Current thinking and research in brief therapy: Solutions, strategies, narratives* (pp. 287–304). Philadelphia: Taylor & Francis.

Weitzenhoffer, A. M. (1989). *The practice of hypnotism: Vol. 1. Traditional and semi-traditional techniques and phenomenology*. New York: Wiley.

Wells, W. (1924). Experiments in waking hypnosis for instructional purposes. *Journal of Abnormal and Social Psychology, 18*, 389–404.

12

HYPNOSIS, MINDFULNESS, AND ACCEPTANCE: ARTFUL INTEGRATION

JOHN C. WILLIAMS, MICHAEL N. HALLQUIST, SEAN M. BARNES,
ALISON S. COLE, AND STEVEN JAY LYNN

Mindfulness refers to purposeful, nonjudgmental attention to the unfolding of experience on a moment-to-moment basis (Kabat-Zinn, 1990/2005). This deceptively simple activity has arguably revolutionized the treatment of many psychological disorders. Mindful awareness of the ebb and flow of experience creates a viable platform for therapy by buffering the impact of self-centered thoughts, cognitive biases, and prior conditioning experiences that contribute to maladaptive behaviors and emotional problems (see Brown, Ryan, & Creswell, 2007, for a review of mindfulness).

Mindfulness can be practiced through formal meditation methods, including focusing attention on breathing, noticing experiences and how they naturally unwind, and withholding judgments and attempts to alter the experiences in any way. Mindfulness can also be practiced more informally throughout the day by cultivating an accepting awareness of internal and external experiences. Although mindfulness is historically linked to Buddhist meditation, it is currently integral to an array of spiritual, philosophical, and, most recently, psychological traditions.

All clinical material has been disguised to protect patient confidentiality.

Mindfulness has influenced Western psychological science for at least 50 years (Perls, 1969). However, over the past few decades, researchers have turned increasing empirical attention to mindfulness, as evidenced by an explosion of psychological and medical research reports on the topic from less than 89 in 1990, to over 600 by the end of 2006 (Brown et al., 2007). Mindfulness is now a core feature of a number of cognitive–behavioral therapies, including mindfulness-based stress reduction (MBSR; Kabat-Zinn, 2003), mindfulness-based cognitive therapy (MBCT; Segal, Williams, & Teasdale, 2002), dialectical behavior therapy (DBT; Linehan, 1993), acceptance and commitment therapy (ACT; Hayes, Strosahl, & Wilson, 1999), and integrative behavioral couple therapy (Christensen, Jacobson, & Babcock, 1995). Moreover, mindfulness-based interventions have been used successfully to treat stress (e.g., Shapiro, Schwartz, & Bonner, 1998), anxiety (e.g., Tacón, Caldera, & Ronaghan, 2004), depression (Ma & Teasdale, 2004; Teasdale et al., 2000), borderline personality disorder (McQuillan et al., 2005), substance abuse (e.g., Bowen et al., 2006), marital distress (e.g., Christensen et al., 2004), chronic pain (e.g., Kabat-Zinn, Lipworth, & Burney, 1985), psoriasis (Kabat-Zinn et al., 1998), and psychosis (Bach & Hayes, 2002; Gaudiano & Herbert, 2006). Finally, researchers and clinicians have used mindfulness interventions to improve treatment adherence (e.g., Gregg, Callaghan, Hayes, & Glenn-Lawson, 2007).

Given the mushrooming literature supporting the integration of mindfulness techniques and traditional therapies, it is perhaps surprising that workers in the field have not seized on the possibility of integrating mindfulness and hypnotic procedures. The current chapter presents a framework for integrating hypnosis and mindfulness in an eclectic approach to psychotherapy. We discuss body scans, breath awareness, and mindful metacognitive sets as methods of enhancing hypnotic interventions. Next, we illustrate this approach with case material. Finally, we examine recent studies on the integration of mindfulness and hypnosis and discuss implications for further research.

INTEGRATING MINDFULNESS AND HYPNOSIS

Hypnosis and mindfulness are similar in that they alter attention in service of therapeutic goals. *Hypnotic methods* can be defined as interventions that encourage patients to focus their attention on imaginative suggestions and their subjective responses to them. *Hypnotic suggestions* generally focus on changing specific behaviors and experiences, in keeping with therapeutic aims and objectives. In mindfulness interventions, suggestions are not paramount. Rather, mindfulness emphasizes general acceptance of the flow of moment-to-moment experience rather than delimited changes in thoughts, feelings, and behaviors.

Mindfulness thus promotes a global shift in attention, in lieu of attachment to any particular experience or goal, other than nonjudgmental attention itself.

Salient differences aside, it is, nevertheless, possible to find common ground between mindfulness and hypnosis in response set theory (Kirsch & Lynn, 1997, 1998), which can serve as a foundation for integrating hypnosis and mindfulness in psychotherapy (see Lynn, Das, Hallquist, & Williams, 2006). *Response sets* are conditioned patterns of associations that facilitate particular cognitions, behaviors, and self-representations. Response sets can be activated by internal or external stimuli, such as suggestions and a variety of environmental cues. Mindfulness and hypnosis can be usefully combined to ameliorate maladaptive response sets and develop novel adaptive response sets.

Mindfulness can deautomatize habitual response sets and bring conscious awareness to maladaptive behavior patterns. Teasdale, Segal, and Williams (2003) suggested that mindfulness trains individuals "to switch out of habitual, relatively automatic, patterns of reaction into a more intentional, considered choice of response" (p. 159). By encouraging nonjudgmental awareness, mindfulness activates self-monitoring and supervisory attentional processes that may bring to light maladaptive response sets and encourage the development of multiple options in situations that were previously tied to a single maladaptive response. For example, by adopting a mindful response set, a patient who frequently responded to criticism with verbal outbursts of anger, can choose among many response options, including expressing anger, acting with deference and forgiveness, and/or accepting the critical remarks as a potentially useful source of feedback. Moreover, mindfulness may facilitate awareness of the immediate reward–consequence contingencies operative in a situation, which mitigates responding in a reflexive, rigid, or unconscious rule-bound manner. Indeed, contingency-governed behavior is associated with greater behavioral flexibility than rule-governed behavior (Hayes et al., 1999).

Whereas mindfulness facilitates the recognition and dissolution of maladaptive response sets in general, hypnotic suggestions can target specific symptoms and maladaptive response sets and, through suggestion, replace them with more adaptive response sets, beliefs, and attitudes. Accordingly, hypnosis and mindfulness techniques can be artfully combined to gain leverage in treating psychological problems (see Lynn et al., 2006, for a more detailed explanation of the integration of hypnosis and mindfulness).

CLINICAL APPLICATIONS

Meta-analyses and qualitative reviews have documented that hypnosis enhances the effectiveness of both psychodynamic and cognitive–behavioral psychotherapies (Kirsch, 1990; Kirsch, Montgomery, & Sapirstein, 1995;

Lynn, Kirsch, Barabasz, Cardeña, & Patterson, 2000). In fact, the mean effect for adding hypnosis to cognitive–behavioral therapy (Cohen's d = .48) rivals the effect size of psychotherapy itself (Cohen's d = .52; Lipsey & Wilson, 1993). As mindfulness and acceptance therapies yield treatment gains similar to more well established cognitive–behavioral therapies (see Baer, 2003, for review), there is reason to believe that hypnosis will likewise enhance the effectiveness of mindfulness training. Indeed, instructions to practice mindful awareness can be thought of as attention-altering suggestions that can be augmented when therapists administer them within a hypnotic context. Relatively traditional hypnotic inductions that emphasize relaxation (see chap. 10, this volume), for example, can be used to establish a hypnotic context (see case material for details on maintaining theoretical consistency during integration). We suspect that clients will reap the most benefits when hypnosis is used in conjunction with mindfulness training early in treatment insofar as mindfulness may require considerable training and practice to implement effectively. Moreover, clinicians can use hypnosis to mitigate stressful situations and promote relaxation more generally, thereby freeing up cognitive resources necessary to master mindfulness skills, as our case example will illustrate.

Mindfulness interventions can be easily integrated into standard hypnotherapy scripts. Clinical findings indicate that integrating mindfulness techniques with hypnotherapy may yield positive therapeutic outcomes beyond either approach used in isolation (Holroyd, 2003). Mindfulness may nicely complement the later stages of hypnotic interventions by sustaining and generalizing treatment gains to real-life settings. Indeed, preliminary evidence indicates that mindfulness training, which can be implemented in a variety of situations, much like self-hypnosis, enhances the persistence of treatment gains (Walrath & Hamilton, 1975).

Enhancing Mindfulness-Based Treatments Using Hypnosis

We now present techniques that can be used to integrate mindfulness and hypnosis in practice. The techniques we describe focus on cognitive, affective, and behavioral dimensions of human experience.

Body Scan

The body scan is a common meditative exercise that facilitates and refines sensitivity to bodily experiences and increases daily awareness of the body. The body scan is often done lying down, but it can also be done while standing or sitting. The client scans the body for sensations beginning with the head or the toes, working slowly to the other end of the body. There is no set time limit, and the goal is not relaxation, although it may ensue. When the mind inevitably wanders, attention is refocused on the body part that was the object of attention when concentration waned. Continued practice enhances the ability to sustain concentration.

Hypnotic suggestions for a body scan could include the following:

> Now that you have found a comfortable position, begin to notice the focus of your attention. Do you notice any sensations associated with the position of your body? Perhaps (if lying down) where the back of your body touches the floor? Or perhaps your mind is occupied with thoughts about the future or the past. For the next [X number of] minutes, you will direct your attention systematically to each part of your body, concentrating in turn on each part, and noticing what sensations you can become aware of. Your only task is to generate an intention to remain focused on this task. Your mind will naturally begin to wander, so simply refocus it on the body part you were attending to when you drifted away. Make a commitment now to bring your attention back to your body. Connect with the present moment, with your own body, and witness your powers of concentration increasing on a moment-to-moment basis.

Posthypnotic suggestions for the body scan could include suggestions to scan the body whenever one walks into a building, through a doorway, or gets into bed at night.

Breath Awareness

Increasing awareness of the inflow and outflow of the breath is one of the most common and effective ways to develop attentional control. MBSR (Kabat-Zinn, 2003) and MBCT (Segal et al., 2002) use attention to the breath as an anchor point to develop the ability to observe, describe, and attend to internal events, a response set that replaces a judgmental stance toward internal experience. Like the body scan, the purpose of breath awareness is to train attention and concentration, and identify internal events while describing them from a neutral, detached point of view. The breath awareness technique directs attention to the physical process of breathing while the participant simultaneously notes all of the internal events that draw attention away from the breath. The task is to notice when this happens, describe the event in neutral terms, then "let it go" by returning attention to the breath. The participant says, "I am having the thought _____; I am having the feeling _____" and then returns to the breath without commenting further on the thought or feeling. Examples of hypnotic suggestions for breath awareness could include the following:

> Now that you are sitting comfortably, direct your attention to the flow of the breath; notice the various parts of the body in which you sense this flow. Notice your abdomen, and see if you can feel any expansion and

contraction as your breath flows in and out. Notice your chest, and see if you can sense it rising and falling. Notice any sensation of airflow in your throat. Notice the sensations of air flowing in and out of your mouth or nose. Now choose the place in which you feel the sensations of the breath most strongly, whether it is the pit of your belly or the very tip of your nose. Let your attention rest on that place. For the next [X number of] minutes, your task will be to focus your attention on the inflow and out-flow of the breath; watch the breath flow in and out, feel the sensations of the flowing breath. You don't need to change how you are breathing, simply watch it. At times your breath may be shallow or deep, fast or slow. While you are doing this, the mind will begin to wander. This is perfectly natural. You may begin to experience thoughts, feelings, or sensations that pull your attention away from the breath. These could be memories about the past, plans for the future, or thoughts about what you are doing. You may find yourself thinking about the breath rather than attending to how it actually feels in this moment. All of this is perfectly natural. When this happens, it is not because you are doing the exercise wrong; it is just what minds do. Your task is to focus on the breath, and whenever you notice that your mind has wandered, simply redirect it to the breath; whatever thoughts, feelings, or sensations drew your attention away, simply notice them. "I was having a thought about _____; I was feeling _____."Just notice what it was, and direct your attention back to the breath, to the pure sensations of the breath.

Posthypnotic suggestions for breath awareness may be put to good use by establishing a mindful response set to certain stimuli, such as talking to one's spouse or boss, when one notices habitual thought patterns arising, or at times when one would typically smoke a cigarette. In addition, posthypnotic sugges-tion may be used to create a habit of mindful breath awareness at specific times of the day to enhance the generalization of mindful awareness to daily life. Therapists can suggest momentary or sustained breath awareness in response to daily stimuli, including brushing one's teeth, sitting down for a meal, get-ting in or out of the car, and leaving the workplace at the end of the day. Of course, suggestions for breath awareness may be provided for any situation in which thought or emotional content are conspicuous and problematic.

Mindful Metacognitive Set

Wells (2000) defined *metacognition* as cognitive processes that are engaged in the appraisal, monitoring, or control of other cognitions. In both formal meditation and mindfulness, a key aspect is developing a specific relationship to internal events. More specifically, mindful awareness cultivates the recogni-tion that internal stimuli (e.g., thoughts, feelings, sensations) are merely events that occur within the self, but they are not the self. That is, we are not what we think, but we are the arena in which our thoughts take place.

The development of a mindful metacognitive set takes practice. It is typical for clients at the beginning of mindfulness practice to become frustrated by their inability to remain focused on the experience of thoughts as "thoughts," rather than as "truths" about the self, others, or situations. Exercises such as the body scan or breath awareness are invaluable aids to developing mindful metacognition. The ability to concentrate on an attentional target (e.g., breath) provides a vivid and instructive contrast to the flow of mental content that distracts from the attentional task.

Therapists can maximize the impact of common metacognitive metaphors by administering them as suggestions in a hypnotic context. Hypnotic suggestions related to metacognitive awareness could include the following: Imagine that your thoughts are written on signs carried by parading soldiers (Hayes, 1987) or that thoughts "continually dissolve like a parade of characters marching across a stage" (Rinpoche, 1981, p. 53). "Observe the parade of thoughts without becoming absorbed in any of them. Imagine that the mind is a conveyor belt. Thoughts, feelings that come down the belt are observed, labeled, and categorized" (Linehan, 1993; Tart, 1986).

Posthypnotic suggestions for mindful metacognition may be used in conjunction with a variety of hypnotic interventions. In treating disorders of eating, smoking, or alcohol abuse, for example, suggestions may be given to refocus attention during a craving episode on thoughts, feelings and sensations that arise, and to label them as such (i.e., "I'm having thoughts about using _____," "I have an uneasy sensation in my stomach.") and observe them as mental events rather than identifying with them or acting on them. Similarly, suggestions to observe thoughts and detach from them can be useful in situations in which the client's thoughts are historically and problematically fused to action, such as anger at a spouse or child escalating to yelling. Suggestions can be given to identify angry feelings when they arise and to focus on the experience of the feeling and the urgency to act rather than reflexively acting on transient impulses.

Formal and Informal Mindfulness Practice

Hypnotic interventions can be developed to increase the practice of formal and informal mindfulness meditation. Kabat-Zinn (1990/2005) noted that the most important part of mindfulness work is to keep the practice alive and delineated formal and informal aspects of mindfulness practice.

Hypnotic interventions can enhance the following formal aspects of meditation practice: (a) watching the breath rather than thinking about it, (b) returning to breath awareness as soon as attention becomes attached to thoughts, (c) not engaging in self-criticism when attention becomes absorbed in thinking, (d) realizing that the goal of meditation is not to attain a particular state of mind or experience, and (e) making a commitment to regularly practicing meditation. Moreover, posthypnotic suggestions can include reminders to meditate every day at a specific place and time.

Informal mindfulness practice centers on developing moment-to-moment awareness throughout the day by tuning into the breath, the body, and/or by noticing what mental content is active. Suggestions for mindful awareness in everyday life include being mindful at certain times of the day (e.g., upon waking, at the end of a stressful day) and at specific intervals (e.g., every hour) and when engaging in activities such as walking up a flight of stairs, exercising, and during conversations.

Enhancing Hypnotic Interventions Using Mindfulness and Acceptance

Mindfulness and acceptance strategies and principles can be used to generate an array of suggestions applicable to various disorders and conditions as well as to reduce stress in general. The next section illustrates how mindfulness and acceptance procedures, derived from DBT (Linehan, 1993) for treating borderline personality disorder, may be included in hypnotic interventions designed to regulate emotions. Because the sudden onset of unpleasant emotions may leave little time for responding mindfully, situations that typically trigger difficult emotions can serve as cues to practice mindfulness. For example, if the client has a difficult relationship with his spouse and experiences tension and conflict when both are home in the evening, then the arrival of the spouse could serve as a cue to become mindful of emotion. The onset of emotion can also serve as a cue for breath awareness and "checking in" to see what one is currently experiencing. Clients should be encouraged to observe their emotional responses and related thoughts and bodily sensations, labeling emotions as they arise (e.g., *anger*, *sadness*), with an eye toward experiencing the emotion as fully as possible while remaining connected to the breath. Clients can take their "emotional temperatures" throughout the day, observe the ebb and flow of emotions, and pay particular attention to positive emotions as they come and go to counteract a bias toward remembering negative emotional experiences.

CASE MATERIAL

The following case of an actual client (i.e., not a composite) was treated by one of us (Hallquist) for 17 sessions over the course of 6 months. Joan was a 40-year-old woman who was on disability because of relapsing-remitting multiple sclerosis. Joan was in the process of divorcing her second husband of 15 years, had moved to a town thousands of miles away from her husband, and was living on her own for the first time. Shortly after separating from her husband, Joan purchased a relatively run-down home, which was all she could afford on her modest disability check. She described feeling highly anxious about her ability to handle daily tasks such as cleaning the house, paying her bills, and renovating her home. She also described deep feelings of loss related to the failure of her marriage, having to move out of their home, and being separated from one of her three daughters, who continued to live with Joan's ex-husband.

Much of each day, Joan engaged in a vicious cycle of rumination about her past and worry about her future. When engaged in worry and rumination, Joan felt nauseated, often did not complete household tasks, and rarely socialized with friends and family. The intensity of her nausea had led Joan to lose over 15 pounds in the 6 months prior to therapy. In addition, Joan reported waking up in the early morning with ruminative thoughts running through her mind, which precluded her going back to sleep. She stated that she frequently felt exhausted and wished that she were able to sleep for longer each night.

Joan had a lengthy history of emotional dysregulation and depression. At the age of 25, she experienced a severe bout of depression that lasted roughly 1 year and resulted in 2 weeks of inpatient hospitalization. In addition, she was quite prone to perceiving others' actions as rejecting of her, and these actions confirmed her negative self-concept. Joan saw herself as a weak, incompetent woman who needed, in her words, a "strong, stable man" to take care of her and her children. She felt that without a steady relationship and a husband who would provide for the family's financial needs, she would be unable to take care of herself, would eventually be abandoned by everyone, and would have to kill herself. Indeed, Joan had attempted suicide after her estrangement from her second husband, and she perceived him as a malevolent man who wished that she were dead. Further, Joan relied heavily on others' opinions to make everyday decisions. She had a handful of friends whom she consulted each day about relatively simple decisions, such as how to arrange her furniture or what bills to pay first.

At the time of the initial interview, Joan met diagnostic criteria for generalized anxiety disorder, major depressive disorder, and dependent personality disorder. She also displayed symptoms of borderline personality disorder, such as "desperate attempts to avoid abandonment" (American Psychiatric Association, 1994). Joan had two major treatment goals: (a) to eliminate her debilitating cycle of worry and rumination and (b) to build the self-confidence that she felt was necessary for her to live an independent and valuable life.

The primary treatment modality used in this case was ACT (Hayes et al., 1999), although more eclectic techniques and conceptualizations were incorporated into the treatment. In brief, ACT emphasizes the importance of accepting thoughts and feelings for what they are: transient mental events that do not necessarily correspond closely to reality. Further, ACT sees much of psychopathology as stemming from experiential avoidance, which is defined as, "the phenomenon that occurs when a person is unwilling to remain in contact with particular private experiences (e.g., . . . emotions, thoughts, or memories . . .) and takes steps to alter the form or frequency of these events and the contexts that occasion them" (Hayes, 2004, p. 14). Attempts to suppress thoughts, although successful in the short-term, may increase the potency and frequency of these thoughts (Wenzlaff & Wegner, 2000). Thus, the main goal in ACT is to increase psychological flexibility, which is defined as the ability to remain in contact with aversive experiences when doing so serves valued ends.

In Joan's case, I conceptualized much of her worry and rumination as stemming from her unwillingness to experience the considerable feelings of loss that accompanied her divorce and her deep fears of independence and isolation. Joan endured a number of potent stressors, including the failure of her marriage, separation from her daughter, financial independence, and the emotional battering she sustained in her marriage. She emerged from the experience feeling as though she had invested so much of herself in pleasing her husband that she no longer knew who she was.

Given Joan's level of distress, I incorporated hypnosis early in the treatment to help her achieve relief from worry and rumination and to increase her willingness to learn mindfulness skills and complete ACT interventions. Consistent with the emphasis of mindfulness therapies on experiential avoidance as a central pathological process, I emphasized the use of hypnosis for distress tolerance and emotional awareness, rather than symptom remission, to minimize avoidance and rumination. The excerpt that follows is from the second therapy session, in which hypnosis was introduced to Joan. As mentioned in chapter 1, discussing the client's reservations and misconceptions of hypnosis is crucial to its effectiveness. In the interest of space, however, the initial discussion of the client's ideas about hypnosis was removed.

> *Therapist:* As I mentioned earlier, I thought that we could incorporate hypnosis into therapy to help you tolerate those times of really strong rumination and worry when you feel overwhelmed. Basically, hypnosis is a skill that you can learn to cope with negative thoughts and emotions without necessarily having to reason through or fight with them.
>
> *Joan:* I don't understand. How can I deal with my emotions without trying to figure out where they came from?
>
> *Therapist:* Well, that's a great question, and I think I can answer it better by helping you experience hypnosis. But to your question, I think of emotions and thoughts as temporary events. They come and go. Like do you ever feel really sad, the sort of sadness that you think will never leave, and then the doorbell

rings or a friend calls, and you feel jarred out of your sadness at least for a few moments?

Joan: Sort of, yeah, I think I know what you mean. Like I was at my sister's house the other day, and I was really ruminating about what an ass my ex-husband is and how low I feel, and we got to playing cards, and I really got into the game. And after a while, I noticed that I was engaged in the game and had forgotten all about my suffering. I was just playing.

Therapist: So, your attention was so focused on the game that you forgot about your suffering. But, Joan, where did your suffering go? Did you figure it out?

Joan: Well, no, I mean it was still there, and as soon as I realized that I had forgotten about it, it came flooding back to me. I just had to touch it, and it was there again, and I wished I had just kept playing.

Therapist: And what happened then, when you started wishing that you hadn't thought about your pain?

Joan: I guess I really focused on it and focused on myself and how terrible my life is right now. And I started playing a lot worse because I couldn't focus on the game. I just kept trying to stop thinking about it.

Therapist: And the more you tried to stop thinking about it, the more it took over, and it felt like you were fighting a war with yourself?

Joan: Exactly.

Therapist: That's a great example of what we were discussing last session: that struggling with thoughts and feelings makes them even bigger and stronger than they would be otherwise. And that's one area where hypnosis can help you out: by focusing your attention on helpful suggestions and taking you out of your internal criticism. In hypnosis, I will be offering you suggestions that focus your attention on your internal experience— whatever that may be—and on becoming more of who you want to be. I will offer positive suggestions to you about your ability to become engaged in your life and I will also suggest that you begin to see your thoughts as thoughts, as transient. But I think it's important to be careful about this because it's easy to hear what I'm saying as, "Hypnosis will make me feel good and not bad." That could easily become just another part of the war with sadness and suffering, like "I have to do hypnosis now because I feel so bad and I want to feel good and I just want these negative thoughts to go away, but they won't." And so on.

But like I've said before, I don't think there's any quick and easy way to get rid of the way you feel, including hypnosis. Using hypnosis as an attempt to not feel bad is just another way of feeding the frenzy of your worry and rumination. And what I'm asking you to do is to put down the weapons—to call a cease fire—because the only person who is dying in this war is you, Joan; your life is being consumed by this fight with your thoughts. Hypnosis is a tool that you can use to help you get out of your head, to set down your thoughts without having to figure them out, to adopt an accepting stance toward yourself and your internal experience, to slow down the stream of words flowing through your mind.

Joan: That sounds like a tool that would be good for me. My thoughts do run away with me and I get so wrapped up in trying to figure my way out of things. I can see the pull to want hypnosis to take away my pain; I'd give anything for my pain to miraculously be taken from me. Anyhow, let's get started. I want to learn more about this.

Therapist: Great! So to begin hypnosis, many people find it easiest to become relaxed and focused with their eyes closed. But if you would become more relaxed and focused with your eyes open, that's fine too. [Joan closes her eyes.] Now, start out by exhaling all the way, really let all the air go out of your lungs, and then take a deep breath in.

The induction continued from there in much the same way as a traditional hypnotic induction. As described earlier, traditional hypnotic inductions (i.e., emphasizing relaxation and focusing of attention) within the integrative framework outlined in this chapter need not be altered significantly. In Joan's case, given her propensity to struggle with thoughts or feelings that differed from what she thought was good, hypnotic inductions tended to be permissive in their suggestions. For example, induction suggestions included, "Perhaps you're finding yourself becoming increasingly relaxed right now, or perhaps you are even more alert. Whatever your experience is, I'd like to suggest that it is just right, even if you don't know that consciously." These suggestions were designed to encourage the client to accept her experience, even if it was not exactly what she wanted.

The following excerpt was drawn from a session in the middle of therapy and serves to illustrate the synthesis of hypnotic suggestions with principles of mindfulness- and acceptance-based psychotherapy. Joan had called her ex-husband to negotiate divorce proceedings, and he had become angry with her for requesting 50% of the couple's wealth, to which she believed she was entitled. Joan had agreed that in-session hypnosis might be useful to help reduce her distress about this encounter to make room for a more in-depth exploration of the events and her responses to her husband. The therapist responded as follows:

I would like for you to connect with a deep intention to experience whatever would best benefit you—you don't have to know this consciously. Your unconscious can assist you in this task today, and, even without knowing it, I'd like to suggest that your unconscious is already working on your behalf, helping you to connect with parts of yourself that you may have closed off, helping you to step up into your life in a meaningful way, on behalf of becoming who you want to be, embracing more of who you are. Take a moment now to take a deep breath in, and let it out. Good. That's it. Deep breath in, and let it out. With each breath you inhale, you can connect even more deeply with your unconscious and the resources that will promote a shift that you are ready to make in your life—even if you don't know it consciously—a shift on behalf of living more fully and becoming more of yourself.

You are aware of all of the losses and struggles that you have faced in the past several years. Your marriage has dissolved and you are thousands of miles away from one of your daughters. Your interactions with your husband recently have been negative and upsetting. I know that you have been struggling to push away thoughts of these losses and that you worry about your finances and your future. As you continue to breathe in and out deeply, just take a moment to notice what sorts of thoughts and feelings arise as I mention the issues you have been struggling with. [*Waits 20 seconds.*] Whatever comes up, just notice it, see if you can allow yourself to experience fully your emotions without struggling to change them. Treat yourself gently, treat yourself with compassion. Bring your mindfulness skills to this exploration. With each breath you exhale, see if you can experience your life as it is now, see yourself as you are now. If you have judgments about yourself or about others, can you just notice those without latching on to them or struggling with them?

I would like to suggest that you are strong enough to contain your experiences as they are without having to push them away. Even if your mind is telling you otherwise, you have the strength right now to experience your emotions. With each breath you exhale, see whether you can let go of a little bit of your resistance to feeling upset about your argument with your ex-husband. Can you be present with your anger and sadness about this argument while also staying present with your breath, noticing each inhale and exhale? Perhaps you are finding yourself becoming more calm or perhaps you are getting more in touch with agitation right now. Whatever you feel right now is just right and is supporting you to become a stronger person, more in touch with your emotions, more independent and self-assured.

In addition to incorporating in-session hypnosis work, Joan was given tapes of hypnotic interventions that she was encouraged to listen to at home.

These tapes emphasized contacting fully her emotions and experiences without trying to change them, practicing mindfulness (i.e., observing her experiences in a nonjudgmental, nonattached way), ego strengthening, and marshalling her resources on behalf of becoming an independent person. Joan was also taught mindfulness meditation beginning in the third session, which included body and breath awareness and an intentional practice of observing the flow of her thoughts without attaching to or struggling with particular experiences (see the discussion earlier for more description about the synthesis of mindfulness meditation and hypnosis). Joan was encouraged to practice mindfulness meditation for 10 minutes each day to develop greater metacognitive awareness of her thought patterns. She reported that she completed mindfulness practice approximately four times per week and found it moderately helpful in breaking up her rumination and worry as well as restoring a sense of calmness.

Over the course of treatment, Joan responded particularly well to the ACT-consistent notion of focusing on her values as a guide for her actions rather than allowing her emotions to determine her activities. For example, she agreed to begin research on what steps would be required to remodel her bathroom, which she stated was in serious disrepair. She completed this research in the presence of significant fear about her ability to afford such renovations, and she also was able to implement a plan that would address the worst problems in the bathroom (a cracked bathtub and a leaking toilet) economically. Joan also made significant strides toward decorating her home, which was a topic about which she had sought excessive reassurance and advice from others.

Joan also began to explore whether there were career options that she would enjoy and that would be compatible with the uncertainty of her multiple sclerosis episodes. She had a long-standing interest in helping others and began to consider that a career in social work would be especially meaningful to her. Joan expressed ambivalence about losing her disability compensation if she were to become employed. Nevertheless, she thought that a job would facilitate her spending less time worrying and ruminating and would restore a sense of purpose to her life. Joan found a program in the local area that would pay for much of her schooling in exchange for 2 years of service with a local agency. Near the end of therapy, she had been approved to participate in this program and expressed great excitement about her career transition.

When Joan terminated therapy after 17 sessions, her rumination and worry had become less frequent and much less distressing. She reported an increased awareness of her proneness to overestimate the likelihood of possible negative outcomes, and she had begun to joke with herself and others about her tendency to "act like Chicken Little and think that the sky was falling." Joan continued to listen to the taped hypnosis interventions regularly and said that she found these particularly calming when she was upset. Her practice of mindfulness continued, although she tended to use this skill only when she was particularly upset because she found the deep breathing calming. Perhaps the most notable change in Joan's behavior was her willingness to engage in activities that were consistent with her values while maintaining awareness of her anxieties surrounding such activities. For example, Joan was anxious about completing the annual paperwork required for her to remain on disability compensation because she feared that her symptoms were not severe enough and she would be denied coverage. In the presence of her anxiety, Joan acknowledged the importance of submitting this paperwork in a timely fashion, and she was able gain some distance from the intensity of her anxiety using ACT strategies, such as thinking of her worries as mere passengers on the bus she is driving.

Although Joan made much progress during therapy, she retained a high degree of negative emotionality, which may have reflected one basic aspect of her personality. She tended to have adversarial interactions with other peers and continued to struggle with her divorce negotiations. Nevertheless, the incorporation of hypnosis, mindfulness, and acceptance interventions in psychotherapy proved particularly useful in this case. Hypnotic suggestions incorporated themes of self-acceptance, self-compassion, mindful awareness, and making contact with painful emotions. ACT-related interventions were also bolstered by themes from hypnotic work, including Joan trusting her unconscious resources to develop a sense of independence and fostering positive expectancies about her ability to engage in valued activities.

RESEARCH AND APPRAISAL

Researchers have devoted attention to both mindfulness and hypnosis, independently. However, we are not aware of any research on the use of hypnosis and mindfulness techniques in conjunction. Nevertheless, extant research indicates that the practice of meditation and the level of facility with meditation do not appear to affect hypnotic suggestibility (Murphy, Donovan, & Taylor, 1997; Rivers & Spanos, 1981; Spanos, Gottlieb, & Rivers, 1980; Spanos, Stam, Rivers, & Radtke, 1980; Spanos, Steggles, Radtke-Bodorik, & Rivers, 1979). Researchers have, in fact, discovered similarities between the subjective experiences correlated with hypnosis and particular types of meditation, especially among highly suggestible participants (see Cardeña, 2005; Holroyd, 2003). People who are trained in either self-hypnosis or meditation tend to use the techniques for the same reasons (e.g., stress reduction, relaxation, refreshing mental attitudes during the work day) and also encounter similar impediments to practice (e.g., difficulty scheduling the time to practice, discomfort with the technique; Soskis, Orne, Orne, & Dinges, 1989). Although workers in the field have drawn attention to similarities across the subjective experiences of mindfulness and hypnosis, some research supports the fact that there are many notable differences between them (see Lynn et al., 2006).

Researchers have also attempted to compare the neuropsychological correlates of mindfulness and hypnosis (see Holroyd, 2003); however, the dependence of neurophysiological activity on the type of meditation being practiced (e.g., concentrative vs. expansive) and the specific hypnotic suggestions being administered precludes generalizing conclusions derived from the available evidence (see Lynn, Kirsch, Knox, Fassler, & Lilienfeld, 2007). Drawing meaningful conclusions from this work is also difficult because researchers' understanding of the specific meaning of neurophysiological activity is still rudimentary. Nevertheless, technical innovations, including brain-imaging methods, promise exciting discoveries regarding the neural underpinnings of hypnosis, mindfulness, and their interaction.

In regard to relative treatment efficacy for stress reduction, Walrath and Hamilton (1975) compared participants trained in transcendental meditation, autohypnosis, or relaxation. All participants were high-suggestible and there were no differences among groups on baseline measures. Results indicated that groups did not differ in terms of autonomic reduction following the procedure (i.e., all showed a marked reduction), though meditators did show a significantly more persistent reduction in heart rate postintervention. Although replication and expansion of this study are necessary, these findings may indicate that the gains associated with mindfulness are more enduring than those associated with hypnosis.

CONCLUSION

There is a long history of therapists integrating hypnosis into traditional psychotherapies and thereby enhancing treatment efficacy (Lynn & Kirsch, 2006). During the last 10 years, many clinicians and researchers have fundamentally shifted the focus of psychotherapy by emphasizing mindfulness and acceptance rather than affective changes. Many people consider this shift to be so revolutionary that they have proclaimed that the development of mindfulness- and acceptance-based therapies represents the advent of the "third-wave" of behavioral therapy (e.g., Hayes, 2004). It seems reasonably safe to predict that clinicians will continue to integrate hypnosis into new mindfulness- and acceptance-based therapies and that traditional hypnosis treatments will benefit from the integration of mindfulness techniques along the lines we have described.

Research evaluating the efficacy of combining mindfulness and hypnosis techniques is in its infancy. At this point, the research base rests on little more than case studies, theoretical speculation, and an array of potential hypotheses. Furthermore, hypnosis researchers and mindfulness researchers continue to struggle with the definition and operationalization of relevant constructs and techniques. The results of hypnosis research are heavily dependent on the specific suggestions administered, and the types of meditative techniques used similarly influence mindfulness research. Accordingly, basic research is fundamental to elucidate the constructs of interest, and consumers of the research would do well to carefully consider the methodology of studies when interpreting the results of research that addresses the following questions: (a) Does the combination of hypnosis and mindfulness practice yield therapeutic gains above and beyond the use of either method in isolation? (b) will hypnosis and mindfulness practice augment the salutary effects of cognitive–behavioral therapies (Lipsey & Wilson, 1993)? (c) what psychological mechanisms mediate treatment gains associated with hypnosis and mindfulness? and (d) is it possible to tease apart the specific effects of mindfulness and hypnosis from nonspecific effects, such as motivation, expectations, therapeutic relationship, and so forth (Roemer & Orsillo, 2003)? We hope that our chapter will spur research that will empirically evaluate the synthesis of these techniques, and prove to be a boon to clinical practitioners.

REFERENCES

American Psychiatric Association. (1994). *Diagnostic and statistical manual of mental disorders* (4th ed.). Washington, DC: Author.

Bach, P., & Hayes, S. C. (2002). The use of acceptance and commitment therapy to prevent the rehospitalization of psychotic patients: A randomized controlled trial. *Journal of Consulting and Clinical Psychology, 70,* 1129–1139.

Baer, R. A. (2003). Mindfulness training as a clinical intervention: A conceptual and empirical review. *Clinical Psychology: Science and Practice, 10,* 125–143.

Bowen, S., Witkiewitz, K., Dillworth, T. M., Chawla, N., Simpson, T. L., Ostafin, B. D., et al. (2006). Mindfulness meditation and substance use in an incarcerated population. *Psychology of Addictive Behaviors, 20,* 343–347.

Brown, K. W., Ryan, R. M., & Creswell, J. D. (2007). Mindfulness: Theoretical foundations and evidence for its salutary effects. *Psychological Inquiry, 18,* 211–237.

Cardeña, E. (2005). The phenomenology of deep hypnosis: Quiescent and physically active. *International Journal of Clinical and Experimental Hypnosis, 53,* 37–59.

Christensen, A., Atkins, D. C., Berns, S., Wheeler, J., Baucom, D. H., & Simpson, L. E. (2004). Traditional versus integrative behavioral couple therapy for significantly and chronically distressed married couples. *Journal of Consulting and Clinical Psychology, 72,* 176–191.

Christensen, A., Jacobson, N. S., & Babcock, J. C. (1995). Integrative behavioral couple therapy. In N. S. Jacobson & A. S. Gurman (Eds.), *Clinical handbook of couples therapy* (pp. 31–64). New York: Guilford Press.

Gaudiano, B. A., & Herbert, J. D. (2006). Acute treatment of inpatients with psychotic symptoms using acceptance and commitment therapy: Pilot results. *Behavior Research and Therapy, 44,* 415–437.

Gregg, J. A., Callaghan, G. M., Hayes S. C., & Glenn-Lawson, J. L. (2007). Improving diabetes self-management through acceptance, mindfulness, and values: A randomized controlled trial. *Journal of Consulting and Clinical Psychology, 75,* 336–343.

Hayes, S. C. (1987). A contextual approach to therapeutic change. In N. S. Jacobson (Ed.), *Psychotherapists in clinical practice: Cognitive and behavioral perspectives* (pp. 327–387). New York: Guilford Press.

Hayes, S. C. (2004). Acceptance and commitment therapy and the new behavior therapies: Mindfulness, acceptance, and relationship. In S. C. Hayes, V. M. Follette, & M. M. Linehan (Eds.), *Mindfulness and acceptance: Expanding the cognitive–behavioral tradition* (pp. 1–29). New York: Guilford Press.

Hayes, S. C., Strosahl, K. D., & Wilson, K. G. (1999). *Acceptance and commitment therapy: An experiential approach to behavior change.* New York: Guilford Press.

Holroyd, J. (2003). The science of meditation and the state of hypnosis. *American Journal of Clinical Hypnosis, 46,* 109–128.

Kabat-Zinn, J. (2003). Mindfulness-based stress reduction (MBSR). *Constructivism in the Human Sciences, 8,* 73–107.

Kabat-Zinn, J. (2005). *Full catastrophe living.* New York: Random House. (Original work published 1990)

Kabat-Zinn, J., Lipworth, L., & Burney, R. (1985). The clinical use of mindfulness meditation for the self-regulation of chronic pain. *Journal of Behavioral Medicine, 8,* 163–190.

Kabat-Zinn, J., Wheeler, E., Light, T., Skillings, A., Scharf, M. J., Cropley, T. G., et al. (1998). Influence of mindfulness meditation-based stress reduction intervention on rates of skin clearing in patients with moderate to severe psoriasis undergoing phototherapy (UVB) and photochemotherapy (PUVA). *Psychosomatic Medicine, 60,* 625–632.

Kirsch, I. (1990). *Changing expectations: A key to effective psychotherapy.* Pacific Grove, CA: Brooks/Cole.

Kirsch, I., & Lynn, S. J. (1997). Hypnotic involuntariness and the automaticity of everyday life. *American Journal of Clinical Hypnosis, 40,* 329–348.

Kirsch, I., & Lynn, S. J. (1998). Social–cognitive alternatives to dissociation theories of hypnotic involuntariness. *Review of General Psychology, 2,* 66–80.

Kirsch, I., Montgomery, G., & Sapirstein, G. (1995). Hypnosis as an adjunct to cognitive behavioral psychotherapy: A meta-analysis. *Journal of Consulting and Clinical Psychology, 63,* 214–220.

Linehan, M. M. (1993). *Cognitive–behavioral treatment of borderline personality disorder*. New York: Guilford Press.

Lipsey, M. W., & Wilson, D. B. (1993). The efficacy of psychological, educational, and behavioral outcomes: Confirmation from meta-analysis. *American Psychologist, 48,* 1181–1209.

Lynn, S. J., Das, L. S., Hallquist, M. N., & Williams, J. C. (2006). Mindfulness, acceptance, and hypnosis: Cognitive and clinical perspectives. *International Journal of Clinical and Experimental Hypnosis, 54,* 143–166.

Lynn, S. J., & Kirsch, I. (2006). *Essentials of clinical hypnosis: An evidence-based approach*. Washington, DC: American Psychological Association.

Lynn, S. J., Kirsch, I., Barabasz, A., Cardeña, E., & Patterson, D. (2000). Hypnosis as an empirically supported adjunctive technique: The state of the evidence. *International Journal of Clinical and Experimental Hypnosis, 48,* 343–361.

Lynn, S. J., Kirsch, I., Knox, J., Fassler, O., & Lilienfeld, S. O. (2007). Hypnosis and neuroscience: Implications for the altered state debate. In G. A. Jamieson (Ed.), *Hypnosis and conscious states: The cognitive neuroscience perspective* (pp. 145–165). New York: Oxford University Press.

Ma, S. H., & Teasdale, J. D. (2004). Mindfulness-based cognitive therapy for depression: Replication and exploration of differential relapse prevention effects. *Journal of Consulting and Clinical Psychology, 72,* 31–40.

McQuillan, A., Nicastro, R., Guenot, F., Girad, M., Lissner, C., & Ferrero, F. (2005). Intensive dialectical behavior therapy for outpatients with borderline personality disorder who are in crises. *Psychiatric Services, 56,* 193–197.

Murphy, M., Donovan, S., & Taylor, E. (1997). *The physical and psychological effects of meditation: A review of contemporary research with a comprehensive bibliography* (2nd ed.). Petaluma, CA: Institute of Noetic Sciences.

Perls, F. (1969). *In and out of the garbage pail*. Boulder, CO: Real People Press.

Rinpoche, B. (1981). Commentary. In Wang-Ch¥ug Dorje, *The Mahamudra: Eliminating the darkness of ignorance*. Dharamsala, India: Library of Tibetan Works and Archives.

Rivers, S. M., & Spanos, N. P. (1981). Personal variables predicting voluntary participation in and attrition from a meditation program. *Psychological Reports, 49,* 795–801.

Roemer, L., & Orsillo, S. M. (2003). Mindfulness: A promising intervention strategy in need of further study. *Clinical Psychology: Science and Practice, 10,* 172–178.

Segal, Z. V., Williams, S., & Teasdale, J. (2002). *Mindfulness-based cognitive therapy for depression: A new approach to preventing relapse*. New York: Guilford Press.

Shapiro, S. L., Schwartz, G. E., & Bonner, G. (1998). Effects of mindfulness-based stress reduction on medical and premedical students. *Journal of Behavioral Medicine, 21,* 581–599.

Soskis, D. A., Orne, E. C., Orne, M. T., & Dinges, D. F. (1989). Self-hypnosis and meditation for stress management. *International Journal of Clinical and Experimental Hypnosis, 37*, 285–289.

Spanos, N. P., Gottlieb, J., & Rivers, S. M. (1980). The effects of short-term meditation practice on hypnotic responsivity. *Psychological Record, 30*, 343–348.

Spanos, N. P., Stam, H. J., Rivers, S. M., & Radtke, H. L. (1980). Meditation, expectation and performance on indices of nonanalytic attending. *International Journal of Clinical and Experimental Hypnosis, 28*, 244–251.

Spanos, N. P., Steggles, S., Radtke-Bodorik, H. L., & Rivers, S. M. (1979). Nonanalytic attending, hypnotic susceptibility, and psychological well-being in trained meditators and nonmeditators. *Journal of Abnormal Psychology, 88*, 85–87.

Tacón, A. M., Caldera, Y. M., & Ronaghan, C. (2004). Mindfulness-based stress reduction in women with breast cancer. *Families, Systems, & Health, 22*, 193–203.

Tart, C. T. (1986). *Waking up: Overcoming the obstacles to human potential.* Boston: New Science Library.

Teasdale, J. D., Segal, Z. V., & Williams, J. M. G. (2003). Mindfulness training and problem formulation. *Clinical Psychology: Science and Practice, 10*, 157–160.

Teasdale, J. D., Segal, Z. V., Williams, J. M. G., Ridgeway, V. A., Soulsby, J. M., & Lau, M. A. (2000). Prevention of relapse/recurrence in major depression by mindfulness-based cognitive therapy. *Journal of Consulting and Clinical Psychology, 68*, 615–623.

Walrath, L. C., & Hamilton, D. W. (1975). Autonomic correlates of meditation and hypnosis. *American Journal of Clinical Hypnosis, 17*, 190–197.

Wells, A. (2000). *Emotional disorders and metacognition.* New York: Wiley.

Wenzlaff, R. M., & Wegner, D. M. (2000). Thought suppression. *Annual Review of Psychology, 51*, 59–91.

13

ENHANCING HYPNOTIZABILITY AND TREATMENT RESPONSE

JEFFREY D. GFELLER AND DONALD R. GORASSINI

Within the context of hypnosis, some people vividly experience perceptual changes and enact behavioral suggestions, whereas others experience little or no success in responding to suggestions. Hypnotizability is the construct most frequently cited as being responsible for these individual differences (Lynn & Rhue, 1991). Whereas there is consensus that individuals vary widely with regard to their hypnotizability, the extent to which hypnotic responsiveness can be modified has been vigorously debated (Bates, 1990; Bertrand, 1989; Diamond, 1977; Gorassini, 2004; Spanos & Flynn, 1989). In this chapter, we assert that hypnotizability can be substantially enhanced in ways that may yield more successful treatment of many conditions. Approaches and strategies that facilitate optimal hypnotic responding are presented and discussed, with particular reference to the treatment of dysfunctional pain. Case material is presented to illustrate these strategies for practitioners who use hypnotic approaches. Before presenting this information, we briefly discuss alternative perspectives regarding the modifiability of hypnotic responsiveness and whether hypnotizability is relevant to clinical outcomes.

All clinical material has been disguised to protect patient confidentiality.

There has been considerable debate among proponents of two alternative paradigms regarding the extent to which hypnotic responsivity can be modified or enhanced. One perspective, termed the *special process view* (Hilgard, 1977, 1979), conceptualizes hypnotic responsiveness as reflecting the ability to passively experience dissociation among various cognitive subsystems (see chap. 6, this volume). This dissociative ability is purported to account for most hypnotic phenomena, including hypnotic analgesia, hypnotic amnesia, and the sense of involuntariness that often accompanies responses to hypnotic suggestions. This dissociative capacity, particularly evident in highly hypnotizable people, is viewed as an enduring trait that resides in the individual and is not amenable to substantial modification. The impressive 10-, 15-, and 25-year test–retest correlations of .64, .82, and .71, respectively, for hypnotic responding (Piccione, Hilgard, & Zimbardo, 1989) are often cited as proof of the traitlike nature of hypnotizability.

An alternative perspective, termed the *social–cognitive skills model* (Spanos, 1982), views hypnotic responding as the by-product of an ability that is determined by numerous intrapersonal, interpersonal, and contextual factors. These include expectancies and attitudes toward hypnosis; cognitive skills, such as vividness of imagery and absorption in imaginings; expectancies and attitudes toward hypnosis; and interpersonal variables, such as the degree of trust and rapport with the hypnotist. Each factor is viewed as potentially modifiable, at least to a limited extent. The cognitive skills model contends that hypnotizability can be substantially enhanced when participants are given facilitative information and training that addresses these factors.

The social–cognitive skills model is likely to appeal to cognitive–behavioral clinicians who view hypnosis as an active coping skill that patients learn in the context of a collaborative relationship with the therapist (see chap. 7). The focus on practice and the enhancement of hypnotic skills moves patients toward independent practice with the technique. Thus, once therapists provide patients with facilitative information and training, the process can be conceptualized as a self-hypnotic approach.

The strategies and techniques presented in this chapter are based largely on the principles derived from the social–cognitive skills model of hypnosis. Before presenting strategies to enhance hypnotizability, the issue of whether the level of hypnotic responsiveness matters significantly with regard to treatment outcome for various conditions deserves consideration. Hypnosis has been used as a means of treatment for many conditions (see Flammer & Bongartz, 2003; Kirsch, Montgomery, & Sapirstein, 1995, for meta-analytic reviews; see also Wadden & Anderton, 1982), including anxiety disorders (Bryant, Moulds, Guthrie, & Nixon, 2005; Clarke & Jackson, 1983; see also chap. 14, this volume); impotence (Crasilneck, 1982, 1990); addictive disorders, such as cigarette smoking (Green & Lynn, 2000; Holroyd, 1980; see also chap. 24, this volume) and alcoholism (Granone, 1971); obesity (Kirsch, 1996; Wadden & Flaxman, 1981; cf. Allison & Faith, 1996); psychophysiological disorders, including asthma (Brown, 2007; Neinstein & Dash, 1982; see also chap. 22, this volume); dermatological conditions, such as warts (Spanos, Stenstrom, & Johnston, 1988; Tasini & Hackett, 1977; see also chap. 22, this volume); and as a treatment for intractable pain stemming from various etiologies (Barber, 1986; Montgomery, DuHamel, & Redd, 2000; see also chap. 21, this volume).

Hypnotizability can play a role in therapeutic success in two ways. First, the subskills making up hypnotic ability can be used to combat symptoms of the various conditions cited. The amalgam of skills that comprise hypnotic ability produce the alterations in subjective experience called for in hypnotic suggestions (e.g., negative hallucinations). These same abilities can contribute to the subjective changes that comprise a therapeutic effect (e.g., analgesia) when one is suggested. If someone scores low in hypnotic suggestibility, it is because she or he fails to use, or fails to use well, the tactics necessary for producing suggested subjective changes, whether for a therapeutic outcome or not. A program of hypnosis enhancement would consist, therefore, of training in which subskills to apply and how best to apply them. As noted, social–cognitive skills theorists propose that these factors are modifiable.

Second, successfully responding to hypnotic suggestions could produce important therapeutic changes beyond the specific abilities responsible for producing subjective alterations. Success at hypnotic tasks could enhance a client's sense of mastery and self-efficacy (Bandura, 1977) and feelings of rapport with the therapist (Gfeller, Lynn, & Pribble, 1987), all of which serve as common factors (Frank, 1974) in therapeutic success. The capacity to produce these effects would thus make hypnotic training a useful adjunct to other forms of therapy.

The empirical literature indicates that hypnotizability is relevant to outcome. However, the relation between hypnotizability and outcome is far from a 1:1 correspondence, and sometimes suggestibility does not predict treatment success at all (Lynn, Boycheva, & Barnes, 2008). Still, in no study reported to date is high hypnotic suggestibility associated with a negative treatment outcome (Lynn & Kirsch, 2006). Moreover, in the following disorders or conditions, the findings regarding hypnotizability and treatment outcome are at least somewhat promising, albeit not entirely consistent: pain-related conditions, smoking cessation, obesity, warts, anxiety, somatization, conversion disorders, and asthma (Lynn, Shindler, & Meyer, 2003). In fact, hypnotic suggestibility seems to be a better predictor of outcome than expectancies in the treatment of conversion disorder (Moene, Spinhoven, Hoogduin, & Van Dyck, 2003).

The available evidence suggests that a patient's level of hypnotizability does not equally affect clinical outcome for each of the conditions noted earlier. Some authors (Soskis, 1986; Wadden & Anderton, 1982) have noted that hypnotizability appears to be most relevant to conditions for which successful intervention can be achieved by altering the patient's subjective experience. Examples of conditions in which altering one's perception and subjective experience can bring about positive outcome include those involving traumatic memories and psychophysiological conditions, such as dysfunctional pain and conversion disorders. For conditions in which successful outcome requires behavioral change (e.g., smoking cessation, weight reduction), level of hypnotizability appears to be somewhat less important insofar as significant alteration of subjective experience by itself does not guarantee alteration of behavior. Rather, motivation to resist impulses to overeat or smoke, for example, may be key. However, as noted earlier, even in these conditions, there may be some relation between hypnotizability and outcome.

What is important for our purposes is that the successful treatment of many conditions may depend less on absolute level of hypnotizability, as measured by a standardized scale of suggestibility, than on nonspecific factors shared by a variety of successful interventions (Wadden & Anderton, 1982). Accordingly, although hypnosis may serve as a useful component in the treatment of conditions requiring behavioral change, the use of adjunctive cognitive and behavioral approaches is clearly warranted.

From a common factors perspective of treatment (Frank, 1974), one's level of hypnotizability may influence outcome when hypnosis is used as an adjunct to other techniques to effect behavior change. More specifically, a patient's experience of significant perceptual alterations during a hypnotic induction may enhance the credibility of the "therapeutic myth" that the hypnotic suggestions provided during treatment will result in expected behavioral changes. An example would be a multicomponent smoking cessation treatment that uses a variety of self-regulatory approaches, including self-hypnosis, as a cognitive strategy to help patients cope with the inevitable desire for a cigarette. In this situation, a patient who has successfully responded to ideomotor suggestions, such as hand levitation, may be more likely to believe that "hypnotic ability" will assist him or her in successfully resisting the urge to smoke during the initial days of abstinence. The successful implementation of self-hypnosis to cope with smoking urges may give patients a sense of mastery and self-efficacy (Bandura, 1977) that will facilitate a successful outcome.

CLINICAL APPLICATIONS

The information summarized previously suggests that hypnotic responsiveness is most relevant with respect to a variety of conditions in which successful outcome can be achieved by altering patients' subjective experience and perceptions. This guideline is clearly applicable with respect to the hypnotic treatment of dysfunctional pain. *Dysfunctional pain* may be defined as pain that has lost its "signal value," meaning that the discomfort experienced by the patient should no longer be perceived as a cue that requires immediate medical attention (Soskis, 1986).

The experimental and clinical studies relating hypnotizability to one's level of pain reduction have documented a reasonably strong and positive relationship between these variables (Friedman & Taub, 1984; Hilgard, MacDonald, Morgan, & Johnson, 1978; Hilgard & Morgan, 1975; Montgomery et al., 2000; Patterson, Hoffman, Palacios, & Jensen, 2007; Spanos, Radke-Bodorik, Ferguson, & Jones, 1979). Therefore, facilitating hypnotizability with patients who experience dysfunctional pain should enhance their ability to effectively manage their discomfort with hypnotic interventions.

As noted previously, the social–cognitive skills model provides a descriptive account of the salient attitudinal, cognitive, and interpersonal factors that facilitate optimal hypnotic responding. For illustrative purposes, we discuss these factors primarily within the context of enhancing hypnotizability among individuals experiencing dysfunctional pain. Nevertheless, the scheme for enhancing hypnotic responsiveness, described shortly, is applicable to a wide range of psychological and psychophysiological disorders.

Attitudes and Expectancies

Discussing patients' general attitudes and expectancies about hypnosis, as well as any past hypnotic experience, is an important component of facilitating hypnotic responsiveness and behavior change (Kirsch, 1985; Kirsch & Council, 1989; Lynn & Kirsch, 2006). Common negative expectancies about hypnosis, such as fearing a loss of control or maintaining a concern that people are gullible or weak-willed if they are "easily" hypnotizable, should be explored.

Negative expectancies specific to the hypnotic treatment of particular disorders should be explored before initiating hypnosis. Asking patients what they expect to experience during hypnosis and how hypnosis may affect their situation often will provide information regarding inhibitory beliefs. The following is a list of inhibitory expectancies commonly encountered when treating patients with dysfunctional pain:

1. The use of hypnosis implies that my pain problem is psychological in nature and not caused by a physical condition.
2. Hypnosis represents an ineffective technique when compared with prescription analgesic medications.

3. My use of hypnosis to manage pain will result in a loss of atten-tion from my family or loss of compensation resulting from the pain condition.
4. I will not be able to notice when my pain level has increased, resulting in further injury.

Beliefs that may potentially limit hypnotic responding merit attention.

The expectation that the effective use of hypnosis implies that a pain problem is primarily psychological in nature can limit a patient's willing-ness to use hypnosis to attenuate pain. Therefore, patients may need reas-surance that the hypnotist accepts that their pain condition is genuine and not psychological in origin (see chap. 25). At the same time, the clinician can provide a model for understanding how hypnosis successfully decreases one's perception of pain severity. The *gate-control theory* of pain (Melzack & Wall, 1982) is a useful model that provides a credible account of how physiological, emotional, and cognitive factors interact to influence pain perception.

The belief that the successful use of hypnosis may result in a loss of fam-ily attention or a loss of compensation stemming from the pain condition may also inhibit optimal hypnotic responding. Accepting patients' reports of pain as genuine does not mean that their expression of pain is unresponsive to external factors such as attention and support from those around them. Addressing this operant component of pain (Fordyce, 1976) by educating family members is often an important means of influencing the social rein-forcement of the patient's verbal and behavioral expression of pain. Failure to address these social contingencies often limits patients' ability to acquire hypnotic skills as a means of managing their pain.

Some patients may be reluctant to experiment with hypnosis because of their belief that its use would impair their ability to discern increases in pain, resulting in further injury or discomfort. This is a genuine concern among pain patients who have overused some form of mental distraction in the past to cope with pain that is exacerbated with physical activity. Therefore, it is important to frame hypnosis as a means of coping with pain increases result-ing from activities such as exercise or a recreational outing and not as a means of allowing patients to overdo a physical activity. Discussing the previously described concept of the signal value of pain and situations where patients need to attend to increases in discomfort is helpful in this regard.

It is impractical and inefficient to exhaustively address every negative attitude that may limit patients' hypnotic ability before exposing them to hypnosis. However, clinicians should be ready to explore inhibitory beliefs with patients who experience limited success with hypnotic interventions.

Cognitive Skill Factors

The social–cognitive skills model emphasizes facilitating a number of cognitive processes to enhance patients' ability to use hypnosis as a means of ameliorating their symptoms or condition. Pertinent cognitive strategies for optimal hypnotic responding are as follows:

1. Portraying hypnosis as a cognitive experience not far removed from many everyday life phenomena.
2. Discussing the concept of goal-directed fantasy or imaginative involvement and its role in hypnotic experience.
3. Elaborating on the importance of absorption and suspension of reality orientation for facilitating optimal hypnotic responsiveness.
4. Explaining hypnosis as an active process to be learned by the patient as a coping skill.

Portraying the hypnotic experience as sharing similarities with many everyday phenomena provides patients with a sense of what to expect during hypnosis. Using examples such as maintaining focused attention while reading a novel or imaginative involvement while daydreaming is helpful in this regard.

The role of *goal-directed fantasy* (Spanos & Barber, 1974) or involvement in imaginings consistent with symptom reduction is another important concept to explore with patients. With regard to the treatment of dysfunctional pain, Chaves (1989) noted the value of eliciting a detailed description of patients' phenomenological experience of their pain (e.g., "My leg feels like it is burning," "My back feels like it is in knots"). This information often suggests idiographic imagery or metaphors that can be readily used by the patient.

Elaborating on the role of absorption, or "staying focused," on imaginings to facilitate optimal hypnotic responding is also important insofar as a failure to remain focused on images that attenuate pain may impede patients' success with hypnosis. Discussing the theatrical concept of "willing suspension of disbelief" provides a heuristic construct to assist patients with appreciating the suspension of reality orientation necessary to attain optimal hypnotic skills.

Presenting hypnosis as an active process that can be mastered to better manage one's pain condition is an essential component in enhancing hypnotizability (Spanos, Robertson, Menary, & Brett, 1986). For example, patients with dysfunctional pain should understand the importance of actively interpreting suggestions for analgesia rather than passively waiting for the analgesia to occur. Thus, if the hypnotic suggestion is given that ice is being applied to the site of pain, the patient should actively focus on imagery consistent with this suggestion to maximize its effectiveness.

The modeling of these cognitive strategies by the hypnotist is a particularly effective means of imparting skills that facilitate optimal hypnotic responding. For example, the hypnotist may demonstrate an ideomotor response such as arm levitation and verbally report his or her goal-directed imaginings that facilitate a sense of lightness or movement in the arm. Similarly, the hypnotist may verbally report his or her subjective experience during attentional focusing and describe how this process results in a diminution of other sensory experiences in the body. Modeling cognitive strategies by the hypnotist also conveys an implicit message that the hypnotist uses the techniques being presented. This message may have a positive effect on rapport between the patient and therapist.

Patients undoubtedly have limits on the extent to which they can acquire and enhance cognitive skills such as goal-directed fantasy and absorption in imaginings. Positive changes, however, can occur with facilitative information and practice. Lazarus (1977) provided a number of structured exercises for enhancing imagery skills. One imagery enhancement exercise that can be readily applied to pain reduction involves picturing in the "mind's eye" a blackboard on which patients imagine themselves writing letters of the alphabet and erasing the letters to conclude the exercise. With several attempts, patients usually report increased clarity of the imagined board and letters. At this point, patients can be given a permissive suggestion to imagine a drawing of their pain on this board using whatever imagery they choose. Erasing the image of their pain from the blackboard often results in a significant decrease in discomfort for a period of time. This imagery exercise can be easily adapted for other applications ranging from defusing traumatic memories to decreasing the urge to smoke. For example, during hypnosis, an ex-smoker who is craving a cigarette may draw a picture of a cigarette on the imaginary blackboard and then "mentally erase" the drawing, resulting in a diminished urge to smoke.

Interpersonal Factors

As in all therapeutic contexts, establishing a positive therapeutic alliance is important to facilitate patients' success with the application of their hypnotic abilities (Gfeller et al., 1987; Sheehan, 1980). The social–cognitive skills perspective views the therapeutic relationship as a collaborative process in which the hypnotist is a participant–observer who assists patients in understanding the nature of hypnosis and exploring the factors that may constrain and enhance their hypnotic ability. Perceiving the clinician as trustworthy and genuine facilitates these goals. Therefore, hypnotic interventions should not be implemented until there is a clear sense that some degree of positive rapport has been established. With patients who are receptive, simply encountering a clinician who demonstrates an understanding of their condition and who expresses a desire to improve their situation is sufficient. However, patients who are less receptive, who express skepticism and inhibitory beliefs regarding hypnosis, often require additional attention from the clinician to establish an interpersonal climate where they feel safe to develop their hypnotic abilities. Exploring patients' inhibitory beliefs is one means of increasing receptiveness to hypnosis. The modeling of hypnotic responding by the therapist also conveys a sense of genuineness that facilitates rapport. Whatever approaches are taken, they should be advanced in the spirit of providing facilitative information to the patient, not as a "hard sell" intended to portray hypnosis as a panacea.

Although hypnotizability is portrayed as a skill that can be enhanced with instruction and practice, few things facilitate the therapeutic alliance more effectively than a positive first encounter with hypnosis. Thus, clinicians should balance optimizing patients' first experience of hypnosis with the hazard of delaying this initial experience through excessive preparation.

CASE MATERIAL

The case of "John," based on a person treated by the first author (Gfeller), is presented to illustrate the application of the various strategies for facilitating hypnotic ability and obtaining a positive therapeutic outcome.

John was a 43-year-old physician who was referred for pain management related to abdominal pain stemming from pancreatic cancer. In addition to abdominal pain, he experienced nausea and anorexia, which resulted in significant weight loss. He had undergone both chemotherapy and radiation therapy, which caused a minimal remission of the cancer. His oncologist had informed him there was little else that could be done to medically treat his condition.

Because John was requiring increasingly large doses of narcotic medication to reduce his abdominal pain, both he and his physician were interested in exploring psychological means to better manage his discomfort. John's personal interest in using alternative methods of pain control stemmed from his displeasure with the sedation he experienced with the analgesic medications. The sedation compromised the quality of time he spent with his wife and their young son. Although he was no longer regularly seeing patients, he continued to consult with colleagues on selected cases from his home and took great pride in maintaining this activity, which was limited when he felt excessively drowsy or fatigued.

During the initial meeting, John briefly summarized his medical treatment for the pancreatic cancer as well as the adverse symptoms he was experiencing. When asked to describe his abdominal pain in detail, he reported the pain to be "gnawing" and "relentless" in nature. When asked whether he used any mental strategies to reduce his discomfort, he acknowledged that his pain sometimes decreased when he was reading or talking with his wife.

Although John indicated that he had never experienced hypnosis, he was somewhat pessimistic that he could be hypnotized because he was "too inquisitive and scientifically minded." I replied that he might initially experience limited success with hypnosis for a variety of reasons, including his scientific mode of thinking and his lack of understanding of what was required of him. However, I had confidence in his ability to use hypnosis once we attended to his inquisitive nature by providing him with information about the nature of hypnosis and how to optimize his hypnotic ability. At this point, I gave John the following information:

> Hypnosis is difficult to define, but one thing I know for certain is that the ability to be hypnotized lies within you; it is not a power that I possess. Successful hypnosis seems to involve the ability to focus your mental attention on a particular sight, sound, or image that you create in your mind's eye. This ability is something akin to the absorption you have experienced when reading or when engrossed in conversation with your wife, experiences you mentioned earlier that resulted in some pain reduction.
>
> People differ in their ability to experience hypnosis. Some take to it like a duck to water; others seem initially uncomfortable with the process and demonstrate limited hypnotic ability. However, a person's degree of hypnotizability is not etched in stone. While you may not take to hypnosis like a duck to water, you can certainly become more proficient with hypnosis, just as you can learn to be a good swimmer.

To determine whether John held beliefs that might impede his responsiveness to hypnosis, I explored his expectations about what hypnosis would be like as well as his perception about how the experience may affect his level of pain. John's comments indicated that he had few misconceptions about hypnosis and that he was not fearful of experiencing a loss of control during hypnosis. However, he expressed two beliefs that could have limited his hypnotizability. First, he conveyed the expectation that somehow the experience of hypnosis would just happen and would not require effort on his part. Second, he was concerned that hypnotic analgesia would be minimal and transient compared with that produced from the potent medications he was taking.

To address the first expectation, we discussed the "involuntary" nature of hypnotic responding, with me demonstrating an ideomotor response (i.e., arm levitation). As I responded, I reported my imaginings that facilitated movement in the arm. Following the demonstration, I elaborated on the experience, noting that although it was clear that I had raised my own arm, I experienced a sense of the arm rising by itself because I was so engrossed in imagining a rope and pulley that was being used to hoist my arm into the air.

John required little prompting to try responding to a similar suggestion. I provided a less difficult suggestion for arm lowering that he performed with ease, indicating afterward that he had imagined someone placing increasingly heavier amounts of weight on his hand, causing it to move downward. Following this, I indicated that his experience of hypnosis would be a similar process that would require his active participation. Hypnosis was not something that I would do to him; rather, being hypnotized was an experience that he would initially create with my assistance and later create entirely on his own.

With regard to John's expectation that hypnotic analgesia would be limited and transient in nature, I indicated that some people are able to use hypnosis to markedly reduce their level of discomfort. Because he was a man of science, I asked that he keep an open mind about how effective hypnosis might be in reducing his pain. I also indicated that just as there were a number of medications one could take for pain, there were also a number of available hypnotic strategies to reduce the experience of pain. We reviewed several possible approaches, including imagined anesthesia, direct diminution of pain, reinterpretation of painful sensations, and dissociation from pain through the use of vivid imagery (see Barber, 1986). John expressed an interest in the dissociative approach, indicating he wanted to "get as far away from my pain as possible." Therefore, we discussed possible scenes or images that would provide such an escape. John indicated that he loved to scuba dive and that he had vivid memories of tropical fish and coral he had encountered while diving. We agreed to use these images during his initial experience with hypnosis.

Although John might have benefited from additional information to facilitate hypnotic responding, these benefits needed to be balanced against the importance of initiating hypnosis and assisting him in reducing his pain. Because we had addressed the identified barriers to hypnotic responding and he had positively responded to an ideomotor suggestion, I believed he was ready to experience hypnosis and suggestions for pain reduction.

I asked John to rate the severity of his abdominal pain on a 1-to-5 scale of increasing discomfort. He reported that his pain level had been a 3 throughout our meeting. I then guided him through a 20-minute hypnotic exercise with suggestions for relaxation and attentional focusing. I suggested that he picture himself slowly descending in scuba gear toward a reef teeming with marine life to deepen his absorption in the imagery he was experiencing. After spending several minutes describing this reef in great detail, I ended the exercise with the suggestion that he would soon be successful at mentally traveling to this setting on his own.

John's response to hypnosis was quite positive. He reported imagining the reef and marine life with vividness and clarity. Most important, he indicated that his pain level had decreased to a 1.5 on the 5-point scale. I asked him to note his pain level over the next few hours to help determine how long this relief lasted. I then scheduled John for an appointment several days later.

At the start of the next session, John indicated that the reduction in pain had lasted only several hours, and he expressed pessimism that hypnosis could result in more lasting relief. I suggested that the duration of relief might well increase as his experience with hypnosis increased. Moreover, he would soon be able to reduce his pain without my assistance. I again guided him through a hypnotic exercise and recreated the imagery of the reef he had visited in his mind's eye several days earlier. However, this time we audiotaped the procedure and John used the cassette tape to experience hypnosis at home during the next week.

At our third session, John indicated that, with the benefit of the tape-recorded exercise at home, he had more successfully managed his pain. In addition, the pain reduction was lasting up to 5 or 6 hours. At this point, I recommended that John begin alternating between using the tape-recorded procedure and self-initiating hypnosis, including any imagined setting that provided him with a sense of comfort.

At the next session, John was visibly pleased. He indicated that he had been successful in reducing his pain using his own "induction." Moreover, he reported that he was using less medication to control his pain. His wife indicated that he was more interactive and seemed less focused on his discomfort.

I continued to see John periodically to assist him with refining his hypnotic abilities and to explore other hypnotic approaches to attenuate his pain. For example, we attempted to use hypnosis to counter the anorexia caused by the cancer and the radiation therapy he had received. Although we had little success in affecting this symptom, his wife reported that John had continued to use hypnosis to reduce his pain until shortly before his death.

RESEARCH AND APPRAISAL

The efficacy of the strategies presented for enhancing hypnotizability, derived largely from the social–cognitive skills model of hypnosis, is supported by approximately 30 studies, conducted in 10 different laboratories, that have documented appreciable gains in hypnotic responding when persons have been provided with the facilitative information and cognitive skills training (e.g., Bates & Brigham, 1990; Gfeller et al. 1987; Gorassini & Spanos, 1986). More than 15 studies have demonstrated that approximately 50% to 80% of initially low hypnotizable persons respond as highly hypnotizable following participation in a multicomponent cognitive skills training procedure (see Gorassini, 2004; Gorassini & Spanos, 1999).

Proponents of the special process view (Bates, 1990; Bowers & Davidson, 1991) have questioned the genuine nature of these increments, suggesting that enhanced hypnotizability represents artificial compliance with experimental demands by research participants. For interested readers, Lynn (2004) provides a cogent discussion of the compliance effects issue from the social–learning cognitive skills perspective. In brief, the research in this area indicates that (a) trained participants' enhanced hypnotic abilities generalize to novel suggestions, including those for pain reduction; (b) trained participants subjective reports are not distinguishable from those of "natural high" susceptible participants who have not experienced cognitive skills training; (c) strong pressures for enhanced responsiveness unaccompanied by specific skills training fails to produce hypnotic enhancement; (d) participants asked to fake high suggestibility show a telltale overplay effect and thus are distinguishable from natural as well as trained highs; and (e) skill training works equally well when participants expect their behavioral and subjective responses to remain known only to themselves, as when they anticipate the experimenter is privy to their responses (for reviews, see Gorassini, 2004; Lynn, 2004). In hypnotic enhancement studies that measured faking directly, a small proportion of high scoring individuals did appear to be faking. Of this group, natural high scorers faked as much as (Gearan, Schoenberger, & Kirsch, 1995) or more than (Burgess, du Breuil, Jones, & Spanos, 1990–1991) skill trained high scorers. In addition, the increases in hypnotic responding produced by skill training have been shown to persist for over 2 years following training (Spanos, Cross, Menary, & Smith, 1988). These findings place some burden of proof on proponents of the special process view to identify characteristics that differentiate natural hypnotic talents from those enhanced through cognitive skills training.

CONCLUSION

We believe the strategies outlined in this chapter will facilitate the successful use of hypnosis, particularly with patients who are viewed as unlikely candidates for hypnotic intervention because of limited hypnotizability. We further contend that the strategies we recommend will be especially effective when treating conditions or symptoms that are ameliorated by altering patients' subjective perceptual experiences. The tactics should be applied flexibly and tailored to address idiosyncratic factors that limit hypnotic responsivity with individual patients.

More generally, the social–cognitive skills model, from which the strategies are derived, provides an alternative perspective for conceptualizing hypnotic phenomena that may resonate with clinicians who are uncomfortable using constructs associated with the special process view of hypnosis (see Lynn & Kirsch, 2006). The model may be particularly appealing to cognitive–behavioral clinicians because hypnosis is viewed as an active coping skill that patients learn to use independently through a collaborative relationship with the therapist. Capafons (2004) provides a valuable synopsis of a cognitive–behavioral introduction to hypnosis that is consistent with the perspectives presented throughout this chapter (see also chap. 7, this volume).

Finally, it should be acknowledged that these techniques, like all tactics of change, have their limitations. Some persons, because of a variety of factors, may have limited success in using facilitative information and cognitive skills training to enhance their hypnotic responsiveness. Those who study hypnotic phenomena will continue to search for factors that constrain and enhance patients' hypnotic skills, providing further insights regarding how to best tailor hypnotic interventions to help patients.

REFERENCES

Allison, D. B., & Faith, M. S. (1996). Hypnosis as an adjunct to cognitive–behavioral psychotherapy for obesity: A metadata-analytic reappraisal. *Journal of Consulting and Clinical Psychology, 64*, 513–516.

Bandura, A. (1977). *Social learning theory*. Englewood Cliffs, NJ: Prentice-Hall.

Barber, J. (1986). Hypnotic analgesia. In A. D. Holzman & D. C. Turk (Eds.), *Pain management: A handbook of psychological treatment approaches* (pp. 151–167). Elmsford, NY: Pergamon Press.

Bates, B. L. (1990). Compliance and the Carleton Skills Training Program. *British Journal of Experimental and Clinical Hypnosis, 7*, 159–164.

Bates, B. L., & Brigham, T. A. (1990). Modifying hypnotizability with the Carleton Skills Training program: A partial replication and analysis of components. *International Journal of Clinical and Experimental Hypnosis, 38*, 183–195.

Bertrand, L. D. (1989). The assessment and modification of hypnotic susceptibility. In N. P. Spanos & J. F. Chaves (Eds.), *Hypnosis: The cognitive–behavioral perspective* (pp. 18–31). Buffalo, NY: Prometheus Books.

Bowers, K. S., & Davidson, T. M. (1991). A neo-dissociation critique of Spanos's social–psychological model of hypnosis. In S. J. Lynn & J. W. Rhue (Eds.), *Theories of hypnosis: Current models and perspectives* (pp. 105–143). New York: Guilford Press.

Brown, D. (2007). Evidence-based hypnotherapy for asthma: A critical review. *International Journal of Clinical and Experimental Hypnosis, 55*, 220–249.

Bryant, R. A., Moulds, M. L., Guthrie, R. M., & Nixon, R. D. V. (2005). The additive benefit of hypnosis and cognitive–behavioral therapy in treating acute stress disorder. *Journal of Consulting and Clinical Psychology, 73*, 334–340.

Burgess, C. A., du Breuil, S. C., Jones, B., & Spanos, N. P. (1990–1991). Compliance and the modification of hypnotizability. *Contemporary Hypnosis, 10*, 293–304.

Capafons, A. (2004). Clinical applications of "waking" hypnosis from a cognitive–behavioural perspective: From efficacy to efficiency. *Contemporary Hypnosis, 21*, 187–201.

Chaves, J. F. (1989). Hypnotic control of clinical pain. In N. P. Spanos & J. F. Chaves (Eds.), *Hypnosis: The cognitive–behavioral perspective* (pp. 242–272). Buffalo, NY: Prometheus Books.

Clarke, J. H., & Jackson, J. A. (1983). *Hypnosis and behavior therapy: The treatment of anxiety and phobias*. New York: Springer.

Crasilneck, H. B. (1982). A follow-up study in the use of hypnotherapy in the treatment of psychogenic impotence. *American Journal of Clinical Hypnosis, 25*, 52–61.

Crasilneck, H. B. (1990). Hypnotic techniques for smoking control and psychogenic impotence. *American Journal of Clinical Hypnosis, 32*, 147–153.

Diamond, M. J. (1977). Hypnotizability is modifiable: An alternative approach. *International Journal of Clinical and Experimental Hypnosis, 25*, 147–165.

Flammer, E., & Bongartz, W. (2003). On the efficacy of hypnosis: A meta-analytic study. *Contemporary Hypnosis, 20*, 179–197.

Fordyce, W. E. (1976). *Behavioral methods for chronic pain and illness*. St. Louis, MO: Mosby.

Frank, J. D. (1974). *Persuasion and healing*. New York: Schocken Books.

Friedman, H., & Taub, H. A. (1984). An evaluation of hypnotic susceptibility and peripheral temperature elevation in the treatment of migraine. *American Journal of Clinical Hypnosis, 24*, 172–182.

Gearan, P., Schoenberger, N. E., & Kirsch, I. (1995). Modifying hypnotizability: A new component analysis. *International Journal of Clinical and Experimental Hypnosis, 43*, 70–89.

Gfeller, J. D., Lynn, S. J., & Pribble, W. E. (1987). Enhancing hypnotic susceptibility: Interpersonal and rapport factors. *Journal of Personality and Social Psychology, 52*, 586–595.

Gorassini, D. R. (2004). Increasing hypnotic responsiveness. In M. Heap, R. J. Brown, & D. Oakley (Eds.), *High hypnotisability: Theoretical, experimental, and clinical issues* (pp. 213–239). London: Brunner/Routledge.

Gorassini, D. R., & Spanos, N. P. (1986). A social–cognitive skills approach to the successful modification of hypnotic susceptibility. *Journal of Personality and Social Psychology, 50*, 1004–1012.

Gorassini, D. R., & Spanos, N. P. (1999). The Carleton Skill Training Program for modifying hypnotic suggestibility: Original version and variations. In I. Kirsch, A. Capafons, E. Cardeña-Buelna, & S. Amigó (Eds.), *Clinical hypnosis and self-regulation: Cognitive–behavioral perspectives* (pp. 141–178). Washington, DC: American Psychological Association.

Granone, F. (1971). Hypnotism in the treatment of chronic alcoholism. *Journal of the American Institute of Hypnosis, 12*, 32–40.

Green, J. P., & Lynn, S. J. (2000). Hypnosis and suggestion-based approaches to smoking cessation: An examination of the evidence. *International Journal of Clinical and Experimental Hypnosis, 48*, 195–224.

Hilgard, E. R. (1977). *Divided consciousness: Multiple controls in human thought and action*. New York: Wiley.

Hilgard, E. R. (1979). Divided consciousness in hypnosis: The implications of the hidden observer: In E. Fromm & R. E. Shor (Eds.), *Hypnosis: Development in research and new perspectives* (pp. 45–85). Chicago: Aldine.

Hilgard, E. R., MacDonald, H., Morgan, A. H., & Johnson, L. S. (1978). The reality of hypnotic analgesia: A comparison of highly hypnotizables and simulators. *Journal of Abnormal Psychology, 87*, 239–246.

Hilgard, E. R., & Morgan, A. H. (1975). Heart rate and blood pressure in the study of laboratory pain in man under normal conditions and as influenced by hypnosis. *Acta Neurobiologica Experimentalis, 35*, 741–759.

Holroyd, J. (1980). Hypnosis treatment for smoking: An evaluative review. *International Journal of Clinical and Experimental Hypnosis, 28*, 341–357.

Kirsch, I. (1985). Response expectancy as a determinant of experience and behavior. *American Psychologist, 40*, 1189–1202.

Kirsch, I. (1996). Hypnotic enhancement of cognitive–behavioral weight loss treatments—another meta-reanalysis. *Journal of Consulting and Clinical Psychology, 64*, 517–519.

Kirsch, I., & Council, J. R. (1989). Response expectancy as a determinant of hypnotic behavior. In N. P. Spanos & J. F. Chaves (Eds.), *Hypnosis: The cognitive–behavioral perspective* (pp. 360–379). Buffalo, NY: Prometheus Books.

Kirsch, I., Montgomery, G., & Sapirstein, G. (1995). Hypnosis as an adjunct to cognitive–behavioral psychotherapy: A meta-analysis. *Journal of Consulting and Clinical Psychology, 63*, 214–220.

Lazarus, A. (1977). *In the mind's eye: The power of imagery for personal enrichment*. New York: Guilford Press.

Lynn, S. J. (2004). Enhancing suggestibility: The effects of compliance versus imagery. *American Journal of Clinical Hypnosis, 47*, 117–128.

Lynn, S. J., Boycheva, E., & Barnes, S. (2008). To assess or not assess hypnotic suggestibility? That is the question. *American Journal of Clinical Hypnosis, 51*, 213–239.

Lynn, S. J., & Kirsch, I. (2006). *Essentials of clinical hypnosis: An evidence-based approach*. Washington, DC: American Psychological Association.

Lynn, S. J., & Rhue, J. (1991). An integrative model of hypnosis. In S. J. Lynn & J. W. Rhue (Eds.), *Hypnosis theories: Current models and perspectives* (pp. 397–438). New York: Guilford Press.

Lynn, S. J., Shindler, K., & Meyer, E. (2003). Hypnotic suggestibility, psychopathology, and treatment outcome. *Sleep and Hypnosis, 3*, 2–12.

Melzack, R., & Wall, P. D. (1982). *The challenge of pain*. New York: Basic Books.

Moene, F. C., Spinhoven, P., Hoogduin, K. A. L., & Van Dyck, R. (2003). A randomized controlled trial of a hypnosis-based treatment for patients with conversion disorder, motor type. *International Journal of Clinical and Experimental Hypnosis, 51*, 29–50.

Montgomery, G. H., DuHamel, K. N., & Redd, W. H. (2000). A meta-analysis of hypnotically induced analgesia: How effective is hypnosis? *International Journal of Clinical and Experimental Hypnosis, 48,* 138–153.

Neinstein, L. S., & Dash, J. (1982). Hypnosis as an adjunct therapy for asthma: Case report. *Journal of Adolescent Health Care, 3,* 45–48.

Patterson, D. R., Hoffman, H. G., Palacios, A. G., & Jensen, M. J. (2007). Analgesia effects of posthypnotic suggestions and virtual reality distraction on thermal pain. *Journal of Abnormal Psychology, 115,* 834–841.

Piccione, C., Hilgard, E. R., & Zimbardo, P. G. (1989). On the degree of stability of measured hypnotizability over a 25-year period. *Journal of Personality and Social Psychology, 56,* 289–295.

Sheehan, P. W. (1980). Factors influencing rapport in hypnosis. *Journal of Abnormal Psychology, 89,* 263–281.

Soskis, D. A. (1986). *Teaching self-hypnosis: An introductory guide for clinicians.* New York: Norton.

Spanos, N. P. (1982). Hypnotic behavior: A cognitive, social psychological perspective. *Research Communications in Psychology, Psychiatry, and Behavior, 1,* 199–213.

Spanos, N. P., & Barber, T. X. (1974). Toward a convergence in hypnosis research. *American Psychologist, 29,* 500–511.

Spanos, N. P., Cross, W. P., Menary, E. O., & Smith, J. (1988). Long term effects of cognitive skill training for the enhancement of hypnotic susceptibility. *British Journal of Experimental and Clinical Hypnosis, 5,* 73–78.

Spanos, N. P., & Flynn, D. M. (1989). Simulation, compliance, and skill training in the enhancement of hypnotizability. *British Journal of Experimental and Clinical Hypnosis, 6,* 1–8.

Spanos, N. P., Radke-Bodorik, H. L., Ferguson, J. D., & Jones, B. (1979). The effects of hypnotic susceptibility, suggestions for analgesia, and the utilization of cognitive strategies on the reduction of pain. *Journal of Abnormal Psychology, 88,* 282–292.

Spanos, N. P., Robertson, L. A., Menary, E. P., & Brett, P. J. (1986). Component analysis of cognitive skill training for the enhancement of hypnotic susceptibility. *Journal of Abnormal Psychology, 95,* 350–357.

Spanos, N. P., Stenstrom, R. J., & Johnston, J. C. (1988). Hypnosis, placebo, and suggestion in the treatment of warts. *Psychosomatic Medicine, 50,* 245–260.

Tasini, M. E., & Hackett, T. P. (1977). Hypnosis in the treatment of warts in immunodeficient children. *American Journal of Clinical Hypnosis, 19,* 152–154.

Wadden, T. A., & Anderton, C. H. (1982). The clinical use of hypnosis. *Psychological Bulletin, 91,* 215–243.

Wadden, T. A., & Flaxman, J. (1981). Hypnosis and weight loss: A preliminary study. *International Journal of Clinical and Experimental Hypnosis, 29,* 162–163.

IV

TREATING PSYCHOLOGICAL PROBLEMS AND POPULATIONS

14

HYPNOSIS AND THE TREATMENT OF ANXIETY DISORDERS

DAVID I. MELLINGER

Approximately 40 million Americans over 18 are afflicted each year with one or more anxiety-related disorders (Kessler Chiu, Demler, & Walters, 2005), and an estimated 12.5 million are debilitated to the point where they seek mental health help (Narrow, Rae, & Regier, 1998). Moreover, in a typical year, between a quarter and a third of the people in the United States exhibit subclinical symptoms of panic, including shortness of breath, racing heart, dizziness, or a sense of unreality (Antony & Swinson, 2000), and approximately 6 million people suffer from panic disorder, marked by recurrent panic attacks and anxiety (Kessler et al., 2005).

Panic is an integral part of many anxious conditions. Daunted by the possibility of panicking in situations where escape could be difficult or embarrassing, the fears of individuals with panic disorder often generalize into the development of situational or social phobias. Social phobia is much more common than specific and situational phobias. People with social phobia become terrified in anticipation of feeling foolish, stupid, or humiliated. Excessive and unreasonable social fears affect an estimated 15 million

---

All clinical material has been disguised to protect patient confidentiality.

Americans, making social phobia one of the most widespread anxiety disorders (Kessler et al., 2005). Fears of specific events such as thunderstorms or objects such as bugs or snakes are also common and plague 1 out of every 11 people. Rather than being focused on a particular situation, event, or activity, the anxiety of people with generalized anxiety disorder (GAD) is interwoven into the fabric of their everyday activities and consists of physical and emotional tension, worrisome thinking, and feelings of apprehension that intensify around potential threats. The 6.8 million people nationwide with GAD as a psychiatric diagnosis (Kessler et al., 2005) worry during an average of 60% of each day, compared with 18% for the rest of the general population (Borkovec, 1999).

Cognitive–behavioral therapy (CBT) has proven to be far more effective than any other treatments for anxiety (Barlow, 2002; Chambless & Ollendick, 2001; Deacon & Abramowitz, 2004). The cognitive–behavioral and hypnotic approaches presented here are cogent means of discouraging avoidance of what is feared, modifying maladaptive thinking styles and fostering the experience of control and mastery over anxious thoughts and feelings.

In recent years, several meta-analytic reviews have documented the effectiveness of CBT for panic disorder (see Deacon & Abramovitz, 2004) and social phobia, showing that gains endure after treatment (Federoff & Taylor, 2001; Feske & Chambless, 1995; Gould, Buckminster, Pollack, Otto, & Yap, 1997; Taylor, 1996). Three meta-analytic reviews have shown the effectiveness of CBT for GAD (Borkovec & Wishman, 1996; Gould, Otto, Pollack, & Yap, 1997; Weston & Morrison, 2001).

Research indicates that hypnosis can contribute to the effectiveness of cognitive and behavioral treatment of anxiety. Schoenberger, Kirsch, Gearan, Montgomery, and Pastyrnak (1997) compared a cognitive–behavioral treatment for public speaking anxiety involving cognitive restructuring and real-life exposure with an intervention identical in every respect, except that participants were given a hypnotic induction and suggestions instead of nonhypnotic relaxation training. Participants in all conditions were then asked to rate their anxiety during an impromptu speech. Compared with no treatment, both treatments resulted in reduction of anxiety, but only the hypnosis group was found to differ from the group that was not treated on both behavioral and subjective measures. Anxiety dissipated more quickly for those participants who were hypnotized than it did for those who were given the nonhypnotic CBT. After reviewing the literature on hypnosis and anxiety, Schoenberger (2000) concluded that cognitive–behavioral hypnotherapy has more salutary effects in the treatment of anxiety than no treatment.

This chapter first illustrates the treatment of anxiety through the integration of hypnotic methods with cognitive–behavioral principles and effective techniques including self-control and mindfulness training procedures. Following this, I examine clinical applications of hypnotic anxiety treatment through several case examples that refer to actual clients treated. Finally, I briefly discuss the literature supporting these interventions and discuss implications for future research.

REVERSE ENGINEERING FOR ANXIETY TREATMENT

The treatment of anxiety with hypnosis and empirically supported methods involves a process of guided discovery: working backward, in effect, from the causes of anxiety reactions to their treatment. This process, called *reverse engineering,* enables scientists to keep devices, from heart defibrillators to tricycles, running smoothly by figuring out how to repair malfunctions while learning in the process what makes them work. Reverse engineering and guided discovery help to demystify the deep sense of dread integral to anxiety disorders by (a) analyzing clients' catastrophic thinking to determine the main factors and actual events that led to malfunction of their danger prevention systems and then (b) selecting the techniques that can systematically reverse the damage and restore healthy functioning (Mellinger & Lynn, 2003).

Catastrophic Thinking

To reverse engineer anxiety, it is first necessary to understand what produces it. The catastrophic thinking characteristic of many anxiety conditions has anxious people edgily predicting frightening events, despite the low probability of their actual occurrence (A. T. Beck, 1976; Ellis, 1962; Ellis & Dryden, 1997). Persons with phobias tend to exaggerate the negative impact of their particular anxiety-provoking situations, whereas those with GAD tend to exaggerate the likelihood that negative events will occur. Regardless of whether phobic avoidance or active worry is triggered, the fears behind the anxiety reaction are generally excessive and deeply disturbing.

Anxiety Expectancy

At the heart of catastrophic thinking is *anxiety expectancy,* a self-confirming response expectancy that takes the form of apprehension of a disconcerting physiological stress reaction (Kirsch, 1985; Reiss & McNally, 1985). Despite the fact that phobic situations and panic attacks are neither imminently nor mortally dangerous, people with phobias are prone to strong vigilance for evidence that validates their fearfulness, so every panic attack can seem to confirm the frightening quality of phobic fears. The expectation of a panic attack in itself is frightening enough to induce panic. In a related way, socially anxious feelings are predicated on the anticipation of encountering negative experiences in situations in which the individual may interact with others or be observed or judged (Heimberg & Juster, 1995). Each time this prophecy of anxious discomfort appears to be fulfilled, the expectancy for future episodes of anxious disturbance is heightened.

The catastrophic images that fill the anxious person's mind arise automatically during negative emotional arousal (A. T. Beck, 1964; J. S. Beck, 1995). Automatic thoughts are spontaneous, dire predictions and frightening images of possible physical, mental, or social harm, often organized into anxiety propositions that link specific events, situations, or activities, with specific feared consequences. For example, a person may develop the anxiety proposition that he could suffer cardiac arrest during a brisk, steep hike in which his heart is pounding, and his fear would generalize to other uphill climbs. Phobic disorders thus appear to be self-confirming expectancy disorders (Kirsch, 1985; Kirsch & Lynn, 1999).

Many people with anxiety disorders have *anxiety sensitivity* (AS) in strong measure (Reiss & McNally, 1985). AS is the predisposition to experience anxious discomfort, so people with high AS are likely to notice and attend to physical sensations. They are prone to misinterpret normal bodily feelings as abnormal and thus react to them with worrisome emotional distress. This tendency to transform harmless physical feelings into negative emotional reactions can lead to avoidance of triggering situations, anxiety expectancies, and the development of anxiety disorders.

Research has shown that the stronger the anxiety expectancy, the stronger the avoidance (Kirsch, 1985; Kirsch & Lynn, 1999). Because avoidance allows escape from what is feared, anxiety is reinforced and becomes more ingrained (Mowrer, 1960) in the form of anxiety propositions. Moreover, because avoidance precludes learning from direct experience that fears are unrealistic or exaggerated, anxiety and hopelessness are inevitable by-products. However, by confronting fears in a systematic, graduated manner and identifying, challenging, and changing the beliefs and expectancies that engender them, it is possible to modify anxiety expectancies and thus better contend with anxiety (Mellinger & Lynn, 2003).

CLINICAL APPLICATIONS

In this chapter, I focus on treatment of panic, social and situational phobias, and GAD. However, the techniques and strategies I present may also be applied to the entire spectrum of phobic conditions. More detailed step-by-step descriptions of nonhypnotic procedures for the treatment of anxiety, similar to the methods described next, can be found in Mellinger and Lynn (2003).

Treatment of Panic and Phobic Anxiety

Treatment of panic and phobias begins with assessment, followed by provision of a working model of the client's anxiety and panic disorder. At this point, training in application of the model centers on reframing the *emergency response*—the sympathetic nervous system response.

The role of panic symptoms in the anxiety condition should be assessed because any anxiety disorder with panic as a significant component can be tackled more directly once panic is controlled. A careful psychosocial assessment should be made of family history of anxiety disorders, social support, and onset of symptoms. Anxious clients should also receive a medical workup that includes an evaluation of thyroid or blood sugar imbalances, arrhythmias, Cushing's disease, transient ischemic attacks, congestive heart failure, hyperventilation, mitral valve prolapse, inner ear conditions, and metabolic conditions, such as Vitamin B2 deficiency (see Ballenger, 1997). In cases of intractable anxiety, medications should be considered (see Mellinger & Lynn, 2003, for a discussion of issues associated with medication).

A behavioral analysis of anxiety begins with identification of the client's unique pattern of physical symptoms of panic (e.g., intensity, frequency, variability); the cues that typically trigger panic; and the catastrophic thoughts, anxiety propositions, and expectancies that contribute to an episode of panic. Assessment can be accomplished through self-monitoring and record keeping in everyday life situations. A full assessment also includes identification of behavioral avoidance patterns as well as safety behaviors, subtle avoidance maneuvers that create the illusion of safety without reducing anxiety, such as drinking liquids, carrying a snack, or using a talisman. A behavioral avoidance test can aid in assessment by establishing, for instance, how close the client can stand to a spider. Self-hypnosis (see chap. 10, this volume) can also be used for exploration by following suggestions of enhanced abilities to imagine feared events and detect feelings as they unfold, as in the following example:

> Now let's go deeper into your fears of being closed in. With complete awareness that you are only imagining, imagine seeing yourself squeezing past the passengers in the other seats of your row in the airplane, fitting yourself into a confining window seat. Imagine just what you are thinking and feeling, first as you prepare to board, when you take your seat, and then after the flight crew has sealed the plane and you await takeoff. Imagine watching yourself try to maneuver past your seatmates to get to the restroom, feeling enclosed in that cramped space as you pull the door shut. As you watch and imagine, analyze your reactions carefully and accurately at each moment as you cope with any discomfort you may feel. Let each image come into focus now, clearer and clearer, every detail coming into view. Note the passage of time, notice anyone else who is

there during your experience. What specific physical panic symptoms did the person you observed feel? At its strongest, how severe was the panic, and how long did it last?

Providing clients with a working model of anxiety and panic is integral to the treatment of anxiety disorders. A description of the sympathetic nervous system response—the emergency response—provides the basis for reinterpreting and thus reverse engineering physical responses. The therapist continues with the client as follows:

The physical portion of panic attacks is known as the emergency response, otherwise referred to as ER. Although uncomfortable, ER symptoms are not a bit dangerous. Note whether the person in the tight space wants to escape or to avoid the anxious feelings. Is he able to persist and go forward despite his unease? No matter how he feels, realize that the ER is really a false alarm, so there is no immediate mortal danger. You can grasp this so very clearly, let this conviction take root deep within you: Despite the anxiety you observe in the person on the plane, you know, even if he doesn't yet, that there is no real danger. Don't confuse these physical symptoms with real danger. This confusion and uneasiness are anxiety's tricks! After you share with me what you experience, I will tell you more about the physical causes of each of the symptoms you identify in the person on the plane.

[*The client describes relevant thoughts, images, and physical reactions. The therapist then continues.*] Focus closely on my words. Let them resonate and stay deep within you for whenever you may need them. From now on, you will be able to rapidly identify any of the physical symptoms you identified that you experience as just anxiety and no more—just your response to what you are afraid of, but they are not dangerous in any way. I repeat, ER symptoms not dangerous in any way. When you state the real cause of the symptom to yourself, this will help you relax and feel at ease. You will know the physical symptom does not mean danger. Each time you recognize a cause of a physical sensation that troubles you, it will be your cue to enter self-hypnosis and to relax . . . relax. Go deeper now, and listen carefully.

You said you identified a tightening of the chest and a strong heart beat as physical symptoms of anxiety. Chest muscles and other muscles tighten in response to a sense of danger, whether real or illusory. The tightening of chest muscles forces the rapid, shallow breathing that is known as panic breathing. Panic breathing quickly increases the body's oxygen supply, but the strong current of air causes dryness in the mouth and throat and creates the feeling of a lump in the throat. The heart beats very strongly to circulate the oxygen-rich blood to the places throughout the body where it is needed most. Scientists have observed that panic is frequently accompanied by altered breathing that usually results in an increased carbon dioxide level that may lead to tingling, numbness, and lightheadedness. But I can reassure you that people do not faint during panic attacks. Numbness and tingling are caused by the decrease of blood flow to the hands and feet, because more blood tends is diverted to the big skeletal muscles during times of fear. Sweating occurs because of the hard physical work the body does to get the heart and lungs all pumped up and the muscles tensed. Heat is the byproduct, and the body's cooling system offsets this by sweating. [A *physiological description of the function of each of the panic symptoms the client reports is provided.*]

Now, go deeper and register what I have told you, feeling comforted that you will be able to understand the true causes of physical symptoms instead of confusing them with real danger. To ensure that you remember, I will prepare a sheet explaining the cause of each physical symptom you identified. Please review this handout to deepen the understanding you will need to contend with panicky feelings.

Self-Control Relaxation Training

A core component of many treatments for anxiety disorders is *self-control relaxation training* SCRT. Because rapid, shallow breathing and physical tension are integral to many anxiety-related symptoms (Fried, 1999), SCRT consists of training in (a) regulating breathing and (b) engaging in body scan exercises, as well as (c) focusing on present-moment sensory awareness. As the following example derived from Mellinger and Lynn (2003) will illustrate, SCRT can help to relieve the physical tension that accompanies anxiety and catalyze the dissipation of disturbing thoughts and impulses.

Now I will teach you a technique that will enable you to change how you breathe in order to relieve panic breathing. Go into your self-hypnosis and relax, relax completely. Slow your breathing and make it regular. Settle your mind on the places in your body where you feel the breathing most strongly. Notice the coolness of the air as you breathe in, the warmth as you breathe out. Note the motion of the air through your airway and listen to the subtly different sounds as you inhale and exhale. Pretend that your breath is like the waves gently washing on a shore. Feel the air flowing in through your airway, expanding your lungs, and then flowing outward. Feel the area beneath your solar plexus expand and thrust out with each in-breath and contract and draw in with each out-breath. Experience the expansions and contractions of your lungs, the flow of your breath, and the sounds of your in-breaths and out-breaths as musical instruments that blend into a symphony of sensations. To help maintain a good rhythm, count slowly back down from 10 to 1, breathing in with each count. As you release each breath, say the word "smooth" to yourself. Feel yourself relax as your breathing slows down and you give yourself suggestions to feel at ease. Practice this exercise at least six times a day at unstressed times. If you detect any tension or anxiety, focus on your breathing, slow and regulate it, and then breathe easier, retaining only as much physical tension in your body as you feel you need. Learn how little tension is needed in your everyday life.

Now let's try something different in your self-hypnosis. Imagine you are in a mildly distressing, anxiety-provoking situation. See it in your mind's eye. Feel the fear starting to creep in. Feel your breathing start to speed up. As you focus on your breathing, notice how the fear releases its grip on you, how your focus on breathing shifts your focus of attention, and intentionally begin slowing your breathing. Good. Breathe as easily and as rhythmically as you can. If you breathe only a few times a minute, that's all right. As you slow your breathing, feel yourself beginning to calm, as you go deeper into your self-hypnosis.

Now, shift your focus to where you are holding tension in your body. With your mind's eye, scan your body carefully from your head to your toes, and notice where there is any extra tension. Locate the tension, let your mind abide with it. Tension, you don't need. Activate your ability to ease up and let go, like we have practiced. If any part of your body feels especially tense, release all the tension you don't need. You may release it quickly, just letting it go, or release it slowly and feel it flow or trickle away, replaced by a sense of being at peace with that part of your body. If you are still anxious, notice what you are thinking. How are you talking with yourself? After you open your eyes, you will be able to tell me about your experiences. After you have learned to ease your tension and your breathing at times when you are not tense, practice the imagination exercise I have taught you with a scene that is somewhat distressing. You are in control; use your self-hypnosis. You can breathe through and relax your body's tightness and ease yourself through any discomfort. Continue your practice until you feel comfortable and fully in control. [Body scan]

OK. Now I'd like to teach you a different way to contend with anxiety as you experience your self-hypnosis deeper and deeper. Focusing your attention on the input from your senses will help you stay in the present to reduce the tendencies to fear the future or dwell on the past. Expand your mind to awareness of thoughts and emotions. Now open another door of your mind and be aware of sounds. Notice high sounds and low, their steadiness or intermittence, the smooth or rough quality. Listen to sounds from within you, from outside, nearby or in the distance. Simply listen and expand your awareness of all the sounds around you. Now notice the textures of whatever has your attention, like the warmth or coolness of the air, its flow against your skin, or the aromas in the air. Just be aware. Feel your body making contact with the surfaces you are resting on. Continue to be aware of your breathing in and out. Abide in the present, notice when your thoughts slip toward anxiety about the future and notice when you can ease them, nudge them back to the here and now. Remember to notice your breathing. When you feel any tension, it's perfectly natural. Focus on your breathing and use the relaxation tools you have learned in your SCRT training. [*Focus on the present moment*]

It's important that you practice SCRT consistently and use your self-hypnosis at times that are minimally stressful so you can sharpen your breathing and awareness skills, but it is imperative to apply it at select times of stress. Prepare by learning to relax on cue. At times of minimal discomfort, practice your self-hypnosis and cue yourself by mentally saying "Relax!" "Ease off," or "Let go," or use your anchor [*see chap. 10, this volume*], and then spend a few moments using your favorite SCRT technique for maximum effect. For instance, when you start to feel antsy in the dentist's waiting room or while thinking about a meeting with your supervisor, take a few calming breaths; tense and then relax your hands; or shift your focus to the sounds, sights, and scents that fill the present. [*Cue-controlled relaxation*]

Between our sessions, practice and optimize the techniques you have learned. Continue to practice and to customize your self-hypnosis for the next couple of weeks or longer, until you find that you can consistently lower your tension level shortly after beginning a practice. Once you have attained this skill, continue to practice cue-controlled relaxation regularly.

After you have become skillful at relaxing, you may want to train in abbreviating your practices while achieving the same calming effect. An initial abbreviated relaxation practice could consist of a few breaths followed by active relaxation of your hands and face. After a number of practices in which you pay careful attention to tensing and relaxing, you will probably be able to achieve results like those of extended practices. [*Shorten practice*]

By this time, self-hypnosis training and practice may have relieved the client's panic and phobic anxiety. SCRT contributes to relief of most anxiety disorders, but additional cognitive restructuring and exposure techniques provide means of contending with two irrational beliefs that can foster persistent worry and a compelling sense of dread. The first is the fear that anxiety is the opening act to a terrible main event. Because clients have already trained in coping with panic and anxiety by this point in treatment, they have a growing conviction that episodes of anxiety are not harbingers of insanity, medical crises, or public humiliation and can learn to challenge these fears with accurate data and scientific explanations. The second error is that despite evidence to the contrary, people generally believe that once a panic attack begins it will be long lasting and severe. Accordingly, the therapist can share the following information with the client:

> People may continue to feel anxious because they persist in worrying or conjuring up frightening images of what they fear; yet you already know and comprehend the real nature of anxiety and panic. When you

experienced self-hypnosis and imagined yourself in an airplane experiencing anxiety, although you were able to observe your anxious discomfort, the anxiety did end before long. No one's panic attack is eternal. Disturbing feelings ebb and flow like waves on a shore. The next time you feel even somewhat anxious, deep in the back of your mind you will know that anxiety is only temporary. It always passes, always. Anytime you need to, anytime you want to, this thought will be available to you. Your moods and feelings change, and anxiety will pass and soon be replaced with a sense of calm and composure. Now let's talk about your last panic attack. What did you tell yourself afterward? How long did it last? Did you remind yourself it was only a temporary mental event? Remember that your anxiety is only a very temporary state of affairs. Let it come . . . and let it go . . . let it come, and let it go.

Reestimation

When apprehensive, people who suffer from panic and phobic conditions often overestimate the probability that things will turn out badly. Participants in Borkovec's (1999) anxiety research program kept journals of their worrisome predictions. They found that 86% of the time things came out better than expected, and the other 14% of the time, though not particularly good, at least left the worriers satisfied with the ways they coped with what happened. By learning to reestimate the likelihood of bad outcomes, people build more objective assessment skills that help modify predictions skewed by anxiety, as the following example illustrates:

> Go deeply into your self-hypnosis and visualize a scene that frightens you when you are very anxious. Rate the likelihood that the event will turn out badly using the following scale: 0% if there's no chance of a bad outcome, 50% for a 50–50 proposition, 100% for a seemingly certain catastrophe. What is your rating? Now rethink your rating based on the following considerations: How often has this kind of situation come out badly before? Do your most worrisome thoughts usually become realities? What is your recent track record with this kind of situation? Do you have convincing evidence that the situation will turn out negatively? What if you drop all clear-cut, demoralizing exaggerators from your self-talk, like "always," "never," "terrible," and "total failure"? Are there other valid ways of looking at the situation or other explanations for what happened before? For example, when you described how humiliated you felt when your friend grinned as you talked about your concerns, is it possible that she was distracted because she was thinking about something else or didn't grasp how upset you really were? Imagine that your dearest friend, someone who really loves you, is keenly aware of your fears. What words of wisdom, comfort, or support could you imagine him or her saying softly to you to help you through the difficult moments? Now I'd like you to arrive at a preferable way to think about your concerns.

Discussion ensued about the difference between envisioning the most feared outcome versus reframing fears and imagining the most realistic outcome. Reasoning with oneself and reestimating the likelihood of catastrophe can lead to a greater appreciation of cognitive errors that evoke anxiety and can provide more realistic perspectives that are likely to relieve anxiety by competing with anxious cognitions. The following four cognitive techniques can be useful in contending with remaining issues:

During the next week, as soon as you notice your anxieties building, ask yourself, "What am I afraid of?" Take note of your fears and note the specific anxiety proposition that underlies each one. Reconsider everything that provokes your anxiety in order to provide a basis for a less fearful, more realistic way of thinking about it. In a previous session, you identified the anxiety proposition that you feared you would be unable to return a defective item to a store because you would become tongue-tied, panicky, and consumed with embarrassment. Listen carefully to the following suggestions and use them as guides for your self-talk now and anytime you have these sorts of anxieties. Your hyperventilation ensures that you will have plenty of oxygen, and your extra strong heartbeat circulates it throughout your body. Your dry mouth and tight throat are products of your strong, rapid breathing and the tension you feel, which is also tightening your neck muscles. Slowing and regulating your breathing and tensing and relaxing your neck muscles will relieve your physical anxiety. You will be able to reassure yourself that dryness of your mouth and tight muscles have never fully silenced or paralyzed you, and never can. You only need say a few simple statements to the store clerk to accomplish your goal. You have experienced anxiety in these situations simply because of your old mental habit of engaging in self-talk that leads your mind to mistake physical symptoms for real danger. You will experience great relief as you realize you can have control over your fears, and you will work hard to achieve this. [Reconsider anxious thoughts]

Let's try something else. Another anxiety proposition you identified earlier was that your mind would fill with scary thoughts when you were at a party with your friends, and you'd think you were going crazy. Being flooded with these frightening thoughts was your worst-case scenario. But now let's take a closer look at the situation. Imagine you are at a party now and this happens. Get a sense of this happening to you: Go deep into your self-hypnosis. Now ask yourself, Would your buddies resent you forever because you acted confused and scared and asked them for reassurance and help during some hard moments? No, you say? It's unlikely to happen? Often when you ask yourself, "What's the worst that can happen?" you realize that what you fear is very different from the realistic outcome. And even if the worst did occur, wouldn't you be able to endure it? Couldn't you actually cope if need be? I think so. Get deeply in touch with your knack for coping effectively, with your real inner strength, and make a tight fist of determination. Anytime you need to, remind yourself of your determination simply by forming a fist or bringing your fingertips together, and you will quickly and easily regain the sense of your inner strength. Strength is within. Your strength is within; tap this strength now. Tap it and make it yours. [*"What's the worst that can happen?"*]

If the worst case situation did happen, you can simply ask yourself, "So what?" If your head filled with frightening images during your anxiety episode and made you feel panicky, say to yourself that your mind and will are strong, strong; they have guided and protected you through the most challenging and frightening of times. You will know deep inside, deep within yourself, that you are only fearful, nothing worse, and that your buddies are more likely to offer help in a congenial way than to belittle or shun you. Even if they were rather put off, would it end your friendship? Even if you had to repeatedly seek their reassurance and support, so what? More and more, you will be able to reassure yourself, calm yourself, and feel more confident that you can and will be able to contend with any anxiety you encounter. There is far more to you as a person than any anxiety you may experience. You are realizing that anxiety does not get to take you over; it cannot define you. Get a sense of yourself as so vastly surpassing your anxiety, not defined by what you fear, as opening the doors wide to your broadening horizons. Get a sense of a new, expanded you, who you can and will be. [*"So what?"*]

During the week, you will have flashes of your new sense of your stronger self. Perhaps you will find yourself thinking of times when you have successfully contended with anxiety, of things working out for you much better than expected. The changes in your thinking may surprise you—how capable you are of transformation, the transformation in the way you think and feel, the way you are as a person. And you will be able to enjoy this transformation as it unfolds. [*Posthypnotic suggestion*]

Now imagine that you have been transformed into what we will call the "new you." Get inside the skin of this new you who embodies how you would like to cope with anxious situations should they recur. The old, socially anxious you probably would be stressed over the most disturbing moments and their bad effects on your self-image. The new you can think of it as a challenge. Get in touch with your strength, your creativity, your resolve to face your stresses with valor. In your imagination, place yourself in another social situation where you have felt very uncomfortable. How would you cope with your anxiety? Reconsider everything that provokes your anxiety in order to provide a basis for formulating a less fearful, more realistic way of thinking. As you become aware of the challenges you will face, you will feel empowered to tackle emergent stressors more effectively. The new you will try out techniques that may help and adopt new, more positive perspectives as you begin socializing differently. Now let this new you talk to me. [*Shaping the new you*]

[*Therapist–client discussion ensues, and the therapist continues.*]

During the week, enter self-hypnosis when you need to and get in touch with the new you. Consult her [or him] for a sense of how to think about situations you fear if they occur. List thoughts that you find raise your anxiety; rate their anxious probability and then reestimate the realistic probability of their occurrence. Note how the considerations and rationales that contributed to your reestimation help to map the way new you would think. Now transform your anxiety propositions into realistic propositions. For example, to combat your fear of a catastrophic physical reaction, you can say to yourself, "This is just a little panic I'm having before my talk, not a sign of heart disease or prelude to humiliation." Add something like, "It will probably last just a few minutes, and I'll feel better soon." Listen carefully to yourself and let this penetrate to a deep level and enhance your valor, for you are much, much stronger than your anxiety propositions make you seem. From this moment on, you will engage in the process of decatastrophizing anxious thoughts and remember to embrace the new you for assistance whenever needed. Treat each incident of heightened anxiety as an opportunity for strategic coping. Be sure to practice your SCRT several times each day, regardless of whether you feel good or bad.

Imaginal and Real-Life Exposure

If SCRT and cognitive restructuring do not sufficiently alleviate the client's anxiety, the next step is to integrate planned exposure with the cognitive practice sessions. Exposure may be to real life or imagined events and situations. Real-life exposure may either be precisely preplanned or "opportunistic"—capitalizing on opportunities for exposure that occur naturally in select environments. A good starting point for overcoming severe avoidance is imaginal exposure therapy (Lazarus, 1977), illustrated by the following example:

Today we will begin to raise your comfort level in social situations by learning to practice imaginal exposure. The assumption underlying this technique is that things we fear in reality, we also fear in imagination; the corollary is that the things we cease to fear in imagination will no longer disturb us in the actual situation.

[*After the client agrees to learn the technique, the therapist continues.*]

Go deep into your self-hypnosis now. Let the specific situation or specific aspect you fear the most come to mind. Just let images and feelings come to you. You may find it interesting to discover that you can keep your anxiety manageable, quite manageable, during this process. When you know what makes you the most uncomfortable, just begin to talk about it and without further thought, rate the intensity of your anxiety.

The client talks about anxieties that trigger a spectrum of different intensities of distress. After he or she comes out of self-hypnosis and discusses the situations with the therapist, they create a hierarchy from the least to the most intense level of discomfort. The situations they choose to work on at first should be readily accessible, involve significant but tolerable anxious distress, and offer the prospect of meaningful satisfaction as an incentive for surmounting them. A deepening procedure like the *staircase technique* can serve as a productive means of boosting the client's capacity to face the intense fears that have produced severe avoidance, as in the example that follows:

> Now enter your self-hypnosis and imagine you are standing at the top of a sweeping stone staircase with 10 steps leading down to a verdant, beautiful garden. In a moment, I will be asking you to descend the staircase. I will guide you with my counting. Each step can take you deeper, closer to realizing your goals. Taking the first step. One. Let your feet relax, feel the spreading calmness. Two. More and more comfortable. Three. Feeling the easing, the calm spreading throughout your body. Four. Deeper and deeper relaxation. Wouldn't it feel good to keep feeling relaxed in an easy, effortless way? You know you don't have to do anything, so that every bit of tension you don't need flows out of your body. Five. Or you can feel even calmer, more deeply relaxed. Six. Discovering a sense of safety, of composure, spreading throughout your body and mind. The calmness is spreading through you. Seven. Nothing to bother, nothing to disturb you. Do you think you are ready to go even deeper? And yet it really doesn't matter how deeply at ease you become, just that you feel comfortable. Eight. Nearing the bottom; soon you will arrive at the place where you feel so secure and calm. Do you feel the instants of stillness between breathing out and breathing in? Can you experience the quiet inside? Nine. You don't even have to think to feel calm and safe and at ease. Ten. You have arrived! So comfortable, so fully at ease.
>
> Now I will talk to you in your place of comfort and security. Now begin to envision the situation you ranked lowest in discomfort. Focus deeply on it, imagine it vividly, and signal me when your anxiety becomes strong. Very good. Now mentally switch off the scene. Relax, relax; go even deeper than you were before. Go to your safest, favorite place now, discover and experience real comfort there, a sense of determination to forge ahead in order to be the new you, the person you know you can be. Now, let's do it again. The idea is to resume vividly visualizing the anxiety-provoking situation, then to switch it off and relax deeply and to repeat the process until you no longer feel any discomfort. After you have succeeded in reducing your discomfort to a minimum, we will move ahead to the next situation on your hierarchy. When you practice on your own between sessions, try to tackle situations that are manageable for you, and we will ascend the steps of your hierarchy together to the most difficult of situations. [*Imaginal exposure*]

Imaginal exposure is beneficial in itself and also as preparation and rehearsal for behavioral or real-life exposure. As in imaginal exposure, a hierarchy is developed and the initial selections for practice are tolerably anxiety provoking. Exposures are broken down into graduated steps, and each activity is practiced until the client's anxiety decreases to a low level before advancing to the next, more challenging, step. Consider an exposure hierarchy related to a client's efforts to feel comfortable enough to ride an elevator up to his fifth floor office. (He has been taking the stairs.)

1. Walking into the building lobby and watching people go in and out of the elevator.
2. Practicing stepping into the elevator and remaining there for between a few seconds to up to 2 minutes while a friend holds the "door open" button.
3. Remaining in the stationary elevator with the door closed and a friend with his finger on the stop button for periods increasing from seconds to 2 minutes.
4. Stepping into the elevator alone and holding the door open button while remaining inside for gradually lengthier periods.
5. Doing Step 3 alone.
6. Riding up and then down one floor with a friend and repeating it 10 times.
7. Riding up one floor alone to where a friend is waiting and then down to the friend, who has taken the stairs. Repeat 10 times.
8. Repeating Step 7 up to an empty landing and then down to where the friend awaits. Repeat 10 times.
9. Ride the elevator up to an empty landing two floors up and then down to where the friend awaits, and repeat 10 times.
10. Continue increasing the number of floors until he has ascended at least five floors and then descending to the floor where the friend waits. Repeat 10 times.
11. Ride up and down at least five floors alone and repeat 10 times.

During these regular exposures, which involve practice in one or more different situations or steps in the hierarchy, have the client (a) enter a wakeful state of self-hypnosis, (b) practice SCRT and cue-controlled relaxation, (c) notice automatic thoughts and anxiety propositions that have been challenged and restructured in therapy, and (d) replace them with flexible coping responses. The client should practice regularly, both in good moods and bad, and should try to remain in each situation until the level of anxious discomfort peaks and then declines.

Treatment of phobias, particularly social phobia, can be augmented by taking advantage of the wealth of opportunities for exposure that arise in the course of everyday life. The following plans for *opportunistic exposure* are based on Mellinger and Lynn (2003).

1. Make brief eye contact and smile at 50 different people.
2. Greet at least 25 people.
3. Ask 20 people directions to the restroom, the nearest pay phone, the nearest service station, or the nearest Italian, Chinese, Thai, or Mexican restaurant.
4. Purchase numerous small items at different stores. Pay with a check or credit card, so you can practice signing your name in front of other people.
5. Make brief comments to, or ask questions of, 25 different people at a supermarket. For example, ask for help choosing ripe produce, inquire about a product a fellow shopper is putting in his or her cart, find out from someone who is examining items which brands he or she prefers, or engage in small talk with fellow shoppers in the checkout line.

During weekly therapy, the results of the exposure practice sessions are reviewed. It is helpful for clients to record what they did, thought, felt, and imagined and the strategies they used to challenge anxious thoughts and alter perspectives on their fears. Success experiences should be highlighted, and the therapist should help identify any remaining anxiety propositions and cognitive errors requiring restructuring. Asking the client to enter self-hypnosis, revisit scenes that aroused the most anxiety and provide commentaries about the experiences can do this. Then each scene can be reimagined with the client implementing more effective ways of coping with the anxiety, such as challenging negative thinking and reinterpreting physical symptoms and ultimately mastering his anxieties in imaginal exposure practice. Cognitive techniques are principally important in facilitation of behavioral exposure, which has the greatest therapeutic impact for clients who are socially or situationally phobic. Imaginal and real-life exposure proceed until all hierarchy items are completed with minimal or negligible anxiety, typically 5 to 10 sessions, unless the symptom picture is complicated by depression, a personality disorder, or other serious psychopathology.

Techniques for Generalized Anxiety

The line between healthy and unhealthy worry can be vanishingly fine. Healthy worry stimulates problem solving and planning is generally of short duration and creates only mild emotional distress. When worry turns unhealthy, the expectation of negative events or outcomes is exaggerated, mental clarity is diminished, and negative thoughts and images may persist long after a problem is solved. Worry accompanies a number of anxiety disorders and may dominate the lives of people with GAD.

Early Cue Detection

The treatment of GAD begins with early detection of worry cues followed by the implementation of strategies aimed at curtailing worry. Worry can be detected early by noticing physical indicators and thoughts or mental images that portend anxious disturbance. Physical indicators may include fidgeting, muscle tension, sweating, or rapid heartbeat, whereas mental indicators include thoughts of being overwhelmed, afraid, or "what if?" thinking, as well as images such as being targeted by harsh criticism, letting down those who count on you, or feeling immobilized by stress.

Mindfulness and Acceptance Can Supplant Avoidance and Suppression

Persons with GAD often scan the environment for threat and fortify themselves against feeling and expressing strong emotions. One way of exposing clients to the gamut of human emotions and training them to refrain from avoidance is through the practice of mindfulness and acceptance. By determining what is avoided and learning to confront what is feared, a sense of effectiveness replaces hopelessness. A high level of acceptance and experiencing of emotions is associated with positive psychotherapeutic outcomes (e.g., Greenberg & Safran, 1989). Techniques that promote mindful acceptance of negative as well as positive experiences as they unfold have an important role in the treatment of GAD (see Borkovec, 2002; Roemer & Orsillo, 2005) as well as social anxiety (Herbert, 2006) and panic disorder (Germer, 2005; Karekla, Forsyth, & Kelly, 2004). Mindfulness techniques may be used as the front line approach for contending with worries that the client has detected early.

Mindfulness training can easily be incorporated into hypnotic treatment to assist clients in accepting and becoming comfortable with evanescent emotional states and to release them from reacting in habitual, maladaptive ways (Lynn, Lama Surya Das, Hallquist, & Williams, 2006). When working on overcoming avoidance of intense emotional experience, we promote the client's mindful acceptance through suggestions for self-hypnosis, as in the following example:

> As you continue to follow your breath, go deeper into your self-hypnosis and observe all of your thoughts, yet be detached from them. Don't ignore any that may bubble up; simply notice them without reacting. Just observe. Realize they are just thoughts, just tapes made over a lifetime of learning. Let them float past, detached, objects floating along a tranquil stream. Imagine your breathing as a pump that makes the stream's water

flow. Even if your thoughts are pleasant and you want to cling to them, just let them go, watch them move downstream, the stream always changing, never the same—the stream of consciousness—thoughts and feelings that you observe, knowing all the while that you can react to any thought or feeling you wish, or just let it flow by, watching another thought or feeling replace it in your ever-changing stream of awareness.

This mindful acceptance technique may be integrated into the practice of early cue detection. I instruct clients to enter self-hypnosis at regular intervals 10 times a day and do a body scan, monitor anxious thinking, ask themselves what they are worried about or afraid of, and then implement an abbreviated version of the mindful acceptance technique. If worry persists, the client can use the following cognitive restructuring techniques, discussed earlier: (a) reestimating the realistic probability of negative outcomes; (b) articulating the most likely, best case, and the worst case scenarios and using the "so what?" technique for the latter; and (c) identifying and restructuring specious and maladaptive thinking. If the subject of the worry is a realistic and immediate problem, the client should engage in brainstorming and devise a detailed coping plan. Hypnotic suggestions can also be useful. Reminders help: that excessive worry does not improve decision making or prevent negative events; that a worrisome thought is only a theory, not a fact; and that the client has successfully negotiated many challenging situations in the past. It also helps to suggest images, such as releasing lingering worries to waft in the breeze, attached to the strings of pretty helium-filled balloons.

Worry Postponement

Worry postponement is a technique that involves making a conscious decision to monitor and postpone worries for an interval of between a few seconds and a part of a day. After lengthier postponements, the worry should be scheduled to be dealt with at a specific time, and when the time arrives, the client should opt either to think actively about it or to postpone it still again until another specific time. Worry postponement may be used repeatedly until the worry is dealt with or fades away.

Worry Periods

Disconcerting, seemingly uncontrollable, recurrent worries are very much a part of GAD (Wells, 1997). When a client identifies these tenacious anxieties, postponement to worry periods—when uninterrupted attention is devoted to worry exposure—can be instrumental in mastering them. Worry periods are instituted daily for at least 20 minutes. A hierarchy of the client's least to most disturbing worries can serve as the agenda, and clients can enter self-hypnosis and practice the cognitive–behavioral techniques I have summarized. After repeated cognitive exposures to what is feared, clients' anxiety generally diminishes as a result of habituation.

Emotional Processing of Interpersonal Feelings

Foa and Kozak (1986) identified the necessity for emotional processing of fear in order to overcome it. A recent innovation in the treatment of GAD is the recognition of the importance of emotional processing of interpersonal feelings. Anxiety about interactions appears to be a factor in most anxieties, and clients with GAD worry about interpersonal matters more than any other (Roemer, Molina, & Borkovec, 1997). In Newman, Castonguay, Borkovec, and Molnar's (2004) integrative therapy for GAD, clients are made aware that they may be so inclined to avoid what they fear from others that they do not endeavor to fulfill their own interpersonal needs, inadvertently bringing about the very situations that engender both anxiety and negative outcomes. For example, by protecting themselves from vulnerability to others by refraining from disclosure of their needs and feelings, clients may be perceived as disinterested and unapproachable. The goal is to shift clients' energies from apprehension and rigidity toward greater openness and spontaneity with others and also to heighten compassionate awareness of themselves and their needs. Newman et al. recommended combining CBT with emotional deepening techniques derived from other traditions such as experiential and gestalt therapies. They further recommended using the following questions to facilitate in-depth exploration of relationships with significant people: (a) "What event happened between you and the other person?" (b) "What emotions did you feel?" (c) "What did you need or hope to get from the other person?" (d) "What did you fear from the other person?" (e) "What did you do?" (f) "What happened next between you and the other person?" and (g) "What emotions did you feel?" (continuing the exploration by returning to the original question).

Hypnosis can be integrated into this framework by inviting clients to enter self-hypnosis while responding to these questions and by observing their own experiences unfolding on a movie or TV screen. Clients are told that they have a start and stop control and a feeling control that can be turned both on and off. For the first run-through, clients are instructed to describe what occurs as they watch the action with the feeling knob turned off. During the subsequent run-through, clients are instructed to turn the feeling knob on and stop the action whenever they sense the "self" they are observing beginning to feel the slightest discomfort. At that point, they can "enter the movie" by doing a body scan and examining the relationship between their anxious feelings and catastrophic thoughts. After gaining a better sense of what they need, want, and fear in relation to the significant other person, they are then asked to turn the feeling control to the point when they can feel the feelings as the scene unfolds so that they can fully experience themselves in the moment with this person. Whenever the client or therapist would like to discuss the events in more depth, clients can "step out of the movie" by shutting off the feeling control. The exercise can be repeated until they can tolerate and accept the spectrum of feelings that arise and grasp the cognitions that trigger distancing behaviors and the nature of emotional retreats. The therapist can also use the technique to foster compassion and empathy by asking clients to focus on the thoughts and feelings they attribute to the person with whom they are interacting and observe the interplay between behaviors and the other's fear- and worry-provoking reactions. Age regression can be used to explore important childhood relationships to enhance understanding of the developmental antecedents of clients' current expectancies and avoidances.

CASE MATERIAL

Julie, a 29-year-old programmer, sought help for generalized anxiety centering on problems with stress in her relationships. Although Julie was self-assured at work, she often felt insecure in her personal life. She had started to date Sal, and as they became more involved, she grew anxious and occasionally panicky. Her anxieties centered on her apprehension that as the relationship deepened she would become increasingly vulnerable to angst and fear of abandonment.

Julie discussed her interest in hypnosis with me, her therapist. I administered the Stanford Hypnotic Clinical Scale (Morgan & Hilgard, 1978–1979; see also chap. 3, this volume) and determined that she was moderately hypnotizable. I introduced her to self-hypnosis and guided her in its use to help contend with her anxiety and cope with her catastrophic fears.

Anxiety and Panic Attacks

Whenever she and Sal drove a distance from her home, Julie would become increasingly anxious; she had a panic attack one evening when they were going to dine out in another part of the city. She and I assessed her anxiety through self-hypnosis, and she spent a session learning to reframe her anxieties and panic. After that, she gave somewhat less credence to her passing notion that Sal was treacherous and no longer believed that her anxiety attacks were destructive. Still, she was bothered by bouts of preoccupation and worried about spending quality time with her new boyfriend.

I proposed that by occasionally exaggerating her vague worries, she was actively expanding her anxious distress. I asserted that the anxious thoughts and anxiety attacks she had been experiencing were mental events that discomfited her without any lasting purpose, comparable with dreading meeting a feared and respected teacher until you are actually in his or her presence, enthralled and fascinated by his or her charisma. Hypnosis could aid her in coping with negative thoughts and emotions without necessarily having to reason through or fight with them. I taught her a technique of hypnotically augmented mindfulness to help relieve her physical tension and anxiety, as follows:

> Emotions and thoughts are just temporary events that come and go if you let them. Imagine you're driving with Sal toward the edge of the city. The air in his car is stale, and you feel uncomfortable. As you leave familiar environs behind, the fear starts to creep in. Feel the fear. Feel your breathing rate changing, quickening. Observing your thoughts, all of the thoughts that bubble up. Simply noticing your thoughts without reacting, realizing that they are just thoughts, just old tapes. Your thoughts are constantly moving, your feelings always changing. Imagine that each thought is a ripple on the water of a stream flowing past you. Imagine your breathing as a pump that makes the water flow: appearing to slow down, then quickening, always flowing. The stream always changing, always streaming with your energy, never the same, the stream of the thoughts and feelings you observe, knowing that you can let any thought or feeling you wish flow by. Letting your fears go—every feeling, negative or positive, just letting them flow past.

Julie practiced revisiting the scene in the car during hypnosis and self-hypnosis, observing the anxieties and tension that would bubble up and practicing mindfulness to help them evaporate or flow away. She also practiced entering self-hypnosis and briefly attaining a mindful state at least five times a day and whenever she noticed herself becoming anxious. After 2 weeks, she became more comfortable with Sal and no longer was prone to panicking.

Active Worry

Julie's active worries often materialized when she would try to discuss the future with Sal. She tried to deal with this by avoiding this topic but felt just as bad. To investigate further how these anxieties affected her feelings and behavior, I asked Julie to enter self-hypnosis and review her recent, anxiety-provoking interactions with Sal as if watching them on a television screen. Following the procedure for hypnotically enhancing the processing of interpersonal feelings outlined earlier, Julie arrived at the realization that Sal would casually disregard her efforts to plan the direction of their relationship together and do whatever necessary to divert their conversations away from her concerns. She would get frustrated, start to think she was tricked and overpowered, slide into feeling unsafe and detached, and become increasingly silent.

Mellinger:	Now go into self-hypnosis. View your conversation with Sal with the "feeling control" on, and let your index finger lift when you start to feel uncomfortable. [*Julie's finger lifts.*] Good. Stop the tape. What just happened?
Julie:	I was telling him about my enjoyable experience taking care of my sister's young kids and how I was interested in buying a house pretty soon, and then we drove past a motorcycle shop, and he abruptly started talking about the high performance bike he'd like to buy himself.
Mellinger:	Go right back into the scene. Let your mind's eye scan your body and notice any tension that you feel. Focus on each of the tense places inside you. Notice what you are saying to yourself. What emotions are you feeling?
Julie:	Frustrated! Why can't he stop acting like a spoiled child and take me seriously!
Mellinger:	It's disturbing to be disregarded when you're talking about your desires and hopes.
Julie:	I'm really hurt. I'm starting to think it's too dangerous to have feelings for him.
Mellinger:	Caring for him is sometimes frightening. Now go back into the scene. Experience your fear and hurt, your tension. Turn up the feeling control as much as you can. Stay with the feelings. Good. Now shut it off. Now imagine someone you deeply trust, who really loves you and considers your well being paramount, advising you how to proceed. Would your loving advisor tell you to close yourself off, to suppress your desires and hopes? Or to vocalize them, to assert yourself, because you're worthy of happiness?

Julie realized that she would prefer to assert herself to Sal, rather than withdrawing. She decided to tell him she wanted to discuss their future and let him know when he frustrated her efforts to do so. Her efforts were successful, and they developed an ongoing dialogue about the direction their relationship was taking.

Fear of Abandonment

Julie's apprehensions resurfaced a few weeks later, paradoxically because she and Sal seemed to be getting serious as a couple. When he invited her to be his guest at his company's gala holiday party at a mountain resort, she felt both pleased and deeply worried. I described it as follows:

Imagine him urging you to attend the party. He's proud of your relationship, so he wants you by his side for this special celebration. He keeps amiably endeavoring to overcome your reluctance. You're really flattered—and nervous! He won't take no for an answer. Your tension mounts. What are you telling yourself, what are you saying to yourself? What's the worst that could happen?

Julie reported her strong fear of humiliation in front of Sal and his associates as well as an underlying dread of isolation and abandonment that was difficult to control. She learned about the nature of unhealthy worry—nebulous, disconcerting, exaggerating the negativity of worst-case scenarios—and she was able to reframe and lessen her fears.

She finally decided she would go to the party but continued to be daunted by her mental image of feeling like a deer in the headlights in front of festive strangers. Because she was unable to feel assured of her ability to cope, I decided to use the staircase technique and hypnotically enhanced imaginal exposure to help enable her to contend with this frightening scenario:

> You told me that you feared being alone and uncared for at the gala and of your dread of becoming so petrified with anxiety that you would humiliate yourself in front of Sal and his friends. Let's look closely at what you envision. Go deeply into your self-hypnosis. Visualize being at the party now and imagine your fear becoming a reality. Experience your isolation. As you watch Sal celebrating, animated, interacting with others, no one even approaches you. You are all alone. Get in touch with your sense of rejection, the tightening inside you. Take some time to really feel this sense and the anxiety. Stay with it. Now go to your place of calm and safety. Relax there; tap your inner strength, feel your calm determination. Go deeper now. Use the staircase technique: Descend the steps, one by one, growing calmer and more and more deeply relaxed with every step. Continuing your descent as you start feeling a pervasive sense of composure. Raise your index finger when you can feel it. [*Julie lifts her index finger.*] Good. Now go down another step, feeling more and more safe and secure, and another, arriving at a very safe, very secure place. Stay with it. Now imagine the anxiety-provoking scene again. Get it vividly in mind, but this time shift your thinking. Imagine actively coping with your fears, feeling like you really can, reassuring yourself, energizing, motivating. Feeling your inner calm, your deep inner vitality. You are at ease, listening to other people with composure, focusing your attention on them, catching people's eyes, breathing smoothly, regularly. Imagine breathing with so little effort, your breath flowing smoothly among other people, around other people, and returning to you, linking you together in a pleasant way. Remaining in the moment, steadfast, your anxiety subsiding like the surf receding from the shore. You're feeling better, safer. You know Sal is there somewhere, but you are enjoying your own presence of

mind. Listening, relaxing, and listening and chatting, paying attention to other people, the sense of connecting with others calms and reassures you at a deep level, and you can talk as well as listen. Now move in your mind's eye to your place of comfort and security. Go there and get relaxed, very relaxed. Are you there? Good. Now once again start to visualize yourself feeling alone and uncared for at the party. Continue to practice imagining scenes where your anxiety is provoked, then move over to your calm place, and then return to the scene to continue mastering your fear. Devote all the time you need to this, until the fear has subsided.

The next four sessions were devoted to imaginal exposure and desensitization, as well as Julie's self-hypnosis between sessions. At the party, Sal was gracious, although not especially attentive, but Julie had a remarkably pleasant experience. Her fears did not turn into reality. Her anticipatory anxiety turned into excitement, and she interacted well and enjoyed the occasion. She savored her feeling of accomplishment. Her relationship with Sal continued to go well, and her anxieties continued to diminish.

RESEARCH AND APPRAISAL

In the previous sections, I reviewed the types and prevalence of anxiety disorders, discussed the clinical applications of CBT for the treatment of the most prevalent of these, and examined the evidence supporting the adjunctive use of hypnosis in the treatment of anxiety disorders. The case report recounted the hypnotically enhanced treatment of a client diagnosed with generalized anxiety disorder using assessment during self-hypnosis, reframing, a mindfulness technique, cognitive therapy of catastrophization, and imaginal exposure and desensitization. I now consider the effects of hypnosis in anxiety disorder treatment and review the literature supporting the clinical application of hypnosis and mindfulness training to generalized anxiety disorder (see chap. 13, this volume).

Impact of Hypnosis on Effect Size

Hypnosis has been used to treat psychological disorders for centuries. A great deal of empirical research has shown CBT to be effective for treatment of anxiety, but relatively few controlled studies have evaluated the effectiveness of hypnosis as an adjunct to CBT for anxiety treatment. Gerschman, Burrows, Reade, and Foenander (1979) found that participants who were highly hypnotizable responded more favorably to treatment of their dental phobias. Moreover, a subsequent study (Gerschman, Burrows, & Reade, 1987) reported a significant positive correlation ($r = .54$) between hypnotizability and reduction of dental phobic anxiety. Van Dyck and Spinhoven (1997) found in their study comparing in vivo exposure alone to exposure plus hypnosis in the treatment of agoraphobia with panic disorder, that cognitive–behavioral hypnotherapy was more effective in the treatment of anxiety than no treatment.

A meta-analysis by Kirsch, Montgomery, and Sapirstein (1985) found 18 studies between 1974 and 1993 comparing CBT with the same treatments augmented by hypnosis. The mean effect size for the difference between hypnosis and nonhypnotic conditions was determined to be $SD = 0.87$, indicating that hypnosis augmented CBT significantly. The largest effects by far were attained in treatments for obesity, and once these were factored out, a value of $SD = 0.53$ was obtained, indicating that clients who received CBT with adjunctive hypnosis improved more through treatment than 70% of those who received CBT only. These finding suggest that hypnosis may enhance the effectiveness of CBT, particularly among clients who are highly hypnotizable.

Response Expectancy

According to the response expectancy model of phobias (Kirsch, 1985; Kirsch & Lynn, 1999), phobic disorders are seen as self-confirming expectancy disorders. Schoenberger et al. (1997) examined the role of expectancy in their research comparing the effectiveness of hypnosis-enhanced CBT and nonhypnotic CBT. Participants in a study of treatment for public speaking anxiety—a form of discrete social phobia—were asked to rate the amount of change they expected in their levels of anxiety. The expectation of change was associated with actual improvement on a number of outcome measures, including anxiety about public speaking situations, fear of negative evaluations by other people, and ratings of anxious discomfort experienced during a brief, impromptu speech. People who expected to improve more had greater success in treatment. Although this expectation could be attributed to individual differences (e.g., greater self-efficacy), participants in the hypnotically enhanced treatment expected to experience significantly greater improvement than did people in the CBT-only condition. This suggests that the addition of hypnosis led to greater improvement in part by strengthening expectancies for improvement.

Nonspecific Effects and Hypnotic Susceptibility

The Kirsch et al. (1995) meta-analysis evaluated the impact of several differences in treatment protocols as possible moderators of the efficacy of hypnosis. The researchers found that neither the relaxation training provided during hypnosis nor the inclusion of hypnotic suggestions accounted for the benefit of adding hypnosis to CBT. Studies of hypnosis in the treatment of obesity were the only ones in this meta-analysis that included assessments of effects sustained at the time of long-term follow-up. Long after visits to the therapist had ended, hypnotic treatments continued to result in better compliance with the treatment program relative to control treatments, and this behavior change was correlated with weight loss. These findings imply that the benefits of hypnosis may continue to increase after treatment for other presenting problems as well, although additional research will be needed to verify this outcome.

Among a group of patients with panic disorder treated in a Hungarian psychiatric clinic, those who improved substantially with nonhypnotic treatment were significantly more hypnotizable than those who demonstrated little or no improvement (Kopp, Skrabski, Mihaly, Buza, & Ratkoczi, 1988). Many researchers have proposed that highly hypnotizable clients should be most responsive to hypnotic treatments. Spiegel, Frischholtz, Maruffi, and Spiegel (1981) found that "hypnotizable patients were over 2.5 times more likely to report some positive impact than those who were found to be nonhypnotizable" (p. 243) when treated in a single 45-minute session involving hypnosis and a problem restructuring strategy.

Studies that have examined the relationship between hypnotizability and therapeutic outcome with hypnosis as an adjunct in treatment have generally reported the relationship to be positive, although the findings are not entirely consistent (Lynn & Kirsch, 2006). However, it may be the case that people who are more suggestible (i.e., hypnotizable) may report positive outcomes in the absence of behavioral changes in everyday life. In discussing hypnotic approaches to treatment of anxiety disorders, Crawford and Barabasz (1993) hypothesized that moderately to highly hypnotizable individuals would respond more strongly to hypnotic approaches because of their skills in imagery and absorption. Lynn and Rhue (1988) asserted that cognitive strategies in which individuals imaginally distance or separate themselves from deeply disturbing events might be used effectively as a creative therapeutic activity. Borkovec (1999) posited that training GAD clients in imagining their fears and solutions could increase the salutary effect of imaginal desensitization. In the case example, the client's creative powers were enlisted when she used the TV screen and controls to heighten her awareness and augment her capacity to express her interpersonal needs; detailed imaginal exposure and desensitization in hypnosis and self-hypnosis helped allay her fear of abandonment.

Given these findings, it follows that clinicians should administer standardized hypnotizability scales, such as the Stanford Hypnotic Clinical Scale (Morgan & Hilgard, 1975), as part of the initial evaluation to determine the appropriateness of the use of hypnosis for anxiety treatment. Still, many of the suggestions that are potentially beneficial to anxious clients do not require especially high suggestibility (e.g., simple imagery, relaxation, imaginative rehearsal).

Imagery and Mindfulness Strategies

Mindfulness strategies, as well as those embodying compassionate self-acceptance, have often been proposed to augment CBT of GAD, although evidence documenting their effectiveness is still limited. Borkovec, Alcaine, and Behar (2004) asserted that meditation practice (e.g., focus on breathing) increases client's attentional flexibility, whereas Roemer and Orsillo (2005) maintained that mindfulness can kindle the capacity to be compassionate with oneself as well. Mellinger (2007) proposed that the metacognitive therapies outlined by both Segal, Williams, and Teasdale (2002) and Wells (2005) train clients to use select mindfulness techniques for reduction of rumination and active worry. In the case reported in this chapter, mindfulness taught hypnotically appeared to be helpful to the client in reducing the perniciousness of her "worry about worry."

CONCLUSION

A number of factors may account for the enhancement of CBT for anxiety disorders with hypnosis: Highly hypnotizable people are more likely to respond to psychological treatment per se; hypnosis is likely to increase the effectiveness of CBT; and hypnosis can readily and usefully be integrated into CBT for panic, social, and situational phobic disorders. Hypnotizability appears to be a factor in improvement in anxiety disorders, perhaps because individuals who are receptive to hypnosis may be more comfortable working imaginatively and also because training of the imagination can facilitate desensitization of worry about worry, arguably a potent factor in the maintenance of generalized anxiety. Imaginativeness may also be a factor in hypnotic use of mindfulness techniques, a factor which Lynn et al. (2006) proposed as a useful enhancement of treatment for GAD, easily incorporated as a means of assisting clients to respond comfortably to evanescent emotional states and releasing them from reacting in habitual, maladaptive ways to active worry.

Further research in a number of directions will help to clarify the role of hypnosis in hypnotically enhanced treatment of anxiety disorders. The roles of response expectancy, hypnotizability, and imaginal ability should be delineated more precisely. A particularly fertile ground is the study of the functions of hypnosis in increasing the effectiveness of CBT for GAD, because attentional variables and augmentation of creative and imaginative mental faculties appear to be significant factors in this disorder.

REFERENCES

Antony, M. M., & Swinson, R. P. (2000). *Phobic disorders and panic in adults: A guide to assessment and treatment.* Washington, DC: American Psychological Association.

Ballenger, J. C. (1997). Panic disorder in the medical setting. *Journal of Clinical Psychiatry, 58,* 13–17.

Barlow, D. H. (2002). *Anxiety and its disorders: The nature and treatment of anxiety and panic.* New York: Guilford Press.

Beck, A. T. (1964). Thinking and depression: II. Theory and therapy. *Archives of General Psychiatry, 10,* 561–571.

Beck, A. T. (1976). *Cognitive therapy and the emotional disorders.* New York: International Universities Press.

Beck, J. S. (1995). *Cognitive therapy: Basics and beyond.* New York: Guilford Press.

Borkovec, T. D. (1999, March). *New developments in the treatment of worry.* Paper presented at the advanced practice symposium of the national conference of the Anxiety Disorders Association of America, San Diego, CA.

Borkovec, T. D. (2002). Life in the future versus life in the present. *Clinical Psychology: Science and Practice, 9,* 76–80.

Borkovec, T. D., Alcaine, O. M., & Behar, E. (2004). Avoidance theory of worry and generalized anxiety disorder. In R. G. Heimberg, C. L. Turk, and D. S. Mennin (Eds.), *Generalized Anxiety Disorder: Advances In Research and Practice* (pp. 77–108). New York: Guilford Press.

Borkovec, T. D., & Wishman, M. A. (1996). Psychosocial treatment of generalized anxiety disorder. In M. Mavissakalian & R. Prien (Eds.), *Long-term treatments of anxiety disorders* (pp. 171–199). Washington, DC: American Psychiatric Press.

Chambless, D. L., & Ollendick, T. H. (2001). Empirically supported psychological interventions: Controversies and evidence. *Annual Review of Psychology, 52,* 685–716.

Crawford, H. J., & Barabasz, A. F. (1993). Phobias and intense fears: Facilitating their treatment with hypnosis. In S. J. Lynn, I. Kirsch, & J. W. Rhue (Eds.), *Handbook of Clinical Hypnosis* (pp. 311–338). Washington, DC: American Psychological Association.

Deacon, B. J., & Abramowitz, J. S. (2004). Cognitive and behavioral treatments for anxiety disorders: A review of meta-analytic findings. *Journal of Clinical Psychology, 60,* 429–444.

Ellis, A. (1962). *Reason and emotion in psychotherapy.* Secaucus, NJ: Lyle Stuart.

Ellis, A., & Dryden, W, (1997). *The practice of rational–emotive behavior therapy* (2nd ed.). New York: Springer.

Federoff, I. C., & Taylor, S. (2001). Psychological and pharmacological treatments of social phobia: A meta-analysis. *Journal of Clinical Psychopharmacology, 21,* 311–324.

Feske, U., & Chambless, D. L. (1995). Cognitive–behavioral versus exposure only treatment for social phobia: A meta-analysis. *Behavior therapy, 26,* 695–720.

Foa, E., & Kozak, M. J. (1986). Emotional processing of fear: Exposure to corrective information. *Psychological Bulletin, 99,* 20–35.

Fried, R. L. (1999). *Breathe well, be well: A program to relieve stress, anxiety, asthma, hypertension, migraine, and other disorders for better health.* New York: Wiley.

Germer, C. K. (2005). Anxiety disorders: Befriending fear. In C. K. Germer, R. D. Siegel, & P. R. Fulton (Eds.), *Mindfulness and psychotherapy* (pp. 152–172). New York: Guilford Press.

Gerschman, J. A., Burrows, G. D., & Reade, P. C. (1987). Hypnotizability and dental phobic disorders. *International Journal of Psychosomatics, 34*(4), 42–47.

Gerschman, J. A., Burrows, G. D., Reade, P. C., & Foenander, G. (1979). Hypnotizability and the treatment of dental phobic behavior. In G. D. Burrows, G. D. R. Collison, & L. Dennerstein (Eds.), *Hypnosis 1979* (pp. 33–39). New York: Elsevier.

Gould, R. A., Buckminster, S., Pollack, M. H., Otto, M. W., & Yap, L. (1997). Cognitive–behavioral and pharmacological treatment for social phobia: A meta-analysis. *Clinical Psychology Review, 8,* 819–844.

Gould, R. A., Otto, M. W., Pollack, M. H., & Yap, L. (1997). Cognitive–behavioral and pharmacological treatment of generalized anxiety disorder: A preliminary meta-analysis. *Behavior Therapy, 28,* 285–305.

Greenberg, L., & Safran, J. (1989). Emotion in psychotherapy. *American Psychologist, 44,* 19–29.

Heimberg, R. G., & Juster, H. R. (1995). Cognitive–behavioral treatments: Literature review. In R. G. Heimberg, M. R. Liebowitz, D. A. Hope, & Fr. R. Schneier (Eds.), *Social phobia: Diagnosis, assessment, and treatment* (pp. 261–309). New York: Guilford Press.

Herbert, J., & Cardaciotto, L. (2005). An acceptance and mindfulness-based perspective on social anxiety disorder. In S. M. Orsillo & L. Roemer (Eds.), *Acceptance and mindfulness-based approaches to anxiety: Conceptualization and treatment* (pp. 214–240). New York: Springer.

Herbert, J., & Dalrymple, K. L. (2006). Acceptance-based behavior therapy for social anxiety disorder: A preliminary treatment manual. Unpublished manuscript, Department of Psychology, Drexel University, Philadelphia, PA.

Karekla, M., Forsyth, J. P., & Kelly, M. M. (2004). Emotional avoidance and panicogenic responding to a biological challenge procedure. *Behavior Therapy, 35,* 725–746.

Kessler, R. C., Chiu, W. T., Demler, O., & Walters, E. E. (2005). Prevalence, severity, and comorbidity of 12-month *DSM–IV* disorders in the National Comorbidity Survey Replication (NCS-R). *Archives of General Psychiatry, 62,* 617–627.

Kirsch, I. (1985). Response expectancy as a determinant of experience and behavior. *American Psychologist, 40,* 1189–1202.

Kirsch, I., & Lynn, S. J. (1999). The automaticity of behavior in clinical psychology. *American Psychologist, 54*, 504–575.

Kirsch, I., Montgomery, G., & Sapirstein, G. (1995). Hypnosis as an adjunct to cognitive–behavioral psychotherapy: A meta-analysis. *Journal of Consulting and Clinical Psychology, 63*, 214–220.

Kopp, M. S., Skrabski, A., Mihaly, K., Buza, K., & Ratkoczi, E. (1988, September). *Psychophysiolgical regulation treatment in two subroups of panic patients*. Paper presented at the meeting of the Fifth International Congress of Psychophysiology, Prague, Czech Republic.

Lazarus, A. A. (1977). "Hypnosis" as a facilitator in behavior therapy. *International Journal of Clinical and Experimental Hypnosis, 21*, 25–31.

Lynn, S. J., & Kirsch, I. (2006). *Essentials of clinical hypnosis: An evidence-based approach*. Washington, DC: American Psychological Association.

Lynn, S. J., Lama Surya Das, Hallquist, M. N., & Williams, J. (2006). Mindfulness, acceptance, and hypnosis: Cognitive and clinical perspectives. *International Journal of Clinical and Experimental Hypnosis, 54*, 143–166.

Lynn, S. J., & Rhue, J. W. (1988). Fantasy-proneness: Hypnosis, developmental antecedents, and psychopathology. *American Psychologist, 43*, 35–44.

Mellinger, D. I. (2007). *Mindfulness and irrational beliefs*. Manuscript submitted for publication.

Mellinger, D. I., & Lynn, S. J. (2003). *The monster in the cave: How to face your fear and anxiety and live your life*. New York: Berkley Books.

Morgan, A. H., & Hilgard, J. R. (1978–1979). The Stanford Hypnotic Clinical Scale for adults. *American Journal of Clinical Hypnosis, 21*, 148–169.

Mowrer, O. H. (1960). *Learning theory and behavior*. New York: Wiley.

Narrow, W. E., Rae, D. S., & Regier, D. A. (1998). *NIMH epidemiology note: Prevalence of anxiety disorders*. Retrieved April 5, 2004, from http://www.nimh.nih.gov/publicat/numbers.cfm

Newman, M. G., Castonguay, L. G., Borkovec, T. D., & Molnar, C. (2004). Integrative psychotherapy for anxiety disorders. In R. Heimberg, D. S. Mennin, & C. L. Turk (Eds.), *Generalized anxiety disorder: Advances in research and practice* (pp. 320–350). New York: Guilford Press.

Reiss, S., & McNally, R. J. (1985). The expectancy model of fear. In S. Reiss & R. R. Bootzin (Eds.), *Theoretical issues in behavior therapy* (pp. 107–121). New York: Academic Press.

Roemer, L., Molina, S., & Borkovec, T. D. (1997). An investigation of worry content among generally anxious individuals. *The Journal of Nervous and Mental Disease, 185*, 314–319.

Roemer, L., & Orsillo, S. M. (2005). An acceptance-based behavior therapy for generalized anxiety disorder. In S. M. Orsillo & L. Roemer (Eds.), *Acceptance and mindfulness-based approaches to anxiety: Conceptualization and treatment* (pp. 213–240). New York: Springer.

Schoenberger, N. E. (2000). Research on hypnosis as an adjunct to cognitive–behavioral psychotherapy. *International Journal of Clinical and experimental Hypnosis, 48,* 154–169.

Schoenberger, N. E., Kirsch, I., Gearan, P., Montgomery, G., & Pastyrnak, S. L. (1997). Hypnotic enhancement of a cognitive–behavioral treatment for public speaking anxiety. *Behavior Therapy, 28,* 127–140.

Segal, Z. V., Williams, J. M. G., & Teasdale, J. D. (2002). *Mindfulness-based cognitive therapy for depression: A new approach to preventing relapse.* New York: Guilford Press.

Spiegel, D., Frischholtz, M. A., Maruffi, B., & Spiegel, H. (1981). Hypnotic responsiveness and the treatment of flying phobia. *American Journal of Clinical Hypnosis, 23,* 239–247.

Taylor, S. (1996). Meta-analysis of cognitive–behavioral treatments for social phobia. *Journal of Behavior Therapy and Experimental Psychiatry, 27,* 1–9.

Van Dyck, R., & Spinhoven, P. (1997). Does preference for type of treatment matter? A study of exposure in vivo with or without hypnosis in the treatment of panic disorder with agoraphobia. *Behavior Modification, 21,* 172–186.

Wells, A. (1997). *Cognitive therapy of anxiety disorders: A practical manual and conceptual guide.* Chichester, England: Wiley.

Wells, A. (2005). Detached mindfulness in cognitive therapy: A metacognitive analysis and ten techniques. *Journal of Rational–Emotive & Cognitive–Behavior Therapy, 23,* 337–355.

Weston, D., & Morrison, K. (2001). A multidimensional meta-analysis of treatments for depression, panic, and generalized anxiety disorder: An empirical examination of the status of empirically supported therapies. *Journal of Consulting and Clinical Psychology, 69,* 875–899.

15

HYPNOSIS AND DEPRESSION

MICHAEL D. YAPKO

This chapter explores the use of hypnosis as a core component of a multidimensional approach to treating depression. It provides a clinical rationale for using hypnosis in a variety of ways, ranging from symptom management to psychoeducation to interrupting depressive cognitive and behavioral patterns. Sample hypnotic suggestions are provided as well as an illustrative case example. Throughout the chapter, hypnosis is framed as a means of absorbing the client in a more functional, self-enhancing frame of mind.

Since my previous chapter on this topic appeared in the first edition of this volume more than 15 years ago, there have been many changes in the way depression is both viewed and treated (Yapko, 2006). Psychologically based treatments of depression have received considerably less attention in the last decade, the so-called Decade of the Brain (Library of Congress and the National Institute of Mental Health, 2000), than have biologically based ones, especially antidepressant medications. Antidepressant medications have been steadily released to the general public, and there are now nearly two dozen available. According to the Pharmaceutical Research and Manufacturers of America, there are nearly two dozen more antidepressants in various stages of

All clinical material has been disguised to protect patient confidentiality.

research and development (NewsRX.com, 2000). The number of people who have taken antidepressants has increased dramatically in just the last 3 to 5 years, and the public's interest in, and desire for, effective antidepressant medications continues to increase. Pharmaceutical companies have been advertising antidepressants heavily on television, radio, and in popular magazines. As a direct result of these widely disseminated advertisements, the general public has been led to believe that depression is a biological disease requiring medication as a primary, or even sole, form of intervention. It is no wonder that the sales of antidepressants have soared (Kravitz et al., 2005).

Despite their still-growing popularity, medications have proven to be controversial. There are some researchers, such as Kirsch et al. (2008), Kirsch and Sapirstein (1999), and Antonuccio, Danton, and DeNelsky (1995), who have boldly questioned whether the use of medications provides any significant contribution to a therapeutic effect beyond placebo. Echoing a similar concern, though with a different viewpoint of the data, a remarkable article in the January 17, 2008, issue of *The New England Journal of Medicine* (Turner, Matthews, Linardatos, Tell, & Rosenthal, 2008) documented the practice of pharmaceutical companies to selectively publish antidepressant trials, thereby misleading people to believe that antidepressants are more effective than they really are. Other researchers studying the negative effects of medications have noted that selective serotonin reuptake inhibitors are the class of drug most commonly found in adverse drug events, a problem often not addressed by the general physician in a primary care environment (Gandhi et al., 2003).

In 2004, the Food and Drug Administration (FDA) placed a so-called black box warning on antidepressants, indicating that their use by children and adolescents may lead to increased suicidal ideation and suicidal behavior in this younger population. To date, Prozac is the only antidepressant approved by the FDA for use specifically with depression in those under age 18. Despite this, pediatricians regularly prescribe an array of antidepressants to children under age 18. In a telling 1999 survey of North Carolina physicians and pediatricians, the majority (72%) reported they had prescribed antidepressants to children. Perhaps shockingly, few of them (only 8%) felt they were appropriately trained to prescribe these drugs to children (Rushton, Clark, & Freed, 2000). It is not difficult to understand the dilemmas (e.g., parental pressures, peer pressures, time pressures) pediatricians face that lead them to prescribe medications they feel poorly trained to prescribe confidently.

Numerous therapeutic efficacy studies have been conducted to assess the relative merits of many different forms of treatment, including various forms of psychotherapy. The general consensus at this time is that there are clear advantages to combined approaches to treatment (March et al., 2004; Scott, 2000). Thus, although studies of drug therapies have received the lion's share of research funding, psychotherapy has been shown to be effective in ways that can complement the use of antidepressant medications. Thus, clinicians do not need to get locked into an "either–or" approach (i.e., medication or psychotherapy as mutually exclusive approaches).

Despite the need for new and diverse approaches to treatment, it seems evident that solely biological approaches to either understanding or treating depression are limited in their usefulness; depression does not just involve biology. Cross-cultural epidemiological research, family studies, studies of individual coping styles, and research into many other psychologically based processes all highlight the fact that depression is determined by many factors, many of which are rooted in both individual and interpersonal psychologies (Hammen, 1999; Just & Alloy, 1997; Kaelber, Moul, & Farmer, 1995; O'Leary, Christian, & Mendell, 1993; Weissman et al., 1996; Yapko, 1996, 1997).

In 1999, the World Health Organization issued a statement declaring depression as the world's fourth greatest cause of human suffering (behind heart disease, cancer, and traffic accidents). They also predicted at that time that depression would continue to increase worldwide and that by the year 2020 it would become the second most common cause of human suffering (Murray & Lopez, 1997). Depression is increasing in prevalence around the world, not just in the United States. Every demographic group is showing significant increases in the rate of depression, despite the mental health profession having developed effective forms of treatment. These data can be interpreted in a variety of ways, but depression experts generally agree that intervention on a purely biological basis alone is not an adequate reply to the growing problem (Breggin, 1999; D. Burns, 1999b; Seligman, 2002). Instead, emphasis can be placed on encouraging people to evolve the kinds of life skills that have been shown in therapeutic efficacy studies not only to reduce depression but also to prevent it (O'Connor, 2001; Seligman, 1995). Given the emphasis most hypnosis practitioners place on self-efficacy, members of the hypnosis community can play a strong role in advocating for both effective treatment using hypnosis as well as a greater investment in strategies of prevention. To do this will take some rethinking as to what mental health professionals know about depression and how hypnosis might be well applied in its treatment.

In the same way that the mental health profession must continually revise its most basic assumptions in light of new data, the hypnosis community must also revise some of its most basic assumptions. To date, controlled research about the use of hypnosis in treating depression has been exceedingly rare (Yapko, 2001). Only one recent study, by Alladin and Alibhai (2007), has provided an empirical basis for supporting the use of hypnosis in treating depressed patient populations. Alladin and Alibhai described their use of a combination of hypnosis with cognitive–behavioral therapy, termed *cognitive hypnotherapy*, with 84 patients with depression randomly assigned to 16 weeks of treatment of either cognitive hypnotherapy or cognitive–behavioral therapy alone. The addition of hypnosis to the treatment was found to significantly enhance treatment results.

With so little research available in the domain of hypnotic treatment for depression, the field of hypnosis has had little to add to the larger conversation about what specifically hypnosis can objectively be said to add to the treatment process. In fact, to the detriment of the field, such research had been actively discouraged by influential hypnosis experts who regularly claimed that not only did hypnosis have nothing to offer in the treatment of depression, but that it could also actually be harmful to patients with depression. (For a detailed discussion of this issue, see Yapko, 1992, 2006.) Thus, much of what clinicians have learned about the potential benefits of applying hypnosis has come from clinicians who regularly use hypnosis in their treatments, rather than from clinical researchers who have conducted the relevant research.

Despite the lack of controlled research involving hypnosis, there is plenty of clinical evidence for its effectiveness (see Lynn, Kirsch, Barabasz, Cardeña, & Patterson, 2000, for a detailed analysis of the literature regarding empirical support for hypnotic interventions). The hypnosis research literature contains hundreds, perhaps thousands, of studies that attest to the merits of hypnosis in helping people to better manage their symptoms and their lives. Hypnosis is commonly described across different clinical populations and disorders as a vehicle for empowering people, which is a fundamental part of treating depression, a disorder characterized by disempowering hopelessness and helplessness (Beck, 1997; D. Burns, 1999a).

The research makes it abundantly clear that depression is much more than a biologically based problem (Joiner, Coyne, & Blalock, 1999; O'Connor, 1997). Thus, helping people recognize that depression arises, in part, because of social and psychological factors can help them to avail themselves of the benefits psychotherapy can provide. After all, no amount of medication (or brain stimulation or brainwave reeducation) can provide people with better problem-solving skills, coping skills, cognitive skills, relationship skills, or a supportive network of friends. Of the various approaches to treating depression that have been evaluated scientifically, there is unequivocal evidence that the therapies that actively encourage people to develop specific life-enhancing skills perform better than other therapies that do not (Jacobson & Gortner, 2000; Thase et al., 1997).

As has been pointed out in a variety of places, hypnosis is not a therapy in and of itself (American Psychological Association, 1999; Yapko, 2003). Rather, hypnosis is considered a vehicle for establishing a therapeutic relationship and then introducing therapeutic possibilities through the clinician's suggestions. Thus, the salient questions revolve around how hypnosis might be used to enhance other, more established, forms of psychotherapy. In this chapter, therefore, I focus on a few ideas as to how hypnosis may best be applied in treatment.

HYPNOSIS IN THE TREATMENT OF DEPRESSION

As the mental health profession's understandings of both hypnosis and depression have deepened in recent years, the early concerns that hypnosis would hurt rather than help the client with depression have markedly diminished. Clinicians have learned, for example, that suicidality is not caused by inadequate ego defenses and that depression is not caused by anger turned inward. Instead, there are specific risk factors evident in one's thinking, behaving, relating, and perceiving that can, under certain conditions, give rise to depressive episodes. As a result, clinicians have many more immediate and well-defined targets for hypnotic intervention than was previously realized. It has been amply demonstrated that psychotherapy can succeed, and succeed well, when people who suffer depression are taught key life skills that empower them to live more personally satisfying lives.

Hypnosis can be used in a variety of ways, ranging from superficial to profound. These include the following (see Barabasz & Watkins, 2005; Lankton & Lankton, 1983; Yapko, 1997, 2003, 2006): (a) symptom management strategies (e.g., enhancing sleep, reducing anxiety), (b) resource accessing and skill-building strategies (e.g., teaching social skills or problem-solving skills), (c) deframing and reframing strategies (e.g., "It's not your genetic destiny, it's a skill you should learn" or "It's not what happened to you, it's how you interpreted its meaning"), and (d) associational and dissociational strategies (e.g., shifting the focus away from feelings to thoughts or from the past hurts to future possibilities). Sophisticated applications of hypnosis can meaningfully address underlying dynamic issues as well as symptoms, serving as a highly efficient therapeutic tool for establishing meaningful therapeutic associations. In this way, hypnosis may be used in conjunction with any other therapy modality one desires to facilitate a more rapid and deeply integrated establishment of the desired therapeutic associations.

A RATIONALE FOR USING HYPNOSIS WITH INDIVIDUALS WITH DEPRESSION

The goal of any therapy, regardless of its emphasis, is to interrupt hurtful self-limiting patterns of the patient's experience and to build adaptive or functional patterns in their place. Recently, a shift in the practice of psychotherapy has been to focus on and amplify positive resources of the patient, to actively structure positive learning, and to encourage dormant positive capacities to develop. Considerable attention has been paid to this new focus in therapy that has come to be called a *positive psychology* (Seligman & Csikszentmihalyi, 2000). Hypnosis as an intervention tool is able to amplify existing resources, reassociate dissociated aspects of experience, and facilitate the establishment of desirable associations on whatever level (e.g., cognitive, relational, physiological, behavioral) the therapist deems appropriate. Hypnosis is a practical vehicle for delivering a positive psychology.

RELATIONSHIP TO OTHER VIEWS OF DEPRESSION

Currently, there are two especially prominent and well-researched psychotherapy models of depression that dominate the clinical field: the cognitive model and the interpersonal model (Beck, 1997; Goodman & Gotlib, 2002; Joiner & Coyne, 1999). Both enjoy considerable support in studies of effectiveness. Each is considered in this section in relation to the implications for treating depression with hypnosis.

Cognitive models of depression take at least two forms. In the model developed primarily by Aaron Beck, which is arguably the best researched treatment model, the emphasis is placed on identifying and correcting the cognitive distortions evident in the patient's quality of thinking (Beck, 1997; Beck, Rush, Shaw, & Emery, 1979; D. Burns, 1999a). Simply put, the patient makes identifiable errors in thinking that fuel the negativity and despair of depression. In fact, the relationship between thought and affect is viewed as a two-way relationship: Cognitive distortions fuel negative emotions, and likewise, negative emotions fuel cognitive distortions. In treatment, the patient is taught to identify and self-correct faulty patterns of thinking. Beck identified many of the most common categories of cognitive distortions and developed rapid and efficient techniques for challenging and clarifying the patient's thoughts.

Martin Seligman (1989, 1990, 1995) developed another cognitive model of depression that focused specifically on the attributional style of the patient. Seligman described one's attributional style as a regularly relied on and highly predictable pattern for determining the meaning of events in one's life and, subsequently, the reactions one forms to those events. Seligman identified specific patterns of attributional style and encouraged clinicians to make use of Beck's cognitive therapy techniques for refuting and clarifying the patient's depressogenic attributions. The skills of flexible thinking; looking for multiple, plausible explanations for an event's occurrence; drawing clear and reasonable conclusions on the basis of objective evidence; and responding appropriately and effectively to the characteristics of the current context are all emphasized as important and desirable outcomes in both cognitive models.

The interpersonal therapy model of depression, originally developed by Gerald Klerman, Myrna Weissman, Bruce Rounsaville, and Eve Chevron (1984), and further developed by others (e.g., Goodman & Gotlib, 1999; Joiner & Coyne, 1999), emphasizes the relationship between depression and the quality of one's interpersonal relationships. The emphasis is on building effective relationship skills to establish mutual support, mutual respect, clarity of personal boundaries, open and honest communication, intimacy, and the other necessary and desirable skills for relating positively and meaningfully to others. As a telling example of the power of relationships to influence mood, there is considerable evidence that distressed marriages lead to a higher incidence of depression and, conversely, that depression leads to greater marital distress (Beach, Sandeen, & O'Leary, 1990; Hammen, 2002; Yapko, 1999). It has also been shown that depression in parents is a strong risk factor for the development of depression in their children, despite the fact that the data suggest only a mild genetic contribution (Silberg & Rutter, 2002). Such evidence provides a compelling rationale for acknowledging the social side of depression; treating biology alone may thus be a disservice to the individual.

It is enlightening to note that both cognitive and interpersonal views of depression focus on interrupting specific dysfunctional patterns and building healthier, more adaptive ones. Neither model, both of which are well supported empirically, focus on abstract issues or presumed psychodynamics. Neither approach emphasizes a focus on analyzing the client's personal history, instead focusing on making well-defined changes in the present. Both views emphasize that therapy should be relatively brief in duration and not long-term. Both require the therapist to be an active teacher and facilitator, not merely a passive source of client support. Both emphasize that the goal of therapy is to change the structure of how the patient thinks and relates and therefore focus only on what the patient thinks or does. The key point both models emphasize is that when the structure of a patient's thought patterns changes for the better, so must the associated content of their thoughts.

These points are highly relevant in formulating skillful applications of hypnosis. Hypnosis is regarded as a tool, a vehicle for dispensing information, building perspective, enhancing skill acquisition, and creating a context for therapeutic change to take place. Thus, one can use hypnosis to highlight to a patient his or her cognitive distortions, offering suggestions for more automatically recognizing and refuting them. Although Beck and Seligman have not spoken of an "unconscious mind" in the way that many practitioners of hypnosis have been inclined to, each has described "automatic thoughts" that must be identified, brought to conscious awareness, refuted and replaced. Hypnosis can play a role in focusing an individual on any specific dimension of internal experience, one chooses, including a cognitive one. Thus, if one wishes to make use of cognitive therapy techniques, hypnosis can be used to help establish therapeutic associations in the patient for more readily identifying and clarifying his or her distorted thoughts and attributions (Alladin, 2006; Yapko, 1992, 2003, 2006).

Similarly, if one chooses to focus on the relational dimension, using the interpersonal model as a conceptual and practical framework, hypnosis is also applicable. Identifying and relating skillfully to other peoples' needs and values, establishing and consistently enforcing one's limits in one's dealings with others, and developing greater awareness of one's own needs and how they might best be met are all examples of skills one might wish to help the patient build using hypnotic suggestions. In short, the ability of hypnosis, applied either formally or informally, to build a strong link between the troublesome context and the skilled response desired in that context is the primary reason why hypnosis can be so easily integrated into virtually any model of treatment.

CLINICAL APPLICATION

There are many different possible targets for therapeutic intervention in the treatment of depressed individuals. Whatever targets a clinician deems appropriate to aim at in treatment, it is vitally important that the client believe that any effort to change his or her responses will likely be successful. Without the belief that things can change in meaningful ways, the depressed client's sense of hopelessness can effectively derail the process of therapy.

The remainder of this chapter focuses on two specific patterns associated with depression that are so central to the treatment process that therapy cannot succeed if they are not skillfully addressed either directly or indirectly: (a) a stable attributional style and (b) perceptual and/or behavioral rigidity. In the remainder of this section, I describe these two patterns and how hypnosis might effectively be used in addressing them.

Stable Attributional Style

Probably the single most important pattern to evaluate and address in the patient with depression is his or her degree of stable attributional style. A stable attributional style is the perception that adverse life conditions are not only unchanging but also unchangeable and are, hence, stable (Seligman, 1989). Beck also described negative expectations as a cornerstone of depression (Beck, Rush, Shaw, & Emery, 1979). These are both ways of describing the fact that the individual with depression is typically unable to project positive changes ahead into the future, thus restricting his or her vision of the future to either an undefined, but negative, impression or an interminable continuation of the currently debilitating circumstances.

The patient with depression is typically absorbed in the belief that his or her experience of depression and the negative life circumstances causing it cannot improve. Thus, it becomes a primary goal in the treatment process to address a patient's stable attributional style for several important reasons. First, the relationship between a stable attributional style and one's level of motivation to attempt to change is apparent: Why should a depressed person try to improve his or her circumstances if he or she believes nothing can change? Second, why should patients with depression continue in the therapy if there is no immediate experiential evidence to suggest that their condition can improve? For example, when a therapist only takes an extensive history (e.g., symptom history, medical history, family history) in a first session, the patient discovers at the outset of treatment that the therapist may do nothing to change his or her direct experience. The absence of any kind of intervention may unwittingly reinforce the patient's stable attributional style.

One of the patterns evident in many patients with depression is a low frustration tolerance, which clinicians must recognize and acknowledge so that the client does not form the rapid and erroneous conclusion that therapy will not help. This is the basis for my strong recommendation that hypnosis, specifically a hypnosis session designed to build positive expectancy, be used as early on in the treatment process as is feasible, perhaps even in the first session. Stated succinctly, the first goal of treatment in addressing depression is to try and shift the person's stable attributional style to an unstable attributional style, encouraging a belief in the client that things can change and that any effort expended can be helpful when expended in a positive direction. As Kirsch (1990) described, changing a client's expectations in a positive direction is a key to effective psychotherapy. This is especially true in treating depression.

Hypnosis may be used to build positive expectancy and facilitate the development of an unstable attributional style. This is the reason for doing even a simple, yet positive, induction process with a patient. Even a brief and superficial hypnosis session has the ability to reduce the client's distress, anxiety, and rumination, thereby demonstrating directly and experientially that his or her symptoms are malleable; it suggests directly that his or her experience can change. The use of hypnosis to build positive expectancy in a particular area of the patient's life can amplify the patient's motivation to change and then guide that motivation in a new and specific direction. Once hypnosis is performed, posthypnotic suggestions to help generalize the positive expectations to other areas of the patient's life as well will need to be given. Otherwise, the typically concrete cognitive style of the depressed patient will lead him or her to restrict the new learning to only the specific context described.

EXHIBIT 15.1
Hypnotically Building Expectancy

1. Identify the patient's dominant temporal orientation (i.e., past, present, future).
2. Identify the patient's primary representational system (i.e., preferred or most heavily relied on sensory system).
3. Identify the patient's cognitive style (i.e., degree of concrete or abstract style, degree of specific or global style).
4. Identify the goal (i.e., specific expectations).
5. Effect induction, building a response set (i.e., a momentum toward acceptance of suggestions).
6. Introduce metaphors illustrating the inevitability of change.
7. Access personal transitions from the patient's history.
8. Identify personal resources evident in past transitions.
9. Identify specific future contexts requiring a new response.
10. Embed the positive resources identified in item 9.
11. Rehearse the new (i.e., behavioral, cognitive, affective) sequence.
12. Generalize positive resources to other selected contexts.
13. Provide posthypnotic suggestions for integration.
14. Effect closure and disengagement.

Exhibit 15.1 suggests a generic sequence for conducting a hypnosis session designed to interrupt negative expectations for the future. The goal of such a session is to impart two important messages at an experiential level: (a) The future is not simply more of the past, and (b) one already has relevant resources that can be skillfully used to resolve difficulties. The hypnotic phenomenon of age progression plays a clear and pivotal role in building positive expectancy. Age progression techniques are those approaches that experientially orient the patient to the future (Yapko, 2003). In the generic sequence outlined in Exhibit 15.1, age progression is used to extend personal resources identified in the past into future contexts where they will be wanted or needed. This emphasis on finding relevant personal resources, even in a patient who is deeply depressed, is a meaningful application of positive psychology. In essence, the hypnotized patient is encouraged to experience positive future consequences in the present that arise from implementing new skills, new behaviors, and new perceptions in the course of daily living. At a stage of treatment as early as the first session, the expected changes need not even be specified by the therapist, but can be described in a general way that only sounds specific, such as in the following example:

> You've described the discomfort that has led you to seek help. . . . You want to feel differently . . . but you really don't know yet that you can feel differently. . . . If you think about it . . . there have been times in your life when you found yourself facing some challenge you didn't think you'd surmount. . . . and you went through periods of feeling uncertain . . . such

as when you were a young child and you weren't sure you could cope with having to go to school . . . and when you were in elementary school and you were unsure you'd be all right in junior high school. . . . There are lots of examples of times when you didn't feel you could go on . . . but you did. . . . You found a way . . . and, even though you don't realize it yet, there will be a way now too for you to take another step in a better direction . . . a way for you to move past this time in your life . . . into a new time in your life that can have so much more of what feels good to you available to you. . . . And, as you will discover . . . when we talk about new possibilities . . . new ways to handle things effectively . . . new ways to approach old problems . . . I think you'll enjoy discovering . . . that some of the best times you will ever have in your life . . . are times that haven't happened yet . . . .

These suggestions impart the message that the client's experience can change in meaningful ways, encouraging a shift from a stable (i.e., things cannot change) attributional style to an unstable (i.e., things can change) one. Age progression can help move distant consequences into the realm of more immediate experience. Through an emphasis on positive future possibilities based on new, more effective courses of action, the chief depressogenic pattern of stable attributional style can be meaningfully addressed in the therapy.

Perceptual and Behavioral Rigidity

No one experiences frustration, disappointment, loss, rejection, and other life adversities only once. Life's difficulties are repetitive, and if depression is one's patterned response to adversity, then depression will be a frequent unfortunate companion. If one has a broad array of resources to use to respond flexibly to the great diversity of experiences life throws at each of us, effectively handling each situation according to its own merits, then depression is less likely. If one responds rigidly to circumstances, usually by applying patterns developed in similar past circumstances to current yet different circumstances, one is likely to respond ineffectively and thereby generate an unwanted and potentially hurtful response. If one globally condemns oneself for being ineffective or incompetent and if one believes one will always be this way, the risk of depression is substantial. Rigidities in thinking, feeling, or behaving can be viewed as the basis for peoples' difficulties in general, and for depression in particular.

Once the seeds of recognition that change is possible have been planted, the patient is likely to experience a shift in perception, developing a glimmer of hope that there will be a way to effectively resolve the problems at hand that led him or her to seek therapy in the first place. With the help of the clinician, the patient can arrive at a state of greater willingness to entertain the possibility of developing meaningful alternatives in perception

EXHIBIT 15.2
Facilitating Flexibility: Generic Hypnotic Structure

1. Effect induction.
2. Establish receptive mind-set.
3. Introduce metaphors that reflect change.
4. Introduce metaphors that reflect rigidity.
5. Access personal ability to adapt (i.e., change with changing times).
6. Identify adaptive resources in current and future contexts.
7. Extend existing resources into current and future contexts.
8. Allow integration of adaptive skills to be applied in ways anticipated during the hypnosis session.
9. Provide posthypnotic suggestions for automatically using the new responses in the appropriate context(s).
10. Effect closure and disengagement.

and/or behavior, the essence of flexibility. Exhibit 15.2 describes a generic hypnotic process for facilitating flexibility in some aspect of the depressed patient's experience.

The use of hypnosis to facilitate flexibility is a means to impart several key messages: (a) There are many right (i.e., effective) ways to accomplish a goal, not only one; (b) if you fail, adapt and try another approach; (c) familiarity aside, find the best (i.e., most effective) response for the circumstances; and (d) change is inevitable and adaptation is an ongoing process. It should be pointed out that the use of hypnosis in itself is a potentially powerful statement from the therapist because it models flexibility in the therapeutic relationship. The boundaries of how the therapist and the patient interact are expanded in the process, indirectly stating, "We can relate to each other meaningfully in a variety of ways."

The patient's beliefs and values are among the most potent factors dictating his or her range of responses to life events. Ultimately, this is why the cognitive elements of the patient's world will need to be addressed somehow through the therapy. When a patient reports "feeling stuck," it is most likely an indication of subjective perceptions, not an objective statement about the lack of possibilities. In this situation, direct hypnotic suggestions to the patient to seek alternative interpretations or alternative solutions is one obvious application of hypnosis. However, the use of metaphorical approaches as an indirect means of suggestion with the hypnotized patient can also be a valuable means of providing important therapeutic messages, embedding them in the metaphor's memorable contexts (Zeig, 1980).

The ability of metaphors, or anecdotes, to impart perspective and build an identification has been well described in the literature (G. Burns, 2001, 2005; Lankton & Lankton, 1989). In the early stages of treatment, when facilitating flexibility is considered a preliminary goal preceding interventions more specifically focused on the patient's individual issues, metaphors may be used to build a momentum of acceptance for ideas and tactics relating to developing flexibility and believing in the inevitability of change. Such metaphors may involve either universal life transitions (e.g., outgrowing childhood fears, learning to manage one's money) or transitions unique to the particular patient, taken directly from his or her own personal history (e.g., having moved from one city to another, having graduated from college). The general goal of facilitating flexibility is one that continues throughout the therapy, with the clinician continually imparting the message that change is possible and that it will always be necessary to develop new responses when old ones no longer achieve the desired effect.

CLINICAL MATERIAL

The use of hypnosis to facilitate experiential learning and to build new adaptive associations can be a powerful aspect of the therapy. In addition to the use of hypnosis in the therapist's office, teaching self-hypnosis and encouraging learning in real-life contexts with experimental behaviors given by the therapist as behavioral task assignments (i.e., "homework") to complete in-between therapy sessions are also considered fundamental to the treatment of depression. There is substantial evidence that when therapists provide structured homework assignments to assist patients in developing salient skills, both the rate and quality of improvement is substantially enhanced (D. Burns & Spangler, 2000). Hypnotic interventions in particular are described in this section as they were used in the treatment of a depressed patient named Roland.

Roland was a 65-year-old man presenting with an incapacitating episode of major depression. He reported sleep disturbance, constant anxiety, negative ruminations, social withdrawal, and continuous feelings of sadness. Roland was on disability at the time I first saw him, unable to continue in his work as a city project engineer. The current depressive episode had its onset 4 months earlier, near the time that he had had surgery for a hernia. Prior to the surgery, Roland had experienced a considerable amount of pain, which he catastrophized and interpreted as evidence that he had cancer. The unequivocal diagnosis of having only a hernia and no cancer provided little relief for Roland who by now had convinced himself that he was "officially old." He was sure the hernia was just the first step on the road of inevitably deteriorating health. Roland began to ruminate constantly about ill health, interpreting every physical sensation as concrete evidence of something being terribly wrong with him. Roland reported that his depression was intense, immobilizing, and incurable, because he "knew" he was old and deteriorating, and no one could do anything about that. He stated in absolute terms his debilitating view that his life was "essentially over," with nothing to look forward to other than continuous deterioration and eventual death. At the time of the hernia surgery, Roland had only 6 weeks to work to reach retirement and attain his retirement benefits. Unless he could return to work and complete those 6 weeks, he would lose his retirement pension. He felt unable to return to work, even for only 6 weeks, and he could not foresee that changing, although he agreed going back to work was a highly desirable goal.

Roland was married to a loving, supportive woman who was seen in one joint session early in the treatment process. He had been seen previously for treatment by two psychotherapists: a psychiatrist who simply prescribed antidepressant medications, to which Rowland did not respond well, and a supportive psychologist, who encouraged him to ventilate his feelings of anger at losing his youth. Roland felt that this latter treatment depressed him even more and soon discontinued that therapy. A friend of his, who was also a therapist, referred him to me. Roland's physical health was deemed well above average for his age and posed no significant limits on what he was physically able to do.

It was immediately clear that Roland's highly intellectual and analytical demeanor was lending itself to the uncontestable ruminations about aging and deteriorating. It was also apparent that Roland expected nothing positive from his imminent retirement and, in fact, had made no plans at all for it. Although, for many individuals, spontaneity is a good thing, Roland's life was a highly structured, duty-bound one. His lack of a plan for retirement, and his lack of a sense of purpose beyond his work, combined with his negative expectations for his health, all served to amplify his depression. They represented appropriate targets for therapeutic interventions using hypnosis.

The goals of Roland's therapy included the following:

1. Facilitating a positive future orientation (i.e., a positive expectancy regarding the future).
2. Facilitating an unstable attributional style relative to personal circumstances.
3. Facilitating a flexible and generative approach to daily living (i.e., expanding his narrow repertoire of activities and finding enjoyable things in which to become involved).
4. Facilitating a positive relationship with his body to interrupt the emerging hypochondriacal one.
5. Facilitating a greater sense of personal value from activities other than work.

Roland was seen for a total of 13 sessions; 10 of these were concentrated over the first 4.5 months of treatment, and the remaining were conducted over the next 3 months. Hypnosis was used formally in 9 of the 13 sessions. Each of the hypnosis sessions was audiotaped, and the tapes were given to Roland to permit him to reinforce the relevant learning as often as he wished. The hypnosis sessions each addressed either the theme of that particular session's content (i.e., something of immediate concern that week) or a goal consistent with the larger aims of treatment (e.g., encouraging flexibility in adapting to his impending retirement). The hypnosis sessions are described as follows.

In the first session, hypnosis was used to promote a general relaxation, both physically and mentally. A key suggestion in that first session was, "There are worthwhile experiences you are capable of having that are beyond logic or rationality." A goal of this session was to promote in Roland a recognition that the things that would make a difference for him were things beyond those he already knew and that although his view of himself and his world was limited to only what he knew currently, that was not all there was. This helped to destabilize his stable attributions about himself and his world while encouraging a legitimate basis for hopefulness. Also, by focusing on physical sensations associated with the hypnosis that were defined as comfortable and pleasant, the idea was seeded that he could begin to experience his body in a more positive manner.

In the next hypnosis session, an idea was elaborated that had been the focus of the previous session, namely that Roland could not fully control his own destiny, that some things were uncontrollable and could be comfortably accepted as such (e.g., the weather, the seasons, the phases of life). This hypnosis session therapeutically reframed his negative focus on aging as a futile attempt to control the uncontrollable. He was given the homework assignment to carry out in-between sessions to try and control the uncontrollable (e.g., try and make it rain, try and make the sun rise in the middle of the night). Roland quickly grasped the concept that no amount of effort could make one younger, so the goal of living each day doing what you can came into clearer focus. These ideas were further developed in the third therapy session. Following this session, Roland went back to work on a half-time basis to begin his final 6 weeks. He was working full-time again within 2 weeks.

Self-exploration was encouraged in the next hypnosis session as a way of discovering what he enjoyed independently of others' expectations or their demands of him. Roland was encouraged to consider as examples people with public personas who, on a personal level, were not as they seemed to be. Roland was thereby indirectly encouraged to recognize that he did not have to live up to an arbitrary image. A metaphor for encouraging exploration at a deeper level was provided by describing swimmers and surfers who had only a surface view of the ocean (a metaphor chosen because

Roland enjoys boating in his native San Diego) in contrast to divers who submerge themselves in the deep ocean and are thereby afforded a "deeper view." This session paved the way for Roland to eventually learn to respond to deeper personal preferences and interests. It was not that Roland had no interests beyond work, it was that he rarely allowed himself to pursue them. There were always other things to do that he felt needed to be done, and simply doing things he wanted to do seemed unacceptably self-indulgent to him. Following this fourth session, Roland signed up for a course in philosophy at a local university and also began taking regular walks on the beach.

In the subsequent hypnosis sessions, the focus was on reinforcing the changes beginning to take place that Roland was aware of, particularly physical ones. Roland reported a marked improvement in his sleep and attributed this to the self-hypnosis procedure he was taught, which he described as "a more satisfying process than just counting sheep." The hypnosis focused on the many physical sensations he was capable of experiencing that were pleasant (e.g., "the loving touch of your wife; the feel of your bed supporting you as you lay in it at night; the soothing sensations of a hot shower"). The goal was to redefine physical sensations as comfortable, not suspect. Sensations described in hypnosis went from external ones to internal ones (e.g., "the feeling of stretching your muscles, the feeling of pleasant hunger that precedes a wonderful meal, the comfort of being tired before a good night's sleep"). This redefinition of physical sensations took place in the seventh session directly following the previous few session's focus on developing more varied interests. In addition, Roland was encouraged to do at least one spontaneous thing each day. He consistently chose to approach strangers in contexts appropriate for engaging them in "small talk." He enjoyed discovering he still had his sense of humor through these interactions.

In the next hypnosis session, which took place in the ninth therapy session, Roland was encouraged to associate retirement with feeling free to pursue personal interests that previously may have seemed too tangential or even trivial. I provided examples of things to absorb his interest but then immediately and deliberately discounted them as trivial. Roland's response was to emerge from the hypnosis session with an irritated statement that my judgments about the trivialities of peoples' hobbies seemed questionable to him because, he stated emphatically, "all that really mattered was that they enjoyed them." Roland then actively defended being able to do as one wished, regardless of another person's judgment. This was important because it established the subjective worth of things that are not explicitly purposeful or meaningful, which Roland had clearly internalized. It was also important because Roland could establish a boundary, defining his interests as legitimate even if someone such as me could question them.

In the next hypnosis session, Roland was encouraged to review all of the changes he had experienced since beginning therapy: His sleep had normalized, he had returned to work and completed his 6 weeks and then formally retired, he had enrolled in and enjoyed a philosophy course, he had established a regular walking and exercise program, he had established enjoyable social contacts with others, he had developed greater spontaneity, and he focused on things he could do and make happen proactively, rather on those he could not do anything about. The major skills acquired through therapy were summarized, and posthypnotic suggestions for retrieving these skills as wanted or needed in the appropriate contexts were provided. This took place in the 10th session. The subsequent hypnosis sessions each reinforced Roland's progress and emphasized remaining more flexible and responsive to balancing his internal needs with external realities. After three monthly follow-up sessions, therapy was terminated. A 1-year follow-up personal interview was conducted to establish that the therapeutic gains had been maintained, which they were.

The emphasis in this case was on how hypnosis sessions were distributed and conducted throughout a complete therapy to illustrate the use of hypnosis in treating depression. Hypnosis was used as a tool to consolidate important skills and establish new and beneficial associations in the patient. Each of the goals of therapy was met by addressing Roland's concerns through a focus on the associated patterns maintaining his symptoms. Hypnosis played a significant role in mobilizing Roland's resources in the direction of positive and lasting change.

Two cornerstones of depression are hopelessness and helplessness. Roland had convinced himself that his future contained little more than progressive deterioration. His selective focus on such a negative expectation drained any motivation to try to go beyond his difficulties. To catalyze successful outcomes, it is essential to facilitate a motivating and compelling vision of the future in treatment. Research clearly indicates that expectancy plays a key role at every stage of treatment (Scott & Watkins, 2004).

Hypnosis by itself is not the curative agent in any therapy. Rather, it is the ability of hypnosis to stimulate the patient's subjective associations on cognitive, affective, and behavioral dimensions of experience. Thus, hypnosis can be used to correct cognitive distortions or suggest a change in behavior. In Roland's case, his distorted belief (i.e., overgeneralization) that a transient episode of pain related to a hernia was the harbinger of disasters to come was a primary focus of treatment. Specifically, the first two sessions encouraged him to adopt the view of negative circumstances as transient, not permanent, and as evidence of a specific, not a global, problem. This served to build hopefulness and a willingness to participate in the treatment process. Thus, hypnosis was used to facilitate the correction of an error in his thinking.

It bears repeating that I do not generally view hypnosis as the therapeutic agent in successful treatments but rather as a catalyst for communicating therapeutic ideas or facilitating therapeutic experiences on an experiential level. The case of Roland highlights the use of hypnosis and directives in the active treatment of patterns of depression.

RESEARCH AND APPRAISAL

The unfounded and obsolete views regarding hypnosis as contraindicated for treating depression have effectively delayed its systematic study (for a detailed discussion of this issue, see Yapko, 1992, 2006). Thus, meaningful relevant research is sparse at best. However, there is research that indicates that hypnotized persons may have easier access to more intense emotions (Barabasz & Watkins, 2005; Nash, 1992), and there is evidence that hypnosis empowers people and enhances treatment in general (Lynn et al., 2000). As mentioned previously, only one recent study (Alladin & Alibhai, 2007) has provided an empirical basis for supporting the use of hypnosis in treating patients who are depressed. Before any substantive research can be done, two important factors need to be taken into account. First, because hypnosis is not a therapy, it can be used as a tool only within the context of some greater structured therapeutic approach. How will the effects of hypnosis in particular be evaluated in relation to the therapy in general? Second, clinicians can distinguish formal hypnotic procedures from the informal use of hypnotic suggestive patterns. How will psychotherapists determine which aspects of hypnosis are the central elements of a meaningful therapeutic intervention?

If one uses a broader definition of *hypnosis* that encompasses the patterns of influential communication evident in any psychotherapy, the necessity of defining indefinable hypnotic experiences diminishes. The use of hypnosis to present important ideas and to structure important experiential learning can be better studied when *hypnosis* is not so narrowly defined as to be limited to a specific type of procedure. However, such a broad definition makes research considerably more difficult.

Despite these difficulties, research investigating the use of hypnosis on patients with depression clearly needs to be done if there is to be any legitimate basis for continuing to encourage its use with such a clinical population. There are at least two possible avenues of research: (a) investigating whether therapies using formal hypnosis sessions to teach specific skills or ideas show better results (e.g., more rapid symptom relief, less relapse) than the same therapies conducted without the use of formal hypnosis and (b) investigating whether therapies using hypnotic communication patterns (e.g., therapeutic metaphors, reframings, paradoxes) in the therapy to teach specific skills or ideas show better results than the same therapies conducted without such methods.

Only the most obvious and standardized of hypnotic methods will be researchable. The subtleties of nuance, nonverbal delivery, implication, and so forth, will likely always evade more objective scrutiny. However, the positive value of substantive research cannot be ignored, because such research holds the key to a more widespread acceptance and use of hypnosis in the treatment of depression.

CONCLUSION

With society's increasing emphasis on individualism, materialism, technology, speed, and other such sociocultural phenomena, it is clear that the prevalence of depression is also increasing, just as the World Health Organization predicted. The role of the therapist is to focus on the patterns with which an individual has been socialized, identifying how those patterns create, maintain, or put the individual at risk of depression. The therapy process is one of pattern interruption and pattern building, differing from one treatment to the next only in the content of the patterns that are addressed and in the choice of therapy model applied to address them. Such an approach strives to expand strengths rather than just reduce pathology. More than a semantic issue, whether one focuses on amplifying the positive or diminishing the negative has profound implications for the ways one will conduct therapy in general and use hypnosis in particular.

There are a number of useful frameworks for conducting therapy with patients with depression. The cognitive and interpersonal approaches in particular have demonstrated their efficacy and are thus often seen as strong allies of hypnosis. There are many excellent reasons to use hypnosis in the treatment of patients with depression, some of which include the following:

- Hypnosis facilitates active and experiential learning.
- Hypnosis catalyzes more rapid integration of relevant learning.
- Hypnosis establishes therapeutic associations in a more focused and concentrated way.
- Hypnosis interrupts one's usual experience of one's self, enhancing an unstable attributional style.
- Hypnosis models flexibility by encouraging experiences beyond one's usual self-limiting parameters.

New understandings of both depression and hypnosis afford therapists the opportunity to approach the treatment of patients with depression in a much more comprehensive way than ever before. Depression is a highly treatable disorder with a high rate of recovery, and a therapist who is skilled in the use of hypnosis can play a powerful role not only in the recovery process but in the prevention of relapses as well.

REFERENCES

Alladin, A. (2006). Experiential cognitive hypnotherapy: Strategies for relapse prevention in depression. In M. Yapko (Ed.), *Hypnosis and treating depression: Applications in clinical practice* (pp. 281–313). New York: Routledge.

Alladin, A., & Alibhai, A. (2007). Cognitive hypnotherapy for depression: An empirical investigation. *International Journal of Clinical and Experimental Hypnosis, 55,* 147–166.

American Psychological Association, Division of Psychological Hypnosis. (1999). *Policy and procedures manual, 4–5.* Washington, DC: Author.

Antonuccio, D., Danton, W., & DeNelsky, G. (1995). Psychotherapy versus medication for depression: Challenging the conventional wisdom with data. *Professional Psychology: Research and Practice, 26,* 574–585.

Barabasz, A., & Watkins, J. (2005). *Hypnotherapeutic techniques* (2nd ed.). New York: Brunner-Routledge.

Beach, S., Sandeen, E., & O'Leary, K. (1990). *Depression in marriage.* New York: Guilford Press.

Beck, A. (1997). Cognitive therapy: Reflections. In J. Zeig (Ed.), *The evolution of psychotherapy: The third conference* (pp. 55–64). New York: Brunner/Mazel.

Beck, A., Rush, A., Shaw, B., & Emery, G. (1979). *Cognitive therapy of depression.* New York: Guilford Press.

Breggin, P. (1999). *Reclaiming our children: A healing plan for a nation in crisis.* Cambridge, MA: Perseus Publishing.

Burns, D. (1999a). *Feeling good: The new mood therapy* (Rev. ed.). New York: Avon Books.

Burns, D. (1999b). *The feeling good handbook* (Rev. edition). New York: Plume.

Burns, D., & Spangler, D. (2000). Does psychotherapy homework lead to changes in depression in cognitive behavioral therapy? Or does clinical improvement lead to homework compliance? *Journal of Consulting and Clinical Psychology, 68,* 46–56.

Burns, G. (2001). *101 healing stories: Using metaphors in therapy.* New York: Wiley.

Burns, G. (2005). *101 healing stories for kids and teens.* New York: Wiley.

Gandhi, T., Weingart, S., Borus, J., Seger, A., Peterson, J., Burdick, et al. (2003). Adverse drug events in ambulatory care. *The New England Journal of Medicine, 348,* 1556–1564.

Goodman, S. H., & Gotlib, I. H. (Eds.). (2002). *Children of depressed parents: Mechanisms of risk and implications for treatment*. Washington, DC: American Psychological Association.

Hammen, C. (1999). The emergence of an interpersonal approach to depression. In T. Joiner & J. Coyne (Eds.), *The interactional nature of depression: Advances in interpersonal approaches* (pp. 21–35). Washington, DC: American Psychological Association.

Hammen, C. (2002). Context of stress in families of children with depressed parents. In Goodman, S. H. & Gotlib, I. H. (Eds.), *Children of depressed parents: Mechanisms of risk and implications for treatment* (pp. 175–199). Washington, DC: American Psychological Association.

Jacobson, N., & Gortner, E. (2000). Can depression be demedicalized in the 21st century: Scientific revolutions, counterrevolutions, and the magnetic field of normal science. *Behavior Research and Therapy, 38*, 103–117.

Joiner, T., & Coyne, J. (Eds.). (1999). *The interactional nature of depression: Advances in interpersonal approaches*. Washington, DC: American Psychological Association.

Joiner, T., Coyne, J., & Blalock, J. (1999). On the interpersonal nature of depression: Overview and synthesis. In T. Joiner & J. Coyne (Eds.), *The interactional nature of depression: Advances in interpersonal approaches* (pp. 3–19). Washington, DC: American Psychological Association.

Just, N., & Alloy, L. (1997). The response styles theory of depression: Tests and an extension of the theory. *Journal of Abnormal Psychology, 106*, 221–229.

Kaelber, C., Moul, D., & Farmer, M. (1995). Epidemiology of depression. In E. Beckham & W. Leber (Eds.), *Handbook of depression* (pp. 3–35). New York: Guilford Press.

Kirsch, I. (1990). *Changing expectations: A key to effective psychotherapy*. Pacific Grove, CA: Brooks/Cole.

Kirsch, I., Deacon, B. J., Huedo-Medina, T. B., Scoboria, A., Moore, T. J., & Johnson, B. T. (2008, February). Initial severity and antidepressant benefits: A meta-analysis of data submitted to the Food and Drug Administration. *PLoS Medicine, 5*(2). Retrieved February 26, 2008, from http://www.plosmedicine.org/article/info:doi/10.1371/journal.pmed.0050045

Kirsch, I., & Sapirstein, G. (1999). Listening to Prozac but hearing placebo: A meta-analysis of antidepressant medication. In I. Kirsch (Ed.), *How expectancies shape experience* (pp. 303–320). Washington, DC: American Psychological Association.

Klerman, G., Weissman, M., Rounsaville, B., & Chevron, E. (1984). *Interpersonal psychotherapy of depression*. New York: Basic Books.

Kravitz, R., Epstein, R., Feldman, M., Franz, C., Azari, R., Wilkes, M., et al. (2005). Influence of patients' requests for direct-to-consumer advertised antidepressants: A randomized trial. *JAMA, 293*, 1995–2002.

Lankton, S., & Lankton, C. (1983). *The answer within: A clinical framework of Ericksonian hypnotherapy*. New York: Brunner/Mazel.

Lankton, S., & Lankton, C. (1989). *Tales of enchantment: Goal-oriented metaphors for adults and children in therapy*. New York: Brunner/Mazel.

Library of Congress and the National Institute of Mental Health. (2000). *Project on the Decade of the Brain*. Retrieved October 21, 2008 from http://www.loc.gov/loc/brain/

Lynn, S., Kirsch, I., Barabasz, A., Cardeña, E., & Patterson, D. (2000). Hypnosis as an empirically supported clinical intervention: The state of the evidence and a look to the future. *International Journal of Clinical and Experimental Hypnosis, 48*, 239–259.

March, S., Silva, S., Petrycki, S., Curry, J., Wells, K., Fairbank, J., et al. (2004). Fluoxetine, cognitive–behavioral therapy, and their combination for adolescents with depression. *JAMA, 292*, 807–820.

Murray, C., & Lopez, A. (1997, May 17). Global mortality, disability, and the contribution of risk factors: Global burden of disease study. *The Lancet, 349*, 1436–1442.

Nash, M. (1992). Hypnosis, psychopathology, and psychological regression. In E. Fromm & M. Nash (Eds.), *Contemporary hypnosis research* (pp. 149–172). New York: Guilford Press.

NewsRX.com. (2000, July 5). Survey finds 103 medicines in development for mental illnesses. *Drug Week*. Retrieved August 12, 2002, from http://www.psycport.com/2000/07/05/eng-newsrx/eng-newsrx_101417_137_708142497577.html

O'Connor, R. (1997). *Undoing depression: What therapy doesn't teach you and medication can't give you*. Boston: Little, Brown.

O'Connor, R. (2001). *Active treatment of depression*. New York: Norton.

O'Leary, K., Christian, J., & Mendel, N. (1993). A closer look at the link between marital discord and depressive symptomatology. *Journal of Social and Clinical Psychology, 13*, 31–41.

Rushton, J., Clark, S., & Freed, G. (2000, June). Pediatrician and family physician prescription of selective serotonin reuptake inhibitors. *Pediatrics, 105*, e82. Retrieved June 30, 2000, from http://pediatrics.aappublications.org/cgi/content/full/105/6/e82

Scott, J. (2000). Treatment of chronic depression. *The New England Journal of Medicine, 342*, 1518–1520.

Scott, J., & Watkins, E. (2004). Brief psychotherapies for depression: Current status. *Current Opinion in Psychiatry, 17*, 3–7.

Seligman, M. (1989). Explanatory style: Predicting depression, achievement, and health. In M. Yapko (Ed.), *Brief therapy approaches to treating anxiety and depression* (pp. 5–32). New York: Brunner/Mazel.

Seligman, M. (1990). *Learned optimism*. New York: Alfred Knopf.

Seligman, M. (1995). *The optimistic child: How learned optimism protects children from depression.* New York: Houghton-Mifflin.

Seligman, M. (2002). *Authentic happiness: Using the new positive psychology to realize your potential for lasting fulfillment.* New York: Free Press.

Seligman, M., & Csikszentmihalyi, M. (2000). Positive psychology: An introduction. *American Psychologist, 55,* 5–14.

Silberg, J., & Rutter, M. (2002). Nature–nurture interplay in the risks associated with parental depression. In S. H. Goodman & I. H. Gotlib (Eds.), *Children of depressed parents: Mechanisms of risk and implications for treatment* (pp. 13–36). Washington, DC: American Psychological Association.

Thase, M., Greenhouse, J., Frank, E., Reynolds, C., Pilkonis, P., Hurley, K., et al. (1997). Treatment of major depression with psychotherapy psychotherapy–pharmacotherapy combinations. *Archives of General Psychiatry, 54,* 1009–1015.

Turner, E. H., Matthews, A. M., Linardatos, E., Tell, R. A., & Rosenthal, R. (2008). Selective publication of antidepressant trials and its influence on apparent efficacy. *The New England Journal of Medicine, 358,* 252–260.

U.S. Food and Drug Administration. (2009). *Antidepressant use in children, adolescents, and adults.* Retrieved August 10, 2009, from http://www.fda.gov/Drugs/DrugSafety/InformationDrugClass/UCM096273

Weissman, M., Bland, R., Canino, G., Faravelli, C., Greenwald, S., Hwu, H.-G., et al. (1996). Cross-national epidemiology of major depression and bipolar disorder. *JAMA, 276,* 293–299.

Yapko, M. (1992). *Hypnosis and the treatment of depressions: Strategies for change.* New York: Brunner/Mazel.

Yapko, M. (1996). Depression: Perspectives and treatments. In *Encyclopædia Britannica: 1997 Medical and Health Annual* (pp. 287–291). Chicago: Encyclopædia Britannica.

Yapko, M. (1997). *Breaking the patterns of depression.* New York: Random House/Doubleday.

Yapko, M. (1999). *Hand-me-down blues: How to stop depression from spreading in families.* New York: St. Martin's Griffin.

Yapko, M. (2001). *Treating depression with hypnosis: Integrating cognitive–behavioral and strategic approaches.* New York: Brunner-Routledge.

Yapko, M. (2003). *Trancework: An introduction to the practice of clinical hypnosis* (3rd ed.). New York: Brunner-Routledge.

Yapko, M. (Ed.). (2006). *Hypnosis and treating depression: Applications in clinical practice.* New York: Routledge.

Zeig, J. (1980). *A teaching seminar with Milton H. Erickson, M.D.* New York: Brunner/Mazel.

16

HYPNOSIS IN THE TREATMENT OF POSTTRAUMATIC STRESS DISORDERS

DAVID SPIEGEL

Hypnosis has been used in the treatment of those who have undergone traumatic experiences for more than 150 years. Early uses involved hypnotic analgesia to help patients through traumatic surgical procedures before the advent of inhalation anesthesia (Esdaile, 1846). Freud began his exploration of the unconscious through the use of hypnosis at a time when he conceptualized and treated hysterical reactions as the aftermath of traumatic experiences in childhood (Breuer & Freud, 1893/1995). More recently, hypnotic techniques were used during World War II to treat what were then called "traumatic neuroses." Despite the growing acceptance of psychoanalysis as a model for psychotherapy in that era, hypnotic techniques were found to be efficient and effective in helping soldiers with acute combat reactions to work through, control, or put aside the effects of traumatic experiences (Kardiner & Spiegel, 1947). With the substantial growth in the recognition of posttraumatic stress disorder (PTSD; American Psychiatric Association, 2000) as a diagnosis has come an increased interest in hypnosis as a tool in psychotherapy.

In this chapter, I outline some of the reasons for this parallel growth and some reasons for the utility of hypnosis in the psychotherapy of PTSD. In

All clinical material has been disguised to protect patient confidentiality.

doing so, I describe dissociation as playing a role during and after traumatic stress that is both adaptive and problematic, helping survivors get through life-threatening situations but delaying or altering their ability to work through and put into perspective their traumatic experiences. I describe hypnosis as a kind of controlled dissociation that can be used to facilitate the processing of traumatic memories, assisting in the management of emotional and somatic reactions to trauma and providing a therapeutic framework for reexperiencing and working through its psychological, psychosomatic, and interpersonal aftermath.

TRAUMA

Trauma is a sudden discontinuity in physical experience that elicits similar discontinuities in mental experience. Most trauma victims report a sharp contrast between their mental states just prior to the trauma (e.g., "I was driving to the airport, and I was so excited about the trip") and during and after it (e.g., "Suddenly this man was in my car with a gun. I couldn't do anything. I can't get him out of my mind. Nothing is the same anymore. I can't enjoy anything"). A more classically dissociative example is that of a young man who was struck by a drunken motorcyclist on the highway and who sustained severe injuries to both legs, which eventually necessitated an amputation. As he lay on the highway in tremendous pain, friends were urging him to get off the road so he would not be hit again. He found himself thinking about a fishing trip with his father at a mountain lake, walked off the road, and felt no pain until several hours later at the emergency room. Such abrupt shifts in mental state may be adaptive and serve the defensive purpose of separating a person from the full impact of the physical trauma as it is occurring. This adaptive defense may help distance individuals from pain and overwhelming fear. It may also work too well in helping people from consciously working through traumatic memories because they remain largely out of awareness.

There is much that is spontaneously dissociative in the nature of the acute response to trauma. This has been recognized in the emphasis on dissociative features in the diagnosis of acute stress disorder, including numbing, depersonalization, derealization, being in a "daze," and dissociative amnesia (American Psychiatric Association, 2000). Furthermore, there are a substantial number of dissociative features in the symptoms of PTSD, especially numbing and amnesia. A neural pathway linking frontal lobe activity to inhibition of the hippocampus has been identified in an experimental model that provides a mechanism for understanding dissociative amnesia (Anderson et al., 2004). This means that hypnosis, a state of artificially induced dissociation (Nemiah, 1985; H. Spiegel & Spiegel, 2004), may be especially relevant and useful in accessing memories of trauma and in helping patients to work them through as part of the treatment of PTSD.

DISSOCIATION DURING TRAUMA

There is evidence that many people dissociate during traumatic experiences (D. Spiegel & Cardeña, 1991). For example, it is not uncommon for rape victims to feel as though they were floating above their body and feeling sorry for the woman being attacked. One young woman who accidentally fell from a third-story balcony described her experience of the event as follows.

> It was as if I was standing on another balcony watching a pink cloud float down to the ground. I felt no pain at all and tried to walk back upstairs. It turned out that I had suffered a broken pelvis.

It is also not uncommon for athletes who have sustained serious injuries during a game to become aware of them only after the game is over, and a study of the responses to the Loma Prieta earthquake provides evidence that two-thirds of a sample of normal students experienced some kind of dissociative symptom (e.g., distortion, unusually intense memories, dissociative amnesia, depersonalization, derealization) in the immediate aftermath of the earthquake (Cardeña & Spiegel, 1993).

The relevance of dissociation to trauma was illustrated longitudinally by J. R. Hilgard (1970), who observed that highly hypnotizable students reported a history of more physical punishment in childhood than did their less hypnotizable peers. Several studies have also shown that psychiatric patients with a history of sexual and physical abuse in childhood scored high on measures of dissociation (Herman, Perry, van der Kolk, 1989).

The diagnosis of PTSD is associated with high hypnotizability (D. Spiegel, Hunt, & Dondershine, 1988; Stutman & Bliss, 1985). Indeed, dissociative disorders have come to be reconceptualized as chronic PTSD secondary to physical and sexual abuse in childhood (Frischholz, 1985; Kluft, 1988; D. Spiegel, 1984). A girl who was a repeated victim of incest by her father used to focus all of her attention on her hand rather than other parts of her body during the sexual assaults. Another patient took herself to an imaginary field full of wildflowers as a way of distancing herself from paternal beatings and sexual abuse. In this sense, dissociation, the disintegration of experience and memory, served as an adaptive defensive function against trauma while it was occurring. This defense, however, can increase the difficulty of integrating and working through these memories subsequent to the trauma. If the traumatic experiences are too easily kept out of consciousness, necessary corrective grief work may be postponed or avoided. For example, it is common for trauma victims to blame themselves inappropriately for events that they could not have foreseen or controlled. This occurs both because people conceptualize true randomness with difficulty and because inappropriately blaming oneself for trauma may be less painful than fully accepting one's complete helplessness at the hands of an attacker or in a natural disaster. Conscious, painful attention to traumatic memories in their aftermath can help to correct these frequent distortions, which may predispose one to the development of PTSD symptoms.

From this viewpoint, trauma can be conceptualized as the experience of being made into an object, devoid of any sense of control. It is indeed helplessness that is the core painful experience defended against by trauma victims. Defenses, such as separating oneself from one's body, are useful in creating a sense of distance from physical helplessness. Psychological control is maintained when physical control is lost. Ironically, in the individuals who develop PTSD, psychological control is lost when physical control returns. These patients now feel victimized by an intrusive reliving of the traumatic event. When the traumatic memory recurs, it often does so in the present tense. Not only is the memory more intense, but the uncertainty of the outcome, the fear of dying, and the fear of being helpless at the hands of the victimizer or force of nature is relived with all of its original intensity. The memory may be kept out of conscious awareness, and dissociative amnesia may develop. However, the message of this amnesia is that the memory is too horrible to be allowed into consciousness and the emotions associated with it are too painful. Indeed, there is an analogy between the major components of hypnosis and the major symptoms of PTSD.

One important component of hypnosis is *dissociation*, which is the compartmentalization of components of experience (H. Spiegel & Cardeña, 1991; H. Spiegel & Spiegel, 2004). Dissociation is a mechanism that is associated with the diminished responsiveness and loss of pleasure in usually pleasurable activities that typifies PTSD (American Psychiatric Association, 2000). Patients with PTSD dissociate content from affect, often demonstrating demoralization without conscious recollection of the details. Thus, a female rape victim with dissociative amnesia for the rape may find herself unable to tolerate any sexual contact with a loving partner, treating him as though he were the assailant.

A second important component of hypnosis is *absorption* (Tellegen & Atkinson, 1974). This is a narrowing of the focus of attention at the expense of peripheral awareness (e.g., getting so lost in a good movie or novel that one enters the imagined world and loses awareness of the surroundings in which the story occurs). This absorption in an event is reminiscent of some of the intrusive reliving of traumatic experiences that individuals with PTSD undergo. They may spontaneously relive the trauma as though it were occurring again in the present tense, dissociating awareness that they did indeed survive the trauma, which is analogous to hypnotic age regression (D. Spiegel, 1986). Thus, they experience it with great emotional intensity and without the comforting recognition that they lived through the event.

A third important component of hypnosis is *suggestibility*, which is a heightened responsiveness to social cues and an exaggerated willingness to uncritically accept social input (Cardeña & Spiegel, 1991). This is similar to the stimulus sensitivity typical of individuals with PTSD. A female rape victim may avoid passing near anything that reminds her of the setting in which the rape occurred (e.g., any elevator or park). Thus, there is much about trauma that seems to elicit spontaneous dissociative processes. Therefore, it is logical that hypnosis should be an especially valuable tool in treatment.

Alterations in consciousness, memory (including amnesia), and identity can occur in both hypnosis and dissociation (H. Spiegel & Spiegel, 2004). Dissociative amnesia is indeed a diagnostic criterion of both acute stress disorder and posttraumatic stress disorder (American Psychiatric Association, 2000). A key difference between hypnosis and dissociation is the controlled and focused aspect of hypnosis, in contrast to the often unbidden and uncontrolled nature of dissociative symptoms. Hypnosis generally involves an induction ceremony, either self-administered or initiated by a clinician, whereas dissociative symptoms occur spontaneously and may be experienced as a loss of control, with amnesia and disorientation (Barrett, 1992).

CLINICAL APPLICATIONS

Because hypnosis is a form of structured and controlled dissociation, there is reason to think that many trauma survivors enter hypnotic-like states during and immediately after trauma. Therefore, on the basis of state dependent memory theory (Bower, 1981), it makes sense that psychotherapy using hypnosis would be especially able to facilitate access to congruent mental states and memories and consequently would be helpful in working through the aftermath of trauma. The fundamental principles of the use of hypnosis in the treatment of PTSD involve inducing controlled access to traumatic memories and helping patients to control the intense affect and strong physiological responses that may accompany memories of trauma while restructuring them. Hypnotic concentration can be applied to help patients work through and grieve aspects of the traumatic experience and place the memories into a new perspective, a form of cognitive restructuring.

The psychotherapy of trauma can be understood as an adaptation of the traditional psychoanalytic principle of remembering, repeating, and working through (Freud, 1914). It is necessary to bring into consciousness memories of the traumatic experience, repeat some of the affective and interpersonal quality of the experience, and then work through the material, putting it into a new perspective that makes it less overwhelming and likely to produce symptoms. Another way to conceptualize this is a form of grief work (Lindemann, 1994). Facing the reality of a traumatic experience means grieving certain fantasies of invulnerability and images of the self. Patients who have traumatic reminiscences often experience themselves as degraded and humiliated by the traumatic experience and as being a parody of their former self, carrying on a kind of almost normal existence in which they pretend that the trauma did not occur. The goal is a redefinition of self that acknowledges the reality of the traumatic experience but puts it into perspective and makes it less damaging to the total view of self. Hypnosis is an effective context within which to perform this psychotherapeutic grief work.

One especially useful way of introducing hypnosis into the therapy is through the use of a clinical hypnotizability scale, such as the Hypnotic Induction Profile (HIP; H. Spiegel & Spiegel, 2004) or the Stanford Hypnotic Clinical Scale (E. R. Hilgard & Hilgard, 1975). This form of initial hypnotic induction has several advantages:

1. It provides useful information about the patient's degree of hypnotizability, which is a stable and measurable trait (E. R. Hilgard, 1965; Orne et al., 1979; H. Spiegel & Spiegel, 2004). About 1 in 5 psychiatric outpatients are not hypnotizable, and 1 in 10 are extremely responsive (H. Spiegel & Spiegel, 2004). Patients' performance on a hypnotizability test provides either a tangible demonstration of their hypnotic ability, which is a good starting point for therapy and is often surprising to patients, or it demonstrates that hypnosis is unlikely to be useful. Furthermore, evidence is discussed in the Research and Appraisal section of this chapter showing that patients with PTSD are, as a group, highly hypnotizable. The testing can thus be useful in differential diagnosis as well. Hypnotizability testing provides, with little waste of time, an opportunity to select alternative facilitators of treatment. Thus, the hypnotic induction can be turned into a rational deduction about the patient's resources for change (H. Spiegel & Spiegel, 1980).

2. The atmosphere of testing enhances the treatment alliance and defuses anxieties about loss of control. The therapist's responsibility is to provide a clinically appropriate setting and instructions for the systematic exploration of the patient's hypnotic capacity. This is not a power struggle in which the therapist tries to "get the patient into a trance" and the patient succumbs

or resists. The therapist is interested in finding out the results of the test, not in proving how successful he or she is at hypnotizing a patient. Thus, the atmosphere becomes something of a Socratic dialogue, in which both discover what the patient already "knows" (i.e., hypnotic capacity) but about which there is little conscious awareness. The hypnotic state can be used as a means of providing a sense of physical comfort and safety that is dissociated from memories of events in which the physical environment was much different.

It is also useful to teach patients from the beginning to enter the state of hypnosis as a state of self-hypnosis so that they feel in control of the transition to this altered mental state. The instructions can be simple:

> All hypnosis is really self-hypnosis. Now that we have demonstrated that you have a good capacity to use hypnosis, let me show you how to use it to work on a problem. While there are many ways to enter a state of self-hypnosis, one simple means is to count from one to three. On "one," do one thing: Look up. On "two," do two things: Slowly close your eyes and take a deep breath. On "three," do three things: Let the breath out, let your eyes relax but keep them closed, and let your body float. Then, let one hand or the other float up in the air like a balloon, and that will be your signal to yourself and to me that you are ready to concentrate. (H. Spiegel & Spiegel, 2004, pp. 87–89)

Once in a state of self-hypnosis, patients can be taught to produce a physical sensation of floating, lightness, or buoyancy. Having them initially imagine that they are somewhere safe and comfortable, such as floating in a bath, a lake, a hot tub, or space, can reinforce their sense of physical comfort. This enhances their sense of control over their body, which is critical when reliving memories of bodily discomfort and damage. Once they have established this physical sense of comfort, they can be told to maintain this state regardless of what other images or thoughts come to them.

There are two basic means of accessing traumatic memories. One involves hypnotic age regression. Participants are instructed to go back and relive earlier periods of their life as if they were occurring in the present. They are told that when given a signal, such as stroking the side of their eyes, their eyes will open and they will experience the event as though it were occurring in the here and now. Later, when given another signal, such as stroking the forehead, their eyes will close and their time orientation will be changed again. The alternative method is to have them picture on an imaginary screen a pleasant scene (to establish their ability to visualize in this manner) and then to imagine a scene taken from the traumatic experience as though they were watching their own videotape of the event. It is often useful to first go back to some comparatively neutral time prior to the trauma as a means of establishing patients' control over this technique before tapping material with strong affective associations.

Then, on the basis of the history obtained, the therapist selects one aspect of the trauma and asks the patient to relive it using hypnotic age regression or to see it as if it were viewed on an imaginary screen (i.e., the screen technique). It is useful to have them view the same traumatic event from a different viewpoint (e.g., taking into account what they did to protect themselves during the trauma). It might have been fighting off an assailant, attempting to help a wounded friend, or simply deciding to remain quiet so as not to further provoke an attacker. It is often useful with either age regression or the screen technique to consolidate this restructured perspective by having patients visualize a split screen: on the left picturing some aspect of what happened to them during the trauma and on the right side concentrating on their efforts to protect themselves during the traumatic experience. This helps them to face what was done to them and yet see it from a restructured viewpoint, in which they recognize and acknowledge their efforts at self-protection at the same time as they admit that there was a period of time during which they were physically helpless. This often reduces the exaggerated and inappropriate guilt that most trauma survivors feel. The guilt provides them with a fantasy that they could have controlled events over which they were, in fact, helpless. The mental discomfort involved in feeling guilty for not having overcome the trauma is the price that is paid for avoiding the confrontation with the fundamental sense of helplessness that accompanies physical trauma.

At the end of the session, instructions to end the hypnotic exercise can be given. It is often useful during this termination phase to say, "You will remember as much of this as you care to remember," as a means of not excessively challenging defenses if the patient wants to keep most or all of the material out of consciousness. It is then useful to debrief patients afterward, discussing their memories of the hypnotic work and what new meaning they have extracted from it. This is also an emotional consolidation phase in the therapy, when patients need time to work through and put into perspective strong emotions that might have been aroused by the hypnotic vivification of the traumatic memories. Patients who are not overwhelmed by the material, who have good general mental health (i.e., are not suicidally depressed or psychotic), or who have supportive resources available should be taught to continue the therapeutic work as a self-hypnosis exercise at home. The instructions can include a repetition of the self-hypnosis induction and then the use of the screen technique to visualize contrasting aspects of the trauma: acknowledging and bearing the patients' helplessness while recognizing their efforts to cope with and master the traumatic situation. This can be practiced once or twice a day.

Such exercises often have the effect of organizing and containing the traumatic memories, confining them to the self-hypnosis exercises and thereby freeing the patient to deal with other issues the remainder of the time. In this sense, the hypnosis is like a more focused version of psychotherapy in general. Irrational feelings are expected to flourish in the transference while the therapist hopes that the patient's outside life will also improve. Hypnosis is used as a special state of concentration through which traumatic memories can be accessed and worked through, just as dissociation is often associated with the initial experience of trauma. The literature reviewed later in this chapter indicates a high frequency of dissociative experiences during and immediately after trauma. Detachment and a narrow focus of attention during life-threatening trauma can help to maintain emotional equilibrium and facilitate coping more likely to result in survival (Butler, Duran, Jasiukaitis, Koopman, & Spiegel, 1996; Christianson & Loftus, 1987).

This approach to the use of hypnosis in treating PTSD can be summarized as the series of eight Cs. These principles are presented in approximate temporal order. That is, they are designed to be a series of steps, beginning with the confrontation of trauma and ending with congruence (i.e., the integration of traumatic memories). Nonetheless, some will occur together, and some may occur before others. The main point of these principles is to try to provide an organizing framework for therapists in their use of hypnosis in working through traumatic memories.

1. *Confront* trauma. The focus of this work is to help patients to link current symptomatology to a previous traumatic experience and work through that experience. This means that the primary goal of this kind of psychotherapy is not to analyze personality development or long-standing genetic reconstruction of symptoms. Rather, the goal is the acute and relatively rapid reversal of posttraumatic stress symptoms. If deeper personality issues then surface, the time to deal with them is after the psychotherapy of PTSD has been completed. To address the personality issues first can have the unfortunate effect of reinforcing inappropriate guilt by implying that if the person did not have the preexisting personality problems, the trauma would not have occurred.

2. Find a *condensation* of the traumatic experience. It is not necessary or even helpful to go through every unpleasant detail of the trauma. It is more helpful to find aspects of the traumatic memory that typify the trauma in the patients' mind and work through them.

3. *Confession*. Patients often have to confess to memories, experiences, and feelings about which they feel deeply ashamed. They

may never have discussed them with anyone else. These memories, experiences, and feelings will be revealed with difficulty. It is also useful to distinguish between genuine guilt over acts performed about which patients have reason to feel ashamed (e.g., soldiers who harmed or killed civilians in combat) and events in which the guilt is inappropriate (e.g., a combat soldier who felt that he should have known where a shell would land so that he might have saved a comrade who was hit).

4. Find *consolation*. Therapists should be responsive and empathic with patients in a professionally appropriate way. Patients will interpret neutrality or silence as rejection. A simple statement of comfort, such as, "I am terribly sorry this happened to you," can go a long way toward reassuring patients that they are not being rejected by the therapist even though they themselves feel that memories associated with these events make them unacceptable as people.

5. Make *conscious* previously repressed or dissociated material. Material stored unconsciously is rarely transformed. One can think of consciousness as a kind of processor that allows information to be examined, parsed, and reassembled. The overwhelming sense of having been shown to be a coward, for example, can be matched with memories of having tried to rescue friends or having used considerable ingenuity in protecting oneself during a traumatic experience, thereby transforming traumatic memory. When the material is stored in the unconscious again, it is stored in restructured form.

6. Mobilize and focus *concentration*. Concentration, because of its intensity and narrowness of focus, provides an opportunity for unearthing memories in considerable detail and then putting them aside again. As a result, many trauma victims fear that they will be flooded with memories and feelings and will never emerge from them again. Hypnosis provides a ceremonial occasion in which the individual can focus intently on the memories with the inference that once they have done so, they can put them aside until the next hypnotic encounter with them.

7. Maintain *control*. Because the key issue in dealing with traumatic memories is helplessness, it is especially important that the process of the psychotherapy gives individuals a sense of heightened control over their memories. This means that structuring the occasion as one of inducing self-hypnosis is particularly important because it gives patients a sense of control and mastery. It is important that the old myth that hypnosis is some-

thing done to one person by another is dismissed and that the hypnotic encounter is viewed as an active collaboration in which the therapist helps patients to assess and use their own hypnotic capacity.

8. Creating *congruence*. The goal is to help patients acknowledge, tolerate, and work through traumatic memories so that they can be integrated into their ongoing view of self without inflicting excessive damage to the self-concept.

There are a variety of other methods that have been used along with hypnosis to treat traumatic experiences. These include *abreaction*, referred to by Freud as the "cathartic method" (Breuer & Freud, 1893/1995); the alteration of traumatic memories (Kardiner & Spiegel, 1947); and the use of positive transference to integrate and alter material that leads to self-rejection (Brende & Benedict, 1980). All of these techniques involve using hypnosis to access traumatic memories and associated strong affects related to the traumatic experience and to transform them in some way in the context of the therapeutic relationship so that they are restored in an altered form that makes them more acceptable to conscious awareness.

The possibility of traumatic transference is an important consideration. Patients will unconsciously and sometimes consciously identify the therapist with the person who or situation that caused the trauma. Therefore, it is especially important that the therapist be sensitive to patients' identification of them with the trauma and work to maintain the therapeutic alliance despite it. Although the therapeutic alliance can be an important tool in the treatment of trauma (Haley, 1974), unacknowledged or ignored fears regarding the therapist and his or her motivation for addressing the traumatic issues can undermine the psychotherapy.

It is important to note that in some states, a victim or witness who is hypnotized either may not testify as to the hypnotically elicited memories or may, in fact, be prevented from testifying in court altogether (Brown, Scheflin, & Hammond, 1998; Scheflin & Spiegel, 1998; Spiegel & Scheflin, 1994). For example, in overturning the murder conviction of Stephen Trochym (February 7, 2007), the Supreme Court of Canada ruled out the use of hypnotically elicited testimony. Therefore, if there is any potential litigation involved regarding the trauma, it is important that patients are informed of potential risks to their testimony and that the patients' attorneys or the district attorney or police be consulted. All encounters in the therapy should be electronically recorded, preferably by videotape. It is also important that the therapist avoid injecting information into the hypnotic recounting of the trauma and to simply set the scene and allow patients to provide all of the associations.

CLINICAL MATERIAL

An Assault Victim

A 32-year-old female nurse was violently assaulted in the early evening as she returned home from shopping. The assailant attempted to drag her up a flight of stairs into her apartment, presumably to rape her. She fought vigorously with him, sustaining, among other injuries, a severe blow to the head. The assailant finally ran away, and she called the police. Because she had not been raped, the police made a cursory investigation and left. She then had a generalized seizure and was taken to the hospital, where it was discovered that she had incurred a basilar skull fracture. By this time, the assailant was long gone. She had little memory of his features and came to me for evaluation several months later to see whether hypnosis would be helpful in refreshing her memory of his appearance. She also experienced symptoms of PTSD, including numbing of responsiveness, intrusive recollection of the trauma, and discomfort in her apartment.

She proved to be moderately hypnotizable, as assessed by the HIP, and was encouraged to use the screen technique and to visualize the traumatic event on the screen. She was able to come to grips in hypnosis for the first time with how dangerous the situation had been. Previously, she had blamed herself for fighting back as hard as she did, thereby sustaining serious injury. She looked at her image of him in hypnosis and said, "He's really surprised that I'm fighting that hard; he doesn't expect me to." She then noticed something else: "I don't think he just wants to rape me; I think he wants to kill me. If he gets me upstairs, he's gonna murder me." I had her picture her efforts to protect herself and the results of those efforts on the right side of the screen. She emerged from the hypnosis with no clearer visual image of what he had looked like because it was dark at the time of the attack. However, she had a transformed sense of her conduct during the assault. She left with the feeling that she had probably saved her life by fighting as hard as she had. Despite having recognized for the first time the extremity of the danger she had been in, she emerged with a much clearer sense of her own instinctive skill at self-preservation and, thus, the traumatic memories became more bearable.

A Vietnam Veteran With Posttraumatic Stress Disorder

A 45-year-old Vietnam combat veteran had been hospitalized for 5 years following a fugue episode in Vietnam (for a more detailed case description, see D. Spiegel, 1981). Despite a prior excellent service record, he was discharged after this episode and had been chronically depressed and suicidal. He had been diagnosed as psychopathic, depressed, and bipolar but had not responded to any psychotropic medications. He related in the interview that he had informally adopted a wounded Vietnamese child who was subsequently killed during the Tet Offensive, and this seemed to have set off the fugue episode, of which he had no conscious memory.

He proved to be extremely hypnotizable on the HIP and relived, with considerable affect, the rocket attack in which the child was killed. He then relived a vivid memory of what had happened during the fugue episode. After seeing the boy's body, he ran into the jungle and engaged in combat with the Vietcong. I then used hypnotic regression to move him to a time when he buried the boy's body and he tearfully dropped imaginary dirt on the boy's casket. He berated himself for not having taken the child somewhere else before the attack: "If I had just taken you over to the hooch, you wouldn't be there, man; it's all my fault." I then asked him to think of a time when he and the child had been really happy together, and he pictured a birthday party he had thrown for the boy several months earlier. He smiled as he relived the boy's delight at the presents he received. The final instruction for the session was picturing on a split screen the boy's grave on the left and that birthday party on the right. I told him that although he had lost the child, no one could take away the happy times they had had together. I told him that he would remember as much as he cared to remember and guided him out of hypnosis. He emerged from 40 minutes of intense abreactive hypnotic age regression with just an image of a grave and a cake.

He practiced this self-hypnosis exercise twice a day and, in conjunction with antidepressant medication, improved substantially over the next several weeks. He discontinued the medication after discharge from the hospital and did well for several months until, in a period of 2 weeks, his wife started going out with another man, his police officer brother was killed in the line of duty, and someone shot his dog. He was rehospitalized but recovered fairly quickly. In the ensuing 14 years, he has done well. Although he has had episodic periods of depression and suicidal ideation that resolve fairly quickly, these periods are related to present circumstances in his life rather than to the traumatic loss, which he feels he has worked through.

Hypnotic Facilitation of Emotion Regulation and Cognitive Restructuring

Both of these cases illustrate the use of hypnosis in helping trauma victims to work through traumatic memories. First, the hypnosis provided focused and controlled access to the memories through the inference that when the hypnosis was over, the memories would be less prominent in consciousness. This helped to make the painful affect associated with the memories more bearable because it implied that their presence in consciousness would be time limited.

Second, the use of the split screen provided an opportunity to acknowledge the reality of the memory while also placing it in a broader perspective.

In the case of the assault victim, the terror she experienced in reliving the danger that she had undergone also helped her to reappraise her own role in resisting the assailant. Whereas previously she had felt guilty about having caused her injury, she was able to change the context of the memory of the assailant by recognizing his intention to harm or kill her, and therefore, her resistance was something that made her feel that she had possibly saved her life rather than gotten herself hurt even more. This made the original memory more tolerable because she had experienced it in a new context.

Similarly, the restructuring with the Vietnam combat veteran helped him to acknowledge and bear the intensity of the loss of this child because he was also able to access memories of happier times with him. This made the loss seem real but not total. This child was no longer alive, but the man's memories of happier times were not canceled by the child's death. Thus, hypnosis can help trauma victims to place their memories into a broader perspective, which makes working through them less overwhelming and more tolerable.

RESEARCH AND APPRAISAL

The Committee on Treatment of Posttraumatic Stress Disorder of the Institute of Medicine (IOM) reviewed the literature and concluded that exposure-based psychotherapies had the strongest evidence base for effectiveness, noting positive but weaker evidence for such treatments as cognitive restructuring, coping skills training, and hypnosis (Institute of Medicine, 2007). One randomized outcome trial indicated that hypnosis is an effective adjunct to treatment for PTSD (Brom, Kleber, & Defares, 1989), and there is accumulating evidence suggesting that hypnosis is highly effective (S. D. Solomon, Gerrity, & Muff, 1992). The IOM report noted that there are elements of exposure in other psychotherapies, and there are interpersonal, cognitive, and coping skills training aspects to exposure-based therapies. Clearly, more randomized prospective trials are needed to examine the efficacy of psychotherapeutic techniques using hypnosis in the treatment of PTSD. However, the broader literature suggests that exposure and reexperiencing traumatic memories facilitated by techniques such as hypnosis could be expected to benefit rather than harm people with PTSD. Hypnosis can help people to access and tolerate reexposure to traumatic memories and can facilitate working through these memories in a supportive psychotherapeutic context.

There are also studies showing that hypnotizability is higher among individuals with PTSD. Stutman and Bliss (1985) showed that Vietnam veterans high in PTSD symptomatology had higher scores on the Stanford Hypnotic

Susceptibility Scale than did Vietnam veterans who do not experience PTSD. D. Spiegel et al. (1988) found that 65 Vietnam combat veterans who were hospitalized with PTSD had extraordinarily high scores on the HIP compared with patients with schizophrenia, affective disorders, and anxiety disorders. They were even significantly more hypnotizable than were a normal comparison population. Thus, the research suggests that patients with PTSD, as a group, are extremely hypnotizable. This is consistent with the theory presented earlier that dissociation is a spontaneous response to trauma and is, in turn, a component of PTSD. Furthermore, it provides systematic data suggesting that as a group, individuals with PTSD should have extremely high hypnotic capacity and therefore be especially able to effectively incorporate hypnosis into their psychotherapy.

More recent research has indicated that dissociative symptoms are common in the aftermath of trauma (D. Spiegel & Cardeña, 1991). In the wake of physical disasters such as earthquakes (Cardeña & Spiegel, 1993), airplane crashes (Sloan, 1988), and tornados (Madakasira & O'Brien, 1987), a substantial proportion of victims reported dissociative reactions, including numbing and depersonalization (Feinstein, 1989; Noyes & Kletti, 1977). Furthermore, the presence of such dissociative symptoms in the immediate aftermath of trauma has been found to predict subsequent PTSD (McFarlane, 1986; Z. Solomon, Mikulincer, & Benbenishty, 1989).

CONCLUSION

Hypnosis is a state of special relevance to the assessment and treatment of PTSD. The phenomena that constitute hypnosis—dissociation, absorption, and suggestibility—are mobilized spontaneously during trauma, during which they may serve as a unique and adaptive defense against overwhelming discomfort. In the aftermath of trauma, however, they may forestall adequate working through of the traumatic experience, thereby predisposing an individual to the development of PTSD. Indeed, many of the symptoms of PTSD are reminiscent of these aspects of hypnotic consciousness. Thus, hypnotic phenomena underlie important aspects of the response to trauma, and recent research shows that patients with PTSD are unusually high in hypnotic capacity. These considerations make hypnosis a natural tool in the diagnosis and treatment of PTSD. It enables individuals to intensely connect with traumatic mental content and to disconnect or dissociate their somatic responses to these memories. Hypnosis therefore provides a means of enhancing control, for both patient and therapist, of access to traumatic memories and dissociation. This type of psychotherapy requires providing a means for restructuring these traumatic memories and therefore facilitating the grief work necessary to come to a new equilibrium. In this way, the special mental state mobilized during trauma may be used in the service of working through and mastering traumatic memories.

REFERENCES

American Psychiatric Association. (2000). *Diagnostic and statistical manual of mental disorders* (4th ed., text rev.). Washington, DC: Author.

Anderson, M. C., Ochsner, K. N., Kuhl, B., Cooper, J., Robertson, E., Gabrieli, S. W., et al. (2004, January 9). Neural systems underlying the suppression of unwanted memories. *Science, 303,* 232–235.

Barrett, D. (1992). Fantasizers and dissociaters: Data on two distinct subgroups of deep trance subjects. *Psychological Reports, 71,* 1011–1014.

Bower, G. H. (1981). Mood and memory. *American Psychologist, 36,* 129–148.

Brende, J., & Benedict, B. (1980). The Vietnam combat delayed stress response syndrome: Hypnotherapy of "dissociative symptoms." *American Journal of Clinical Hypnosis, 23,* 38–40.

Breuer, J., & Freud, S. (1995). Studies in hysteria. In J. Strachey (Ed. & Trans.), *The standard edition of the complete psychological works of Sigmund Freud* (Vol. 2, pp. 183–251). London: Hogarth Press. (Original work published 1893)

Brom, D., Kleber, R. J., & Defares, P. B. (1989). Brief psychotherapy for posttraumatic stress disorders. *Journal of Consulting and Clinical Psychology, 57,* 607–612.

Brown, D. P., Scheflin, A. W., & Hammond, D. C. (1998). *Memory, trauma treatment, and the law.* New York: Norton.

Butler, L. D., Duran, R. E., Jasiukaitis, P., Koopman, C., & Spiegel, D. (1996). Hypnotizability and traumatic experience: A diathesis–stress model of dissociative symptomatology. *American Journal of Psychiatry, 153,* 42–63.

Cardeña, E., & Spiegel, D. (1991). Suggestibility, absorption, and dissociation: An intergrative model of hypnosis. In J. F. Schumaker (Ed.), *Human suggestibility: Advances in theory, research, and application* (pp. 93–107). New York: Routledge.

Cardeña, E., & Spiegel, D. (1993). Dissociative reactions to the San Francisco Bay Area earthquake of 1989. *American Journal of Psychiatry, 150,* 474–478.

Christianson, S., & Loftus, E. (1987). Memory for traumatic events. *Applied Cognitive Psychology, 1,* 225–239.

Esdaile, J. (1846). *Hypnosis in medicine and surgery.* New York: Julian Press.

Feinstein, A. (1989). Posttraumatic stress disorder: A descriptive study supporting DSM–III–R criteria. *American Journal of Psychiatry, 146,* 665–666.

Freud, S. (1914). Remembering, repeating, and working through. In J. Strachey & A. Freud (Eds.), *The standard edition of the complete psychological works of Sigmund Freud* (Vol. 12, pp. 145–156). London: Hogarth Press.

Frischholz, E. J. (1985). The relationship among dissociation, hypnosis, and child abuse in the development of multiple personality disorder. In R. P. Kluft (Ed.), *Childhood antecedents of multiple personality* (pp. 100–126). Washington, DC: American Psychiatric Press.

Haley, S. A. (1974). When the patient reports atrocities. *Archives of General Psychiatry, 30,* 191–196.

Herman, J. L., Perry, J. C., & van der Kolk, B. A. (1989). Childhood trauma in borderline personality disorder. *American Journal of Psychiatry, 146,* 490–495.

Hilgard, E. R. (1965). *Hypnotic susceptibility.* New York: Harcourt, Brace & World.

Hilgard, E. R., & Hilgard, J. R. (1975). *Hypnosis in the relief of pain.* Los Altos, CA: William Kauffman.

Hilgard, J. R. (1970). *Personality and hypnosis: A study of imaginative involvement.* Chicago: University of Chicago Press.

Institute of Medicine. (2007). *Treatment of posttraumatic stress disorder: An assessment of the evidence.* Washington, DC: National Academies of Press.

Kardiner, A., & Spiegel, H. (1947). *War stress and neurotic illness.* New York: Hoeber.

Kluft, R. P. (1988). The dissociative disorders. In J. A. Talbot, R. E. Hales, & S. C. Yudofsky (Eds.), *Textbook of psychiatry* (pp. 557–585). Washington, DC: American Psychiatric Press.

Lindemann, E. (1994). Symptomatology and management of acute grief. 1944. *American Journal of Psychiatry, 151*(Suppl. 6), 155–160.

Madakasira, S., & O'Brien, K. F. (1987). Acute posttraumatic stress disorder in victims of a natural disaster. *Journal of Nervous and Mental Disease, 175,* 286–290.

McFarlane, A. C. (1986). Posttraumatic morbidity of a disaster: A study of cases presenting for psychiatric treatment. *The Journal of Nervous and Mental Disease, 174,* 4–14.

Nemiah, J. C. (1985). Dissociative disorders. In H. Kaplan & B. Sadock (Eds.), *Comprehensive textbook of psychiatry* (4th ed., pp. 942–957). Baltimore, MD: Williams & Wilkins.

Noyes, R., Jr., & Kletti, R. (1977). Depersonalization in response to life-threatening danger. *Comprehensive Psychiatry, 18,* 375–384.

Orne, M. T., Hilgard, E. R., Spiegel, H., Spiegel, D., Crawford, H. J., Evans, F. J., et al. (1979). The relation between the Hypnotic Induction Profile and the Stanford Hypnotic Susceptibility Scales, Forms A and C. *International Journal of Clinical and Experimental Hypnosis, 27,* 85–102.

Scheflin, A., & Spiegel, D. (1998). Working with repressed memory and avoiding lawsuits. *The Psychiatric Clinics of North America, 21,* 847–867.

Sloan, P. (1988). Posttraumatic stress in survivors of an airplane crash-landing: A clinical and exploratory research intervention. *Journal of Traumatic Stress, 1,* 211–229.

Solomon, S. D., Gerrity, E. T., & Muff, A. M. (1992). Efficacy of treatments for posttraumatic stress disorder: An empirical review. *JAMA, 268,* 633–638.

Solomon, Z., Mikulincer, M., Benbenishty, R. (1989). Combat stress reaction: Clinical manifestations and correlates. *Military Psychology, 1*, 35–47.

Spiegel, D. (1981). Vietnam grief work using hypnosis. *American Journal of Clinical Hypnosis, 24*, 33–40.

Spiegel, D. (1984). Multiple personality as a posttraumatic stress disorder. *Psychiatric Clinics of North America, 7*, 101–110.

Spiegel, D. (1986). Dissociating damage. *American Journal of Clinical Hypnosis, 29*, 123–131.

Spiegel, D., & Cardeña, E. (1991). Disintegrated experience: The dissociative disorders revisited. *Journal of Abnormal Psychology, 100*, 366–378.

Spiegel, D., Hunt, T., & Dondershine, H. E. (1988). Dissociation and hypnotizability in posttraumatic stress disorder. *American Journal of Psychiatry, 145*, 301–305.

Spiegel, D., & Scheflin, A. (1994). Dissociated or fabricated? Psychiatric aspects of repressed memory in criminal and civil cases. *International Journal of Clinical and Experimental Hypnosis, 42*, 411–432.

Spiegel, H., & Spiegel, D. (1980). Induction techniques. In G. D. Burrows & L. Dennerstein (Eds.), *Handbook of hypnosis and psychosomatic medicine* (pp. 133–147). Amsterdam, the Netherlands: North-Holland.

Spiegel, H., & Spiegel, D. (2004). *Trance and treatment: Clinical uses of hypnosis.* Washington, DC,: American Psychiatric Press.

Stutman, R. K., & Bliss, E. L. (1985). Posttraumatic stress disorder, hypnotizability, and imagery. *American Journal of Psychiatry, 142*, 741–743.

Tellegen, A., & Atkinson, G. (1974). Openness to absorbing and self-altering experiences ("absorption"), a trait related to hypnotic susceptibility. *Journal of Abnormal Psychology, 83*, 268–277.

17

HYPNOSIS AND THE TREATMENT OF DISSOCIATIVE IDENTITY DISORDER

GEP COLLETTI, STEVEN JAY LYNN, AND JEAN-ROCH LAURENCE

According to the *Diagnostic and Statistical Manual of Mental Disorders* (*DSM–IV*; 4th ed.; American Psychiatric Association, 1994), *dissociative identity disorder* (DID; formerly called multiple personality disorder) is characterized in part by the presence of two or more distinct identities (i.e., a relatively enduring pattern of perceiving, relating to, and thinking about the environment and self) or *personality states* (i.e., temporary patterns of behavior) that recurrently assume control over the individual's behavior. These alternate personality states, or *alters*, often exhibit psychological features that differ markedly from those of the primary, or *host*, personality and are identified by different names, ages, and genders.

This dramatic presentation has assured that DID is arguably the most perplexing of all psychological disorders. Occasionally noticed in the early years of animal magnetism (Laurence & Perry, 1988), it was only with the resurgence of interest in hypnosis and hysteria at the end of the 19th century in Europe that the question of alter personality became a focus of psychological theories. Indeed, from the time of Janet's (1889) landmark writings on

All clinical material has been disguised to protect patient confidentiality.

what he labeled "psychological disaggregation," DID has attracted more than its share of puzzlement and controversy. After psychoanalytic theory nudged dissociation theory out of favor, experimentalists later in the century cast doubt on dissociation (i.e., the compartmentalization of conscious experience into separate streams of awareness; Rosenberg, 1959; White & Shevach, 1942). Nevertheless, dissociation was rehabilitated by Hilgard's neodissociation theory (1977), which lent legitimacy to the study of dissociation and fueled fascination with dissociative conditions. Although Hilgard's theory was founded on the misinterpretation of his own role as hypnotist in eliciting a "dissociative response," and on the angular stone of his theory, the amnesic barrier, which could never be substantiated (Laurence, 2006), an explosion of reports of cases of "multiple personality disorder" in the 1980s followed on the heels of media attention garnered by movies such as *Sybil* (Petrie, 1976) and promoted widespread acceptance of the belief that DID was the direct consequence of childhood sexual abuse and trauma.

This hypothetical causal relation between sexual abuse and DID was not, however, part of the early history of dissociation. Theorists such as Janet, Azam, and Richet conceptualized dissociation as an intricate interaction between psychopathology (mostly hysteria) and social demands, a reflection of the then current zeitgeist (Carroy, 1993; Ellenberger, 1970). In a similar way, the contemporary link between DID and traumatic abuse can be seen as the end result of the ongoing social focus on victimization. Not surprisingly, this viewpoint increasingly met with skepticism in the 1990s and early 21st century, as concerns about the validity of recovered memories of childhood trauma raised questions about whether dissociated identities were "discovered" or created by suggestive psychotherapeutic procedures such as hypnosis and addressing different alter personalities by name (see chap. 2, this volume).

Controversies about DID persist to this day and pivot around whether DID is a socially constructed and culturally influenced condition rather than a spontaneously occurring response to early trauma (Merskey, 1992). Proponents of the posttraumatic model (Gleaves, 1996; Gleaves, May, & Cardeña, 2001; Ross, 1997) contend that DID arises from a history of severe abuse in childhood: To cope with attendant emotional pain, the personality compartmentalizes or "dissociates." In contrast, proponents of the sociocognitive model (Spanos, 1996; see also Aldridge-Morris, 1989; Lilienfeld et al., 1999; McHugh, 1993; Merskey, 1992; Sarbin, 1995) contend that DID results from media influences, including television and film depictions of DID, therapist cueing (e.g., suggestive questioning regarding the existence of possible alters, hypnosis), and entrenched sociocultural expectations regarding the symptoms of DID. As Lynn, Fassler, Knox, and Lilienfeld (2007) observed, therapists who repeatedly ask leading questions such as, "Is there another part of you with whom I haven't yet spoken?" may gradually elicit previously latent alters that ostensibly account for their patients' otherwise enigmatic behaviors (e.g., self-mutilation, rapid and intense mood shifts).

In this chapter, we propose that following a functional analysis, empirically supported methods can be used to treat the emotional dysregulation and manifold symptoms that accompany the typical presentation of DID and that hypnosis can be a valuable treatment adjunct when not used for the purpose of memory and/or alter recovery. The case study we present, of an actual patient we treated, illustrates the multifaceted treatment of a person with a characteristic presentation of dissociative symptoms treated with eclectic cognitive–behavioral methods using hypnosis as an ancillary treatment.

CLINICAL APPLICATIONS

The persistence of controversies swirling around DID has not precluded an emerging consensus in several areas. First, there is little dispute that some people display symptoms consistent with a diagnosis of DID, although the genesis of these symptoms is controversial. The estimated prevalence of DID varies from virtually nonexistent (e.g., Piper, 1997; Rifkin, Ghisalbert, Dimatou, & Sethi, 1998) to as much as 1% to 2% (e.g., Ross, 1997). Second, there is an emerging consensus that suggestive techniques such as hypnosis should not be used to recover childhood memories of trauma and/or to identify alter personalities. And third, there is consensus that DID is, in the great majority of cases, not feigned or a result of malingering.

These points of agreement aside, there is a dearth of systematic research on the treatment of DID, and controlled outcome studies are not available to inform recommendations regarding what treatments are effective for patients reporting dissociative experiences. However, the symptoms of DID are often comorbid with a variety of disorders with a broader treatment base, including borderline personality disorder, anxiety, depression, and schizoaffective disorder (see Lynn et al., 2007). Indeed, Ellason, Ross, and Fuchs (1996) reported that patients with DID qualify for an average of 8 Axis I disorders and 4.5 Axis II disorders.

Dissociation as Avoidance

Therapists who treat DID must confront the question: How do people come to see themselves as possessing multiple dissociated selves? In our clinical experience, dissociative symptoms often serve as cue-controlled avoidance maneuvers triggered by internal prompts (e.g., memories, automatic cognitions) and external cues, including aversive events and context-generated suggestions (e.g., therapists, television). In extreme cases, avoidance seemingly promotes a retreat to an "alternate personality," imbued with particular experiences, beliefs, or emotions at great variance from the host personality. For instance, the thought, "What I did was monstrous," can be transformed into "I am a monster," and further metamorphize into, "My monster alter was responsible for what I did." In this manner, an overall sense of a "good self" that fears and avoids conflict can be preserved. The sense of an altered self in DID can arise from attempts to understand puzzling and confusing thoughts, emotions, and behaviors that coalesce in the belief that the personality is fragmented into distinct indwelling entities.

Dissociative responding is, of course, one of many potential avoidance strategies that are perpetuated through negative reinforcement. Whereas strong negative affect can trigger negative emotions and avoidance (dissociation), disturbing cognitions can likewise trigger negative affect and attendant avoidance (dissociation). Accordingly, a dissociative response provides negative reinforcement insofar as it mitigates dysphoria and disturbing thoughts.

Dissociation, Imagination, and Fantasy

Dissociation can also be understood in terms of the use of imagination and attention-regulating strategies that operate to create a credible feeling of distance or separation from aversive events outside the realm of personal control or from feelings that generate guilt, anger, or anxiety (Lynn, Rhue, & Green, 1988). For example, Bowers (1991) observed that "Fantasized alternatives to reality . . . can become increasingly complex and differentiated with minimal involvement of executive level initiative and control" (p. 168). Bowers further noted that, "When a seriously disturbed individual is also fantasy-prone, 'multiple personality' may be the result" (p. 168). Young (1988) observed that "multiple personality reflects the gradual crystallizing of a fantasy that is amalgamated with dissociative defenses" (p. 15).

Enacting different alters may become a viable way of coping with everyday conflicts and stressors. Indeed, fantasy-prone persons report that they (a) had imaginary playmates during childhood and pretended they were different people and (b) engaged in fantasy when faced with aversive events (Lynn & Rhue, 1988). In addition, research supports at least a modest association between imaginative abilities and dissociative experiences and symptoms in children and adults (see Lynn, Neufeld, Green, Sandberg, & Rhue, 1996; Rauschenberger & Lynn, 1995, 2002–2003). Dissociative experiences can be predicted at least as accurately by absorption and fantasy-proneness abilities as by the report of trauma (Pekala, Angelini, & Kumar, 2001).

To complicate matters, the same abilities, absorption and fantasy-proneness, have been linked to the ability to confabulate and to create false memories in normal individuals and clinical patients (Jang, Paris, Zweig-Frank, & Livesley, 1998; Laurence, Nadon, Nogrady, & Perry, 1986). As emphasized in the *DSM–IV*, "care must be exercised in evaluating the accuracy of retrieved memories, because the informants are often highly suggestible. . . . There is currently no method for establishing with certainty the accuracy of such retrieved memories in the absence of corroborative evidence" (pp. 480–481). Actual or created memories reinforced by repetition can then serve as a trigger to further dissociative experiences, leading to a consolidation and even an exacerbation of the dissociative symptoms (Laurence & Perry, 1988). Because of the high rate of comorbidity in patients reporting dissociative experiences, the memory narratives of the patients must be evaluated with great care. The confabulatory tendencies may lead to dissociative responses, which in turn serve to validate the memories. Dissociation thus exacts a dear cost: It precludes learning more adaptive means of accepting, reinterpreting, or mastering negative thoughts and emotions, and it is resistant to extinction because it is repeatedly associated with tension reduction.

The Rationale for Hypnosis

Given that imaginative abilities are associated with both hypnotic responding and dissociation (Lynn & Sivec, 1992), it is not surprising that patients with dissociative disorders (i.e., DID and dissociative disorder not otherwise specified) score higher on measures of hypnotic suggestibility than patients with schizophrenia, anxiety disorder, mood disorder, and college student control participants (Frischholz, Lipman, Braun, & Sachs, 1992). Moreover, patients with posttraumatic conditions seem to be more hypnotically suggestible than most other patient populations (Bryant, Guthrie, & Moulds, 2001; Spiegel, Hunt, & Dondershine, 1988; Stutman & Bliss, 1985). Higher levels of hypnotic suggestibility among patients with PTSD are associated with therapeutic success (Cardeña, 2000; Cardeña, Maldonado, van der Hart, & Spiegel, 2000), and higher levels of hypnotic suggestibility are associated with avoidance symptoms (Bryant, Guthrie, Moulds, Nixon, & Felmingham, 2003). Accordingly, highly hypnotizable and dissociative individuals may be more likely to develop posttraumatic and dissociative conditions than individuals with other psychiatric conditions (Butler, Duran, Jasiukaitis, Koopman, & Spiegel, 1996). Nonetheless, a prospective study measuring hypnotic suggestibility before exposure to trauma is required before any final conclusion can be reached (Lynn & Cardeña, 2007).

The link between dissociation and imagination, as well as the relatively high suggestibility of individuals with dissociative and posttraumatic stress disorders, implies that hypnosis may play an integral role in treating DID and avoidance-related symptoms. Hypnosis holds considerable promise as a means of catalyzing exposure-based treatments that assist patients in overcoming avoidance of anxiety-eliciting stimuli and in maintaining a present-centered, solution-focused treatment orientation (Lynn & Cardeña, 2007; Lynn & Kirsch, 2006). Because patients with DID share many features with patients with borderline personality disorder, tactics found to be effective with patients with borderline personality disorder (e.g., cognitive–behavioral methods, mindfulness training, relaxation; Linehan, 1993) may prove useful in treating DID. Hypnosis can augment the efficacy of cognitive–behavioral treatments (Kirsch, Montgomery, & Sapirstein, 1995) and may play a useful role in mindfulness training (Lynn, Lama Surya Das, Williams, & Hallquist, 2006). Thus, hypnosis promises to be a valuable adjunctive method with many patients with DID. More specifically, in patients with DID, hypnosis can be used to (a) promote self-regulation and relaxation and the acceptance of painful emotions; (b) challenge cognitive distortions and minimize the need to resort to different alters to cope with conflicting emotions; (c) facilitate exposure to anxiety-eliciting stimuli; (d) allow for a cognitive–emotional restructuring of memories; and (e) solve problems, anticipate, and rehearse future interactions through age progression.

Education is essential to helping patients understand how they came to adopt the view that they possess multiple personalities (e.g., sociocultural and suggestive influences in therapy, fantasy proneness and role enactment). However, it is imperative to impress on such patients that no matter how fragmented the personality seems to be, it is impossible for a person to truly house more than one personality (Spiegel, 1993). Nevertheless, for some patients, their phenomenological experience of multiplicity is so compelling they cannot be disabused easily of the erroneous idea that they harbor multiple personalities. In such cases, hypnosis can be used to present images and metaphors that legitimize the integration of conflicting personalities (e.g., streams coming together to become a strong river). Kirsch and Barton (1988) suggested that when information gathering is rendered problematic by shifting alters, the metaphor of a "hidden observer" (i.e., "central switchboard," "executive center") can be used to obtain historical information. However, it is essential that the patient understand the metaphorical nature of this suggestion and not reify another alter. A single "problem list" that does not relegate specific issues and difficulties to discrete alters can be generated to create a viable treatment agenda (Lynn et al., 2007).

Treatment Considerations

Lynn et al. (2007) suggested that given the probable importance of sociocultural influences in the presentation of DID, clinicians should assess patients' exposure to information about DID conveyed by movies, books, magazines, the Internet, and, often most important, previous therapists. The use of suggestive procedures (e.g., dream interpretation, guided imagery, journaling of incidents of abuse) should be noted. Information regarding abuse and neglect should be obtained in any complete assessment. However, the credibility of reported memories should be carefully evaluated and corroborated, if possible, because dissociative individuals are likely to be fantasy-prone and score highly on measures of hypnotic suggestibility. It is important that both constructs have been related to false memory risk (Eisen & Lynn, 2001).

DID symptoms are associated with borderline personality disorder, as well as self-defeating and passive–aggressive (i.e., negativistic) personality disorders (Ellason et al., 1996). Accordingly, a careful assessment of suicidality is warranted, along with an evaluation of self-mutilating behavior, which has also been linked with dissociation (Vanderhoff & Lynn, 2001). Medication evaluation is also appropriate in many cases of DID.

To formulate a diagnosis in patients with dissociative symptoms, we recommend that clinicians administer widely used measures of dissociation, including the 28-item Dissociative Experiences Scale (Bernstein & Putnam, 1986), and at least one structured interview, such as the Structured Clinical Interview for DSM–IV Dissociative Disorders (Steinberg, Cicchetti, Buchanan, Hall, & Rounsaville, 1993) or the Dissociative Disorders Interview Schedule (Ross, Heber, & Norton, 1989). To avoid the appearance of a sole emphasis on dissociative symptoms, and to glean information across multiple domains of both abnormal and normal-range personality, we recommend administering the Minnesota Multiphasic Personality Inventory—2 (MMPI–2; Butcher, Dahlstrom, Graham, Tellegen, & Kaemmer, 1989) and the Neuroticism–Extroversion–Openness Personality Inventory (NEO-PI; Costa & McCrae, 1985).

CLINICAL MATERIAL

The patient we describe in the case that follows is a 45-year-old Caucasian female who is currently disabled and living alone most of the year but is sometimes accompanied by her daughter, who attends college nearby, or by members of her family of origin, all of whom live within driving distance. She has never married, has raised her daughter as a single parent, and has remained close to her own parents throughout her adult life. Indeed, extended family have always been of great importance, and she frequently puts the needs of others before her own, which has proved highly problematic in terms of her achieving independence and freedom from guilt.

Prior Treatment History

The patient has a long and complicated treatment history. She first presented for treatment at a university psychological clinic in 1992 at the suggestion of her physician who was alarmed by her behavior during a pelvic examination in his office. He had known the patient for some time already and had never seen her behave as she did during the visit that precipitated his referral. He was in the midst of performing a pelvic exam when there emerged dramatic changes in her demeanor, from someone calm and collected to someone scared and vulnerable one moment, angry and aggressive the next, and vacillating between the two emotional states in rapid succession. Neither of these presentations was consistent with the appropriately mature and composed manner of all prior office visits. Hence, he referred the patient for psychotherapy.

The patient was reluctant, but eventually scheduled the appointment. However, she did not share with the therapist any of the information about her visit to the doctor or the doctor's referral; nor did she give the therapist permission to confer with anyone about her situation. Instead, she gave as her reason for treatment the fact that she was experiencing severe stress related to emerging medical concerns that interfered with her job performance. Although she claimed that she was depressed because she felt her job was in jeopardy, she denied any other concerns and said she just needed to find a way to cope. Her initial diagnosis was an adjustment reaction to life circumstances; however, it quickly became apparent that much more was involved.

The therapist at the time, a graduate student in a university-based clinic, reported that the patient was angry about having a problem she could not solve on her own, that she was impatient and "wanted a quick fix so she could be on her way." She was slow to trust, evasive, and revealed little information when asked about her life history. Moreover, the therapist noted that her mood and behavior would fluctuate dramatically both within and between sessions.

An attempt to use a behavioral problem solving approach to improve the patient's ability to cope was partially successful, but progress was sporadic at best, and new problems kept emerging. As treatment progressed, there were sudden bouts of anger and anxiety in session for no apparent reason, and at one point, the patient started to reveal far more serious problems from her past, the first of which was being raped 7 years prior to treatment onset. This was eventually followed by the revelation of other past traumas from childhood (i.e., the death of a sibling, sexual abuse). The emotional outbursts in session continued. In fact, they escalated whenever any cue or trigger, however peripheral, reminded the patient of her past experiences. The diagnosis was changed to posttraumatic stress disorder.

Crisis phone contacts occurred between sessions. The patient would often call the therapist with an urgent need to talk but often speaking in a different voice, sometimes sounding like a frightened child or an angry adult, frequently apologizing for her behavior afterward, only to do it again repeatedly. It was at this point that the therapist came to realize that this might be a patient who meets the criteria for DID. It was sometime after this time, during the 3rd year of therapy, that one of the coauthors of this chapter (Colletti) assumed responsibility for treating the case, as the previous therapist had completed his graduate studies and was no longer available to provide services.

Work With Current Therapist

Colletti's treatment of the patient proceeded with the understanding from the outset that this was a complex case of an individual in need of intensive psychotherapy for what appeared to be a combination of problems involving posttraumatic stress and serious ongoing life stressors, not the least of which were as yet undiagnosed serious medical problems and severe, chronic pain. Finally, her dissociative episodes and the presence of extreme characterological problems served to complicate the clinical picture.

At the outset of treatment with Colletti, the patient experienced anxious and irritable moods, intense anger, and verbal aggressiveness. She was slow to trust and required numerous sessions to process her feelings about the loss of her former therapist. She reported difficulty negotiating relationships, especially intimate ones with her family of origin, and experienced extreme emotional lability and flashback-like experiences in session that were clearly cue-driven and dissociative in nature and were often followed by amnesia, disorientation, and problems concentrating. In addition to her trauma history, she also recounted an incident when, at the age of 5 or 6, she had a serious and painful eye injury and was molested by her treating optometrist. She also had an abortion while in college and experienced the death of a neonate under her care as a nurse in the context of a live abortion incident. In addition, an unplanned pregnancy resulted in the birth of her daughter and the attendant consequences of being a young mother. In session, the patient often would startle at minor noises. Her problems were suggestive of borderline personality and posttraumatic stress disorder, accompanied by dissociation, while DID was considered as a potential diagnosis.

The patient's medical history was significant. More specifically, she had had surgery for cervical cancer, repeated kidney stones and infections, peripheral muscle weakness and pain, chronically abnormal blood values (i.e., erythrocyte sedimentation rate), cysts on her bladder, and ovarian cysts, all of which were documented in writing and in conversations with a number of her physicians. Years later, a team of medical specialists confirmed a diagnosis of lupus, following an evaluation at the Cleveland Clinic. The patient's numerous medications required careful monitoring for interaction effects.

Initial Treatment Strategy

The initial goal was to provide emotional stabilization and containment of negative affect so that the patient could function outside of session without experiencing repeated crises. Cognitive–behavioral approaches, including activity scheduling for depressed mood, progressive muscle relaxation, and rational disputation of thoughts, were instituted. Recurrent maladaptive thoughts that were addressed throughout the course of her therapy included the following: (a) "Someone will learn I feel weak and afraid"; (b) "It is dangerous to trust others because you will most certainly be hurt, and because that is so, it is equally dangerous to let others see your vulnerability"; (c) "To be weak or incapable of doing something is unacceptable"; (d) "No matter what I do to help myself, I will never get well"; and (e) "I must protect those I love, but I am mentally, or physically, unable to do it." In addition, role-playing and rehearsal of situations in which the patient modeled appropriate assertive responses in the context of family demands was implemented.

Over the next few years, the patient's day-to-day functioning improved significantly, yet ranged from competently performed to impaired, fluctuating between these two extremes mostly as a function of whether or not she experienced a crisis. Effective parenting was perhaps the only area of functioning that consistently remained unimpaired and preserved throughout crises. Serious medical problems persisted, often resulting in severe and chronic pain, frequent hospitalizations, and demoralization in terms of her inability to pursue fulfilling activities, including her career of nursing.

Dissociation persisted in session and out of session. For example, it became clear that the patient reported hearing "voices in her head" and experienced herself as "splitting off" into an angry and aggressive adult "protector" or defender of others and childlike aspects of herself that required protection. She also reported considerable confusion and disorientation at times of high stress, emotional numbing, and an urge to retreat by way of not concentrating on ongoing activities and situations. Not surprisingly, she reported disturbing periods of amnesia. Dissociative episodes were likely to occur before or during the many medical procedures she endured. At this time, she appeared to meet the criteria for DID, and it became increasingly obvious that it was necessary to confront more directly her dissociative symptoms.

Cotherapy

In 1999, Colletti began to attend weekly clinical hypnosis seminars in which another coauthor of this chapter (Lynn) presented an approach to dissociation that was based on combining empirically supported techniques and hypnosis to treat specific symptoms and problems in living. During this time period, Lynn provided emergency coverage for Colletti and conducted a phone session with the patient who "hit if off" with Lynn. At the invitation of Colletti, and with the patient's agreement, Lynn became a cotherapist. Lynn attended sessions two to three times a month, and individual sessions occurred four to six times a month. Lynn taught the patient hypnotic and self-hypnotic techniques and implemented cognitive–behavioral interventions and exposure therapy in the context of the avoidance-based theoretical framework regarding dissociation described earlier. The dual therapist approach provided enhanced opportunities to (a) share expertise and provide consultation and emergency coverage, (b) improve treatment planning, (c) better identify exaggerated transference reactions in response to one or both therapists, and (d) speak in front of the patient to discuss different viewpoints and possibilities, thereby alleviating or "loosening" dichotomous thinking.

The Dissociative Trap

Early in therapy, the therapists shared with the patient the following conceptualization of what they called the *dissociative trap*. During circumstances that posed an emotional threat by reminding her of past upsets, the patient dealt with unmanaged emotions by assigning them to one specific "way of being." That is, she relegated them to a coordinated set of cognitions and behavior patterns suggestive of separate identities that could be characterized as a childlike identity and an angry, aggressive adult. Rarely constructive, and often disabling, this rigid, locked-in, stimulus-bound pattern precluded adaptive coping, no matter how important it was to be able to respond in a more flexible, situationally appropriate manner. It is important that the therapists consistently emphasized the point that although she might have felt at times that she housed distinct personalities, she truly embodied only one personality, even though she felt considerable conflict, anxiety, and a need to numb and escape her present circumstances and justify her actions that seem ego alien at times. It bears mentioning that the diathesis for her dissociative symptoms appeared to be a history of fantasy versus reality-based coping in childhood, of which she became aware as she spoke of the anger she felt regarding her sister's death (i.e., when the patient was 5 years old) and her own guilt at not somehow preventing it. At this time in her life, she reported, she felt as if she began to think of herself as split into angry and excessively protective "parts."

The Treatment Agenda

The therapists then created an agenda, with the patient's input, that included the following goals: (a) to provide education regarding the need to dissociate; (b) to develop a unified positive sense of identity; (c) to validate her feelings and the idea that conflict is inevitable and can be managed; (d) to assist her in accepting responsibility for her behavior; (e) to facilitate positive treatment expectancies, self-control abilities, and her ability to accept positive feedback; (f) to increase assertiveness and improve social interactions with a focus on respect for others and reciprocity in relationships; (g) to restructure maladaptive thinking patterns, attitudes, and beliefs; (h) to enhance decision-making skills; (i) to deepen her capacity to experience and accept the gamut of emotions in the present without engaging in experiential avoidance; (j) to assist her in working through grief and loss issues, including the death of her father; (k) to help her to experience and accept expressions of care and concern extended by others to her; and (l) to help her cope with medical evaluations and treatment procedures. The treatment was guided by the belief that if the therapists attended to her experiential avoidance and the defensive operations that motivated it, it would be possible to reduce, if not eliminate, her dissociative responses and obviate her need to compartmentalize her experiences in terms of "multiple personalities."

Applications of Hypnosis

The treatment continues to this day (430 sessions, as of this writing), and it has been successful in achieving the latter objective. Hypnosis, incorporated into a broader cognitive–behavioral approach, has played a key role in addressing many of the treatment goals. Early in her work with Lynn, it became apparent that the patient displayed an ability to readily experience a variety of hypnotic suggestions for relaxation, peace, and internal calm. The following is a verbatim transcription from an early session:

> Please sit back and begin to let go of the tension that you have accumulated throughout the day, simply letting go of everything you don't need, creating an internal space for you to feel good about yourself, comfortable and at ease. Take a nice deep, deep breath and hold on as long as you can. And as you breathe in, feel the tension of the breath. You know that tension can be a part of life, but you can let it go. But for now, hold onto the tension as long as you can; experience it, create it. And you know you can release it when you feel your lungs are just about ready to burst. Yes, let go and feel how good it can be. You can only experience the tension for a relatively brief period of time before you let it go, and it is replaced with another feeling. Do the same thing once more, hold and release. Feel the tension you don't need now moving out of your body through your fingertips, relaxing your entire upper body, your entire upper body. Feel the relaxation now and the sense of security. Now feel the tension draining out of your lower body, relaxing your entire lower

body, even your ankles and toes. Feel the relaxation now and the sense of security; nothing to bother, nothing to disturb. Experience yourself soothing yourself, calming yourself, feeling more calm and at ease. When you feel yourself holding on too tightly, just breathe and release; let it go, yet holding on to what you need to feel whole and secure, whole and secure. Let thoughts come and let them go. Let feelings come and let them go, as you experience each present moment in its entirety, in its fullness, letting each moment come and go. Thoughts are only thoughts. Feelings are only feelings. You do not have to act on a thought, unless you want to. You don't have to act on an experience, unless you want to. For now, just experience. Let it come and let it go. Stay with it. You can do it. Sense a deep inner calm, peace, and relaxation, comfort and security, and as you do this more and more, you get that glimmering sense, that bright sense of optimism, hope, and acceptance of the totality of your being, your feelings, your thoughts, and of all the possibility it brings.

The patient was taught to produce these and other suggested experiences through self-hypnosis outside sessions and throughout the day by taking several deep diaphragmatic breaths and experiencing contact with her moment-to-moment experience and a sense of serenity and calm. Self-hypnosis was also used in "trigger situations" associated with dissociative reactions. For instance, she would use self-hypnosis when she began to ruminate and become disoriented when she started to think about threats to her (a) daughter's safety and security, (b) physical integrity during medical examinations, and (c) personal autonomy when she felt undermined by individuals in authority she dealt with around disability issues. At the first hint of a flashback, she used a variety of self-regulation techniques and strategies to "stay in the present" (e.g., holding a marble given to her by Lynn, looking at a newly minted coin), including a body scan in which she would "get in touch with and connect" with different parts of her body and say to herself, "That was then, this is now."

The therapists also created an induction that helped her to sleep when she experienced intermittent bouts of insomnia (i.e., typically, waking during the night). These involved her returning her anxious thoughts to her breathing as she imagined herself walking down a staircase, experiencing increasing comfort and relaxation. Hypnosis played an important role in exposure sessions in which she imaginally relived past and anticipated future (through age progression) stressful experiences such as medical examinations and surgical procedures she came to dread. Hypnotic suggestions were provided for her to stay in contact with the imaginal material presented while maintaining a coherent sense of self-awareness.

During the past 2 years, the therapists increasingly facilitated a problem-solving approach in which she assessed and evaluated different possible outcomes of decisions, used self-hypnosis to imagine herself responding in a variety of scenarios as she maintained contact with her feelings, and modified her behaviors as the situation demanded to best achieve her objectives. In a related manner, hypnosis appeared to enhance her comfort during role-playing in which she "interacted" with family members and her daughter to resolve conflicting feelings and gain confidence in her ability to encounter others appropriately.

In addition to these hypnotically augmented interventions, the therapy relied on behavioral activation that encouraged her to be involved in as many activities as her physical limitations allowed. At the same time, the therapists encouraged her to carefully select, limit, and schedule activities. They also encouraged her to assert herself and to refuse excessive demands imposed by others. The therapists rationally disputed (through Socratic method) recurrent negative thinking patterns and the idea that her worth depended on what she could accomplish in a given day. The latter tact was often boosted with posthypnotic suggestions that emphasized her gaining awareness of moments of optimism, positive accomplishments, and possible ways of reframing her experiences.

Treatment Outcome

The treatment was almost entirely successful in eliminating startle reactions, flashbacks, and dissociative responses, including amnesia and disorientation, in response to aversive stimuli. In session, the patient no longer speaks in a different voice or behaves as if she were a person of a different developmental level; this reportedly occurs only rarely outside of session, and only during a crisis. In addition, the patient exhibits improved anger management, impulse control, and the ability to evaluate alternative behaviors in situations that require problem solving. She reminds herself to use self-hypnosis and other coping skills in trigger situations, and she takes considerable pride in doing so. She believes that hypnosis has made a difference in her life. It is notable that she can now tolerate negative affect and accept herself even when she displays anger. The frequency of crises is dramatically reduced, as is the need for intersession contact with Colletti. She has succeeded in raising a child who is now a young adult involved in a healthy relationship and looking forward to attending graduate school.

Unfortunately, serious medical problems persist, and the patient is often unable to pursue pleasurable activities because of severe chronic pain and infrequent, yet highly disturbing, hospitalizations. The therapists now talk about her engaging in *adaptive dissociation* in which she can experience a sense of detachment from aversive medical procedures without experiencing amnesia or a fragmentation of self. Although her daily functioning has clearly improved in most areas, her physical disabilities, chronic pain, and interactions with the medical community suggest the need for ongoing treatment. Nevertheless, as the patient's confidence has blossomed over the past few years, her sense of neediness and dependency has diminished, and the therapists intend to discuss "weaning" her to fewer sessions a month in the near future. Before closing, it bears mention that in hindsight it would have been useful to conduct a more formal evaluation of dissociative symptoms using paper and pencil and structured interviews when dissociative symptoms first became apparent. And as noted earlier, omnibus measures of psychological functioning such as the MMPI or NEO-PI would also have yielded potentially valuable information.

RESEARCH AND APPRAISAL

Anecdotal reports suggest that many treatments, including psychoanalysis, family and couples therapy, videotaped sodium amytal (i.e., so-called truth serum) interviews, and cognitive–behavior therapy, can be helpful in the treatment of DID (Caddy, 1985). Unfortunately, there are no well-controlled comparative outcome studies of different interventions for treating DID. Accordingly, there is a pressing need for research to provide a compelling empirical basis for selecting among treatments. At the present time, there is no empirical basis for assuming that techniques that rely on memory recovery are any more effective than cognitive–behavioral methods grounded in modifying current maladaptive cognitions, emotions, and behaviors. Indeed, the available evidence implies that caution should be exercised in using methods that rely on recovery of purportedly dissociated or repressed memories (see Lilienfeld et al., 1998). Therefore, we recommend that practitioners avoid such interventions and, instead, use empirically supported methods to treat both comorbid conditions (e.g., depression, borderline personality, anxiety, PTSD) and symptoms within and across so-called alters (see Lynn et al., 2007).

Although researchers have not yet examined the addition of hypnosis to empirically supported procedures specific to the treatment of DID, hypnosis does appear to be a viable catalyst with both psychodynamic and cognitive–behavioral therapies (Kirsch, 1990; Kirsch et al., 1995). Moreover, Lynn and Kirsch (2006) have documented that hypnosis can be a useful adjunct in the treatment of conditions often associated with DID, including flashbacks and other posttraumatic symptoms, depression, and anxiety. Accordingly, there is a strong rationale for the use of hypnosis in treating the manifold symptoms of DID, which makes the need for controlled outcome studies comparing hypnotic and nonhypnotic interventions all the more pressing.

CONCLUSION

In the case reported in this chapter, hypnosis appeared to be integral to treatment. The patient was highly responsive to suggestions and looked forward to hypnosis sessions and learning new ways to accept, confront, and master painful emotions. As treatment nears an end, the patient can take comfort in the fact that she has a portable means of coping well beyond the session and therapy hour; she can continue to use the self-hypnosis techniques she has practiced now for years and can refine them on her own and with occasional assistance from her therapists, if needed.

In closing, we call for empirical studies that can enrich researchers' and clinicians' understanding of the role that hypnosis can play in (a) facilitating controlled exposure to strong emotions in treatment as well as stabilizing and managing affect outside of the treatment setting, (b) achieving insight and translating self-understanding to adaptive everyday actions, and (c) assisting in developing and maintaining a positive and integrated sense of self across diverse emotional and behavioral contexts.

REFERENCES

Aldridge-Morris, R. (1989). *Multiple personality: An exercise in deception.* Hillsdale, NJ: Erlbaum.

American Psychiatric Association (1994). *Diagnostic and statistical manual of mental disorders* (4th ed.). Washington, DC: Author.

Bernstein, E. M., & Putnam, F. W. (1986). Development, reliability, and validity of a dissociation scale. *The Journal of Nervous and Mental Disease, 174,* 727–735.

Bowers, K. S. (1991). Dissociation in hypnosis and multiple personality. *International Journal of Clinical and Experimental Hypnosis, 39,* 155–176.

Bryant, R. A., Guthrie, R. M., & Moulds, M. L. (2001). Hypnotizability in acute stress disorder. *American Journal of Psychiatry, 158,* 600–604.

Bryant, R. A., Guthrie, R. M., Moulds, M. L., Nixon, R. D., & Felmingham K. (2003). Hypnotizability and posttraumatic stress disorder: A prospective study. *International Journal of Clinical and Experimental Hypnosis, 51,* 382–389.

Butcher, J. N., Dahlstrom, W. G., Graham, J. R., Tellegen, A., & Kaemmer, B. (1989). *The Minnesota Multiphasic Personality Inventory—2: Manual for administration and scoring.* Minneapolis: University of Minnesota Press.

Butler, L. D., Duran, R. E., Jasiukaitis, P., Koopman, C., & Spiegel, D. (1996). Hypnotizability and traumatic experience: A diathesis–stress model of dissociative symptomatology. *American Journal of Psychiatry, 153,* 42–63.

Caddy, G. R. (1985). Cognitive behavior therapy in the treatment of multiple personality. *Behavior Modification, 9,* 267–292.

Cardeña, E. (2000). Hypnosis in the treatment of trauma: A promising but not fully supported, efficacious intervention. *International Journal of Clinical and Experimental Hypnosis, 48*, 225–238.

Cardeña, E., Maldonado, J., van der Hart, O., & Spiegel, D. (2000). Hypnosis. In E. B. Foa, T. M. Keane, & M. J. Friedman (Eds.), *Effective treatments for PTSD* (pp. 247–279). New York: Guilford Press.

Carroy, J. (1993). *Les personnalités doubles et multiples: Entre science et fiction* [Double and multiple personalities: Between science and fiction]. Paris: Presses Universitaires de France.

Costa, P. T., Jr., & McCrae, R. R. (1985). The NEO Personality Inventory manual. Odessa, FL: Psychological Assessment Resources.

Eisen, M. L., & Lynn, S. J. (2001). Dissociation, memory, and suggestibility in adults and children. *Applied Cognitive Psychology, 15*, S49–S73.

Ellason, J. W., Ross, C. A., & Fuchs, D. L. (1996). Lifetime Axis I and Axis II comorbidity and childhood trauma history in dissociative identity disorder. *Psychiatry: Interpersonal and Biological Processes, 59*, 255–266.

Ellenberger, H. F. (1970). *The discovery of the unconscious.* New York: Basic Books.

Frischholz, E., Lipman, J., Braun, B., & Sachs, R. G. (1992). *Psychopathology, hypnotizability, and dissociation.* Unpublished manuscript.

Gleaves, D. H. (1996). The sociocognitive model of dissociative identity disorder: A reexamination of the evidence. *Psychological Bulletin, 120*, 42–59.

Gleaves, D. H., May, M. C., & Cardeña, E. (2001). An examination of the diagnostic validity of dissociative identity disorder. *Clinical Psychology Review, 21*, 577–608.

Hilgard, E. R. (1977). *Divided consciousness: Multiple controls in human thought and action.* New York: Wiley.

Janet, P. (1889). *L'automatisme psychologique* [The psychological automatism]. Paris: Félix Alcan.

Jang, K. L., Paris, J., Zweig-Frank, H., & Livesley, W. J. (1998). Twin study of dissociative experience. *The Journal of Nervous and Mental Disease, 186*, 345–351.

Kirsch, I. (1990). *Changing expectations: A key to effective psychotherapy.* Pacific Grove, CA: Brooks/Cole.

Kirsch, I., & Barton, R. D. (1988). Hypnosis in the treatment of multiple personality: A cognitive–behavioural approach. *British Journal of Experimental and Clinical Hypnosis, 5*, 131–137.

Kirsch, I., Montgomery, G., & Sapirstein, G. (1995). Hypnosis as an adjunct to cognitive behavioral psychotherapy: A meta-analysis. *Journal of Consulting and Clinical Psychology, 63*, 214–220.

Laurence, J. R. (2006). Lorsque science et croyance s'affrontent: Dissociation, amnésie dissociative et faux souvenirs [When science and beliefs clash: Dissociation, dissociative amnesia and false memories]. In. D. Michaux (Ed.), *Hypnose et Dissociation Psychique.* Paris: Imago.

Laurence, J. R., Nadon, R., Nogrady, H., & Perry, C. (1986). Duality, dissociation, and memory creation in highly hypnotizable subjects. *The International Journal of Clinical and Experimental Hypnosis, 34*, 295–310.

Laurence, J. R., & Perry, C. (1988). Hypnosis, will, and memory: A psycho-legal history. New York: Guilford Press.

Lilienfeld, S. O., Lynn, S. J., Kirsch, I., Chaves, J. F., Sarbin, T. R., Ganaway, G. K., & Powell, R. A. (1999). Dissociative identity disorder and the sociocognitive model: Recalling the lessons of the past. *Psychological Bulletin, 125*, 507–523.

Linehan, M. (1993). *Cognitive–behavioral treatment of borderline personality disorder*. New York: Guilford Press.

Lynn, S. J., & Cardeña, E. (2007). Hypnosis and the treatment of posttraumatic conditions: An evidence-based approach. *International Journal of Clinical and Experimental Hypnosis, 55*, 167–188.

Lynn, S. J., Fassler, O., Knox, J., & Lilienfeld, S. O. (2007). Dissociation and dissociative identity disorder: Treatment guidelines and cautions. In J. Fisher & W. O'Donohue (Eds.), *Practitioner's guide to evidence-based psychotherapy* (pp. 248–257). New York: Kluwer Academic.

Lynn, S. J., & Kirsch, I. (2006). *Essentials of clinical hypnosis: An evidence-based approach*. Washington, DC: American Psychological Association.

Lynn, S. J., Lama Surya Das, Hallquist, M., & Williams, J. (2006). Mindfulness, acceptance, and hypnosis: Cognitive and clinical perspectives. *International Journal of Clinical and Experimental Hypnosis, 54*, 143–166.

Lynn, S. J., Neufeld, V., Green, J., Rhue, J., & Sandberg, D. (1996). Daydreaming, fantasy, and psychopathology. In R. Kunzendorf, N. Spanos, & B. Wallace (Eds.), *Hypnosis and imagination* (pp. 67–98). Amityville, NY: Baywood Publishing.

Lynn, S. J., & Rhue, J. W. (1988). Fantasy-proneness: Hypnosis, developmental antecedents, and psychopathology. *American Psychologist, 43*, 35–44.

Lynn, S. J., Rhue, J. W., & Green, J. P. (1988). Multiple personality and fantasy proneness: Is there an association or dissociation. *British Journal of Experimental and Clinical Hypnosis, 5*, 138–142.

Lynn, S. J., & Sivec, H. (1992). The hypnotizable subject as creative problem solving agent. In E. Fromm & M. Nash (Eds.), *Contemporary perspectives in hypnosis research* (pp. 292–333). New York: Guilford Press.

McHugh, P. R. (1993). Multiple personality disorder. *Harvard Mental Health Newsletter, 10*(3), 4–6.

Merskey, H. (1992). The manufacture of personalities: The production of multiple personality disorder. *British Journal of Psychiatry, 160*, 327–340.

Pekala, R., Angelini, F., & Kumar, V. K. (2001). The importance of fantasy-proneness in dissociation: A replication. *Contemporary Hypnosis, 18*, 204–214.

Petrie, D. (Director). (1976). *Sybil* [Motion picture]. United States: Lorimar Productions.

Piper, A. (1997). *Hoax and reality: The bizarre world of multiple personality disorder*. Northvale, NJ: Jason Aronson.

Rauschenberger, S. L., & Lynn, S. J. (1995). Fantasy proneness, *DSM–III–R* Axis I psychopathology, and dissociation. *Journal of Abnormal Psychology, 104*, 373–380.

Rauschenberger, S. L., & Lynn, S. J. (2002–2003). Fantasy-proneness, negative affect, and psychopathology. *Imagination, Cognition, and Personality, 22*, 237–253.

Rifkin, A., Ghisalbert, D., Dimatou, S., & Sethi, M. (1998). Dissociative identity disorder in psychiatric inpatients. *American Journal of Psychiatry, 155*, 844–845.

Rosenberg, M. J. (1959). A disconfirmation of the descriptions of hypnosis as a dissociated state. *International Journal of Clinical and Experimental Hypnosis, 7*, 187–204.

Ross, C. A. (1997). *Dissociative identity disorder: Diagnosis, clinical features, and treatment of multiple personality*. New York: Wiley.

Ross, C. A., Heber, S., & Norton, G. R. (1989). The dissociative disorders interview schedule: A structured interview. *Dissociation, 2*, 169–189.

Sarbin, T. R. (1995). On the belief that one body may be host to two or more personalities. *International Journal of Clinical and Experimental Hypnosis, 43*, 163–183.

Spanos, N. P. (1996). *Multiple identities & false memories: A sociocognitive perspective*. Washington, DC: American Psychological Association.

Spiegel, D. (1993, May 20). Letter to the Executive Council, International Study for the Study of Multiple Personality and Dissociation. *International Society of the Study of Multiple Personality and Dissociation, 11*, 15.

Spiegel, D., Hunt, T., & Dondershine, H. E. (1988). Dissociation and hypnotizability in posttraumatic stress disorder. *American Journal of Psychiatry, 145*, 301–305.

Steinberg, M., Cicchetti, D., Buchanan, J., Hall, P., & Rounsaville, B. (1993). Clinical assessment of dissociative symptoms and disorders: The Structured Clinical Interview for *DSM–IV* Dissociative Disorders. *Dissociation, 6*, 3–15.

Stutman, R. K., & Bliss, E. L. (1985). Posttraumatic stress disorder, hypnotizability, and imagery. *American Journal of Psychiatry, 142*, 741–743.

Vanderhoff, H., & Lynn, S. J. (2001). The assessment of self-mutilation: Issues and clinical considerations. *Journal of Threat Assessment, 1*, 91–109.

White, R. W., & Shevach, B. J. (1942). Hypnosis and the concept of dissociation. *Journal of Abnormal and Social Psychology, 37*, 309–328.

Young, W. C. (1988). Observations on fantasy in the formulation of multiple personality. *Dissociation, 1*, 21–22.

18

HYPNOSIS IN THE TREATMENT OF ANOREXIA NERVOSA

MICHAEL R. NASH AND ELGAN L. BAKER

Anorexia and bulimia nervosa are exceedingly complex disorders that frequently involve dramatic dissociative features (Beaumont & Abraham, 1983; Russell, 1979). Dissociation of aspects of interoceptive experience and body image, as well as archaic, enmeshed modes of object relating within the family figure prominently in most cases of severe anorexia. Because hypnosis itself may involve a dissociative experience (Hilgard, 1977) as well as a regressed mode of relating (Fromm & Nash, 1997), it is not surprising to find that (a) hypnosis may be particularly helpful in the treatment of patients with an eating disorderss, and (b) even in the experimental laboratory, certain classes of patients with an eating disorders may be more responsive to hypnosis than one would otherwise expect. We provide information about the prevalence of the disorder and a brief summary of the literature, after which we present a treatment paradigm that explicitly addresses key aspects of anorexia nervosa from a developmental, ego-psychological conceptual framework.

CLINICAL APPLICATIONS

Prevalence rates for anorexia nervosa range from .5% to 1% (Craighead, 2002). Anorexia is diagnosed when there is a refusal to maintain body weight at or above a minimally normal weight for age and height (e.g., body weight less than 85% of that expected), along with an intense fear of gaining weight or becoming fat. "Fear of fatness" is accompanied by a disturbance in the way in which body weight or shape is experienced. Concerns about body shape can become so paramount that anorectic women stubbornly deny the seriousness of their low body weight and strongly resist pressures from family and others to gain weight. Some estimate the mortality rate for anorexia at 10%, one of the highest mortality rates for all psychiatric conditions, with a 5% mortality rate over each decade of follow-up (Sullivan, 1995). Amenorrhea (i.e., the absence of at least three consecutive menstrual cycles) also must be present to warrant a diagnosis of anorexia, which may either be of the food restricting or the binge-eating/purging type (Lynn & Kirsch, 2006).

Although references to hypnosis in the treatment of anorexia nervosa are relatively few, they are scattered across a century of distinguished clinical work. Whether the therapy was carried out at the Salpêtrière Clinic in 19th-century France (J. Janet, 1888) or at the Menninger Clinic in America (Brenman & Gill, 1947), strategies of treatment are remarkably similar.

In his 1906 American lectures, Pierre Janet outlined the major symptom picture of "hysterical anorexia" as it was viewed at the Salpêtrière Clinic: self-starvation, binge eating and purging, resistance to treatment, late adolescent onset, family disturbance, dissociation of sensations, and profound underlying psychological conflict (reported in P. Janet, 1924). Earlier, P. Janet had described his brother's hypnotic treatment of a 25-year-old female anorexic patient, Marcelene, who was hospitalized and tube fed following severe weight loss and self-induced vomiting (J. Janet, 1888; P. Janet, 1925). Marcelene had experienced this disorder for several years but had become acutely emaciated and weak. Over several hypnotic sessions, J. Janet was able to restore Marcelene to a normal pattern of food intake by suggesting increased attention to her tactile and visceral sensations. This seemingly indirect approach was undoubtedly a clinical application of P. Janet's assertion that hysterical pathology was dissociative in nature. The treatment process was stormy, with frequent relapses. At first, Marcelene would eat only while hypnotized; on termination of a session, she reported spontaneous amnesia for the proceedings and returned to her anorexic–bulimic patterns. The therapist was eventually able to extend treatment effects across time by suggesting to Marcelene that she remain hypnotized throughout the year but that she should otherwise behave and feel perfectly normal. The patient quickly regained her strength and normal body weight. However, periodic relapses around menstruation and stressful events necessitated frequent "booster" sessions administered by the therapist.

In his other work with patients with acute anorexia, P. Janet emphasized that hypnosis was only a part of a much more comprehensive treatment plan (P. Janet, 1925): The patient should be temporarily isolated from the family; meals should be presented in a simple, routine manner and taken only with a nurse in attendance (the same nurse at all meals); confrontation and pleading should be avoided; and the patient should receive a graduated diet that would "reeducate the appetite and the alimentary functions" (P. Janet, 1925, p. 810). It was only in this supportive inpatient context that hypnosis could be effectively used with the acutely anorexic patient.

Brenman and Gill (1947) reported the case of a 14-year-old anorexic girl who weighed 70 pounds at the time of her admission to the Menninger Clinic. A peculiar hopping compulsion complicated her symptomatology. The patient was particularly resistant to treatment and seemed psychotically inaccessible at times. Accordingly, hypnosis focused on establishing a safe holding environment. During hypnosis, the therapist administered indirect suggestions that eventually led to a complete cessation of the hopping behavior. Following several weeks of comprehensive inpatient care and permissive therapy, the patient's food intake increased markedly. Brenman and Gill speculated that her dramatic response to the suggestions that she stop hopping reinforced her belief that the hypnotist was indeed magically powerful. This in turn led to an experience of increased security and safety in the therapeutic relationship. Although the patient refused subsequent treatment with hypnosis, she became increasingly communicative and responsive to the insight-oriented psychotherapy. Treatment gains proved stable over a long-term follow-up.

Several contemporary clinicians have offered brief reports on their work with patients with anorexia. Crasilneck and Hall (1975) treated 70 cases of anorexia nervosa with hypnosis; marked improvement was reported in more than half of the cases. During the acute stages of anorexia, direct suggestions for increased food intake were given (e.g., increased hunger, enjoyment of eating). Instructions for self-hypnosis were also included. Following medical stabilization, Crasilneck and Hall involved the patients in an uncovering therapy that focused on the unconscious conflicts that presumably precipitated the condition.

Kroger and Fezler (1976) also briefly described using hypnosis in the treatment of anorexia. Direct suggestions were given for reduced level of anxiety, increased appetite, and pleasant food-related memories. Kroger and Fezler offered several standard images of ingesting appealing food as a means of inducing hunger. For patients who reported an inability to eat because of feeling full, the therapist suggested vivid recall of past hunger: sensations of lightness and emptiness in the stomach.

Thakur (1980) also used direct suggestions for healthier eating habits, increased weight gain, and a more realistic body image. In addition, general feelings of interpersonal competence and assertiveness were suggested. Spiegel and Spiegel (2004) used similar direct suggestions with patients with anorexia and emphasized the importance of hypnosis in the early diagnostic process.

Ambrose and Newbold (1980) reported two separate cases of anorexia in young boys who presented with gender confusion and fears of pregnancy. Direct suggestions of increased attention to their own masculinity and reassurance of their male characteristics quickly produced positive results.

Milton Erickson (Erickson & Rossi, 1979) described the successful month-long intensive treatment of an anorexic 14-year-old girl. Using indirect suggestions and paradoxical strategies, Erickson conducted the therapy in four phases:

1. *Distracting frames of reference.* Lectures on oral hygiene and absurdly precise instructions for mouth care were presented.
2. *Depotentiating masochistic defenses.* The patient was instructed to rinse her mouth daily with cod liver oil. Punishment for failure was eating food. The patient, of course, failed.
3. *Therapeutic double bind.* The patient was instructed to oversee her parents' weight gain.
4. *Emotional catharsis.* The therapist provoked the patient by accusing her of being a liar and a coward.

Erickson and Rossi (1979) characterized this type of treatment as essentially involving trance, but it is clear that Erickson's therapy also incorporated the supportive, familial, and dynamic interventions cited as being essential by other clinicians.

Gross (1983) provided a detailed description of the hypnotic treatment of a patient with anorexia. Gross treated 50 cases of anorexia on a large adolescent psychiatry unit. Although the hypnotic procedures were tailored to the specific dynamics of the patient, Gross identified six core symptoms that seemed amenable to hypnotic treatment, augmented by self-hypnosis:

1. *Hyperactivity.* Suggestions for relaxation, slowed respiration, and heart rate were administered. Pleasurable feelings were associated with beautiful beach and park settings.
2. *Distorted body image.* Photographs of the patient's own emaciated body were compared with a more healthy body image.
3. *Defect in interoceptive awareness.* Suggestions were given that directed attention to visceral cues, specifically hunger and satiety. Association of hunger with moderate food intake also was suggested.

4. *Family enmeshment.* Suggestions were given for self-assertion and self-esteem. Age progression suggestions were used to facilitate self-sufficiency outside of the family in the future.

5. *Repressed traumatic event.* Age regression suggestions were used to explore underlying dynamics associated with the onset of anorexic symptoms.

6. *Overt and covert resistance to therapy.* Hypnosis was sometimes represented as a means of weight control rather than being explicitly associated with weight gain. Suggestions encouraged an association between better eating habits and improved vocational or athletic performance.

Operating from a psychoanalytic object-relations perspective, Hornyak (1996) focused on an especially resistant type of patient with anorexia: The patient who presents with a profound deficit in false-self organization. Hornyak observed that this deficit expresses itself in disruptions of interoceptive awareness, affect regulation, and a peculiar disconnect between self and body. Hypnosis is used throughout the often-lengthy treatment with these patients. In the initial phases, hypnosis supports self-regulation and mastery of tension states. Imagery and ego-supportive hypnotic strategies help the patient identify emotions before they are enacted. Eventually, however, the therapist encounters more entrenched defenses characterized as agitated defiance. Supportive hypnotic techniques are used here to preserve the therapeutic alliance in the face of attack. As the preambivalent hate–adore cycle recedes, more adaptive object relations emerge. Passive dependent yearnings are more directly satisfied and eating is no longer burdened with desperation. In the final phases of therapy, hypnosis supports autonomy and mature separation.

There have been a number of other approaches to using hypnosis in treating patients with an eating disorder, most notably from cognitive–behavioral (Vanderlinden & Vandereycken, 1988), ego-state (Torem, 1987), and strategic (Yapko, 1986) perspectives. Lynn, Rhue, Kvaal, and Mare (1993) proposed the use of a graded series of suggestions to reduce the resistance so often encountered in patients with anorexia. The suggestions move from relaxation and daydream to imagination of outcomes and role-play conflict. Similarly, Lynn, Kirsch, Crowley, and Campion (2006) integrated hypnotic techniques into Fairburn's cognitive–behavioral therapy approach (Fairburn, Marcus, & Wilson, 1993), articulating three stages of treatment: (a) supplanting disordered eating behaviors with healthier patterns, (b) successfully interrupting maladaptive eating patterns with a behavioral analysis of alternatives, and (c) consolidating treatment gains. Hypnosis and self-hypnosis techniques are used through all stages.

Marianne Barabasz (2000) articulated a hypnotic approach to eating disorders that uses an essentially cognitive therapy framework (Beck &

Freeman, 1990). With the patient, Barbarasz carefully charts thoughts, behaviors, and feelings to identify the cognitive precursors to dysfunctional eating behaviors. These beliefs are then gradually challenged in the context of hypnosis; self-hypnosis is figural in this approach. During the early phases of therapy, hypnosis is used to promote relaxation, both during the therapy session and in day-to-day life. As the patient progresses, self-hypnosis begins to replace problematic eating behaviors as a response to stressors. Hypnosis is then used to strengthen healthy functional beliefs and alternate coping strategies.

THE BAKER–NASH APPROACH

Our treatment approach was used successfully with a group of 36 women (ages 17–31) who presented with a primary diagnosis of anorexia nervosa. Most of the patients were seen initially on an inpatient basis and then followed in outpatient psychotherapy in a treatment program that combined individual and group psychotherapy, along with occasional use of psychotropic medication. We outline here the hypnotherapeutic strategies used with the patients.

Typically, hypnosis was introduced as part of a multifaceted intervention based on the proposition that the eating disorder had become a metaphor to symbolize a variety of intrapsychic and interpersonal struggles. Many of the struggles centered on self-pathology, control and power conflicts, and difficulties with the adequate differentiation and integration of a cohesive sense of mature identity. These structural and dynamic difficulties operate with differing valences for different patients. Those who present with anorexia nervosa are a relatively heterogeneous group. Therefore, different aspects of the treatment approach were emphasized more or less with different patients depending on their individual needs and specific treatment responses.

1. Hypnosis was introduced to patients as a means of gaining enhanced self-control associated with various opportunities for increased security and mastery. Hypnosis was not introduced as an opportunity to gain control over eating habits or to restore patients' weight. Most patients were more responsive to the specific conscious introduction of hypnosis as an adjunct to the therapeutic regimen because they were ambivalent about mutually participating in activities designed to alter their eating habits or increase their weight level. Most of the patients readily verbalized feelings of being anxious, apprehensive, and out of control in their lives and were generally willing to participate reciprocally in a program designed to facilitate an increased sense of potency and security. When hypnosis was introduced, the general idea was emphasized that hypnotic ability is something that rests in each individual

and can be enhanced through training and practice; therefore, the emphasis was on the development of hypnotic talent as being representative of the growth of the patients' own capacities for self-control.

2. Structured and permissive induction techniques were used with patients with anorexia. A structured rather than purely permissive induction was indicated to help modulate the regressive experiences that often accompany the trance and that may be frightening or even retraumatizing for many patients with anorexia. This permissive approach helps to avoid control struggles and associated resistance around power dynamics and competition. Most patients responded well to an induction that combined relaxation and fantasy, which is also useful for early instruction in self-hypnosis.

3. Early applications of hypnosis were specifically designed to enhance the patients' sense of personal power, to increase their capacity for autonomous functioning, to support the working alliance, and to provide a generalized sense of ego support leading to increased mastery and positive expectations for behavioral success. For this reason, instruction in self-hypnosis was introduced early in the treatment, and patients were taught to use self-hypnotic strategies to manage feelings of anxiety or insecurity between sessions. Hypnosis was also used for tension reduction, with specific suggestions being made to help patients to become increasingly aware of their generalized tension level and to learn to manage this through a variety of relaxation strategies. Direct and indirect suggestions were used to provide the patients with a sense of comfort, thereby supporting the ego's emerging capacity for mastery. Directed and structured imagery and fantasies are often useful in indirectly suggesting to patients improved functioning and to support most positive attitudes regarding capacities for self-control and adaptation.

4. Once patients had learned to use self-hypnosis for relaxation and once hypnotic suggestion and imagery had been established to stabilize and support the working alliance between the therapist and the patient, hypnotherapeutic interventions were directed more specifically at a number of arenas of difficulty that are more directly associated with core pathological features of anorexia nervosa. Many of the patients had a good deal of difficulty with accurately perceiving sensory stimulation from their bodies. For this reason, many of them were unaware of sensory cues typically associated with physiological functioning. For some patients who presented with more severe forms of preelectral structural pathology, this defect appeared to have been related to a more generalized problem with boundary management and maintenance. They defensively avoided awareness of sensory stimulation because this evoked insecurity and anxiety associated at a primitive level with a lack of adequate boundary differentiation and integration. For many of these patients who were more borderline-level, attention to physical functioning began to arouse concerns about the deterioration of body boundaries and

merger with the external environment. For these patients, sensory focusing was preceded by general work on boundary support and management. Both guided imagery and specific sensory exercises were used during hypnosis to support the integrity of boundaries and to communicate through indirect and direct suggestions that body and ego boundaries are constant and dependable.

In addition, many patients had learned to defensively dissociate body and body-related experiences from the conscious perception of self and their intellectualized phenomenological experience of the world. The patients often described, either directly or symbolically, a sense of a split between their "body selves" and their "mind" or "spiritual selves." When this was the case, the hypnotherapeutic work also needed to address the reintegration of these various phenomenological arenas. Imagery and suggestion were used to reestablish a sense of communication between the mind and body that could not be interrupted by anxiety. When anxiety began to intrude on this work, suggestions for calm and relaxation, as well as fantasy designed to reestablish a soothing and comfortable environment, were interspersed with work directed at reintegration until patients were able to maintain a sense of comfort and continuing security while attempting to reconnect physical and mental representations of self and others.

This approach relies on the therapeutic action of a relaxation-based desensitization paradigm. When this work was successful or when the patients were less severely disturbed and therefore not in need of attention to boundaries and unmodulated dissociative experiences, the hypnotherapeutic work directly supported patients' improved awareness of their body-based sensory phenomenology. They were taught during hypnosis to more accurately label and attend to muscle tension and related skeletal and visceral sensations. This was related to their experiences of hunger as well as to the careful differentiation of a variety of affective experiences. Patients were encouraged in the trance to recapture the affect associated with being in a variety of different fantasized situations and to learn to deal with this emotional experience adaptively.

Frequently, patients reported that they began to find themselves unable to eat or to experience hunger in family situations that were emotionally charged (i.e., with anger and anxiety). These situations were revivified in the trance, and patients were taught to differentially recognize their affective responses to these situations and to reduce the associated tension. Patients then managed these feelings through more adaptive coping strategies rather than through the restriction of food intake, withdrawal, or dissociation accompanied by distortions in body experience and body image. This pattern of affective differentiation and abreaction was often accompanied by a generalized decrease in tension and improvement in the symptoms associated with distorted eating behaviors and body image.

5. Body image distortions were also addressed more directly in hypnotherapy. Patients were asked to represent their conscious and preconscious body images in hypnosis by projecting them onto screens or drawing them on blackboards. Age regression techniques were used to uncover the roots of these distortions in malevolent interactions with family members and the associated development of distorted self and object representations. We found that the distortions are often related to split-off aspects of the self-representation that cannot be integrated into a conscious sense of self because they evoke a negative sense of vulnerability and associated negative affect. Once the roots of these distortions have been explicated and explored, interpretative work can be done regarding them in the trance and during nontrance verbal, insight-oriented psychotherapy sessions.

We used directed imagery and fantasy in hypnosis to confront these distortions, to help patients to become increasingly aware of them, and to suggest their amelioration. For instance, distortions in body image drawn on an imaginary blackboard during the trance can be corrected by erasing and redrawing the aspects of the image of the physical self that are particularly distorted. Frequently, patients became anxious and uncomfortable, but relaxation was introduced to restore a sense of comfort and calm. When this had been accomplished, patients could then return to working on correcting distortions in the represented body-image without the intrusion of undue anxiety.

It appears that this work resulted in some generalization of an improved self-image external to the trance. However, more important, patients seemed to be able to learn to think about their physical self and to begin to explore their representations of their body without the same degree of defensiveness and anxiety that characterized attempts at this work prior to the specific use of hypnotic imagery and exploration. Age progression was used to suggest the eventual integration of an adequate and reality-based self-representation and the incorporation of this integrated, accurate, physical representation into the conscious sense of self. This was represented through progressive physical changes or, more symbolically, through natural images of differentiation, integration, and growth, structured through evolving hypnotic fantasy.

6. This work on distortions in body image and the correction of these was closely associated with a more general consideration of the integration of an appropriate and mature sense of personal identity. Because many patients with anorexia experience considerable conflicts around individuation and independence as a result of their prolonged enmeshment in their families, severe generalized distortions in identity maturation are frequently seen. These were explored in hypnosis and corrected through the use of direct or indirect suggestions and through the use of specific images and fantasies. It was often useful to suggest specific hypnotically induced dreams during the trance to help clarify, for the therapist and the patient, the conflicts that were associated with

defects in identity integration. Once these had been clarified, they were further explored in regular psychotherapy sessions and addressed through hypnotic imagery.

7. Hypnotic work was also used to explore the relation between negative affect expression and distorted attitudes toward eating, food, and unusual eating behaviors. The relation between these eating behaviors and their role in controlling or avoiding unacceptable affective experiences were established and connected during the trance through suggestion and imagery. Once this had been done, the unacceptable affect was ventilated and abreacted, resulting in an emerging sense of mastery over those feelings. Dreams and imagery were often useful for this, as were more direct hypnotic abreaction techniques.

8. As aspects of body imagery and general identity integration were corrected, patients' general capacity for mastery was enhanced. Work in hypnosis was used to further address concerns related to separation, individuation, integration, and adaptation. Rehearsal in fantasy, age progression, and guided imagery were used to provide patients with a more positive sense of their ability to tolerate the affect associated with maturation and to deal with their increasing stability and individuated integrated identity. Within the context of exploring these issues, we also used an insight-oriented approach in individual therapy and group treatment, with which these patients were usually simultaneously involved.

The use of directed hypnotic experience, imagery, and fantasy, as well as specific suggestions, does not necessarily correct defects in patients' internal representational world, nor does it resolve all aspects of the dynamic conflicts seen in patients who present with anorexia nervosa. However, it does provide an opportunity to address some of the issues that interfere with successful, traditional psychotherapeutic work with these patients, particularly the defensive use of denial and dissociation, which are central to distortions in body image and general self-concept. Until these have been addressed, successful psychotherapeutic work with these patients is significantly compromised.

RESEARCH AND APPRAISAL

Our hypnotherapeutic approach was used successfully with a group of women whose primary diagnosis was anorexia nervosa. Most of the patients were seen initially as inpatients and then were followed in outpatient psychotherapy in a treatment program that combined individual and group psychotherapy and occasional psychotropic medication. Our work suggests that this sort of hypnotherapeutic approach, when used in conjunction with insight-oriented individual and group therapy and occasional conjoint sessions with families (when the patients are still living at home), is a successful treatment approach. Patients' experiential participation, with an emerging sense of mastery and self-control, avoids many of the struggles that emerge around control issues when patients project parental transferences onto their therapist and attempt to maintain their distorted eating behaviors in an effort to maintain some sense of personal control through manipulating the environment.

Follow-up data at 6 and 12 months indicated that 76% of the patients had a remission of symptoms and stabilized their weight gain at an acceptable level. These data were compared with those from a group of 31 women who were treated identically without the use of the hypnotherapeutic paradigm described earlier. Only 53% of the women in this latter group achieved the same level of symptom remission and weight stabilization. The use of medication and days of inpatient and outpatient therapy were essentially the same for both of the groups.

These results, although preliminary, suggest that the introduction of hypnosis into the treatment paradigm improved participants' treatment responses. Undoubtedly, the therapeutic effects of hypnosis were related to the specific impact of the techniques used and the more generalized and non-specific effects of hypnosis in improving the patients' sense of self-mastery and reinforcing the quality of the therapeutic alliance, which is frequently associated with the clinical application of hypnotic techniques. These preliminary data were obtained from a clinical treatment program rather than from an actual controlled study. Therefore, the patients in the two groups were not matched or randomly assigned to the treatment conditions. The differences in the therapeutic use of hypnosis were a function of which therapist was primarily involved in the patients' treatment; therefore, other therapist-related effects could also account for the differences in treatment outcome. However, a post hoc analysis suggested that most aspects of the patients' treatment in the two groups were constant and were therefore indicative of some positive effect that might have been specifically attributable to the use of the hypnotic treatment approach. Further controlled investigation is, of course, necessary to support this preliminary conclusion.

CONCLUSION

This hypnotherapeutic paradigm provides a more direct avenue for addressing the problems in identity formation that are so frequently encountered with patients with anorexia nervosa. More than simply providing an opportunity for learning adaptive behaviors or for exploring and interpreting the structural and dynamic etiologies of core conflicts, the hypnotherapeutic approach described engages patients experientially in examining, exploring, modulating, and correcting these areas of difficulty. This experientially based use of hypnosis appears to be particularly important in dealing with arenas of structural defect and is also useful in circumventing the extreme defensive denial and control struggles that form the basis for resistance to both behavioral and psychodynamic approaches to psychotherapeutic intervention. For this reason, it appears to augment the patients' ability to use psychotherapy and benefit from treatment in a fashion that is generalized and maintained at a significant level of success.

REFERENCES

Ambrose, G., & Newbold, G. (1980). *A handbook of medical hypnosis*. London: Bailliere Tindall.

Barabasz, M. (2000). Hypnosis in the treatment of eating disorders. In L. Hornyak & J. Green (Eds.), *Healing from within: Hypnosis, imagery methods and women's health care*. Washington, DC: American Psychological Association.

Beaumont, P. J. V., & Abraham, S. F. (1983). Episodes of ravenous overeating or bulimia: Their occurrence in patients with anorexia nervosa and with other forms of disordered eating. In P. L. Darby, P. E. Garfinkel, D. M. Gamer, & D. V. Coscina (Eds.), *Anorexia nervosa: Recent developments in research* (pp. 149–157). New York: Alan R. Liss.

Beck, A. T., & Freeman, A. (1990). *Cognitive therapy of personality disorders*. New York: Guilford Press.

Brenman, M., & Gill, M. (1947). *Hypnotherapy*. Madison, CT: International Universities Press.

Craighead, L. W. (2002). Obesity and eating disorders. In M. M. Antony & D. H. Barlow (Eds.), *Handbook of assessment and treatment planning for psychological disorders* (pp. 300–340). New York: Guilford Press.

Crasilneck, H., & Hall, J. (1975). *Clinical hypnosis*. New York: Grune & Stratton.

Erickson, M., & Rossi, E. (1979). *Hypnotherapy: An exploratory casebook*. New York: Irvington Publishers.

Fairburn, C. G., Marcus, M. D., & Wilson, G. T. (1993). Cognitive behavior therapy for binge eating and bulimia nervosa: A comprehensive treatment manual. In C. G. Fairburn & G. T. Wilson (Eds.), *Binge eating: Nature, assessment and treatment* (pp. 361–404). New York: Guilford Press.

Fromm, E., & Nash, M. R. (1997). *Psychoanalysis and hypnosis*. Madison, CT: International Universities Press.

Gross, M. (1983). Hypnosis in the therapy of anorexia hysteria. *American Journal of Clinical Hypnosis, 26,* 175–181.

Hilgard, E. (1977). *Divided consciousness: Multiple controls in human thought and action*. New York: Wiley.

Hornyak, L. M. (1996). Hypnosis in the treatment of anorexia nervosa. In S. J. Lynn, I. Kirsch, & J. W. Rhue (Eds.), *Casebook of clinical hypnosis* (pp. 51–73). Washington, DC: American Psychological Association.

Janet, J. (1888). Un cas d'hysterie grave [A serious case of hysteria]. *Revue Scientifique, 1,* 616.

Janet, P. (1924). *The major symptoms of hysteria.* New York: Macmillan.

Janet, P. (1925). *Psychological healing* (Vol. 2). New York: Macmillan.

Kroger, W., & Fezler, W. (1976). *Hypnosis and behavior modification: Imagery conditioning.* Philadelphia: Lippincott Williams & Wilkins.

Lynn, S. J., & Kirsch, I. (2006). *Essentials of clinical hypnosis.* Washington, DC: American Psychological Association.

Lynn, S. J., Kirsch, I., Crowley, M., & Campion, A. (2006). Eating disorders and obesity. In S. J. Lynn & I. Kirsch (Eds.), *Essentials of clinical hypnosis: An evidence-based approach* (pp. 99–120). Washington, DC: American Psychological Association.

Lynn, S. J., Rhue, J. W., Kvaal, S., & Mare, C. (1993). The treatment of anorexia nervosa: A hypnosuggestive framework. *Contemporary Hypnosis, 10,* 73–80.

Russell, G. (1979). Bulimia nervosa: An ominous variant of anorexia nervosa. *Psychological Medicine, 9,* 429–448.

Spiegel, H., & Spiegel, D. (2004). *Trance and treatment: Clinical uses of hypnosis* (2nd ed.). New York: Basic Books.

Sullivan, P. F. (1995). Mortality rates in anorexia nervosa. *American Journal of Psychiatry, 152,* 1053–1054.

Thakur, K. (1980). Treatment of anorexia nervosa with hypnotherapy. In H. Wain (Ed.), *Clinical hypnosis in medicine* (pp. 446–493). Chicago: Yearbook.

Torem, M. (1987). Ego-state therapy for eating disorders. *American Journal of Clinical Hypnosis, 30,* 94–103.

Vanderlinden, J., & Vandereycken, W. (1988). The use of hypnotherapy in the treatment of eating disorders. *International Journal of Eating Disorders, 7,* 673–679.

Yapko, M. D. (1986). Hypnotic strategic interventions in Texas of anorexia nervosa. *American Journal of Clinical Hypnosis, 28,* 224–232.

19

CLINICAL HYPNOSIS WITH CHILDREN

JUDITH W. RHUE

Hypnosis with children holds the potential to benefit many young patients experiencing diverse physical and emotional problems. The therapeutic application of hypnosis calls on the skill, flexibility, imagination, and creativity of the practitioner to enter the world of the child, while assuming an accepting and guiding role. The ultimate goal of this endeavor is to empower the troubled child to deal more effectively with the emotional or physical concomitants of an identified situation or illness.

Despite its potential, widespread acceptance of potentially valuable hypnotherapeutic techniques is limited by a paucity of well-controlled research proving its effectiveness and by widely held myths and misconceptions embraced by the public and many health care professionals. Images from stage hypnosis or movies that portray hypnotized individuals as zombielike creatures controlled by the malevolent "hypnotist," as well as other popular negative stereotypes (e.g., people lose consciousness or fall asleep during hypnosis, hypnotizable people are gullible), no doubt deter many who could benefit from exploiting the potential value of hypnosis.

All clinical material has been disguised to protect patient confidentiality.

In this chapter, I delineate a far different picture of the status of hypnosis. I provide an overview of the history of hypnosis with children, discuss theoretical and measurement issues, review the clinical application of hypnosis to an array of childhood disorders, present case material, and address the available research, which will serve to counter popular stereotypes about hypnosis.

HISTORICAL PERSPECTIVES

Various forms of hypnosis with children date back to ancient times, and although no formal idea or measure of hypnotizability was recognized, the use of suggestion was documented in various ancient writings. In their influential book on hypnotherapy with children, Olness and Kohen (1996) noted that healing techniques based on faith and suggestion are described in both the Old and New Testaments of the Bible. They cited Mead's (1949) work in which she noted that in primitive cultures, children enter naturalistic "trance" states when participating in potentially painful rites or ceremonies. Mesmer, in the late 1700s, applied his theory of animal magnetism to some children he treated (Tinterow, 1970), as did John Elliotson, a physician who defended animal magnetism in England. The English surgeon James Braid, who coined the term *hypnosis*, observed that children were particularly sensitive to the procedure. In the late 1800s, Liebault and Bernheim commented on the ease of hypnotizing children and contended that children were able to experience *somnambulism*, the deepest level of experiencing hypnotic suggestion (Bramwell, (1903/1956).

More modern interest in using imaginative and hypnotic techniques with children developed in the 1960s and 1970s with the research and writings of icons in the field, including J. R. Hilgard (1970), Fromm (1972, 1979), Erickson (1958), Gardner (1974, 1977), Boswell (1962), and Singer (1973, 1974). Notably, J. R. Hilgard (1974, 1979) examined hypnotizability in children and documented the positive relation between childhood imaginative experiences and high hypnotic ability in adult life. She argued that children could readily use hypnosis because of its similarity to their natural behaviors. Gardner and Olness (1981; Olness & Gardner, 1988), and more recently Olness and Kohen (1996), coauthored comprehensive and scholarly books on research and clinical applications of hypnosis with children while also engaged in clinical practice and teaching hypnotic techniques for children in professional settings.

HYPNOTIC SUSCEPTIBILITY SCALES FOR CHILDREN

For the purposes of research, and in some cases clinical application, several hypnotic suggestibility scales for children were developed, beginning in the 1960s. Previous research had indicated that children, particularly those between

8 and 12 years of age, were more hypnotizable than adults (Hull, 1933; Messerschmidt, 1933), but methodological problems limited the validity of these findings (London, 1962). To better test children's hypnotic ability, London (1963) developed the Children's Hypnotic Susceptibility Scale in a two-part format paralleling that of the Stanford Hypnotic Susceptibility Scales, Forms A and B (Weitzenhoffer & Hilgard, 1959). Developed specifically for clinical use with children, the Stanford Hypnotic Susceptibility Scale for Children (Morgan & Hilgard, 1979) has only seven items and can be administered in approximately 20 minutes. Because the scale has problems discriminating moderately hypnotizable and highly hypnotizable children, Zeltzer and LeBaron (1984) modified the scale with mixed results (Plotnick, Payne, & O'Grady, 1989).

DEVELOPMENTAL AND THEORETICAL PERSPECTIVES

There is some consensus that children's hypnotic responsiveness is multifaceted and strongly tied to individual differences and developmental processes. Research using standardized scales of suggestibility indicates that children under age 3 exhibit little testable hypnotic ability, with age 4 often representing the lower boundary for testing. Beyond age 4, hypnotic ability, measured by standardized scales, increases throughout early and middle childhood, peaking at around the ages of 12 to 14. Thereafter, hypnotic ability declines somewhat over the course of adolescence, remains largely unchanged through midlife, and declines in older adulthood (Olness & Gardner, 1988).

Despite the lack of measurable hypnotic ability, clinical reports suggest that hypnotherapeutic procedures can be successfully applied with preschool children (Antitch, 1967; Cullen, 1958; Gardner, 1977; Kohen & Wynne, 1997; Kuttner, 1991; LaBaw, 1973). In attempting to explicate a hypnotic process for toddlers and preschool children, J. R. Hilgard and Morgan (1978) described a process of *protohypnosis*, in which the child is involved in external distraction, such as that from sounds or story, rather than internal distraction through self-controlled fantasy.

One view of younger children's hypnotic responsiveness posits it as qualitatively different from that of adults because until middle childhood children (a) do not understand complex, paradoxical hypnotic instructions; (b) are unable to produce self-directed, internal fantasy; and (c) often do not engage in eye closure or relaxation (Olness & Kohen, 1996). According to Piaget, children do not develop well-articulated cognitive schemas until around age 12 (Piaget & Inhelder, 1969). Prior to that age, they do not filter and critically evaluate information in the same way as do adults. However, this lack of criticality may also allow children the freedom to readily experience fantasy and suggested events, possibly explaining their greater hypnotic responsiveness.

Similarly, Cowles (1998) presented an existential–phenomenological model of children's hypnotic abilities based on their cognitive flexibility, uncritical thinking, and their freedom to experience alternative realities and "magical" phenomena. Similarly, Stevens-Guille and Boersma (1992) suggested that children who are deeply involved in hearing a fairy tale are experiencing hypnotic-like phenomena (in their terms, "trance") by virtue of their fixation of attention, the loosening of their usual frame of reference, and their relating the story to their own lives.

Vandenberg (1998) asserted that hypnotic responsivity does not attain a mature level similar to that of adults until late childhood and argued that clinical observations suggest that children, despite not understanding complex instructions, more easily engage in imaginative hypnotic suggestions than do adults. He hypothesized that children possess hypnotic abilities that may not be readily apparent because measures of hypnotic responsiveness rely on verbal skills not developed until age 4 or 5. Evidence for nonverbal precursors of hypnotic ability in early life includes reports that infants can be soothed and distracted during painful procedures by rocking, vocalization, and sounds. More recently, Vandenberg (2002) asserted that new measures, which take young children's developmental abilities into account, must be constructed to accurately assess their hypnotic ability.

In their research on the hypnotizability of children, Poulsen and Matthews (2003) investigated the relationship between waking suggestibility and hypnotizability in a small sample of child psychiatric patients and reported high correlations between nonhypnotic and hypnotic suggestibility. They interpreted their findings as supporting hypnotic responsiveness as falling on a continuum of suggestibility and noted that hypnotic susceptibility scales are valid and stable measures of imaginative suggestibility.

The current developmental and theoretical perspectives can be summarized, as follows:

1. Hypnotic ability peaks during childhood as measured by standardized scales.
2. The experience of hypnosis for young children differs qualitatively from that of adults.
3. Infants and preschool children may benefit from "hypnotic-like" or "protohypnotic" techniques, such as rocking, soothing sounds, and so forth.

INDUCTION CONSIDERATIONS WITH CHILDREN

The type of induction and suggestions used with children varies according to the age and personality of the child and calls into play the creativity and flexibility of the therapist in pursuing imaginative, creative, and often story-oriented hypnotherapeutic techniques. Infants and preverbal children often respond positively to sensorimotor approaches involving touch and body positioning (Hall, 1999). Young children often do not require relaxation to benefit from hypnotic procedures, and some actually prefer an active–alert form of hypnosis. Storytelling provides an excellent medium for the use of suggestions, analogies, and lessons in living, woven into the rhythmic fabric of the story (Rhue & Lynn, 1993).

I consider these approaches with children to be hypnotic in nature. As a rule, child hypnotherapy sidesteps the standard markers of a hypnotic induction, including direct suggestions for eye closure, relaxation, and sleepiness. Rather, visualization, empowerment symbols and images, and elements of cognitive and behavioral interventions can be played out, altered, and replayed in the nonthreatening and malleable format of hypnotic storytelling. In this manner, suggestions and metaphors are used in keeping with the child's naturally occurring use of make-believe and magical thinking.

Therapists who undertake hypnotherapy with children should approach the clinical setting with an appreciation for salient differences in the dynamics of hypnosis with adults and children and be prepared to interact with children in a spontaneous, flexible manner. Childhood through the preadolescent years is a period marked by imaginative involvement and pretend play, which may foster responsiveness to imaginative suggestions (E. R. Hilgard, 1981; Tellegen & Atkinson, 1976). Children may focus their attention and experience altered perceptions and heightened receptiveness to suggestions, even with eyes open and their bodies in motion.

CLINICAL APPLICATIONS

Clinical applications of hypnosis with children emerged in force in the 1970s, although many early reports involved case studies, or small controlled studies. Since then, the number of studies of clinical hypnosis has expanded, particularly with regard to medical conditions. Next, I review a number of current clinical applications of hypnotherapy with children, although my account is by no means exhaustive. Rather, I focus on seminal, innovative, and relatively recent studies in the clinical treatment of childhood disorders and medical conditions.

Pain Management

Acute Pain

Jones (1977) described a noncontrolled study of the use of hypnosis with a few children who underwent a difficult procedure for scoliosis. He reported that the children needed less anesthesia than usual and managed intraoperative tests successfully, although he provided no statistical evidence to support these claims. During the 1980s, researchers reported that they successfully applied hypnosis to reduce the pain of invasive medical procedures, including bone marrow aspirations and lumbar punctures (J. R. Hilgard & LeBaron, 1982; Kuttner, 1989; Zeltzer & LeBaron, 1982). Other hypnosis research with children during that decade focused on reducing pain from cancer and its treatment (J. R. Hilgard & LeBaron; Katz, Kellerman, & Ellenberg, 1987; Kuttner, Bowman, & Teasdale, 1988; LaClave & Blix, 1989; Olness, 1981; Wall & Womach, 1989; Zeltzer & LeBaron, 1982).

More recently, Liossi and Hatira (1999) conducted a randomized controlled study comparing hypnosis, cognitive–behavioral skills, and a no-treatment control group in reducing anxiety and depression in child and adolescent patients with cancer undergoing bone marrow aspirations. Although a local injection of lidocaine anaesthetizes the skin and tissues, it does not lessen the pain associated with the suctioning of the marrow. Patients receiving hypnosis and cognitive–behavioral strategies reported less pain and anxiety than patients in the control group, and patients receiving hypnosis reported less anxiety than those receiving cognitive–behavioral treatments. Hypnosis and cognitive–behavioral strategies were deemed viable treatments for preparing pediatric patients with cancer for bone marrow aspirations. The same researchers (Liossi & Hatira, 2003) conducted a randomized controlled study using hypnosis to reduce procedure-related pain in pediatric oncology patients. Patients were assigned to one of four groups in which standard medical treatment was accompanied by direct hypnosis, indirect hypnosis, attention control, or standard treatment alone. Direct and indirect hypnosis were equally effective, and both were more effective in reducing pain than the control groups.

To evaluate the reduction of pain and anxiety during a common radiologic procedure voiding cystourethrography (VCUG), researchers (Butler, Symons, Henderson, Shortliffe, & Spiegel, 2005) conducted another controlled randomized study, assigning children to receive either hypnosis or routine care. Hypnosis consisted of imagery-based self-hypnosis with the therapist present, whereas routine care consisted of a hospital-provided recreation therapy program and assistance during the procedure. The parents of children in the hypnosis group rated their children's experience as less traumatic, the staff rated the children as less distressed, and the procedure was rated as less difficult and time consuming, implying that hypnotic relaxation may improve care in children undergoing VCUG.

Chronic Pain

The use of hypnosis to treat chronic childhood pain has been described in books and numerous studies and articles over the past 15 years (Dinges et al., 1997; Lambert, 1999; Olness & Kohen, 1996; Walco, Varni, & Ilowite, 1992).

Anbar (2001) reported the resolution of functional abdominal pain (i.e., pain in the absence of an identifiable physiologic cause) in four of five pediatric patients after a single session of instruction in self-hypnosis. Zeltzer et al. (2002) examined the feasibility and acceptability of a combined acupuncture and hypnosis intervention for children experiencing a variety of illnesses causing chronic pain. The combined intervention proved highly acceptable to children and parents, and children became more positive about treatment. Both groups also reported improvements in pain ratings and pain-related dysfunction following treatment. Despite methodological limitations (e.g., lack of control group, no way to parcel out role of acupuncture vs. hypnosis, dependence on self report), this work points to the possible usefulness of combining hypnosis and acupuncture to treat chronic pain.

Asthmatic and Pulmonary Symptoms

Hackman, Stern, and Gershwin (2000) reviewed 20 studies that used hypnosis to treat asthma, although only 6 of the studies focused exclusively on pediatric patients. Studies were categorized on the basis of the degree of randomization and control. Kohen (1996) reported that 70% of children presenting with asthma attained more than 50% reduction in symptoms when treated with relaxation–mental imagery exercises in a self-hypnosis paradigm practiced at home. Ferreiro (1993) reported on hospital treatment of 50 children arriving at the hospital during acute asthma attacks and found that 80% required no medication after hypnosis and remained symptom free for 15 days, based on airway resistance measurements.

In another study, self-hypnosis was used to enhance a sense of self-control and mastery and reduce anxiety in 49 patients with cystic fibrosis who ranged in age from 7 to 49 (Anbar, 2000). Patients learned and used self-hypnosis for a variety of illness-related symptoms, suggesting that patients with cystic fibrosis may benefit from self-hypnosis. Anbar later used self-hypnosis as a complement to medical therapy in 254 pediatric patients at a pulmonary center. Although many of the findings were based on patient self-report, the overall level of improvement across the treated patients suggested the value of additional research. Most recently, Anbar and Hummell (2005) described the use of a teamwork approach to clinical hypnosis at a pediatric pulmonary center and discussed the successful implementation of the methods by varied professionals on a pulmonary team.

Emergency Room Medicine

Although hospitals and urgent care departments rarely provide researchers with the opportunity to conduct controlled hypnosis research with children, hypnotic procedures can be highly beneficial to young patients in these settings. Unfortunately, many physicians receive no training in hypnosis or its benefits during medical school and demean hypnosis as an alternative form of medicine or associate it with stage performances. Despite these barriers, some recognition of the usefulness of hypnosis in emergency medicine has emerged, as documented in case reports and articles in medical journals. Iserson (1999) cited four cases of pain from forearm fractures successfully reduced using hypnosis for analgesia, when no other form of pain medication was available. Iserson also suggested that there are a variety of situations in the emergency department where patients who are fearful or in pain could benefit from hypnotic procedures.

Migraine

Olness and Kohen (1996) reported that the prevalence of juvenile migraines ranges from 5% to 10% of children and stress the importance of careful diagnostic evaluation prior to any treatment intervention. Olness, MacDonald, and Uden (1987) conducted a randomized controlled study that compared hypnotherapy with propranolol and placebo for children with migraine. Results indicated that hypnotherapy surpassed the drug and placebo therapies in reducing migraine frequency. Several uncontrolled clinical studies have used self-hypnosis for headache pain with success (Labbe & Williamson, 1983; Werder & Sargent, 1984).

In a recent case report, hypnosis was used to treat stress-related migraine headaches experienced by a 9-year-old girl after she underwent a liver transplant and subsequently developed aplastic anemia (Kukuruzovic, 2004). She was treated with seven sessions of hypnotherapy over a 12-week period, with a focus on helping her to regain the perception of control over her body, particularly around a weekly change of the catheter-dressing site. By the last session, she reported she was migraine free for 9 weeks.

Tics

Some type of tic behavior is demonstrated by 25% of children; this reaches problematic levels in about 15% of children. Although clinicians and researchers have used hypnosis to treat tics for a number of years, many of the reports involve case studies with limited follow-up (Young, Montano, & Goldberg, 1991). Dillenburger and Keenan (2003), for example, reported the case of a 13-year-old girl who received a hypnotic induction to reduce tic suppression, allowing therapists to observe multiple tics, which had previously been difficult to evaluate. Hypnosis was also used to facilitate self-induced relaxation techniques and to institute competing responses when tics occurred as part of a comprehensive habit reversal program, which also included awareness training, self-monitoring, social support, and contingency management. Over 15 weeks of treatment, with parental monitoring at home, the child's tics were eliminated and remained absent, based on parental reports at an 18-month follow-up. However, because some children refrain from tics in the presence of therapists or researchers, evaluation and treatment can be difficult.

Warts

Over the past 60 years, hypnosis has been reported in numerous small and single case studies for the treatment of children's warts (Clawson & Swade, 1975; Surman, Gottlieb, & Hackett, 1972; Tasini & Hackett, 1977). Larger research studies involving both children and adults have examined the efficacy of hypnotherapy for treating warts, the role of placebo effects (Spanos, Stenstrom, & Johnston, 1988), level of hypnotizability (Chandrasena, 1982), and variations in patients' cognitive processes and expectations (Kirsch, 1985; Spanos, 1990).

Goldstein (2005) reported on an adolescent girl who was successfully treated with hypnosis on two separate occasions. When first seen, the patient had a 7-year history of plantar warts treated with topical agents, with a vacillating course of treatment. After three hypnotherapy sessions, the warts remitted, but 7 years later the patient reported an outbreak of warts on her fingers. After one session, the patient reported that the new warts disappeared, an observation confirmed by a dermatologist. Although a single case study, this report is noteworthy because it addresses the often-presented alternative hypotheses (i.e., spontaneous regression, expectation, high suggestibility) for apparently successful hypnotic treatment of warts. The long-standing nature of the plantar warts first treated seems to negate a spontaneous regression, and the fact that the patient exhibited low expectations and only adequate hypnotic ability reduces the viability of alternative explanations.

Vocal Cord Dysfunction

Anbar and Hehir (2000) used self-hypnosis with an 11-year-old boy in conjunction with a fiber-optic laryngoscopy to confirm a definitive diagnosis of vocal cord dysfunction (VCD). After first using self-hypnosis suggestions in place of a nasal anesthetic, the nasopharyngeal laryngoscope was inserted. Because of the difficulty of reproducing an attack in a controlled setting, hypnotic suggestions were used to provoke an attack, thus confirming the VCD symptoms during the laryngoscopy. Albeit a case study, this report represents the first description of hypnotic suggestion to verify the diagnosis of VCD.

Attention-Deficit/Hyperactivity Disorder

In a series of studies and reports, Barabasz and Barabasz (2000) and their colleagues reported on the use of Barabasz's *instant alert* hypnosis, also known as *instantaneous neuronal activation*, in conjunction with neurotherapy (i.e., brainwave/electroencephalogram [EEG] biofeedback) in treating children with attention-deficit/hyperactivity disorder (ADHD). *Neurotherapy*, which focuses on modifying the beta/theta brainwave ratio as the key to increasing attention, has emerged as an alternative habilitative ADHD treatment for cases in which stimulant or medication-based therapy is not appropriate. Under this treatment paradigm, the slower EEG theta waves, purportedly characteristic of poor attention control, are inhibited, whereas beta waves associated with learning and vigilance are increased through EEG biofeedback. In conjunction with neurotherapy, the authors used alert hypnosis to enhance the production of beta waves, as compared with neurotherapy alone, and found that children who received the combined treatment showed greater improvement than children treated with neurotherapy alone. Barabasz and colleagues have replicated the finding of improvement with combined treatment (Anderson, Barabasz, Barabasz, & Warner, 2000; Warner, Barabasz, & Barabasz, 2000), although both studies involved small numbers of patients who were treated by the same therapist and lacked adequate control groups. Clearly, additional research is warranted.

Habit, Behavioral, and Emotional Problems

Trichotillomania

Trichotillomania (TTM) is characterized by chronic hair pulling that results in hair loss and a sense of pleasure or tension release when pulling the hair. Hypnosis and hypnobehavioral techniques (i.e., combining relaxation with suggestions for behavior change) have been successfully used with children in a number of case studies (Cohen, Barzilai, & Lahat, 1999; Rowen, 1981; Zalsman, Hermesh, & Sever, 2001). To evaluate four different treatments (i.e., medication, hypnotherapy, punishment, and habit reversal) for TTM, Elliott and Fuqua (2002) had students rate the acceptability of the treatment modalities, while varying the age of the patient and the severity of her symptoms. All four interventions were rated as acceptable, but hypnosis and habit reversal were rated as more acceptable than punishment or medication. This study appears to be the first to systematically evaluate the acceptability of widely used treatments for trichotillomania.

Encopresis

Soiling is most frequently viewed socially as a problem after the age of 4, when most children have achieved success in toileting. However, because soiling problems may be related to constipation or other physical problems, a diagnostic workup should be conducted before the problem is viewed as primarily psychological in nature. With soiling problems that are long-standing, a multimodal approach involving hypnotherapy, behavior change techniques, medication monitored by a physician, and parent training may be most efficacious. Linden (2003) reported successfully treating a child with encopresis using "playful metaphors" as part of play therapy, with questionable similarity to more formal approaches.

Enuresis

Enuresis is a common problem that affects between 5 and 7 million children over age 5 in the United States. The disorder often reflects a maturational delay rather than a specific organic cause, which accounts for only about 5% of cases. Studies and case reports (Edwards & van derSpuy, 1985; Walker, Kenning, & Faust-Campanile, 1989) have cited the successful application of hypnosis, with treatment lasting from 4 to 20 weeks and follow-up visits scheduled for 6 months or 1 year. Kohen, Olness, Colwell, and Heimel (1984) reported data on over 250 children treated with hypnosis for enuresis, with 44% achieving complete dryness and 31% achieving significant improvement. Banerjee, Srivastav, and Palan (1993) compared imipramine with hypnotherapy and found that both treatments were equally successful within 3 months (72% vs. 75% dry); although at the 6-month follow-up, the hypnosis treatment group fared better (69% dry vs. 24% dry). Gottsegen (2003) reported four cases of one-session cures of nocturnal enuresis using hypnotic techniques, including "light trance," suggestions, and visualization.

Coping With Difficult Experiences

Children can use hypnotic-like techniques, including fantasy and imaginative involvement, to cope with unpleasant experiences (Kohen, 1986; Kuttner, 1989). Rhue and Lynn (1987) reported that many of the high fantasy-prone participants that they studied reported using fantasy and imaginative techniques to mentally isolate themselves from instances of physical and/or sexual abuse as children. Rhue and Lynn (1993) have described imagination-based techniques as therapeutic tools that may help young patients resolve the traumatic aftereffects of sexual abuse or traumatic loss.

Hypnosis has also been used successfully to treat children with sleeping problems (Ford, 1995; Hammond, 1990; Olness & Gardner, 1988; Wester & O'Grady, 1991), some of whom have experienced traumatic losses (Raphael, 1983; Raphael, Field, & Kvelde, 1980). Hawkins and Polemikos (2002) described a qualitative methodology they employed with a small group of children they taught to use self-hypnosis to manage their sleep difficulties.

The authors used children's self-reports, caregivers' reports, and a measure of sleep disturbance to conclude that self-hypnosis can treat children's sleep difficulties.

School Refusal

In an innovative study of hypnotherapy applied to school refusal, Aviv (2006) reported that 8 of 12 adolescents treated with self-hypnosis reinforced by cell phone at home, or on the way to school, maintained full-time school attendance, whereas 3 other children showed partial improvement.

Conversion Disorder

Case studies have documented the successful treatment of conversion disorders with hypnosis. Bloom (2001) cited two such case studies in which adolescents experienced paralysis. He highlighted the limitations of treating different individuals with conversion disorder with the same hypnotherapeutic approach, or what he called *reusability*. He emphasized the importance of the therapist focusing on the unique qualities and needs of each patient when formulating a hypnotherapeutic approach.

Dissociative Expression and Automatic Word Processing

Anbar (2001) described six patients (ages 12–21) treated with *automatic word processing*, a form of dissociation produced by hypnosis and computer technology. This treatment modality was developed to provide patients at a pulmonary care center with a forum for hypnotic expression leading to insights and therapeutic progress with respect to a variety of disease-associated symptoms and anxiety.

CLINICAL MATERIAL

Tommy, a Caucasian male of 13, was referred to a therapist by his family physician because of headaches and associated anxiety symptoms, first apparent approximately 10 months earlier. Tommy's parents had just finalized their divorce proceedings following a year of financial and emotional upheaval. Although his parents tried to minimize the repercussions to Tommy, he was unhappy about the divorce and continued to hope that his parents would reconcile. Tommy's physician completed an extensive physical workup that failed to discern any physical basis for the headaches. Referral to a neurologist and additional testing similarly produced no organic cause. Medication designed to reduce headache symptoms was the suggested treatment. Because both Tommy's mother and father were reluctant to begin a regime of medication, the primary care physician suggested that hypnotherapy might be helpful.

Approach to Therapy

The therapist's goal is to tailor therapy to the needs of the child, empowering the child through the intertwining of self-hypnosis, direct and indirect suggestion, and behavioral techniques. In concert with this approach, the initial visit "opens the door" for the therapy that follows and should be structured with care. To this end, I scheduled the initial visit at a time when both Tommy's parents were available. Although considerable disharmony existed between the parents, both were invested in helping Tommy adjust and move forward. They signed a release allowing the therapist to exchange information with the physician regarding Tommy's treatment, thus providing a team approach to his care. In the initial visit, I met first with Tommy, then with his parents, and terminated the visit with a brief meeting with all three to review the structure, techniques, and goals for therapy.

Initial Interview With Tommy

As is the case with many children and adolescents, Tommy was unsure of what would happen during therapy and what he was supposed to do. I explained that therapy is a partnership in which two people work together to solve a problem and asked Tommy whether he was willing to work with me. When he agreed, I described self-hypnosis as a skill he could learn to better manage his headaches by focusing his mind and his imagination. Tommy acknowledged that the only hypnosis he had seen was on TV where the hypnotized person did "stupid things like barking like a dog." He also expressed concern about "getting lost in it" and being unable to "get back." I reassured Tommy that he would not "get lost" any more than he did in the theater when he watched an absorbing movie, nor would he bark like a dog unless he wanted to, in which case he could do so without any self-hypnosis. However, like learning other skills, I told him it might come quickly or he might need practice. I also emphasized the responsibility that came with learning self-hypnosis, explaining that he could not "use it" on other people or try to teach it to other kids as a game. Together, we reviewed the therapy goals, confidentiality, and the fact that he would sometimes be meeting with his parents to help them understand and support his changes and learning. With Tommy's agreement, I asked him to begin by describing himself.

Tommy, a thin boy with dark hair and glasses, stated that he was "skinny," but "tougher and smarter" than people gave him credit for being. In describing his social and academic experiences, Tommy reported that, until this year, his grades ranged from A's to C's and that he never played sports but loved to play computer games, particularly military, Star Wars, and other strategy games. Tommy felt that he was "not very popular" with his peers, although he stated that he had one good friend. He believed that his dad was disappointed that he didn't play football or soccer and commented that his dad often told him to "shut down the computer, and stop playing those stupid games." As the discussion moved to the topic of his headaches and anxiety, Tommy reported that many of his headaches started when his parents argued, although now, merely thinking about his parents arguing could produce a headache. Tommy revealed that his headaches and anxiety got better when he lay down in his room with the door closed and listened to music.

When the headaches occurred during the school day, he would request to be sent home. Although the school was reluctant to excuse him, on two occasions when he was sent back to class, Tommy felt increasingly anxious, the headache progressed, and he vomited. Tommy's grades had declined sharply during the past 6 months, and he often felt too upset to study. As a stressor in addition to his parents' divorce proceedings, Tommy had begun middle school in the fall. Coming from a small elementary school, the middle school represented a dramatic change, integrating many students from diverse backgrounds, leaving Tommy feeling isolated. Some of the bullies around school made fun of his headaches, and Tommy wanted the headaches to stop.

I used terminology that reflected his interest in Star Wars and military strategy and which paralleled his way of describing things. I noted that we had already developed an alliance and had gathered information for a battle plan. I told him that during the next session we would lay out a strategy for battling the headaches. The idea that we would create a "battle plan" to "conquer" the headaches was intriguing, and Tommy expressed enthusiasm for "challenging" the headaches and "fighting them."

Initial Parent Visit

In the visit with Tommy's parents, I explained self-hypnotic techniques and how they could help Tommy control his headaches, also providing his parents with an overview of current clinical applications of hypnosis. Although Tommy would be seen individually, his parents would be updated at the end of every six sessions regarding self-hypnosis techniques, during which time I would enlist insight and feedback from them and provide suggestions for how they could facilitate Tommy's efforts.

Sessions 2 Through 6

Tommy identified school as the place where he felt most upset and anxious when a headache occurred. He hated leaving school but was afraid that if he stayed, he would vomit publicly again. I asked Tommy to close his eyes, visualize the headache, and describe its appearance, thus giving it form.

Tommy stated that the headache was short, round, and covered with tangled dark blue hair. It had a wide black mouth filled with razor-sharp teeth, and it was extremely cold. I suggested that Tommy freeze the image, immobilizing the headache, thus rendering it temporarily harmless. I then suggested that Tommy practice focusing his energy and strength, as the Jedi warriors from Star Wars were taught to do. With enough practice, a young warrior could call on "the Force" to defeat his enemies, wielding a light saber powered by the Force to defend and defeat with deadly accuracy and strength. Much of the session focused on building the image of a light saber, and when Tommy was able to do so, I asked him to practice developing the image of the light saber at home for a few minutes each day.

Over the next four sessions, Tommy continued to work on visualizing the light saber while feeling strong and calm. He practiced visualizing himself building guard towers to detect the onset of anxiety "attackers," allowing him to repel their assault and reinforce his feelings of calm and strength. I spent a few minutes of each session talking with Tommy about his computer games, his feelings about his parents, his headache symptoms, and school. Tommy reported that he rarely saw his parents argue anymore, although he continued to have two to three headaches per week, particularly as the time approached for him to spend the week with the other parent.

At the onset of a headache, Tommy began to use the self-hypnotic techniques he had learned, although he also still went to his room to lie down and listen to his music. He wanted to be able to control his headaches without leaving school or vomiting. By the sixth session, Tommy had stopped lying down when he felt headache symptoms, instead focusing his power through self-hypnosis. He reported less anxiety about the headaches and that the battle had turned in his favor.

At the end of the sixth session, I met with Tommy's parents to obtain their feedback and to update goals and plans for the remaining six sessions. Although meeting with parents may be controversial for some, this can be justifiable if the therapist does not reveal information from the child but rather solicits the parent's help and support by evaluating change to date, and focusing on what remains to be done. Tommy's parents felt that Tommy was making good progress based on his grades and the fact that he had fewer headaches and his mood had improved. I reviewed some of the techniques that Tommy would be practicing and encouraged his parents to continue to support his efforts.

Sessions 7 Through 12

I focused on helping Tommy develop the self-confidence and skill necessary to handle headache symptoms that might occur in school. With Tommy's input, we developed a "battle plan" for school that Tommy would implement at the first sign of a headache. He would begin by visualizing the image of the headache, then "freezing" it, and finally blasting it with the Force. Then, he was to think the words "calm" and "alert" while still maintaining attention in class. Tommy and I practiced this by me playing the part of the teacher and asking Tommy to solve math problems or answer history questions. At times, both Tommy and I would laugh but would then return to the scenario with seriousness. Despite some difficulty with dividing his attention, Tommy's sense of control and mastery increased.

When Tommy experienced some mild headache symptoms in school, he reported "blasting" them with enthusiasm. As school progressed, Tommy grew taller and heavier and appeared to cope well. He took an advanced computer course, in which he excelled, his grades improved, and he developed friendships. His headache and anxiety symptoms subsided, and he attended school regularly. Whether it was because of his physical or emotional maturation, the bullies left him alone. Tommy, his parents, and I agreed that the 12th session would be our termination point, although he could return to therapy if the headaches recurred.

Case Review and Issues

Tommy's case illustrates how a therapist can draw on events, activities, hobbies, images, and symbols to actively involve a child or young adolescent in therapy. Empowered through the use of an imagery-based self-hypnotic therapy, Tommy built confidence in his ability to cope with his headaches and anxiety. I felt that he needed to perceive control over some aspect of his life, making self-hypnotic techniques the vehicle of choice. Given the number of issues in his life that he could not control, using a more traditional, therapist-dominated hypnotherapy might have proved counterproductive by perpetuating a situation in which Tommy did not feel in control. No formal assessment of Tommy's hypnotic ability was performed, and I viewed it as an unimportant issue in this case, insofar as Tommy responded well to suggestions. Moreover, Tommy's love of strategy-based computer games suggested an ability to focus and become absorbed in vivid imagery.

The cooperation of Tommy's parents, and their willingness to put aside their personal issues and animosities, made the therapy go smoothly and increased the likelihood of success. Whereas some therapists do not have regular meetings with parents, I have found that building a positive relationship and using parental feedback proves helpful in therapy. Certainly, any progress that can be made in the therapy setting can be unraveled in moments by a threatened or disaffiliated parent. Therapists should avoid the role of mediator but attempt to be clear with all involved about the "ground rules" of therapy.

Although the door was left open for Tommy to return to therapy, no follow-up visit was scheduled, and on the basis of sporadic encounters with Tommy's parents, he remained headache-free and successful in school.

RESEARCH AND APPRAISAL

Over the past half century, interest in the use of hypnosis with children has widened. J. R. Hilgard's (1970, 1974) and Singer's (1973) writings on the antecedents of childhood hypnotizability and its relationship to creativity and imagination documented the pathways and correlates of childhood hypnotizability. London (1965) and Morgan and Hilgard (1978–1979) determined that hypnotizability emerges at ages 3 to 4, followed by increases up to around 12 years of age, with mild declines to around age 16 and relative stability thereafter.

Several books during the 1980s and 1990s addressed issues of hypnosis research with children and the clinical application of hypnosis to childhood disorders (Gardner & Olness, 1981; Kohen & Olness, 1993; Olness & Gardner, 1988; Olness & Kohen, 1996). Similarly, a number of edited hypnosis volumes (Lynn, Kirsch, & Rhue, 1996; Rhue, Lynn, & Kirsch, 1993; Wester & O'Grady, 1991; Wester & Smith, 1984) addressed the application of hypnosis to childhood problems.

Recent years have witnessed a slight upswing in the number of research articles published in the arena of hypnosis with children, although many of these are case studies or studies that lack control groups or adequate numbers of participants. Milling and Costantino (2000) described and appraised the controlled studies of child clinical hypnosis in a number of areas. Their mission was threefold: (a) to summarize the findings of controlled outcome studies of child clinical hypnosis, (b) to assess the methodological strengths and weaknesses of the small body of research, and (c) to evaluate the child clinical hypnosis outcome studies against criteria advanced by Chambless and Hollon (1998) for empirically supported therapies (ESTs).

To meet the third criteria, and be designated efficacious, there must be at least two between-group design experiments conducted by at least two different investigative teams, demonstrating that the intervention is superior to a no-treatment control condition, an alternative treatment, or a placebo, or that the treatment is as effective as a previously established treatment. With only one between-group design study that meets these criteria, a treatment may be deemed possibly efficacious. With two different teams providing evidence of results superior to a placebo or to a treatment of previously established efficacy in studies that control for nonspecific processes, a treatment may be deemed efficacious and specific. Milling and Costantino (2000) reviewed studies that used a between-subjects design with a hypnotic intervention compared with at least one alternative hypnotic or nonhypnotic intervention and/or a placebo, attention, or no-treatment control condition with all participants no older than 18 years of age. The authors grouped the surveyed studies into five content areas: learning problems, basic physiological processes, general medical problems, nausea and emesis from chemotherapy, and acute pain.

On the basis of their assessment of the small number of studies that met the criteria to be included in the review, the authors concluded that child clinical hypnosis research was in an early stage of development with few controlled studies that included basic research prerequisites such as random assignment. Further, they noted that the available research focused on hypnotic interventions to treat acute pain or the side effects of chemotherapy, with no controlled hypnosis research for children's emotional or behavioral problems. The authors also observed that the child clinical hypnosis research has not developed sufficiently to conclude that any child hypnosis intervention qualifies as efficacious or efficacious and specific on the basis of EST criteria. Finally, the lack of a treatment manual, or an equivalent, to structure treatment implementation prohibits independent replication and fails to meet the criteria for qualifying for any kind of EST status. The authors advocate for experimental rigor and careful documentation of procedures.

Certainly, the clinical literature on hypnosis with children reflects many attempts in good faith to describe case interventions with a variety of disorders and group data from hypnotic interventions, particularly with patients undergoing pain and chemotherapy. Unfortunately, even the positive outcomes reported from many of these studies are inadequate to validate the status of an empirically established treatment using the current standards. It remains a challenge to the hypnosis researchers working with child populations to design and administer research protocols that document the efficacy of hypnotic interventions.

CONCLUSION

Hypnosis holds the potential to benefit many children who experience a spectrum of physical and emotional disorders. It appears that the hypnotic responsiveness of children is multi-faceted and that developmental processes occurring during childhood influence its manifestation. Induction techniques vary with regard to the developmental level of the individual child and call on the skill, flexibility, imagination, and creativity of the therapist. Clinical reports bear witness to the successful application of hypnotherapeutic procedures even with young children where sensorimotor or story-oriented hypnotherapeutic techniques are used.

Successful applications of hypnotherapeutic interventions include those dealing with pain management, asthma treatment, migraine headache, and emergency room medicine, as well as a variety of behavioral and emotional problems. Although research articles in the arena of hypnosis with children have increased in recent years, many of these are case studies or studies lacking control groups, sufficient numbers of participants, and follow-ups. In order for hypnotherapy with children to gain greater acceptance and visibility, more rigorous experimental design and documentation is vital in future research.

REFERENCES

Anbar, R. D. (2000). Self-hypnosis for patients with cystic fibrosis. *Pediatric Pulmonology, 30,* 461–465.

Anbar, R. D. (2001). Self-hypnosis for the treatment of functional abdominal pain in childhood. *Clinical Pediatrics, 40,* 447–451.

Anbar, R. D., & Hehir, D. A. (2000). Hypnosis as a diagnostic modality for vocal cord dysfunction. *Pediatrics, 106,* e81.

Anbar, R. D., & Hummel, K. E. (2005). Teamwork approach to clinical hypnosis at a pediatric pulmonary center. *American Journal of Clinical Hypnosis, 48,* 45–49.

Anderson, K., Barabasz, M., Barabasz, A., & Warner, D. (2000). The efficacy of Barabasz's instant alert hypnosis in the treatment of ADHD with neurotherapy. *Child Study Journal, 30,* 51–62.

Antitch, J. L. (1967). The use of hypnosis in pediatric anesthesia. *Journal of the American Society of Psychosomatic Dentistry & Medicine, 14,* 70–74.

Aviv, A. (2006). Tele-hypnosis in the treatment of adolescent school refusal. *American Journal of Clinical Hypnosis, 49,* 31–40.

Banerjee, S., Srivastav, A., & Palan, B. M. (1993). Hypnosis and self-hypnosis in the management of nocturnal enuresis a comparative study with imipramine therapy. *American Journal of Clinical Hypnosis, 36,* 113–119.

Barabasz, A., & Barabasz, M. (2000). Treating ADHD with hypnosis and neurotherapy. *Child Study Journal, 30,* 25–42.

Bloom, P. B. (2001). Treating adolescent conversion disorders: Are hypnotic techniques reusable? *The International Journal of Clinical and Experimental Hypnosis, 49,* 243–265.

Boswell, L. K. (1962). Pediatric hypnosis. *British Journal of Medical Hypnotism, 13,* 4–11.

Bramwell, J. M. (1956). *Hypnotism: Its history, practice and theory.* New York: Julian Press. (Original work published 1903)

Butler, L. D., Symons, B. K., Henderson, S. L., Shortliffe, L. D., & Spiegel, D. (2005). Hypnosis reduces distress and duration of an invasive medical procedure for children. *Pediatrics, 115,* 77–85.

Chambless, D. L., & Hollon, S. D. (1998). Defining empirically supported therapies. *Journal of Consulting and Clinical Psychology, 66,* 7–18.

Chandrasena, R. (1982). Hypnosis in the treatment of viral warts. *Psychiatric Journal of the University of Ottawa, 7,* 135–137.

Clawson, T. A., Jr., & Swade, R. H. (1975). The hypnotic control of blood flow and pain: The cure of warts and the potential for the use of hypnosis in the treatment of cancer. *American Journal of Clinical Hypnosis, 17,* 160–169.

Cohen, H. A., Barzilai, A., & Lahat, E. (1999). Hypnotherapy: An effective treatment modality for trichotillomania. *Acta Paediatrica, 88,* 407–410.

Cowles, R. S. (1998). The magic of hypnosis: Is it child's play? *Journal of Psychology: Interdisciplinary and Applied, 132,* 357–366.

Cullen, J. (1958). The breakdown of perceptual skills in neurosis and psychosis. *Bulletin of British Psychological Society, 36,* 34.

Dillenburger, K., & Keenan, M. (2003). Using hypnosis to facilitate direct observation of multiple tics and self-monitoring in a typically developing teenager. *Behavior Therapy, 34,* 117–125.

Dinges, D. F., Whitehouse, W. G., Orne, E. C., Bloom, P. B., Carlin, M. M., Bauer, N. K., et al. (1997). Self-hypnosis training as an adjunctive treatment in the management of pain associated with sickle cell disease. *International Journal of Clinical and Experimental Hypnosis, 45,* 417–432.

Edwards, S. D., & van derSpuy, H. I. (1985). Hypnotherapy as a treatment for enuresis. *Journal of Child Psychology and Psychiatry, 26,* 161–170.

Elliott, A. J., & Fuqua, R. W. (2002). Acceptability of treatments for trichotillomania: Effects of age severity. *Behavior Modification, 26,* 378–399.

Erickson, M. H. (1958). Pediatric hypnotherapy. *American Journal of Clinical Hypnosis, 1,* 25–29.

Ferreiro, O. (1993). Hypnosis—its use in acute attacks of bronchial asthma. *Hypnosis, 20,* 236.

Ford, R. (1995). Hypnotic treatment of a sleeping problem in an 11-year-old boy. *Contemporary Hypnosis, 12,* 201–206.

Fromm, E. (1972). Ego activity and ego passivity in hypnosis. *International Journal of Clinical and Experimental Hypnosis, 20,* 238–251.

Fromm, E. (1979). The nature of hypnosis and other altered states of consciousness: An ego-psychological theory. In E. Fromm & R. E. Shor (Eds.), *Hypnosis: Developments in research and new perspectives* (2nd ed., pp. 81–103). Hawthorne, NY: Aldine.

Gardner, G. G. (1974). Hypnosis with children. *International Journal of Clinical and Experimental Hypnosis, 22,* 20–38.

Gardner, G. G. (1977). Hypnosis with infants and preschool children. *American Journal of Clinical Hypnosis, 19,* 158–162.

Gardner, G. G., & Olness, K. (1981). *Hypnosis and hypnotherapy with children.* Orlando, FL: Grune & Stratton.

Goldstein, R. H. (2005). Successful repeated hypnotic treatment of warts in the same individual: A case report. *American Journal of Clinical Hypnosis, 47,* 259–264.

Gottsegen, D. N. (2003). Curing bedwetting on the spot: A review of one-session cures. *Clinical Pediatrics, 42,* 273–275.

Hackman, R. M., Stern, J. S., & Gershwin, M. E. (2000). Hypnosis and asthma: A critical review. *Journal of Asthma, 37,* 1–15.

Hall, H. (1999). Hypnosis and pediatrics. In R. Temes (Ed.), *Medical hypnosis: An introduction and clinical guide* (pp. 79–93). New York: Churchill Livingstone.

Hammond, D. C. (1990). *Handbook of hypnotic suggestions and metaphors.* New York: The American Society of Clinical Hypnosis.

Hawkins, P., & Polemikos, N. (2002). Hypnosis treatment of sleeping problems in children experiencing loss. *Contemporary Hypnosis, 19,* 18–24.

Hilgard, E. R. (1981). Imagery and imagination in American psychology. *Journal of Mental Imagery, 5,* 5–65.

Hilgard, J. R. (1970). *Personality and hypnosis: A study of imaginative involvement.* Chicago: University of Chicago Press.

Hilgard, J. R. (1974). Imaginative involvement: Some characteristics of the highly hypnotizable and the nonhypnotizable. *International Journal of Clinical and Experimental Hypnosis, 22,* 138–156.

Hilgard, J. R. (1979). *Personality and hypnosis: A study of imaginative involvement* (2nd ed.). Chicago: University of Chicago Press.

Hilgard, J. R., & LeBaron, S. (1982). Relief of anxiety of pain in children and adolescents with cancer: Quantitative measures and clinical observations. *International Journal of Clinical and Experimental Hypnosis, 30,* 417–442.

Hilgard, J. R., & Morgan, A. (1978). Treatment of anxiety and pain in childhood cancer through hypnosis. In F. H. Frankel & H. S. Zamanskey (Eds.), *Hypnosis at its bicentennial: Selected papers.* New York: Plenum Press.

Hull, C. L. (1933). *Hypnosis and suggestibility.* Oxford, England: Appleton-Century-Crofts.

Iserson, K. V. (1999). Hypnosis for pediatric fracture reduction. *The Journal of Emergency Medicine, 17,* 53–56.

Jones, C. W. (1977). Hypnosis and spinal fusion by Harrington instrumentation. *American Journal of Clinical Hypnosis, 19,* 155–157.

Katz, E. R., Kellerman, J., & Ellenberg, L. (1987). Hypnosis in the reduction of acute pain and distress in children with cancer. *Journal of Pediatric Psychology, 12,* 379–394.

Kirsch, I. (1985). Response expectancy as a determinant of experience and behavior. *American Psychologist, 40,* 1189–1202.

Kohen, D. P. (1986). Application of relaxation/mental imagery (self-hypnosis) in pediatric emergencies. *International Journal of Clinical and Experimental Hypnosis, 34,* 283–329.

Kohen, D. P. (1996). Relaxation/mental imagery (self-hypnosis) for childhood asthma: Behavioral outcomes in a prospective, controlled study. *Australian Journal of Clinical and Experimental Hypnosis, 24,* 12.

Kohen, D. P., & Olness, K. (1993). Hypnotherapy with children. In J. W. Rhue, S. J. Lynn, & I. Kirsch (Eds.), *Handbook of clinical hypnosis* (pp. 357–381). Washington, DC: American Psychological Association.

Kohen, D. P., Olness, K. N., Colwell, S. O., & Heimel, A. (1984). The use of relaxation–mental imagery (self-hypnosis) in the management of 505 pediatric behavioral encounters. *Journal of Developmental Behavioral Pediatrics, 5,* 21–25.

Kohen, D. P., & Wynne, E. (1997). Applying hypnosis in a preschool family asthma education program: Uses of storytelling, imagery, and relaxation. *American Journal of Clinical Hypnosis, 39,* 169–181.

Kukuruzovic, R. (2004). Hypnosis in the treatment of migraine. *Australian Journal of Clinical and Experimental Hypnosis, 32,* 53–61.

Kuttner, L. (1989). Management of young children's acute pain and anxiety during invasive medical procedures. *Pediatrician, 16,* 39–44.

Kuttner, L. (1991). Special considerations for using hypnosis with young children. In W. C. Wester II & D. J. O'Grady (Eds.), *Clinical hypnosis with children* (pp. 41–49). Philadelphia: Brunner/Mazel.

Kuttner, L., Bowman, M., & Teasdale, M. (1988). Psychological treatment of distress, pain, and anxiety for young children with cancer. *Journal of Developmental & Behavioral Pediatrics, 9,* 374–381.

LaBaw, W. L. (1973). Adjunctive trance therapy with severely burned children. *International Journal of Child Psychotherapy, 2,* 80–92.

Labbe, E., & Williamson, D. A. (1983). Temperature, biofeedback in the treatment of children with migraine headaches. *Journal of Pediatric Psychology, 8,* 317–326.

LaClave, L. J., & Blix, S. (1989). Hypnosis in the management of symptoms in a young girl with malignant astrocytoma: A challenge to the therapist. *International Journal of Clinical and Experimental Hypnosis, 37,* 6–14.

Lambert, S. A. (1999). Distraction, imagery, and hypnosis: Techniques for management of children's pain. *Journal of Child and Family Nursing, 2,* 5–15.

Linden, J. H. (2003). Playful metaphors. *American Journal of Clinical Hypnosis, 45,* 245–250.

Liossi, C., & Hatira, P. (1999). Clinical hypnosis versus cognitive behavioral training for pain management with pediatric cancer patients undergoing bone marrow aspirations. *The International Journal of Clinical and Experimental Hypnosis, 47,* 104–116.

Liossi, C., & Hatira, P. (2003). Clinical hypnosis in the alleviation of procedure-related pain in pediatric oncology patients. *The International Journal of Clinical and Experimental Hypnosis, 51,* 4–28.

London, P. (1962). Hypnosis in children: An experimental approach. *International Journal of Clinical and Experimental Hypnosis, 10,* 79–91.

London, P. (1963). *Children's Hypnotic Susceptibility Scale*. Palo Alto, CA: Consulting Psychologists Press.

London, P. (1965). Developmental experiments in hypnosis. *Journal of Projective Techniques and Personality Assessment, 29*, 189–199.

Lynn, S. J., Kirsch, I., & Rhue, J. W. (1996). *Casebook of clinical hypnosis*. Washington, DC: American Psychological Association.

Mead, M. (1949). *Male and female: A study of the sexes in a changing world*. New York: Morrow.

Messerschmidt, R. (1933). The suggestibility of boys and girls between the ages of six and sixteen years. *Journal of Genetic Psychology, 43*, 422–437.

Milling, L. S., & Costantino, C. A. (2000). Clinical hypnosis with children: First steps toward empirical support. *International Journal of Clinical and Experimental Hypnosis, 48*, 113–137.

Morgan, A. H., & Hilgard, J. R. (1978–1979). The Stanford Hypnotic Clinical Scale for Children. *American Journal of Clinical Hypnosis, 21*, 148–169.

Olness, K. (1981). Imagery (self-hypnosis) as adjunct therapy in childhood cancer: Clinical experiences with 25 patients. *The American Journal of Pediatric Hematology/Oncology, 3*, 313–321.

Olness, K., & Gardner, G. G. (1988). *Hypnosis and hypnotherapy with children* (2nd ed.). San Diego, CA: Harcourt Brace Jovanovich.

Olness, K., & Kohen, D. P. (1996). *Hypnosis and hypnotherapy with children*. New York: Guilford Press.

Olness, K., MacDonald, J., & Uden, D. (1987). Prospective study comparing propranolol, placebo, and hypnosis in the management of juvenile migraine. *Pediatrics, 79*, 593–597.

Piaget, J., & Inhelder, B. (1969). *The development of physical number concepts in children: Maintenance and atomism*. Oxford, England: Ernst Klett.

Plotnick, A. B., Payne, O. A., & O'Grady, D. J. (1991). The Stanford Hypnotic Clinical Scale for Children—Revised: An evaluation. *Contemporary Hypnosis, 8*, 33–49.

Poulsen, B. C., & Matthews, W. J. (2003). Correlates of imaginative and hypnotic suggestibility in children. *Contemporary Hypnosis, 20*, 198–208.

Raphael, B. (1983). *The anatomy of bereavement*. New York: Basic Books.

Raphael, B., Field, J., & Kvelde, H. (1980). Childhood bereavement: A prospective study as a possible prelude to future prevention intervention. In C. Chiland (Ed.), *Yearbook of the International Association for Child and Adolescent Psychiatry and Allied Professions* (Vol. 6). New York: Wiley.

Rhue, J. W., & Lynn, S. J. (1987). Fantasy proneness and psychopathology. *Journal of Personality and Social Psychology, 53*, 327–336.

Rhue, J. W., Lynn, S. J., & Kirsch, I. (Eds.). (1993). *Handbook of clinical hypnosis*. Washington, DC: American Psychological Association.

Rowen, R. (1981). Hypnotic age regression in the treatment of a self-destructive habit: Trichotillomania. *American Journal of Clinical Hypnosis, 23,* 195–197.

Singer, J. L. (1973). *The child's world of make-believe: Experimental studies of imaginative play.* Oxford, England: Academic Press.

Singer, J. L. (1974). Daydreaming and the stream of thought. *American Scientist, 62,* 417–425.

Spanos, N. P., Stenstrom, R. J., & Johnston, J. C. (1988). Hypnosis, suggestion, and placebo in the treatment of warts. *Psychosomatic Medicine, 50,* 245–260.

Spanos, N. P., Williams, W., & Gwynn, M. I. (1990). Effects of hypnotic placebo and salicylic acid treatments on wart regression. *Psychosomatic Medicine, 52,* 109–114.

Stevens-Guille, M. E., & Boersma, F. J. (1992). Fairy tales as a trance experience: Possible therapeutic uses. *American Journal of Clinical Hypnosis, 34,* 245–254.

Surman, O. S., Gottlieb, S. K., & Hackett, T. P. (1972). Hypnotic treatment of a child with warts. *American Journal of Clinical Hypnosis, 15,* 12–14.

Tasini, M. F., & Hackett, T. P. (1977). Hypnosis in the treatment of warts in immuno-deficient children. *American Journal of Clinical Hypnosis, 19,* 1052–1054.

Tellegen, A., & Atkinson, G. (1976). Complexity and measurement of hypnotic susceptibility: A comment on Coe and Sarbin's alternative interpretation. *Journal of Personality and Social Psychology, 33,* 142–148.

Tinterow, M. M. (1970). *Foundations of hypnosis: From Mesmer to Freud.* Oxford, England: Charles C Thomas.

Vandenberg, B. (1998). Infant communication of the development of hypnotic responsivity. *The International Journal of Clinical and Experimental Hypnosis, 46,* 334–350.

Vandenberg, B. (2002). Hypnotic responsivity from a developmental perspective: Insights from young children. *The International Journal of Clinical and Experimental Hypnosis, 50,* 229–247.

Walco, G. A., Varni, J. W., & Ilowite, N. T. (1992). Cognitive–behavioural pain management in children with juvenile rheumatoid arthritis. *Paediatrics, 89,* 1075–1079.

Walker, C. E., Kenning, M., & Faust-Campanile, J. (1989). Encopresis and enuresis. In E. J. Marsh & R. A. Barkley (Eds.), *Treatment of childhood disorders.* New York: Guilford Press.

Wall, V. J., & Womack, W. (1989). Hypnotic versus cognitive strategies for alleviation of procedural distress in pediatric oncology patients. *American Journal of Clinical Hypnosis, 31,* 181–191.

Warner, D., Barabasz, A., & Barabasz, M. (2000). The efficacy of Barabasz's alert hypnosis and neurotherapy on attentiveness, impulsivity, and hyperactivity in children with ADHD. *Child Study Journal, 30,* 43–49.

Weitzenhoffer, A. M., & Hilgard, E. R. (1959). *Stanford Hypnotic Susceptibility Scale, Forms A and B.* Palo Alto, CA: Consulting Psychologists Press.

Werder, D. S., & Sargent, J. D. (1984). A study of childhood headache using biofeedback as a treatment alternative. *Headache, 24*, 122–126.

Wester, W., & O'Grady, D. J. (1991). *Clinical hypnosis with children.* New York: Brunner/Mazel.

Wester, W., & Smith, A. (Eds.). (1984). *Clinical hypnosis: A multidisciplinary approach.* Philadelphia: Lippincott Williams & Wilkins.

Young, M. H., Montano, R. J., & Goldberg, R. (1991). Self-hypnosis, sensory cueing, and response prevention: Decreasing anxiety and improving written output of a preadolescent with learning disabilities. *American Journal of Clinical Hypnosis, 34*, 129–136.

Zalsman, G., Hermesh, H., Sever, J. (2001). Hypnotherapy in adolescents with trichotillomania: Three cases. *American Journal of Hypnosis, 44*, 63–68.

Zeltzer, L., & LeBaron, S. (1982). Hypnosis and nonhypnotic techniques for reduction of pain and anxiety during painful procedures in children and adolescents with cancer. *Journal of Pediatrics, 101*, 1032–1035.

Zeltzer, L., & LeBaron, S. (1984). Assessment of acute pain and anxiety in children and adolescents by self-reports, observer reports, and a behavior checklist. *Journal of Consulting and Clinical Psychology, 52*, 729–738.

Zeltzer, L., Tsao, J. C. I., Stelling, C., Powers, M., Levy, S., & Waterhouse, M. (2002). A Phase I study on the feasibility and acceptability of an acupuncture/hypnosis intervention for chronic pediatric pain. *Journal of Pain and Symptom Management, 24*, 437–446.

20

WHEN TWO IS BETTER THAN ONE: HYPNOSIS WITH COUPLES

STEPHEN KAHN

Using hypnosis with couples is a relatively new application that has grown considerably in the last 10 years and is one that can be effectively implemented with many family therapy approaches. The model I present incorporates elements of three therapeutic approaches: systemic, cognitive–behavioral, and family of origin dynamic work. More specifically, it is rooted in a systems perspective, uses some cognitive–behavioral techniques, and incorporates family of origin issues (i.e., dynamics from childhood) as they impinge on the creation and maintenance of symptoms. Pinsof (1995) advocated a similar integrative approach to psychotherapy beginning with immediate behavioral work, moving to systemic approaches, and finally contending with family of origin concerns, if the latter is required. His approach resembles the three-stage model outlined next, although Pinsof does not use hypnosis in treatment.

To introduce this model, I briefly review the relevant approaches and discuss the specific role of hypnosis in couples therapy. I then delineate a stress model approach to understanding relationship dynamics. A composite

---

All clinical material has been disguised to protect patient confidentiality.

case study illustrates how the model can be applied in clinical practice. I close with a review of research that affects this work.

THREE APPROACHES TO TREATMENT

Using a *systemic* approach with couples involves viewing the couple (and/or the family) as a total and open system, with each member being inter-related. Positive and negative behaviors are the outcome of their interactions. Thus, blame cannot be assigned to a particular individual, because each participant is part of the system and therefore part of the problem. A couple's level of function is approached by viewing symptoms as part of a system in which normative life transitions and adverse life events create dysfunctional interaction patterns. Symptoms cluster around the poles of enmeshed versus disengaged, maladaptive versus adaptive coping, and flexibility versus stability. When either extreme of these dyadic poles dominates, dysfunction occurs. Symptoms are ameliorated through altering the system's structure, increasing appropriate boundaries, and clarifying and changing reinforcement patterns to engender new outcomes (Walsh, 2002).

Behavioral and *cognitive–behavioral* approaches are also used in hypnosis with couples. Misplaced attention and communication deficits create symptoms that can be ameliorated through couple skills training and alternative reinforcement strategies. Dysfunctional couple systems are conceptualized as resulting from stressful life events and poor coping skills. Adaptive changes in the system are achieved through altering a couple's coping strategies, exchanging information, and enhancing positive personality characteristics that aid adaptation.

Family of origin approaches view unresolved issues in the individual's original family (i.e., from childhood) as related to current symptoms. To grow beyond symptoms, it becomes necessary to complete developmental tasks that enhance the trust and nurturance necessary for bonding and individuation, promoting movement toward a highly functioning, fully differentiated couple (Bowen, 1978). Treatment resolves early conflicts and losses through insight into, and empathy for, historical struggles.

WHY USE HYPNOSIS WITH COUPLES?

Using hypnosis with couples has distinct advantages. The hypnotic relationship heightens the interaction, facilitates the therapeutic alliance, deepens meaning, and enhances outcome for the couple, just as it does in individual therapy. In addition, hypnosis facilitates overcoming resistances and providing greater freedom for the creative unconscious. More specifically, hypnotic techniques such as age regression, hypnotic imagery, time distortion, dissociation, and archaic involvement (i.e., transference) can be effectively used to assist couples.

Primitive and deeply hurtful fighting that couples engage in may be conceptualized as a form of spontaneous *age regression,* in which adults behave as if they were children. Mature adults often devolve into squabbling children in a marital skirmish, even in an office setting. Hypnosis uses age regression to manage primitive emotions and create a deeper interpersonal connection with a constructive interdependence. The heightened attention that hypnosis fosters can assist partners in focusing on adaptive cognitions, as well as pinpointing emotions that partners elicit in one another.

Hypnotic imagery that taps unconscious processes and resources can generate new perspectives and interpersonal connections, transforming negative images of partners into more positive images. Primitive images formed during childhood, termed *imagoes* by Hendrix (1995), can be more successfully managed and manipulated through hypnosis. Hypnotic rehearsal and posthypnotic suggestion (PHS) can aid couples in completing homework assignments and generalizing treatment gains beyond the session. Rehearsing a different, more positive reaction to one's partner in response to old triggers and using PHS can greatly reduce quarrelling.

The following hypnotic phenomena can be used specifically to enhance couples' ability to internalize new perspectives: (a) *Time distortion* can deepen a couple's connection (i.e., by creating a long-standing, stable connectedness) and decrease the pain from recent fighting (i.e., by relegating it to the distant past); (b) *dissociation* can generate distance from the usual triggers that create conflict, helping couples to observe rather than become bitterly entangled; (c) *negative hallucination* can eliminate triggers of negative responses (e.g., if irritating facial expressions are cause for battle, negative hallucination can attenuate the problem); (d) enhanced *affect availability* can promote emotional expressiveness, awareness of feelings, and the availability of positive relationship memories; and (e) *archaic involvement,* or transference, along with rapport and mutuality, can fortify the therapy alliance, decrease resistance, and enhance cooperation.

Although this chapter focuses on a traditional heterosexual couple, the approach described herein also can be used with gay and lesbian couples. This approach is not recommended for physically violent couples or couples in which one or both partners are severely disturbed. As with most other therapeutic interventions, if couples have been estranged for a significant period of time and there is little positive affect or communication, the probability of success is minimized. Accordingly, the earlier in the relationship that interventions are implemented, the greater the likelihood of a favorable outcome.

STRESS AND COUPLES: THE MODEL

This model delineates a specific kind of stress, *co-stress*, which affects many contemporary couples, and outlines interventions for both stress and co-stress. Using this model, I describe how relationships function, how they can break down, and how hypnosis can be used to ameliorate relationship problems. The theory is taken from the literature on hardiness and stress management, particularly the role of stress and its consequences (Kobasa, 1979; Kobasa, Maddi, & Kahn, 1982; Maddi, Kahn, & Maddi, 1998), but it is adapted to couples (see Figure 20.1).

Let us briefly look at stress on the individual level. Individual stress impinges on everyone in different forms (Antonovsky, 1979; Kobasa, Maddi, & Kahn, 1982). As society and social roles have increased in complexity, stress has increased apace. Stressors can be large, small, acute, or chronic in nature, but they clearly affect individuals' quality of life and, consequently, the life of the couple. As can be seen in Figure 20.1, using terms borrowed from physics, stressors lead to *strain* (i.e., weakening of the object's cohesion), which over time leads to some type of *breakdown* (i.e., destruction of basic structure), such as physical illness, psychological dysfunction, or both.

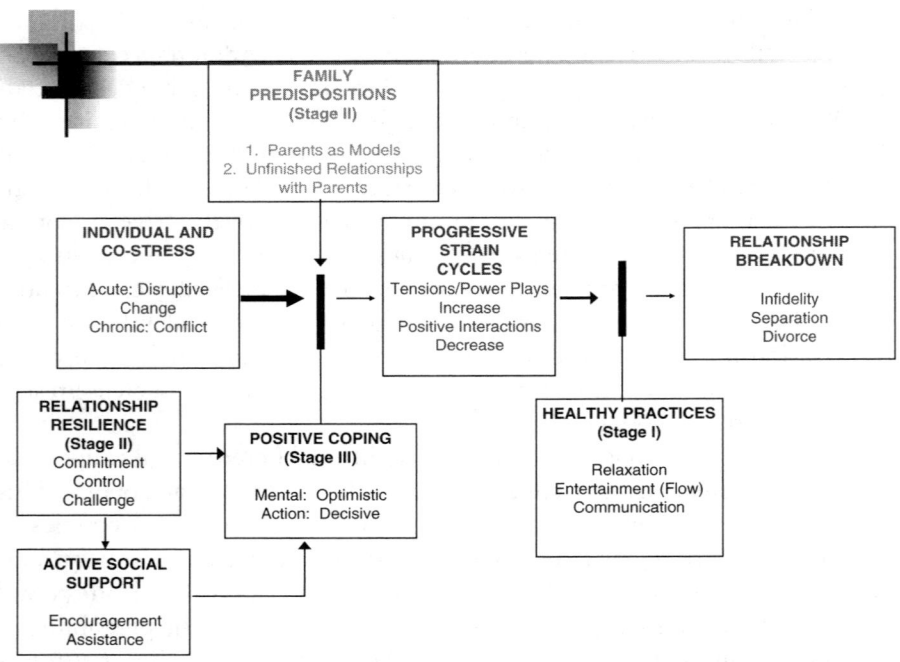

Figure 20.1. Stress factors and resilience in couples.

Individual stresses are changes that require adaptation and range from daily hassles, such as having a flat tire, to being fired from a job or losing a loved one. Stress can be positive (e.g., the birth of a child) or negative (e.g., the death of a spouse; Antonovsky, 1979; Holmes & Rahe, 1967; Kobasa & Maddi, 1979) and may be reflected in body and mind as muscle tension, increases in adrenaline, psychological bracing, rumination, and so forth. Breakdown often involves a predisposition for a particular illness, such as headaches or depression. It is triggered when the ongoing strain causes a particular organ system or adaptive pattern of living to cease functioning appropriately, usually in a catastrophic way (e.g., hospitalization).

This entire process occurs on the level of the dyad when particular stresses impinge on a couple (i.e., co-stress). The primary purpose of becoming a couple is to establish intimacy, mitigate loneliness, and create a better life. Co-stress (i.e., couples cocreated stress) militates against this primary goal by undercutting the fabric of the relationship. Within couple relationships, co-stress is unintentionally created by differences in socialization across genders on the basis of the Western sociocultural milieu. Examples of conditions that create co-stress include the following:

1. Gender differences in communication styles and perceptions of social interactions (Gilligan, 1982; Gray, 1992; Tannen, 1990)
2. Socioeconomic pressures that create the so-called dual-career couple in which both partners need to work yet have limited energy and time, resulting in less support for each other.
3. Differing role pressures that devolve into role conflict and couple conflict.

In Figure 20.1, the second level of boxes indicates what often happens to a couple. Ongoing stress and co-stress create strain cycles in the relationship, which lead to relationship breakdown. When co-stress occurs, it decreases intimacy in a cyclical way. The relationship becomes an exquisitely choreographed dance in which both partners, consciously or unconsciously, participate in keeping one another at arm's length. This, in turn, engenders greater co-stress. These cycles can be static or dangerously progressive, with more vulnerability and pathology increasing the likelihood that the cycles will progress with no positive resolution. On an emotional level, the relationship feels under siege and becomes less resilient, and the feeling of connection required to maintain the relationship erodes. Behaviorally, positive reaction cycles decrease and negative cycles increase, reducing intimacy.

Gottman's (1994) research demonstrated that the ratio of positive to negative interactions must be no lower than 5:1 if a relationship is to survive. Unless the couple works to change the situation, cycles of negative interactions will continue and ultimately increase in frequency and intensity, producing the so-called angry marriage (Maslin, 1995). A common cycle occurs when one partner, usually the male, responds to some irritant with an angry outburst. The other partner typically responds by withdrawing and communicating less, further aggravating the situation, eventually causing another angry outburst by the first partner. If such a cycle is left unchecked, it tears the core fabric of the relationship, depletes the couple's sense of goodwill and positive connection, and can ultimately lead to a major rupture or breakdown in the relationship. As destructive patterns become entrenched, the couple becomes disillusioned about ever resolving their problems. At such times, an affair or angry separation can precipitate divorce.

Each couple has a unique way of processing stress and co-stress based on the template for doing so passed down from the family of origin (i.e., family predisposition; see Figure 20.1). This grid delineates specific stresses that determine whether strain cycles will increase or decrease. If a family provides a positive model of dealing with co-stress, it will facilitate positive coping. Conversely, negative family models are more likely to engender ineffective coping. When this occurs, a relatively small amount of co-stress can mushroom into a highly aversive event and trigger intense strain cycles or behavioral avoidance. For example, if parents bicker constantly, but the mother responds with silence, and later reacts in a passive–aggressive manner, this coping style may be adopted by the offspring, regardless of gender.

Another way the family of origin can influence how a couple deals with co-stress is sometimes referred to as "unfinished business" with parents. Parenting is inevitably imperfect and can wound even the best-adjusted children. Accordingly, many people seek an intimate relationship (often unconsciously) to salve childhood wounds (Hendrix, 1995) and reenact childhood scenarios in the present relationship. For instance, if one parent (i.e., usually the opposite-sexed parent) is distant and emotionally unavailable, the offspring will often seek out a partner who is less distant and strive to achieve a different relational outcome. Indeed, in the couple relationship, the offspring presumably has more control over the partner, thus creating the potential for a better outcome.

CLINICAL APPLICATIONS

Resilience in this chapter is defined as the ability to bounce back from difficulties in a couple's relationship and use the stress as an opportunity to create positive change in the relationship. The term *relationship resilience* is used to refer to the specific variables of commitment, control, and challenge discussed next. Interventions that mitigate the effects of stress and co-stress before they result in strain and breakdown may be implemented in three stages. The three stages are (a) symptom reduction, (b) resilience training, and (c) increasing intimacy. Each stage is comprised of one or more parts and builds on the prior stage, using the strengths in the relationship.

Stage 1: Symptom Reduction

Symptom reduction occurs on a behavioral level by reducing strain before it can lead to relationship breakdown. Healthy couple practices create and enhance a sense of connection by forging (a) a common feeling of being able to relax together, (b) enjoyment of the other person, and (c) new styles of communication. The second and third stages in the resilience model create longer, more enduring changes focused on ameliorating stress and co-stress more directly.

Interventions in the symptom reduction stage are designed to unite couples and dampen the effects of strain cycles that drive them apart, withering the sense of love and connection. A couple that has little sense of connection will respond to stress in a regressive manner. When the connection is strong, couples cope with stress in a resilient manner, bouncing back from adversity more readily. Within the first two sessions, after discussing their history and encouraging the couple to analyze their strengths and weaknesses, it can be helpful to facilitate a sense of togetherness by inviting them to experience the soothing and relaxing effects of hypnosis.

The first strategy for symptom reduction involves treating the couple as a unit, using *simultaneous hypnosis for togetherness*. Using imagery that appeals to both partners facilitates a deeper simultaneous experience of hypnosis. The imagery can be recorded and experienced on a daily basis, thereby enhancing a positive emotional connection. In subsequent sessions, the therapist can strengthen the emerging, yet fragile interpersonal bond by suggesting that the couple (a) imagine themselves doing things together that they enjoy and imagine they can "dial up" a positive affect (Brown & Fromm, 1986), focusing on pleasant sensations in their bodies as this occurs and (b) imagine threads of light connecting them, with feelings of enjoyment and affection flowing along these threads. To further increase the depth of their connection, age regression can take the couple back to the early days of their romantic involvement, when the feelings of connection were strong and undeniable. The couple can bring these feelings to the present and visualize themselves going about their daily activities as they call these images forth.

Another strategy for symptom reduction involves *enhancing communication* and may require four or five sessions. It is important to keep destructive cycles from continuing by asking couples to suspend their fights rather than bringing their arguments into the session. If they feel their viewpoints are respected and are being addressed, many couples are able to follow this directive. Various strategies for communicating (e.g., active listening) can be taught

(B. Guerney, Brock, & Coufal, 1986). Effective communication strategies are used to deconstruct arguments in the session, helping each individual to achieve empathy and understand what his or her partner experiences during ongoing strain cycles. Couples can then be asked to rehearse the new style of communication during hypnosis and enhance the connection they feel by engendering positive affect. Practicing active listening in the context of positive interactions can further cement the relationship, particularly when rehearsed during hypnosis.

Finally, after the predictable patterns of strain cycles are identified, each partner can rehearse a different response early in the cycle to disrupt and ameliorate the negative interactional patterns. This process can be aided by the following dissociation technique to defuse reactivity: *dissociating the observing ego from the experiencing ego*.

Brown and Fromm (1986) used the technique of dissociating the observing ego from the experiencing ego to manage anxiety and defuse reactivity. The technique involves merging the sense of "I" into the *observing ego* by creating, metaphorically speaking, a part of the person that can watch an overwhelming situation from a distance. Couples that become reactive to each other's behaviors and bicker constantly can learn to go into the observing part and watch themselves repeat the same cycles. Because positive connective emotions have been created in previous sessions, the couple is asked to dissociate in the office, where they are not directly experiencing the stressor that provoked relational difficulties. Later, the couple can attempt this exercise during a stressful situation, such as during an argument. This hypnotic intervention is most effective when couples practice it together. However, if the couple is extremely volatile, or the observing ego is not readily accessible, it may be necessary to do this work separately (Daitch, 2007). It may be impossible to defuse couples' reactivity if participants feel acutely vulnerable, which often stems from past relationships, particularly with parents. Accordingly, it may be necessary to postpone the technique until some of the Stage 2 work that follows can be accomplished.

Stage 2: Resilience Training

Hypnotic intervention in this second stage (see Figure 20.1) increases relationship resilience by increasing commitment, control, and challenge for the couple. These three variables differentiate individuals who are distressed when faced with highly aversive circumstances from individuals who are able to bounce back (Kobasa et al., 1982).

With respect to couples, *commitment* is defined as the ability to enjoy one's partner and to deeply invest in that person and the relationship. The opposite of commitment is *alienation*, which encompasses avoiding one's partner, "a dead feeling," and an inability to invest in life as a couple. *Control* is expressed when individuals are empowered by the relationship, which facilitates autonomy and higher functioning. The opposite of control, *powerlessness*, locks the couple into power struggles or continued fighting. Many couples describe powerlessness as feeling "stuck." *Challenge* helps a relationship to feel strong and vital, as each partner experiences growth, understanding, and intimacy as they face life's vicissitudes together. The opposite of challenge is *stagnation*, in which the relationship stays the same, resulting in a feeling of being "suffocated." When a relationship is resilient, it is able to bounce back from stress and co-stress.

Resilience training involves changing the family of origin grid (see Figure 20.1) that filters the stress before it engenders strain. As noted earlier, predispositions to stress that arise from the family of origin can cause a minor stress to become a major one. Altering deleterious family of origin predispositions and increasing resilience can require as many as 15 sessions, depending on the emotional damage sustained during childhood. It is helpful to start with positive modeling for dealing with stress because it gives the couple a chance to capitalize on the resilience they have already gained through therapy. Parental relationships often provide many negative models for coping with stress, but they also provide positive role modeling. Even when the parents' marriage ended in divorce, many individuals are able to recall positive experiences. When couples experience hypnosis simultaneously, they can visualize their own parents together enjoying themselves, or they can imagine a situation in which the parents surmounted a challenge as a team. Observing parents going through the process of coping with adverse circumstances, from beginning to end, and seeing the bond between them grow, can be a valuable gift. The bond can be visualized as threads of light with positive beams of energy flowing between them. It often helps to suggest that the parents hand this bond to the couple as a gift. The couple can then experience the bond as sensations that connect them, fortifying their sense of resilience.

Positive modeling can also be exploited by suggesting that the couple visualize their parents demonstrating reciprocal affection. During hypnosis, they can then imagine themselves expressing to their partner the affection they observed. This exercise increases partner commitment because as partners experience enjoyment from doing these things for each other, even in imagination, their bond solidifies. Moreover, control is enhanced because partners can see themselves carrying on a healthy tradition of connection from their parents, which provides a sense of empowerment. Finally, challenge is increased because the couple's repertoire of relating to each other positively expands.

After the positive sense of the parents' marriage has been passed on, the therapist is in a position to help the couple to confront the effects of negative modeling, which are invariably more difficult to modify. Images of parents' negative interactions with each other often seem strongly imprinted. It may be the case that Gottman's (1994) 5:1 ratio applies, such that 5 positive interactions are needed to balance 1 negative interaction in the child's memory. Wallerstein and Blakeslee (1995) suggested that children of divorced parents are more likely to experience difficulties in relationships and are more likely to divorce than children of parents who are not divorced. In such cases, the positive bond of resilience must come through sources other than the parents' relationship. The following split-screen technique should only be used where the therapist can ascertain that the couple has a resilient relationship.

In the split screen technique (Brown & Fromm, 1986), the couple visualizes images associated with a current positive sense of connection on the right side of the "internal screen," which is then enhanced by positive images from the parents' relationship. On the left side of the screen, the couple visualizes negative images associated with their parents' marriage, such as fighting with the consequent negative reactions in the adult child. At some point, the split between the two sides of the screen dissolves, and the images and emotions are merged to create a new sense of parenting. The parental precursors to the couple's relationship can now be felt in a more neutral way. Often, an overarching positive sense emerges. It may be necessary to work hypnotically with each partner individually, with the other partner present or, if needed, in individual sessions. Work done individually should be conveyed to the partner in the next session.

It is often helpful to the couple to work on unfinished business with parents. Again, positive interactions with parents are recalled and enhanced hypnotically. These positive interactions are linked to the positive connections created from earlier exercises and can be used in the split screen or to shrink the internalized image of a powerful and overbearing parental imago (Hendrix,1995). By these means, the internalized parent becomes less of an ongoing influence, thereby reducing the intensity of strain cycles and creating the opportunity for positive cycles to emerge.

Stage 3: Increasing Intimacy

The last stage of work involves positive coping (see Figure 20.1) that entails encountering and coping with stress as a couple, using the relationship as a resource and capitalizing on techniques from Stages I and II. When facing the stress or co-stress of everyday life, a couple's sense of connection can be eroded by pressure from conflicting roles and from trying to cope with the myriad of tasks demanded of dual-career families. Half a century ago, men and women's roles were clearly delineated, with the male being the breadwinner and the female administering the home. In more recent times, these roles have blurred, and the demands of everyday life have increased, resulting in tension and frustration for couples. These forms of co-stress create an environment that places undue hardship on most couples. In this milieu, it is not surprising that the divorce rate is over 50%. The first technique in Stage III helps partners to become conscious of their own needs to more effectively cope with the difficulties of everyday life and their dual roles.

Focusing for Individuation and Negotiating for Individual Needs

The focusing technique (Gendlin, 1996) is used during hypnosis to deepen its effect. Each partner mentally goes to his or her own special place for relaxation and then asks, "What keeps me from feeling good right now?" Developing the images or phrases that answer this question promotes insight, and setting the images aside promotes relaxation. Then the question can be asked, "What do I really need?" or "What are my deepest needs?" Each partner is encouraged to deeply experience the response by focusing his or her attention on bodily reactions. The couple is encouraged to do this once or twice a day between sessions. Once they are aware of their needs, they implement a joint action plan to fulfill them. The couple is helped to prioritize their needs and their commitment to address them as they arise.

Negotiation is needed when partners' individual needs conflict. Each conflict is viewed as having the potential to increase resilience. Simultaneous hypnosis can be induced, and the therapist can suggest that "a new way to include both people's needs will come up in your mind." Once a solution is apparent, the resulting possibilities can be rehearsed in hypnosis. Feeling an increased sense of resilience (i.e., commitment, control, and challenge) is an important part of this phase of treatment. Talking about resilience and experiencing it during hypnosis is conducive to helping the couple resolve conflict and enhance their relationship.

Separating Parental Imagoes From the Present-Day Relationship

Stress and co-stress can trigger a response from negative parental imagoes (Hendrix, 1995) that interfere with coping. Using the technique described, partners can separate themselves from these imagoes during stressful circumstances rather than in a quiet place removed from conflict. In self-hypnosis, the individuals can imagine splitting their anger into two parts. One part represents the angry self, which reacts to present circumstances, whereas the archaic part, which often is the greater source of the rage, can be dismissed and confronted in the next session.

This dissociation can also be accomplished with one partner imagining the other split into the same two parts. The optimum method uses simultaneous hypnosis in the office, with a recording of suggestions for the couple to listen to at home together. After a number of practice sessions, either partner can stop an argument and take a time out. After about an hour, each partner can use both types of separation and then return to the issue if it has not been resolved. Seeing ones' partner's reactions as stemming from the archaic parts of their personalities, which reflect unresolved issues with parents, facilitates empathy and understanding.

Cognitive work with couples (Beck, 1968) can also be used to isolate and challenge distorted thoughts. Phrases such as "S/he doesn't care about me" or "We are angry with each other all the time" can be changed to "S/he is not considering me but will do so when s/he is less anxious." Each partner's thoughts are different, but in simultaneous hypnosis, they can go through the cognitive exercises and ban their own particular phrases from their lexicon. Using the image of a bright red stop sign and then rephrasing more adaptive thoughts can all be done during hypnosis.

Restructuring Stress and Co-Stress Through Coupling

When stress and co-stress become overwhelming, couples can use their resilience and problem-solving skills to reframe problems, buffer stress, and reduce its impact. To bolster the idea that "two are better than one" in contending with difficult situations, the couple identifies the problem they are facing, prioritizes their goals, and rejects less valued options. Future progressions during simultaneous hypnosis can be used to first visualize the resolution of the problem and then to celebrate the solution. Therapists can give suggestions for the couple to move backward in time to the present to see how they resolved the problem as a team, thereby enhancing their sense of resilience.

Enlisting Social Support

Social support is crucial in dealing with stress and co-stress (Kobasa, Maddi, & Kahn, 1982; Lieberman, Yalom, & Miles, 1973; Maddi, Kahn, & Maddi, 1998; Stroebe, 2000). Social support systems can assist partners in providing much-needed perspective on aversive events and in crystallizing perceptions of connection (e.g., "Your spouse may have been angry, but he really is committed to you and the family") rather than focusing on the partner's negative qualities. When outside support is needed for difficult times in the relationship, this support can be visualized in hypnosis for extra encouragement.

CLINICAL MATERIAL

This case study represents an amalgamation of work with different couples. Although the therapy may impress the reader as a more or less linear process, there were times when it was necessary to return to earlier stages of treatment because the couple would fall back into habitual ways of relating.

When Roger, a 42-year-old business executive, and Janet, a 38-year-old lawyer, first presented for treatment, they complained bitterly about their lack of mutual consideration, rudeness, and hostility. Roger was given to violent outbursts, which he said he later regretted but which Janet experienced as deeply hurtful. "He always goes for the jugular," she said resentfully. Janet felt powerless against the outbursts and so angry and hurt that she would withdraw and not talk to him. They went "round and round" in the office, as if I were not in the room. Finally, Janet stopped talking, her exasperation taking the form of her usual withdrawal, which left Roger frustrated and fuming.

Pointing out the process seemed to help them step back from it long enough to move toward discussing why they had such short fuses around each other. Careerwise, both were doing well, and both enjoyed their two young children. There were no significant stresses (e.g., death of family members, career problems) in their lives, but they both felt overwhelmed by all that they had to do on a daily basis. Roger felt unappreciated for all that he did for the family and wanted acknowledgement and support for his work. Janet felt Roger did not understand her, and her sense of alienation led to her thinking about a separation. When asked, however, both were quite willing to work on the relationship and to give the therapy a try for at least 10 sessions.

In the second session, I obtained background information (e.g., family of origin; information about relationships with their parents, both past and present; information about their parents' marriages). Roger's parents had experienced a particularly bitter divorce. I described how the marriage worked as a system, with no one being the "bad guy," and how we would build on the strengths of their marriage. Both agreed to do the homework, which consisted of stopping the arguments using a "T" sign to take a timeout and following an amended version of timeout rules (Heitler, 1995). I enjoined them to save their arguments for the next session, when we could process them more fully. I also suggested that we do a simultaneous hypnosis session next week, and both agreed.

At the start of the third session, Roger and Janet stated they were pleased that they had largely stopped fighting, and Roger had written out several issues he wanted to discuss. With a brusque tone, Roger related the times he felt angered by Janet's withdrawal and lack of appreciation, which left him infuriated. In the past, he would harshly berate her. However, he had been able to keep his demeaning criticality at bay over the past week. Janet remained withdrawn in a protective mode, believing that Roger could blow up again at any time. She would keep to herself after the children were in bed, making few attempts at communicating. Over the week there was no reason to use the timeout sign, insofar as they avoided each other.

Using a shortened version of active listening, with me as the mediator/ model (L. Guerney & Guerney, 1994), I asked them each to say how they were feeling at that moment without referring to the other, thereby interrupting their usual pattern of communication (Parsons-Fein, 2004). Roger, on the verge of yelling, said he was furious and felt outraged. Speaking of an earlier situation, he said, "She has no business humiliating me that way." After Roger repeated what he said with a lowered tone of voice, less affect, and from his subjective point of view (e.g., "When you said those things, I felt humiliated"), I asked Janet to simply repeat the same words. Roger visibly relaxed, which, I pointed out, was the result of having his feelings heard. It was then Janet's turn. She stated that she felt hurt and blamed and seemed to be on the verge of leaving the session. I commended her for staying and repeated what she had stated but with less urgency. Roger repeated what she said after I did. This seemed to help Janet to feel heard and to calm down. I then asked them to temporarily put aside distressed feelings so that they could feel more connected.

We ended with a 15-minute hypnosis session, which I recorded on a CD and gave to them. After a long induction/deepening relaxation, they mentally traveled to a special place where they each could be themselves alone, a place where they experienced a strong sense of self and felt good about themselves. It was their place alone, without their partner present. Time distortion extended their experience of the special place as if they had been there for hours. I suggested their positive feelings would surround and protect them and melt into their skins as a kind of insulation. Near the end of the induction, they were told they could choose whether they wanted their partner to join them in their special place (i.e., in their imagery) but only if they felt ready. Roger was able to invite Janet into his special place. I assigned them this activity to do together twice daily. Each time they did the exercise, they would decide whether they would invite the other to join them in their special place.

In the fourth session, both Janet and Roger reported that they felt better about the relationship and that they had completed the assignment, with Janet inviting Roger into her safe place a number of times. However, they had fought in the middle of the week, which rekindled old bitterness. Roger had undergone financial setbacks in his business and complained about Janet's spending on "frivolous" items. Janet had tried to spend more quality time with their children and had consequently purchased more things for them. She defended her actions, escalating the usual strain cycle, and Roger responded by yelling at her.

Janet withdrew for almost 2 days but then began to feel less angry. She reported that listening to the recording each day was helpful. Again, I emphasized listening to the other's feelings and attempting to react positively. They noted that they did not use the timeout signal when their fight escalated; both stated they had forgotten to do so in the heat of the argument. We made a new hypnosis CD that incorporated the first recording in a shortened form and began with suggestions for relaxation and a sense of personal space, accompanied by feelings of connection. The recording then asked them to visualize the beginning scene of a fight in which they could feel their anger building. At that moment, they each would dissociate to the observing ego, and it would automatically occur to them to give the timeout signal and then to relax and listen to their partner's feelings stated in subjective "I" terms, rather than in accusatory language. The recording ended with them feeling connected again, able to maintain this bond in rocky times.

Over the next four sessions, Janet and Roger learned to dissociate to their observing egos so that they could step back and listen to the other's feelings. Their readiness to progress to the next stage was evident in the fact that during the previous 4 weeks, they were able to avert a number of fights. I discussed continuing to strengthen their relationship by using resilience (i.e., the three Cs), thereby adopting a new attitude toward the relationship. Each time they avoided a fight, I suggested they understand their partner's vulnerability (i.e., deepening commitment), feel a new sense of control and self-efficacy, and gain confidence that their relationship would grow, bringing them closer (i.e., challenge).

At this point, Janet and Roger were ready to venture into family of origin concerns (i.e., Stage 2). Often, couples decide that they have the tools necessary to manage their relationship and want to discontinue therapy at this point. It is helpful to review areas of improvement and note that the couple can choose to gradually discontinue therapy or strive to gain greater understanding of the root causes underlying their difficulties and achieve greater intimacy. Continued efforts may obviate the need to return to therapy in the future, although the couple must decide for themselves. Roger and Janet chose to continue their work.

In the next six sessions, we explored family of origin issues, using a genogram (McGoldrick & Gerson, 1986). Roger felt that his issues with his parents were most salient. He started the discussion and was able to focus on what he remembered most about his 18 years with them. He recalled how rocky his parents' relationship was and that his parents divorced within a year after he left for college. Roger was the youngest of three children, with two much older siblings. He had never asked but suspected that he was an "accident," that the birth control his parents used after the birth of their second child had failed. Roger's father was distant emotionally, although they enjoyed a "generally good" relationship. However, his father would occasionally have an angry outburst at his wife. Roger's relationship with his mother was less fortunate. He stated, "She is a hard person to get along with, highly critical and difficult to please." However, they now have a more congenial relationship.

Janet was an only child from an intact family. Her difficulties centered on her father, who dominated her mother and controlled the household. His narcissism and her mother's resentful capitulation to his needs left Janet frustrated with both. Neither parent would tolerate her frustration nor allow her to express dissatisfaction. She grew up protectively withdrawing from her parents to keep her feelings in check.

Before pursuing these difficult emotions with each partner's parents hypnotically, we spent a session discussing some of the positive attributes that both had witnessed in their parents' marriages. Roger remembered his parents curled up together in an easy chair enjoying each other. Janet recalled a time when her parents were working on a project together and thoroughly enjoyed each other while they worked. We created the same situations in simultaneous hypnosis, with both receiving their respective gifts from their parents and translating what they received into a connection between the two of them in the present (i.e., the things they would do with each other that would engender the same sense of bonding). This activity encouraged the couple to delve into their unfinished business with their parents with some sense of a positive legacy.

Over the next few sessions, Roger began to understand (and we clarified further) how unfinished business with his parents seeped into his relationship with Janet. His feelings of being unwanted and unappreciated, and the criticism he experienced during childhood left him vulnerable to what he perceived as Janet's lack of appreciation. His father's distance contributed to his sense of isolation when Janet withdrew. His father's maladaptive angry outbursts had become one of Roger's only ways to cope with his sense of isolation. Roger had recognized these tendencies before but never in such sharp perspective, and he never had spoken about them with Janet.

After Janet gained a new understanding of how difficult Roger's childhood was, she began to respond with more empathy when he became angry. We discussed how this insight and Janet's empathy contributed to the three Cs of resilience. While they worked on these family of origin issues, both Roger and Janet were able to maintain their gains, experience diminished strain cycles, and continue to build resilience. Each session ended with hypnosis that touched on maintaining their connection but also used newfound insights to forge a deeper connection. Visualizations included Roger imagining himself as a hurt child, with Janet soothing the child and helping him to heal. This was done with only Roger in hypnosis and Janet observing or speaking in soothing tones to him.

Janet kept putting off talking about her parents' marriage and her relationship with them in favor of focusing on Roger's family. We decided to devote a complete session to Janet and understanding the link between the way she grew up and how her withdrawal mechanisms served a defensive function. In the session, it became obvious to her that her withdrawal from Roger was a means of coping with his frustration, in a manner similar to the situation with her parents. Hypnotic age regression helped her to be able to feel and to express more of her own needs in relation to past circumstances.

In the same way that she supported him, Roger encouraged her and listened intently as she expressed herself.

After Roger and Janet felt that they understood and could empathize with each other's conflicts from childhood, we made a new CD for them to listen to together in simultaneous hypnosis. Both were able to experience hypnosis easily with a short induction. Following a brief time in their own special individual spaces, they created a new place for them to be together by focusing on the emotions they felt toward the other after deepening their resilience. Together, they regressed in age to different points in their own life by traveling to where they could use the sense of connection to empower the small child and help him or her grow big while the parental image grew small. Both felt a sense of release from the past.

Over the course of treatment, the couple's relationship had grown much stronger. Nevertheless, there still were occasional skirmishes and outbursts, but they occurred less frequently. Janet and Roger would deconstruct each episode at home so that both would feel understood. Most of their difficulties were triggered by the co-stress of managing a dual-career household with young children.

Although some aspects of daily coping were addressed throughout treatment, dealing with stress and co-stress became the primary focus of treatment in Stage 3. Again, it is not uncommon for couples to terminate therapy at the end of Stage 2, because the symptoms (i.e., strain cycles) and the underlying issues (i.e., family of origin) have been addressed. Nevertheless, intimacy may be solidified by completing the last stage of treatment, which often includes "fading out" sessions by meeting less often. This contingency needs to be discussed with patients, pointing out that although many important issues were addressed successfully, it is possible to achieve a deeper level of intimacy. Roger and Janet decided they would like to begin phasing out sessions but that they would continue for at least four more.

Stage 3 begins with couples learning to become aware of their individual needs and vulnerabilities. Such recognition was easier for Roger because he was clear about his frustration with his wife's lack of appreciation. He felt a strong sense of isolation because at work he made a number of daily decisions that were crucial to his business. At home, he felt isolated from his wife, who was overwhelmed by her work and child-rearing tasks (about two thirds of these were Janet's). Roger felt that his making meals, taking care of bills, and maintaining their house more than made up for Janet's larger share of child-care responsibilities. Janet stated that she needed small amounts of peaceful time alone.

In simultaneous hypnosis, I suggested that the couple focus on their own needs separately from the family and their spouse. After the induction, I used the Gendlin (1996) focusing technique to examine their physical reaction to the phrase "What keeps me from feeling good right now?" Roger felt an emotional hunger in his chest, and the next question, "What is my deepest need?" brought up a wish to have an "arms around" loved feeling. Janet reported a pushing away feeling in her chest. Staying with this feeling, it evolved into an image of being pecked by large blackbirds. Her deepest need was to soothe the wounds left by the birds. Next, each imagined how his or her need could be met. Roger simply wished for Janet to put her arms around him, whereas she wanted to be soothed. It was easy for her to put her arms around him (they were on the couch together) while still in hypnosis. With an affect dial and time distortion, the soothing feelings were magnified and prolonged.

As Janet removed her arms, I suggested that Roger continue to feel her loving physical presence. Janet, in turn, wanted Roger to give her a sense of soothing. He did so by simply placing his hand on the wounds where she felt them in her body. Again, the affect dial technique and time distortion were used to enhance the experience. After I terminated their hypnosis, we discussed how this powerful session helped deepen their connection by increasing commitment (i.e., feeling valued by the other), control (i.e., feeling empowered by support and soothing), and challenge (i.e., both knew more about the other's needs and how they differed as well as how to fulfill them). The assignment for the following 2 weeks was to do the focusing exercise and determine whether each partner could fill the other's needs and to become more aware of the other's vulnerabilities. During hypnosis, they were also to spend some time focusing on their burgeoning sense of resilience.

In the meeting 2 weeks later, we discussed the progressive increase in resilience that was evident across sessions. Occasional irritable exchanges still occurred, but nothing disrupted their sense of connection. These exchanges occurred most often when either Roger or Janet felt unable to meet the other's needs. During simultaneous hypnosis, we addressed the conflict in needs by looking for a solution that would suit both partners. Roger felt a strong, almost demanding, immediacy to have his needs met. I suggested that Janet express her recognition of Roger's needs to feel appreciated and loved and say in a loving way that she would address them, albeit not immediately. Roger had difficulty with this but ingeniously created an image of the emotions shrinking and seeing himself in past times and in the future, with Janet showing her affection for him in various ways. I suggested that social support (i.e., Roger's friends) could also be visualized to help him cope more effectively. Janet, at times, needed to be alone to repair herself. Roger's exercise facilitated his ability to be alone with his needs. I suggested to Janet that she visualize taking time for herself when she could relax, visualize herself far away, and experience time distortion so that she could feel as though she was away (e.g., on a vacation) for weeks. She responded to these suggestions and smiled with satisfaction when realerted. Both Janet and Roger felt good about the way we addressed their needs, and we agreed to meet in 3 weeks.

Janet expressed frustration with Roger when they returned 3 weeks later. Roger had slipped back into criticizing her, which had resulted in a fight followed by anger and withdrawal. During simultaneous hypnosis, each visualized an angry image of the other and then allowed the parental image or influence to separate itself from the present image. When each was able to do this, they could begin to see that it was not the person from the present who knew them and loved them that was causing the intensity of the conflict.

I suggested that the parental image should melt into the background (i.e., as a symbol of the past), leaving a much less "extreme" present-day partner. In hypnosis, Janet and Roger's more rational "selves" could then resolve the conflict. I gave a posthypnotic suggestion that whenever a fight would begin that they take a few minutes to perform this imagery exercise. Before I dehypnotized them, I suggested that they project themselves into the future when they could see themselves starting a similar fight with all the attendant feelings. Instead of the conflict progressing, they would visualize the other's parental image separating itself and melting into the background, thus defusing the distress. I reminded them that the next session 3 weeks later would be the last one.

Both Roger and Janet arrived at their last session in good spirits but apprehensive about the future. We discussed how their feelings were not unusual for people ending therapy but that their confidence in their growth and resilience would soon overshadow such feelings. I reassured them that they were always able to return but that I did not expect that they would need to. We created a final CD of them experiencing deeply their connection and resilience in the present. We then enacted an age progression so that they could experience their resilience growing even stronger in the future as they saw themselves resolving conflicts resulting from stress and co-stress. They left the session feeling positive and able to handle whatever would come their way. When I called them almost 3 months later to ask how they were, both responded that "things were going well" and that they would call me if anything changed and they required help.

RESEARCH AND APPRAISAL

Clinical outcome research is difficult to undertake, and when it comes to couples, it is perhaps even more difficult. The well-disguised communication between partners in a couple is so subtle and provocative that it eludes even the best of couples' clinicians, even after many sessions. It is not surprising that there is little clinical research on couples, much less on using hypnosis with couples.

Because hypnosis is an adjunctive method rather than a treatment in itself, in practice, it necessarily is integrated into more encompassing treatment approaches. Moreover, hypnotherapy with couples is informed by research developments in the broader field of couples work. John Gottman (1994, Gottman & Silver, 1999) was the first researcher to study couples in their natural habitat and not rely on retrospective data. He distinguished three types of couples that were viable (see Table 20.1). The first type is the *validating* couple, characterized by warmth and support. The second is the *volatile* couple, characterized by arguing or passion. The third is the *avoidant* couple that minimizes conflict and communication but holds an optimistic view of the relationship. These couples all displayed a ratio of five positive interactions to one negative.

In nonviable couples, Gottman discovered that the interaction ratio was closer to one positive for every negative, allowing him to predict divorce with 95% accuracy. Gottman identified two types of nonviable couples: (a) the *hostile/engaged* couple, in which partners are able to function together yet are highly critical or withdrawn and (b) the *hostile/detached* couple, in which partners barely respond to communications and withdraw into isolation.

Gottman distinguished four negative types of marital interactions, which he called the four horsemen of the Apocalypse: (a) *criticism* (e.g., complaining about the other in a malicious manner), (b) *defensiveness* (e.g., avoidance of responsibility while often blaming the other), (c) *contempt* (e.g., overt disgust, particularly in facial expressions), and (d) *stonewalling* (e.g., respond-

TABLE 20.1
Types of Couple Relationships—Four Horsemen: Criticism,
Defensiveness, Contempt, Stonewalling

Types of relationships	Stage 1: Expression	Stage 2: Persuasion	Stage 3: Resolution	Description
Validating*	Communication	Respect	Compromise	Warmth
Volatile (Intensity)*	Squabbling and engagement	Winning	Win/lose	Intense anger and passion
Avoidant (Conflict minimizers)*	Minimal	Minimal	"Agreeing to disagree" and accentuating the positive	Calm
Hostile/ engaged**	Attack (critical)	Defensiveness	Withdrawal	Parallel lives
Hostile/ detached**	Attack (contempt)	Defensiveness	Stonewalling	Isolation

*Ratio of positive to negative interactions is less than 5:1
**Ratio of positive to negative interactions is 1:1.

ing little, if at all; as if stone walls to each other). In martial interactions, the process tends to move from criticism and defensiveness to contempt and finally to stonewalling, although all types of negative interactions are evident in deteriorating relationships.

Gottman developed a series of interventions focused on minimizing the four types of destructive interactions and replacing them with more positive styles. Although Gottman's cognitive–behavioral approach did not use hypnotherapy, he assigned a relaxation exercise (with little imagery) for men who became overwhelmed easily. Notably, Daitch (2007) incorporated some of Gottman's methods in her hypnotic interventions with couples and provided many clinical examples of work with couples using a hypnotic set of tools geared to regulating affect in the couple exchange. Although her work focused on individual mastery, it has many far-reaching implications for enhancing work with couples. Her recommendation to adopt a stage or tier model calls to mind the three stages delineated in the resilience model described earlier.

Using hypnosis with couples is an innovative and somewhat uncharted clinical application. Since the 1970s, a number of clinicians have reported case studies in which they used hypnosis with a particular couple without reference to either the theoretical underpinnings of their work or to the specifics of exactly how they achieved corrective outcomes. For instance, Marriot (1985) used hypnosis to change the balance of power in the relationship; Protinsky (1988) described the use of a variety of techniques, including age regression and age progression, negative hallucination and dissociation in couples work; and Somer (1990) illustrated the use of soothing techniques in simultaneous couple hypnosis to help both partners cope with rape of one of the partners. From case studies, Baddeley (1992) derived nine working principles for the use of hypnosis with couples, and Calof (1983) discussed what he calls *conjoint* (i.e., simultaneous) hypnosis with couples, which he attributes to Araoz (1978). Calof also advocated using hypnosis in groups and mixing family of origin work and intrapsychic work with Ericksonian hypnosis.

Whereas general theories abound regarding couples work, there is a paucity of theories about hypnosis with couples to guide treatment. Although he does not present a well-elaborated theory, Kershaw's (1992) writings describe how both partners create a "hypnotic dance, a mutually created sequence of behaviors and emotions that is stimulated . . . by the best and worst relationships carried from one's family of origin" (p. xvi). This dance can be assessed and reworked so that it is more satisfying to the couple. The first step is to observe how couples cocreate the hypnotic dance and then to interrupt typical interactional patterns and determine how hypnosis is being used maladaptively (e.g., using age regression to pinpoint the individual's most vulnerable moments growing up), which then becomes the central focus of treatment. The therapist uses symbols and metaphors associated with symptoms to change interactions and create new patterns of hypnotic involvements. Braun (1984), Combs and Freedman (1990), and Ritterman (1983) each wrote about hypnosis techniques oriented to work with families, with Ritterman and Combs and Freedman illustrating how to use Ericksonian strategies.

Daniel Araoz (1978) wrote about hypnotic techniques in couples work and suggested using hypnosis simultaneously with both partners. Later, taking a systematic approach, Araoz and Negly-Parker (1988) wrote a volume about couple and family work that was based on their qualitative research (i.e., a five-question open-ended survey) with 50 families treated by either one or both authors. They interviewed 10 families in depth, delineated hypnotic strategies that appeared to be helpful even after termination, and developed a systematic treatment organized around four principles. The first principle is to use *unconscious dynamics* and the imagination to increase awareness of negativity engendered by past experiences and to transform negative thinking into ego-strength and positive coping. *Suggestibility*, the second principle, focuses on negative self-suggestions that engender dysfunction and replace such suggestions with positive suggestions. This leads to the third principle, that of *positivism*, which builds on personal resources to achieve attainable, concrete goals. The fourth principle, *psychosomatics*, uses the emerging understanding of how physical reactions are stimulated by emotional upheaval to promote insight and change core beliefs.

Araoz and Negly-Parker (1988) divided treatment into three stages. The beginning stage involves reframing couple interactions as part of a complex system with each partner becoming empowered to influence outcome through active changes in attitudes and behaviors. Setting up new concrete goals and enhancing healthy interactions is bolstered through using hypnotic rehearsal strategies. The middle phase of treatment helps incorporate these healthy changes both at the individual as well as at the systemic level. In the ending stages of therapy, new ways of functioning are consolidated as the couple reworks old problems and tackles new ones as the techniques become a part of their *modus operandi*.

Daitch (2007) provided many clinical examples of work with couples using a hypnotic set of tools assimilated in three stages, geared to regulating affect in the couple exchange. Parsons-Fein (2004) used many Ericksonian strategies to interrupt old patterns of interacting and replace them with positive ones stimulating growth and intimacy.

Although the extant literature has proved valuable in generating new and potentially effective techniques, it is only recently that forays into the arena of family therapy have become more systematized and subject to empirical scrutiny (Araoz & Negley-Parker, 1988; Daitch, 2007; Kershaw, 1992; Parsons-Fein, 2004). Indeed, sufficient anecdotal evidence has been amassed so that systematic approaches can lend viability and legitimacy to using hypnosis with couples. However, there is a pressing need for randomized controlled outcome studies that examine the benefit of adding hypnotic procedures to cognitive–behavioral and other approaches to working with couples

CONCLUSION

The systematic application of hypnosis to working with couples has become more rigorous and scientific in the last 15 years. In addition to anecdotal evidence, there have been theoretical advances as well as actual qualitative studies that have shown the efficacy of using hypnosis to advance treatment. The model delineated here combines current theories of couples work into a resilience model. Three stages of intervention were outlined that buffer the effects of stress before they strain the relationship and result in breakdown. To reduce strain, hypnotic methods of enhancing communication and connection between partners and reducing reactivity are introduced. The next stage involves working through dysfunctional family of origin issues using a number of hypnotic techniques relying primarily on age regression. The third stage involves tackling current stresses as a couple and increasing intimacy. Whereas this approach has been used as a complete method of treatment, it relies on components that have been proven effective in other work. It remains to empirically validate the entire approach.

REFERENCES

Antonovsky, A. (1979). *Health, stress, and coping.* New York: Jossey-Bass.

Araoz, D. (1978). Clinical hypnosis in couple therapy. *Journal of the American Society of Psychosomatic Dentistry and Medicine, 25,* 58–67.

Araoz, D., & Negley-Parker, E. (1988). *The new hypnosis in family therapy.* New York: Brunner/Mazel.

Baddeley, M. (1992). The use of hypnosis in marriage and relationship counseling. *Australian Journal of Clinical Hypnotherapy & Hypnosis, 13,* 87–92.

Beck, A. T. (1968). *Love is never enough.* New York: HarperCollins.

Bowen, M. (1978). *Family therapy in clinical practice.* New York: Jason Aronson.

Braun, B. G. (1984). Hypnosis and family therapy. *American Journal of Clinical Hypnosis, 26*(3), 182–186.

Brown, D., & Fromm, E. (1986). *Hypnotherapy and hypnoanalysis.* Hillsdale, NJ: Erlbaum.

Calof, D. L. (1983). Hypnosis in marital therapy: Toward a transgenerational approach in Ericksonian psychotherapy. In J. K. Zeig (Ed.), *Ericksonian psychotherapy: Clinical applications* (pp. 71–91). New York: Brunner/Mazel.

Combs, G., & Freedman, J. (1990). *Symbol, story, & ceremony*. New York: Norton.

Cooper, C. (1984). Conjoint group self-hypnosis for couples' enrichment (Doctoral dissertation, University of South Carolina, 1984). *Dissertation Abstracts International*, 45. (6-A), 1641, University Microfilms International.

Daitch, C. (2007). *Affect regulation toolbox practical and effective hypnotic interventions for the over-reactive client*. New York: Norton.

Figley, C. R. (1989). *Treating stress in families*. New York: Brunner/Mazel.

Gendlin, E. (1996). *Focusing*. New York: Bantam Books.

Gilligan, C. (1982). *In a different voice: Psychological theory and women's development*. Cambridge, MA: Harvard University Press.

Gottman, J. M. (1994). *Why marriages succeed or fail*. New York: Simon & Schuster.

Gottman, J. M., & Silver, N. (1999). *The seven principles for making marriage work*. New York: Three Rivers Press.

Gray, J. (1992). *Men are from mars, women are from Venus*. New York: HarperCollins.

Guerney, B., Jr., Brock, G., & Coufal, J. (1986). Integrating marital therapy and enrichment: The relationship enhancement approach. In N. Jacobson & A. Gurman (Eds.), *Clinical handbook of marital therapy* (pp. 151–172). New York: Guilford Press.

Guerney, L., & Guerney, B. G., Jr. (1994). Child relationship enhancement family therapy and parent education. In C. E. Schaefer & L. J. Carey (Eds), *Family Play Therapy*, Northvale, NJ: Jason Aronson.

Heitler, S. (1995). *The angry couple: Conflict-focused treatment, a viewer's manual*. New York: Newbridge Professional Programs.

Hendrix, H. (1995). *Getting the love you want: A guide for couples*. New York: Harper-Perennial.

Holmes, T. H., & Rahe, R. H. (1967). The Social Readjustments Rating Scales. *Journal of Psychosomatic Research, 11*, 213–218.

Kershaw, C. (1992). *The couple's hypnotic dance: Creating Ericksonian strategies in marital therapy*. New York: Brunner/Mazel.

Kobasa, S. C. (1979). Stressful life events, personality, and health: An inquiry into hardiness. *Journal of Personality and Social Psychology, 37*, 1–11.

Kobasa, S., Maddi, S., & Kahn, S. (1982). Hardiness and health: A prospective study. *Journal of Personality and Social Psychology, 42*, 168–177.

Lieberman, M., Yalom, I., & Miles, M. (1973). *Encounter groups: First facts*. New York: Basic Books.

Maddi, S., Kahn, S., & Maddi, K. (1998). The effectiveness of hardiness training. *Consulting Psychology Journal, 50*, 78–86.

Marriott, J. A. (1985). The use of hypnosis in changing the balance of power in a relationship: A case study. *Australian Journal of Clinical Hypnotherapy & Hypnosis, 6*, 29–33.

Maslin, B. (1995). *The angry marriage*. New York: Skylight Press.

McGoldrick, M., & Gerson, R. (1986). *Genograms in family assessment*. New York: Norton.

Parsons-Fein, J. (2004). *Loving in the here and now*. New York: Tarcher/Penguin.

Pinsof, W. (1995). *Integrative problem-centered therapy*. New York: Basic Books.

Protinsky, H. (1988). Hypnotic strategies in strategic marital therapy. *Journal of Strategic & Systemic Therapies, 7*, 29–34.

Ritterman, M. (1983). *Using hypnosis in family therapy*. San Francisco: Jossey-Bass.

Somer, E. (1990). Brief simultaneous couple hypnotherapy with a rape victim and her spouse: A brief communication. *International Journal of Clinical and Experimental Hypnosis, 38*, 1–5.

Stroebe, W. (2000). *Social psychology and health* (2nd ed.). Buckingham, England: Open University Press.

Tannen, D. (1990). *You just don't understand*. New York: Ballantine Books.

Wallerstein, J., & Blakeslee, S. (1995). *The good marriage: How & why love lasts*. New York: Houghton Mifflin.

Walsh, F. (1993). *Normal family processes*. New York: Guilford Press.

V

HEALTH AND SPORT PSYCHOLOGY

21

HYPNOSIS FOR PAIN CONTROL

DAVID R. PATTERSON, MARK P. JENSEN, AND GUY H. MONTGOMERY

Although hypnosis has been used for pain control for more than a century (Esdaile, 1957), recent years have marked a tremendous upsurge in research and clinical use of hypnosis to reduce pain (also known as *hypnoanalgesia*). There are at least four reasons for this renewed interest. First, there has been an impressive increase in the number of quality studies demonstrating the effective applications of hypnosis for pain control over the past decade. In meta-analyses (Montgomery, David, Winkel, Silverstein, & Bovbjerg, 2002; Montgomery, DuHamel, & Redd, 2000), as well as narrative reviews of controlled studies (Patterson & Jensen, 2003), hypnosis has been shown to be an effective technique for pain control for the majority of patients.

Second, coinciding with professional provider interests in hypnosis, Americans in general are consuming complementary and alterative medicine (CAM) at a record pace. People in the United States have demonstrated a burgeoning fascination with approaches to health care that fall outside of the mainstream of conventional medicine, and hypnosis is no exception (Eisenberg

This research was supported by grants from the National Institutes of Health (R01AR054115-01A1 and R01GM42725-09A1).
Clinical material has been disguised to protect patient confidentiality.

et al., 1993). Although we would argue that hypnosis has been accepted by many (although certainly not all) in the medical community as a conventional treatment for pain since at least the 1950s (Crasilneck, Stirman, & Wilson, 1955), some professionals still categorize hypnotic analgesia under the CAM umbrella.

Third, recent compelling evidence that the use of hypnosis can reduce institutional costs may also contribute to renewed interest in hypnosis. For example, Lang and colleagues demonstrated that hypnosis can reduce the cost of perioperative procedures (e.g., insertion of catheters) from $638 per patient to $300 (Lang et al., 2000; Lang & Rosen, 2002;). Montgomery et al. (2007) reported as preliminary data that the savings associated with the use of hypnosis to control postsurgery side effects in patients who have had surgery for breast cancer may be even more substantial.

Fourth, our understanding of both the physiological correlates and psychological mechanisms of hypnosis continues to improve, facilitating the development of hypnotic techniques. For example, sophisticated radiologic techniques have been applied to better understand the relationship between hypnotic analgesia and brain activity (Rainville, Duncan, Price, Carrier, and Bushnell, 1997). On the psychological side, expectancies, contextual effects, response to hypnotizabilty scales, and other cognitive processes have been associated with hypnotically based pain control (Montgomery, Weltz, Seltz, & Bovbjerg, 2002; Patterson & Jensen, 2003). Overall, this body of research has raised the legitimacy of hypnosis in the eyes of the scientific community and has begun to elucidate the underpinnings of this powerful technique.

An issue that has plagued the literature on hypnosis for pain control is that important patient variables that can influence the impact of hypnotic suggestions have often been neglected. In particular, the distinction between acute and chronic pain has seldom been emphasized (Patterson & Jensen, 2003) when, in fact, treatments for these two types of pain could hardly be more disparate. Acute pain usually results from an open wound or tissue damage. Patients experiencing this type of pain have actual nociceptive input arising from damaged tissue signaling that something is wrong and that the brain interprets as "pain."

Acute pain is often associated with medical procedures such as surgery, injury, childbirth, or invasive treatments. Acute pain can be responsive to pharmacologic interventions such as opioid analgesics or anesthetic blocks (Patterson & Sharar, 2001), but these pharmacologic interventions are rarely 100% effective and typically come with their own set of side effects (Kehlet & Dahl, 2003). Chronic pain, in contrast to acute pain, is of longer duration and is usually defined as pain that lasts longer than 3 months (Jacobson & Mariano, 2001; Patterson & Sharar, 2001). Chronic pain is rarely associated with a specific identifiable lesion. Although patients with chronic pain almost always initially experience some type of tissue or structural damage, that component is usually absent by the time they present to a psychologist for treatment (Jacobson & Mariano, 2001). Chronic pain tends to respond poorly to biomedical-focused treatments. The literature on back pain, for example, indicates, in general, that 30% of patients improve after surgical interventions, 30% remain the same, and 30% actually become worse as a result (Turk & Okifuji, 1998).

Whether acute or chronic, pain almost always involves suffering (Fordyce, 1988). The aversive nature of pain can disrupt almost every aspect of daily living (Katz, 2002; Niv & Kreitler, 2001). Patients experiencing pain are approximately 4 times more likely to experience depression or anxiety, and are more than 2 times as likely to have problems with work (Gureje, Von Korff, Simon, & Gater, 1998). Furthermore, pain places an economic burden on individuals, families, and institutions to the overall detriment of society (Loeser, 1999). Four billion workdays may be lost in the United States because of pain each year, with a potential economic impact of $55 billion (Sternbach, 1986). Physicians have reported that their pain management strategies are often inadequate (Loeser, 2001), that they can be reluctant to prescribe opioid analgesics on a long-term basis (Auret & Schug, 2005), and that most pharmacologic interventions are accompanied by their own set of side effects. These include, but are not limited to, respiratory depression, nausea, constipation, urinary retention, cognitive failures, hallucinations, delirium, myoclonus and grand mal seizures, and hyperalgesia (Bruera & Pereira, 1997; Schulz-Stubner, 2000).

However, the limitations of pharmacotherapy for pain control highlight the need for validated nonpharmacological approaches. Based on established models of pain that include central control constructs (Melzack & Wall, 1973), nonpharmacologic approaches to pain management such as hypnosis can be of significant clinical benefit to patients, either as an adjunct or alternative to existing treatments.

CLINICAL APPLICATIONS

Because of their inherent psychological and biological differences, psychological treatments for acute and chronic pain can differ dramatically. For this reason, this chapter is divided into applications of hypnosis for acute and chronic pain. There are multiple robust theories of hypnosis, some of which explain some clinical aspects of hypnoanalgesia better than others (Kihlstrom, 1992; Lynn & Rhue, 1991), and in this chapter we borrow from them accordingly. Much of the material below is discussed in more detail in Patterson (in press) and Jensen and Patterson (2008).

Acute Pain Conceptualization

As mentioned, acute pain is almost always short-lived (i.e., days or weeks, rather than months or years), is associated with tissue damage, and is often associated with events such as medical procedures or accidents. These characteristics of acute pain affect how hypnosis can be applied to acute pain conditions. It is also important to understand that because of the potential intensity of suffering associated with acute pain and the possible perceived lack of control over this pain, patients often experience anxiety in addition to their acute pain (Chapman & Bonica, 1983). Patients undergoing medical procedures may know that an episode of acute pain is forthcoming, and it is not surprising that anticipatory anxiety is common in this population (Montgomery & Bovbjerg, 2004). In events in which patients suddenly experience acute pain without warning, such as traumatic injury, it is likely that they will experience fight–flight protective mechanisms in the anxiety response associated with survival. Such distress can lead to increased pain, making the pain event worse and potentially initiating a vicious cycle (Chapman, 1985; Chapman & Bonica, 1983; Chien, 1967; Mackersie & Karagianes, 1990). Often the role of hypnosis in the treatment of acute pain or in preparing patients for pain associated with upcoming medical procedures is to reduce current and anticipatory anxiety, in addition to ameliorating the pain itself.

There are several characteristics of acute pain that indicate how hypnosis can best be applied. A primary characteristic in this respect is the predictable onset of some types of acute pain. Because acute pain is associated with many medical procedures (e.g., dental care, elective surgery), it is often possible to prepare patients and apply hypnosis well before the procedure itself. Acute pain, such as that from trauma or infection, can also occur without warning, and hypnosis can be effective in such circumstances as well. Another quality of acute pain is that greatly reducing symptoms, or even eliminating them, generally does not create a secondary (e.g., psychodynamic, behavioral, cognitive dissonance) problem for the patient. Whereas with patients with chronic pain there is a greater chance that the pain may serve a psychological or social need, potentially even including issues of social and financial disincentives for improvement, reducing acute pain typically does not present such complications.

Understanding the patient's emotional state at the time he or she experiences acute pain can provide useful guidelines for applying hypnosis. For example, some patients with acute pain may present dependency, fragile coping mechanisms, and/or extreme vulnerability; specifically, they may view themselves as being in a vulnerable position in the health care system where having greater dependence on health care workers can be an adaptive form of coping. Other patients may be used to a high degree of control in their lives in general, and such tendencies may be amplified with the stress of illness and health care. In addition, clinicians should be aware that with high levels of acute pain or pain medication, some patients may show a greater tendency toward dissociation (Patterson, Adcock, & Bombardier, 1997; Spiegel, 1991; Spiegel, Hunt, & Dondershine, 1988; Spiegel, Koopman, & Classen, 1994). If the acute pain they are experiencing is a result of physical trauma, then elements of dissociation, in some patients, may be present. With acute pain, it can also be anticipated that some patients will have sensoriums (i.e., cognitive processing) altered by the presence of medications or the hospital environment (Patterson et al., 1993). Psychological reactions to trauma and hospitalization, as well as the influence of pharmacologic agents, all have a potential impact on how patients may respond to hypnosis, in a negative way for some and a positive manner for others; we unfortunately lack systematic studies to predict how patients will react to hypnosis under such circumstances.

In considering acute pain, it can be helpful to consider whether patients are *monitors* or *blunters* in the manner in which they process threatening information (Patterson, 1995; Thompson, 1981). Patients who cope by monitoring may show a tendency to be hypervigilant during procedures and an unwillingness to use hypnotic techniques that involve removing oneself from the situation through imagery or fantasy. Blunters, however, may welcome hypnotic interventions that encourage a form of distraction or cognitive removal from the situation.

Whether working with patients who have either acute or chronic pain, it is important to understand the critical impact of patients' expectations for pain on their experience of pain. Kirsch (1990) defined expectations for nonvolitional outcomes (such as pain) as *response expectancies*. Response expectancies have been shown to be a significant contributor to pain in both clinical (Montgomery & Bovbjerg, 2004) and experimental (Montgomery & Kirsch, 1996, 1997) studies. In addition, intervention studies have supported expectancy change as an underlying psychological mechanism for the clinical effects of hypnosis (Montgomery, Weltz, et al., 2002; Schoenberger, Kirsch, Gearan, Montgomery, & Pastyrnak, 1997). Consequently, managing patients' expectancies in the context of applied hypnosis can be extremely useful clinically. For example, one should help patients set reasonable and achievable expectancies for pain reduction. The achievement of these goals should increase patients' expectancies of continuing to achieve in, and benefit from, hypnosis. One should not oversell the intervention, but rather create a context where success is achievable. Also, debunking myths about hypnosis (e.g., "You could make me rob a bank," "It is like taking a powerful drug") with the patient is extremely useful. Debunking puts patients at ease and lets them know that their personal experience of hypnosis will be safe and that the goal of the intervention session is to benefit them clinically.

Inductions for Acute Pain

In our view, the nature of hypnotic suggestions used for pain is far more important than the specific induction used. However, several of the aforementioned qualities of acute pain indicate that some types of induction techniques may be more useful and appropriate than others. As mentioned, patients experiencing acute pain may be frightened and/or dependent. Most patients are typically highly motivated to reduce acute pain and may therefore be more cooperative with hypnotic approaches than they might be otherwise. Consequently, brief, direct inductions are often sufficient, or even preferable, to longer inductions because available time to conduct hypnosis interventions may be brief because of medical scheduling. It is also the case with this patient population that, secondary to cognitive limitations, they lack the attention span for induction techniques of any great length (Patterson, 1996).

Posthypnotic Suggestions

Because acute pain often occurs at predictable times in response to procedures, preprocedure hypnosis with posthypnotic suggestions is often particularly useful with this patient population (Patterson, Everett, Burns, & Marvin, 1992; Patterson & Ptacek, 1997). In the case of acute pain associated with medical procedures, hypnotic inductions can often occur at some point before the procedure while the patient is relatively free from both pain and pain medications. Hypnosis can be taught to patients during a window of time when they are free of medical distractions. During the hypnosis session, posthypnotic suggestions can be provided to address postprocedure pain. For example, the patient might be told the following:

> At this time, you may be aware of how completely comfortable and relaxed you feel. Wouldn't it be interesting if you find that whenever you find yourself entering the surgical suite [in labor/entering the procedure room], that you find that this sense of comfort and relaxation becomes even greater.

It is not always practical for the clinician performing hypnosis to be present during the medical procedure. Through the use of posthypnotic suggestions, the patient can be prepared for a procedure even when the clinician is absent. Ideally, such suggestions would be reinforced by either a trained clinician attending the procedure (i.e., often, for example, a nurse) or some other individual (e.g., a technician, a family member) who is skilled at reinforcing the posthypnotic suggestions. For example, if nothing else, it would be useful for a nurse present at the time of the procedure to state, "Now just begin to slow down your breathing and use everything you learned earlier when you were working with hypnosis." Furthermore, patients can be taught to enter hypnosis on their own so that they have a distraction or safe haven from the aversive stimuli associated with planned medical procedures.

Suggestions for the Patient in the Intensive Care Unit

Patients in the intensive care unit (ICU) often experience acute pain, either by virtue of the trauma or illness that put them there, or because of frequent medical procedures. Patients in the ICU face a number of physiological, environmental, and medical challenges (Bone et al., 1995; Patterson et al., 1993). Consequently, they tend to show limited attention, fatigue, and sleep deprivation (Jaffe & Patterson, 2004). For this patient population, concerns about mortality and intense anxiety are to be expected. It should also be kept in mind that, for this population, feeling some pain can be cognitively reframed as a signal that the patient is alive and has survived the surgery. If this tactic is used by a patient, it is only logical that suggestions for feeling no pain when in the ICU should be avoided (Patterson, 1996). In addition to suggestions for reduced pain (e.g., "You will feel far more comfortable than you would have anticipated as a result of our conversation"), patients in the ICU should also be given suggestions that facilitate healing, relaxation, increased overall well-being, improved sleep, and a rapid recovery.

Whether they are in the intensive care unit or not, some patients in acute pain will be in an emotional state of crisis for the reasons discussed earlier. As a result of heightened anxiety or pain associated with this emotional state, the clinician may have difficulty capturing the patient's attention to initiate hypnosis. As an example, the patient may be screaming or crying out in pain in his or her hospital room. With such patients, it is important to model calmness. The patients' attention must first be captured; this might involve using their name and speaking directly and clearly to them. When the patients' attention has been captured, clinicians can then begin to speak more slowly and model calmness to begin the induction. Even though patients in the ICU might be highly distracted, fatigued, and a challenge with respect to capturing attention, they can also be highly cooperative once they are involved in hypnosis.

Finger Signaling

A particularly useful technique with patients who are experiencing acute pain at the time of the induction is the use of finger signaling, an approach that is clinically based and admittedly lacking in empirical support. Finger signaling works well with quick inductions because it allows the clinician to gain feedback from the patient about key suggestions. Ideally, these suggestions are put in a way that allows for an ease of response and automaticity in behavior (Barabasz & Watkins, 2005; Fromm & Nash, 1997). Rather than stating, "I would like you to raise your finger when you become relaxed," a suggestion that would evoke a subjective sense of dissociation might be the following:

> At the time you feel that you have become adequately relaxed, your mind will allow you to know this by allowing this finger [*a finger is touched*] to feel itself jerking up like there is a string attached to it.

Finger signals can be used to establish: (a) that the patient has become adequately relaxed, (b) that they have internalized a desired suggestion (e.g., "When you know that from now on you will feel far more comfortable and will be doing what you need to do to heal, your mind will allow you to understand this by once again by feeling this finger elevate"), and (c) that they are ready to end the hypnosis session. This final point is particularly useful in working with brief inductions because patients often enjoy the experience of hypnosis, and bringing them back too abruptly can lessen the beneficial experience for them (Barabasz & Watkins, 2005).

On the basis of clinical experience, patients occasionally do not respond to suggestions for finger signals during an induction. In this case, it is fine to continue with an induction in the absence of a finger signal. In fact, one of us (Patterson) has found that patients who fail to show a finger signal are often the ones who seem to benefit the most from the hypnotic induction. In any case, the rare failure of a patient to respond to a finger signal does not have to be regarded as a failure of the induction; the lack of response can be ignored until posthypnotic query (if not a dialogue during hypnosis), and patients can be provided with suggestions for relaxation or analgesia in spite of its absence.

Chronic Pain Conceptualization

There are at least five psychologically-based mechanisms that can result in suffering or pain behavior in the absence of nociception (i.e., tissue damage), and they are frequently present in patients with chronic pain. First, this group often has psychological disorders that, when treated, might alleviate the pain (Chibnall & Duckro, 1994; Geisser, Roth, Bachman, & Eckert, 1996; Romano & Turner, 1985); certainly, appropriate treatment of depression and anxiety symptoms will reduce suffering. Second, many patients with chronic pain often hold specific beliefs about their pain that are maladaptive, for example, that the source of their pain requires (only) a biomedical solution, that pain is a signal of harm or physical damage, and that they are necessarily disabled by pain (Jensen, Turner, Romano, & Lawler, 1994); effective treatment involves modifying such thoughts (Turner & Romano, 2001). Third, somatization and somatosensory amplification are associated with chronic pain and are associated with a tendency to experience higher levels of pain (Barsky, Goodson, & Lane, 1988; Wilson, Dworkin, Whitney, & LeResche, 1994).

Fourth, operant and learning factors (e.g., social reinforcement in the form of unemployment compensation or attention from a solicitous spouse) can maintain pain behaviors in persons with chronic pain well after a lesion is healed (Fordyce, 1976). Finally, chronic pain is thought to be maintained, at least in part, by deactivation, guarding, and changes in body mechanics (Fordyce, 1976). Classic treatment involves systematic increases in strength and mobility, as well as multidisciplinary treatment, with goals of returning patients to work, decreasing physician visits, lessening dependence on pain medication, and increasing functional activity (Turk & Okifuji, 1998).

When applying hypnosis to chronic pain, it is important that a sufficiently specialized physician evaluate the patient to determine the extent to which *neuropathic pain* (i.e., pain due to constriction of, or damage to, nerves) versus *nociceptive* pain (i.e., pain due to the transmission of pain signals along otherwise healthy nerves) is contributing to the patient's pain, as well as to determine what biomedical treatments, if any, are indicated. If pain has a primary neuropathic component, the nature of suggestions and the patient's response will be quite different than if the pain is primarily due to nociception. The relative impact of guarding (i.e., changing body mechanics to protect areas in pain) and disuse syndrome (i.e., associated weakness or dysfunction of local muscles and tendons that result from guarding) in addition to the psychological factors described previously should be kept in mind when designing a treatment plan.

Although it is impossible to make absolute generalizations, the factors that impact pain and disability will usually influence the effectiveness of treatments used. For example, an appropriate focus of treatment for most neuropathic pain problems is the pain experience itself, and training in self-hypnosis to teach patients how to reduce the experience of pain (and any associated secondary effects, such as its effects on mood, sleep, and overall well-being) is usually indicated. Nociceptive-based pain problems tend to be more complex and may result from ongoing discomfort due to weakened muscles or tendons or from psychological factors that increase the chances that "normal" sensory information will be interpreted as pain (i.e., that the gating mechanisms for nociceptive input in the spine are largely open; Melzack & Wall, 1965). For the latter patients, a careful evaluation should be made of all of the factors that are likely contributing to pain and a treatment plan developed that addresses these factors, in collaboration with the patient.

Inductions for Chronic Pain

On the basis of clinical experience, there are some considerations in choosing inductions for patients with chronic pain. As a group, and when compared with persons with acute pain, patients with chronic pain tend to be less motivated for, and more resistant to, any type of psychologically based treatment, including hypnosis (Fordyce, 1976). Some patients might interpret effective hypnosis as "proving that the pain had always been in their head" despite years of attempts to demonstrate to health care providers that the pain they experience was "real" (Fordyce, 1988). As a consequence, more time will often have to be invested into building rapport, dispelling myths, and educating patients with chronic pain about hypnosis than those with acute pain. Also, hypnosis should be regarded by both the patient and interventionist as much more of a skill that is taught as opposed to a technique or intervention that is "done to" the patient. The primary goal will usually be to teach patients to use hypnosis and self-hypnosis effectively in their day-to-day life.

For patients with chronic pain, induction techniques that minimize resistance are often preferable. For example, although direct, brief inductions are often effective with patients in acute pain, patients with chronic pain might benefit more from induction techniques that provide them with more choices. Similarly, lengthier inductions that facilitate deep relaxation will generally be better received by such patients and are frequently easy for many patients to respond to.

Lifestyle Changes

As we have described, many treatments for chronic pain involve a focus on increasing activity. A clinician well versed in a biopsychosocial conceptualization of pain might use hypnosis as a means to motivate the patient to engage in more such adaptive behavior. For example, the clinician might say to the patient, "You can feel more confident in your ability to do whatever it takes to become stronger, knowing that over time this will increase your comfort. You can feel proud and enthusiastic about making real changes in your life." When the patient comes to understand that participation in an exercise program (either home-based or through physical therapy) is in his or her long-term best interests, he or she may find that this part of the treatment regimen has been strengthened with such suggestions.

Changes in lifestyle can also be linked to core values of the patient as hypnotic suggestions. Core values are thought to be central sources for motivating change in patients. For example, one woman may wish to manage her chronic pain because it will allow her to be more active with her grandchildren. The hypnotic suggestion might be, "As you picture the joy that you experience when you are with your grandchildren, you will find that it becomes easy to perform stretches each and every day." Or, similarly,

> You will find that at a very deep level, you know what it takes to make
> you comfortable enough to spend time with your grandchildren. You will
> find that you are able to do what it takes quickly and effortlessly.

Using a number of options, we might add the following:

> You may find your visits to the health club fun and entertaining, or you may find that you are able to exercise on a regular basis without even thinking about it, or you find that you take the stairs wherever you go.

Ericksonian Suggestions for Pain Relief

Some of the most creative and extensive suggestions for pain relief have been described by Erickson, who developed many of these strategies for managing his own severe pain that was secondary to his experience with polio (Erickson & Rossi, 1980; Patterson & Jensen, 2003). In reviewing his work, it is interesting to note that Erickson usually provided successive approximations in attempting to reduce pain. In other words, he did not try to take away all of a patient's pain with a given hypnotic session; he tried to move the patient toward reduction on a pain relief continuum over time. Erickson was known to say that clinicians place too much pressure on themselves by trying to take away all of a patient's pain. If a student is able to raise a test grade from 70 to 85, he or she would likely be extremely satisfied with that, yet clinicians may not be satisfied with a "mere" decrease of 15 out of 100 points in their patients' pain. References to Erickson's work with pain control can be found in Erickson, 1980; Erickson and Rossi, 1981; Erickson, Rossi, and Rossi, 1976. A gradual approach to modifying patient beliefs and expectations for pain is also consistent with response expectancy theory (Kirsch, 1990).

In discussing hypnotic suggestions for pain relief, Erickson reported that *hypnotic anesthesia* (i.e., complete loss of sensation) could be accomplished indirectly by building psychological and emotional situations that are contradictory to the experience of pain. However, he warned that anesthesia through hypnosis is seldom attained. He had similar views about suggestions for direct abolition of pain. In the rare circumstances when they are successful, they are often limited in duration. *Hypnotic analgesia* (i.e., reduction of pain but not with a loss of sensation) can be partial, complete, or selective. This is often achieved by introducing sensory modifications into the patient's subjective experience (e.g., relaxation, numbness, warmth, heaviness). *Amnesia* involves suggestions to forget about pain, and also can be selective, partial, or complete. An amnesic suggestion might be, "You may find yourself so involved in this pleasant activity that you forget everything else." *Displacement of pain* involves moving it from one body area to another. The area of the body to which pain is moved can be one that is less threatening or functionally limiting. For example, a patient who experiences neuropathic pain shooting up his hand and forearm might be given the suggestion that the pain has moved up to his shoulder. Theoretically, being able to move the pain to another area of the body demonstrates that he or she is able to control it better. *Hypnotic time distortion* involves altering the duration of time the patient is in pain. Again, the patient can be given a series of options, as follows:

> You may look back in time and realize that instead of being in pain for several hours, the amount of time is reduced to 1 hour or maybe just 15 minutes; I don't know how much time you will choose to start with.

In *reinterpretation of the pain experience*, pain is reinterpreted as another less unpleasant sensation. In one of his more famous cases, for example, Erickson had his patient reinterpret intractable abdominal pain as an irritating mosquito bite. Reinterpretation fits well into a cognitive–behavioral framework in which patients are encouraged to view their pain as "hurt" rather than "harm." *Hypnotic dissociation* was used by Erickson to disorient the patient in terms of time (e.g., reorienting patients to a time earlier in the illness when pain was less severe) or the body (e.g., inducing patients to experience themselves apart from their bodies). A final type of suggestion used by Erickson for pain reduction was *metaphors*, or suggestions embedded in a story. One of his more famous uses of metaphor was to embed suggestions for pain control in a discussion he had with a farmer about gardening. The farmer, being unwilling to discuss his pain, appeared to find comfort in an extended monologue from Erickson about how tomatoes can flourish in certain circumstances. This particular metaphor is quite elaborate and is recommended reading for clinicians interested in the use of pain metaphors (Haley, 1973).

Regression With Finger Signals

A particularly powerful technique for hypnotic pain control is to regress the patient or, simply put, to have the patient remember a period in his or her life during which he or she did not experience chronic pain. The use of finger signals can be useful in this regard. The patient might be told the following:

> In a moment you will find yourself going back in time and experiencing a series of very pleasant images, feelings, or symbols. Anything you experience is fine as long as the memories that you have are pleasant ones. When you arrive at a particularly pleasant and vivid image of how you felt before you developed chronic pain, you will find this [*indicated by touch*] finger pulling up automatically, as if a string was tied to it. [*When the patient shows twitching of the finger, he or she is reinforced for this behavior.*] Good! Now, I want you to experience the feelings you have with this memory. How does your body feel? Truly immerse yourself in those feelings. At the time you find your body filled with those feelings, you will feel your finger pulling up in the air once again. I want you to remember how your body feels without pain, so that you can bring these sensations with you to the present day.

The patient is eventually brought out of hypnosis with the suggestion that the preferable feelings that have been evoked will remain with the patient long after the session has ended.

A Specific Protocol for Self-Management of Chronic Pain

If the clinician determines that training the patient to use hypnosis specifically to reduce his or her experience of pain is appropriate, then the following is a specific protocol that we tend to use with most patients as a first approach. This protocol is discussed in more detail in Jensen and Patterson (2008) and Patterson (in press). Of course, this approach should be modified as needed to fit with patients' needs. Often, we start with a relaxation induction (e.g., suggesting to the patient that he or she focus on relaxing muscles, tendons, and nerves in each area of the body, starting with the left and right feet and moving to the upper legs; then moving to the right and left hand and moving to the upper arms; then relaxing the shoulders, chest, stomach, and pelvis, and finally all of the muscles in the head and face), because many people, even those with low to moderate hypnotic ability, experience suggestions for relaxation as pleasant and this provides an opportunity for early success. Other inductions (e.g., "pleasant place" imagery, age regression, ideomotor inductions) can and should be tried to give the patient an opportunity to experience different options for experiencing hypnotic phenomena. From these, one or two might be selected that that patient enjoys the most, and, with minor variations to maintain the patient's (and the clinician's) interest, can be used throughout treatment.

In the first two sessions, following the induction, we then provide a series of different suggestions for analgesia and comfort and also assess perceived pain intensity after each suggestion. This allows the patient to experience a variety of hypnotic analgesia phenomena, provides the clinician with a sense of which suggestion(s) the patient responds the best to, and provides the patient with positive feedback in regard to hypnotic pain relief. We often start with the following suggestions: extremely deep relaxation (e.g., "When it feels as if you are as relaxed as you can be, you can feel yourself becoming even more relaxed, heavier, and heavier, more and more relaxed"), sensory substitution (e.g., "You may be surprised to experience any sensations that used to be uncomfortable as a different kind of sensation. I am not sure what it will be. Perhaps a heaviness, a warmth, an interesting numbness, a pleasant tingling"), decreased pain (e.g., "Any feelings of discomfort are getting smaller and smaller, almost as if they are getting further and further away, smaller, less intense, so easy to ignore"), imagined analgesia (e.g., "Imagine any areas that are sometimes uncomfortable to be infused with a powerful anesthetic that eliminates all feelings of discomfort. This anesthetic can last for hours, even days. And the more you use it, the more powerful it becomes"), and decreased unpleasantness (e.g., "You know that pain intensity and pain unpleasantness are two different things. It is possible to experience a little pain intensity and have it bother you a lot, and it is also possible to experience significant pain intensity and have it bother you very little. Because the old, chronic pains really do not tell you anything you need to know, they do not have to bother you at all; this makes them so much easier to ignore"). Following a series of such suggestions, we provide posthypnotic suggestions for practice and for increasing the beneficial effects of self-hypnosis with practice (e.g., "Anytime you want to feel this way again, all you ever have to do is close your eyes, take a deep breath, and then let it go, and the feelings will return again. You might want to practice this many times between now and the next session, for a few minutes each time, or for a few times for many minutes. I don't know how often you will practice, but the more you practice, the better you will be at using these skills to increase your comfort and the longer your comfort will stay with you").

Usually, after the first two sessions, the specific suggestions that the patient seems to enjoy the most and respond to the best become clear, and these are included in the subsequent sessions, along with the posthypnotic suggestions for maintenance of gains, and for ease of practice. We also often ask patients to select some suggestion that they wish to experience to improve the overall quality of their life, which may, or may not, be directly related to pain. For this additional suggestion, patients often request improved sleep, improved overall well-being, or increased confidence. We include this as a way to increase the patient's sense of control over the treatment and the content of the hypnotic suggestions used. We make a tape of the next set of sessions (at least two, often more) and provide these to the patient, asking him or her to listen to the tape at least once every day, but more often if possible. We suggest when giving them the tape that the more they listen and the more they practice, the more effective treatment will be. Our protocol usually involves 10 sessions, but we have, on occasion, provided much fewer if the patient requests it, sometimes because he or she feels he or she is not benefiting and at other times because the patient's pain has been reduced to virtually nothing within just a few sessions. We also sometimes provide more than 10 sessions if, in our opinion, the patient would make additional progress with additional treatment.

CLINICAL MATERIAL

We present two case reports and a case series in this chapter. In one we describe the use of hypnosis with acute pain, the second with chronic pain, and a third focuses on preparing patients for upcoming surgery. These case reports are followed by practical clinical suggestions for working with patients prior to surgery.

A Young Man Who Needed Spinal Taps

This case involved a 20-year-old man treated at a Level I trauma center in Seattle. This case was not published and did not include the use of a hypnotizability scale. One night while he and his roommate were intoxicated, they became involved in an argument. His roommate chose to settle the argument by striking the patient in the neck with an axe. It was the patient's good fortune that the trauma did not cause a spinal cord injury. However, the patient contracted spinal meningitis, the treatment for which in our particular hospital involved serial spinal taps. At the time the psychology service was asked by surgery to see the patient, we already had six consults to perform that afternoon and a window of 10 minutes in which to see the patient. The presenting complaint was that the patient was combative during his spinal taps in such a manner that it was making it impossible to administer them. In asking the patient what the issue was, he complained that the pain of the lumbar punctures was too great. The idea of hypnosis struck us as the only possible psychological technique that could be used to address this problem within the allotted window of 10 minutes. Foregoing most of the rapport building and explanations of hypnosis that would be typically involved, the patient was asked whether he would be willing to try hypnosis to help with the lumbar punctures. He agreed, and a quick induction was performed.

The induction involved directive, fast-paced statements to the patient as follows:

> You will listen to my voice, and as I count from 1 to 5, you will find yourself becoming more and more deeply relaxed, deeper and deeper. When I reach 5, you will find yourself in a profoundly relaxed state, much like when you are asleep, but you will still be able to hear my voice.

The patient was given the posthypnotic suggestion that whenever staff members began to turn his body so that he could receive his lumbar puncture, he would feel his body go limp and comfortable, as follows:

> At this point, you may notice how profoundly relaxed and comfortable you are feeling. At some point in the future, you will feel a nurse or a doctor rolling you over so you can have your spinal tap. At the point that this happens, all of the comfort and relaxation that you are experiencing now will rush back, quickly and automatically. The act of turning over on your side will become a signal to become profoundly relaxed.

The principles behind the posthypnotic suggestions relied primarily on conditioned learning. The patient felt threatened by the lumbar punctures, and the appearance of a doctor and/or nurse with the intention of performing a lumbar puncture elicited anticipatory anxiety. A behavior was chosen that was almost certain to take place immediately prior to the threatening procedure (i.e., rolling on the stomach) and rather than having it be a stimulus for anxiety, it was made instead a cue for returning to a profoundly relaxed state. Patients are taught to allow themselves to be extremely relaxed, and a posthypnotic suggestion is tied to a part of the medical procedure.

For the first puncture performed, the hypnosis seemed to have little or no impact. However, for some unexplained reason, when the patient was rolled over for the second procedure, the staff noted that he became limp and cooperative. For the remainder of his approximately one dozen lumbar punctures, the patient was completely compliant. The staff described him as becoming completely relaxed with an ecstatic grin on his face whenever he was rolled over. The patient reported that he had begun to hypnotize himself and to give himself suggestions for improved healing and sleep. He was discharged with resolved health problems and no residual problems from his infection or trauma.

A 33-Year-Old Man With a Below-Knee Amputation

This young Native American man had a 10-year history of a left leg below-knee amputation and a subsequent infection associated with a foot injury from a motorcycle accident. He was married with a solid and supportive relationship with his wife and was currently attending community college, working toward a career in restaurant management. He presented with multiple pain problems, including occasional phantom and residual limb (i.e., "stump") pain, as well as low back and left hip pain. He described the left hip pain as most bothersome, rating the pain as 7 out of 10, on average, and as interfering significantly with his daily life, including his mobility and ability to complete house and school work and recreational activities. (Sleep interference was rated as only 3/10, pretreatment.)

He attributed his hip and low back pain to gait disturbances associated with his need to wear a prosthesis when he walked, and this was confirmed by an evaluating physician. However, both the patient and physician felt that the patient's prosthesis had been adjusted as much as it could be and that the patient had a strong desire to continue to use the prosthesis for walking (and exercise) rather than to use a wheelchair.

The results of the Stanford Clinical Hypnotizability Scale (1959) indicated a high degree of hypnotic skill for this patient (i.e., his score was 5/5). Although he reported that his severe pain made him discouraged at times, he denied most symptoms of depression and anxiety. He did not have a history of invasive biomedical treatments for pain (never having had a nerve block or surgery for pain), and although he had tried opioids in the past, he did not find them helpful and had limited current pain medications to over-the-counter analgesics. His understanding of pain appeared consistent with that of the evaluating physician, suggesting a lack of illness conviction.

On his own, he used distracting strategies for managing pain, although he had never had any formal training in hypnosis. He also reported using a large number of other adaptive pain coping strategies: ignoring pain, activity pacing, relaxation, and participation in a regular exercise and stretching program. He reported that he rarely used maladaptive strategies, such as pain-contingent rest, guarding, activity restriction, and asking for assistance.

Following the first session, in which the patient had been given a series of suggestions for pain control (i.e., as in the protocol described earlier), he reported that he had, on his own, envisioned his body filling with a "white light" during the suggestions for decreased pain and that this was also associated with feeling greater control over his experience. This creative use of hypnosis treatment is often seen in individuals, such as this patient, who have a lot of natural talent and, along the lines of Erickson's approach, should be used in subsequent treatments.

The next day, when the patient came for the second session, he expressed surprise and excitement that he had been pain-free for 5 hours after the first session, despite (or perhaps contributing to) the fact that he did more walking than usual with his prosthesis. He also stated spontaneously that he had felt "more calm" in the past 24 hours than he had felt in years. His presession pain level was 1 out of 10, which was reported to move to 0 out of 10 after the induction. The same suggestions were given in the second session as in the first (i.e., to give the patient and me a chance to observe again which ones seemed most pleasant and effective). In discussion with him, we agreed that two of the suggestions seemed particularly useful (i.e., decreased pain by envisioning the white light and decreased unpleasantness of pain), and we decided to focus on these suggestions for subsequent sessions.

The next two sessions were audiotaped, so that the patient could practice with a tape if he so chose. (Some prefer to practice on their own without a tape, though most do both.) The patient underwent six more sessions, each using the same suggestions that were selected after the second session, although they were worded somewhat differently each time to maintain the interest and focus of the patient. After each session, the patient's pain intensity was 0, though presession pain intensity varied from 0 to 3 during these sessions, and he was pain-free for some hours (varying from 3 to 48) after the sessions. He reported an increased ability to use self-hypnosis (in his case, initiating each practice session with an indrawn breath and then allowing the posthypnotic suggestions for comfort to have their effects while envisioning the white light he spontaneously envisioned during the first session) over time and with continued practice.

After treatment, the patient reported his average pain to be 2 out of 10 and reported substantial improvement (i.e., a decrease) in the impact of his pain on his day-to-day activities, especially his mood (i.e., from pretreatment at 3/10 to 0/10), and interference with enjoyment of life (i.e., from 5/10 to 0/10). He also commented that he felt he had much more control over his pain. At 3 months posttreatment, average pain remained at a 2 out of 10 level, and the negative impact of pain also was maintained. By 6 months, his average pain had dropped to 1 out of 10. He stated at that time that, whenever his pain started to become annoying or more intense, he practiced self-hypnosis on his own (i.e., without the tape) approximately every other day, usually three times a day for 10 minutes each time. Almost always, this practice resulted in a substantial decrease in pain that usually lasted for 3 to 4 hours before he felt the need to use self-hypnosis again.

All of the improvements were maintained to 12 months posttreatment (i.e., on average 1/10 pain with little negative impact), although it is interesting to note that the patient's pattern of self-hypnosis practice had changed by that time. He reported at 12 months follow-up that he was now practicing self-hypnosis on a daily basis, usually twice per day and usually 5 minutes each time. Although he reported the same marked decrease in pain with this practice, he stated that pain relief lasted about 2 hours with this regimen.

Common Elements in Preparing Patients for Surgery

Over the course of my and my collaborators' work with surgery patients at Mount Sinai, we have to date seen over 400 cases. Rather than present a single case, I (Montgomery) report on a common patient profile; that is, the patient who desires to remain alert and to be an active and directive participant in his or her medical treatment.

One key element in preparing a patient for the use of hypnosis in conjunction with surgical procedures is debunking myths concerning hypnosis. On hearing that hypnosis is being considered as part of the treatment plan, some patients immediately go on the offensive. That is, they raise numerous questions and express preconceived beliefs and misconceptions about hypnosis (e.g., "It is mind control"). They almost dare the hypnotist to engage them in hypnosis. This behavior can range from reasonable concern to provocative anger. It is important that the interventionist respect the patient's autonomy and refuse to engage in a power struggle. It is also of primary importance to counter these beliefs with accurate information about hypnosis (e.g., "Hypnosis is not mind control, but a technique you can use to help yourself feel better"), which serves to put patients at ease and set realistic treatment expectations (Kirsch, 1990). Some patients even stridently deny their ability to be hypnotized (e.g., "I am too strong willed to be hypnotized"); however, once hypnosis is framed as a tool that they can use and that is under their control, they are typically put at ease and become willing participants in the hypnosis session. As in any clinical situation, patients interpret hypnosis through the lens of their personality characteristics, schema, and expectancies. It is up to the interventionist to frame hypnosis in a way that is useful for patients. And, as in any clinical situation, it is the interventionist's responsibility to address patients' issues in a way that makes them comfortable with the overall treatment plan.

A second key element in preparing patients for hypnosis is managing therapeutic expectancies. Many patients have past experiences with hypnosis or other related techniques (e.g., meditation), and the interventionist should assess patients' reactions to these experiences before beginning anew. For example, patients are not uncommonly disappointed in their past responses to hypnosis (e.g., "I felt relaxed, but I don't think I was in a trance, so I don't think it worked"). They are waiting for a dramatic experience. It is important to clarify with patients that there is no one right way to experience hypnosis and that hypnosis can be useful regardless of their particular reaction. On a related note, we do not use the word *trance* with patients because it sets unrealistic expectancies that can contribute to a sense of failure on their part. Instead, we work therapeutically to initially set expectancies for achievable goals. Once patients achieve these goals through hypnosis, these responses (e.g., less pain) are self-reinforcing (Kirsch, 1990).

A third key issue to address prior to surgery is the tension patients often express between wanting to relax and wanting to remain alert and in control in order to participate in their surgical treatment (e.g., they want to be able to speak with their treatment team, including anesthesiologists and surgeons). This tension is easily relieved through educating patients that they are the ones in control of their hypnotic experience. If they choose, they can remain alert for discussions of medical procedures and feel relaxed, calm and peaceful during and after surgical procedures. Patients can be instructed that they can end their hypnotic experience whenever they so choose.

RESEARCH AND APPRAISAL

The existing literature supports the view that hypnosis is a useful nonpharmacologic pain management technique. Although hypnosis has been used as a psychological technique for treatment of a broad range of disorders and illnesses (e.g., phobias, depression, anorexia nervosa, multiple personality disorder, psychotic disorders, posttraumatic stress disorders, obesity, smoking, somatization disorders; Rhue, Lynn, & Kirsch, 1993), it is perhaps best known as a pain management technique. Interest in hypnosis for pain control and pain reduction may in part be due to long-standing dramatic reports of pain relief with hypnosis during highly aversive medical procedures (Esdaile, 1957), as well as the breadth of patients hypnosis has been effectively used with. For example, in clinical studies hypnosis has been demonstrated to relieve pain in patients with headache (Spinhoven, Linssen, Van Dyck, & Zitman, 1992; ter Kuile et al., 1994; Van Dyck, Zitman, Linssen, & Spinhoven, 1991), burn injury (Patterson et al., 1992; Patterson & Ptacek, 1997; Wakeman & Kaplan, 1978), heart disease (Weinstein & Au, 1991), arthritis (Haanen et al., 1991; Horton & Mitzdorf, 1994), cancer (Katz, Kellerman, & Ellenberg, 1987; Spiegel & Bloom, 1983; Syrjala, Cummings, & Donaldson, 1992; Wall & Womack, 1989), dental problems (Stam, McGrath, & Brooke, 1984), traumatic medical procedures (Butler, Symons, Henderson, Shortliffe, & Spiegel, 2005), eczema (Hajek, Radil, & Jakoubek, 1991), and chronic back problems (Melzack & Perry, 1975; Spinhoven & Linssen, 1989). Hypnosis has also been shown to be highly effective for ameliorating aversive side effects following surgical procedures, including pain, negative affect, and recovery (Montgomery, David, et al., 2002). Potential advantages of hypnosis include a sense of mastery and control, reduced distress (Montgomery, David, et al., 2002), and feeling pleasant and relaxed in stressful medical settings (Montgomery et al., 2000).

Despite long-standing clinical use and empirical reports on hypnosis, systematic attempts to quantify the effectiveness of hypnotic suggestion for pain relief have been relatively rare. Meta-analysis (Hunter & Schmidt, 1990; Smith, Glass, & Miller, 1980) provides an established quantitative methodology for evaluating the effectiveness of hypnosis for pain relief across study samples in the published literature. More specifically, *meta-analysis* is the organization and integration of previously published data through calculation of effect sizes. An effect size is a standardized estimate of the magnitude of a study effect that permits direct comparisons of effects across studies. In addition, statistical analyses of effect sizes can provide a better understanding of cumulative research findings for an area, or subject, of research interest than traditional narrative review articles (Hunter & Schmidt, 1990).

In a meta-analysis of the use of hypnotic suggestion for pain control, Montgomery et al. (2000) found strong empirical support for the effectiveness of hypnosis. In that paper, an analysis of between-group studies indicated that the average participant in hypnotic suggestion treatment groups had greater analgesic responses than 75% of participants in control groups. Effects of hypnotic suggestion for pain relief did not differ in regard to whether the pain in question was due to clinical issues or experimental stimuli. Essentially, hypnosis worked equally well in clinical and laboratory contexts. It is interesting to note that when levels of hypnotic suggestibility were taken into account, hypnosis was effective for the vast majority of patients. Once patients were divided into high, medium, and low levels of hypnotic suggestibility, the results revealed that although the high suggestibility group experienced less pain than the low suggestibility group, pain relief in the medium suggestibility group did not differ from that revealed in the high or low suggestibility groups. These data further support the view that the role of hypnotizability is more clearly established in a laboratory, as opposed to clinical studies (Patterson & Jensen, 2003).

A more recent meta-analysis of the use of hypnosis with patients who have undergone surgery is equally supportive of hypnoanalgesic effects (Montgomery, David, et al., 2002). Whether the pain outcome studied was self-reported pain (weighted effect size $D = 1.69$, 95%; CI $= 0.56$, 2.82) or pain medication use (weighted effect size $D = 1.17$, 95%; CI $= 0.41$, 1.93) hypnosis was effective for controlling patients' surgery-related pain.

Patterson and Jensen (2003) complemented these meta-analyses in a narrative review of randomized controlled studies of hypnosis for clinical pain. As was the strategy with this chapter, they divided the review based on whether the studies focused on acute or chronic pain. They reviewed 17 studies on acute pain and 12 on chronic pain. In the acute pain studies (e.g., for cancer procedures, childbirth, burn wound care), hypnosis appeared superior to control conditions and generally more effective than alternative treatments. The chronic pain studies, the majority of which were done with headache pain, showed that hypnosis was also more effective than control treatment and had an impact that was equivalent to relaxation training or autogenic training. In both acute and chronic pain studies, when measures of hypnotizability (i.e., suggestibility) were included, increased hypnotic suggestibility was usually associated with greater reports of pain reduction and improved outcome. However, regardless of level of suggestibility, most patients benefited from hypnosis.

Recent articles continue to support the use of hypnotic suggestion to control pain in a variety of populations. For example, Palsson, Turner, Johnson, Burnelt, and Whitehead (2002) demonstrated the effectiveness of hypnosis in patients with irritable bowel syndrome. In that study ($N = 18$), hypnosis was reported to be effective in reducing abdominal pain, and the type of hypnotic suggestions used (i.e., pain specific vs. not) was not a critical factor for achieving patient benefit. In pediatric patients with cancer undergoing lumbar puncture procedures ($N = 80$), Liossi and Hatira (2003) reported that hypnosis was superior to attention control as well as superior to standard care control conditions in terms of pain control. Pediatric patients reported less pain during lumbar punctures when using hypnosis. Furthermore, whether hypnotic procedures were made using direct or indirect approaches, there was no difference in clinical outcome. Benefits due to hypnosis appeared to decrease once patients were shifted from "live" to "self" hypnosis, perhaps suggesting the importance of the therapeutic relationship and/or guidance when working with pediatric patients. A third study not only supports the use of hypnosis for pain control but also suggests that the effects of hypnosis for pain reduction are not limited to western cultures. Harandi, Esfandani and Shakibaei (2004) demonstrated that Iranian burn patients randomly assigned to a hypnosis intervention had significantly less procedural pain than a control group.

Despite a growing empirical literature and clinical interest in using hypnosis to alleviate pain, methodological problems in some studies could potentially dampen enthusiasm for hypnosis and thus inhibit the translation of hypnotic techniques from the research setting to standard clinical practice. One methodological problem is that many of the studies in the literature have small sample sizes. As the health psychology field in general moves toward more stringent criteria for the reporting and evaluation of clinical studies (e.g., Consolidated Standards of Reporting Trials Guidelines; Moher, Schulz, & Altman, 2001), studies of the efficacy of hypnosis for pain control should follow suit. A second problem is that the operational definitions of hypnosis appear to vary widely across studies to the point that it is unclear what construct is being referred to. For example, Gay, Philippot, and Luminet (2002) compared a hypnosis intervention, a relaxation intervention, and a control condition. On the basis of previous published meta-analyses (Kirsch, Montgomery, & Sapirstein, 1995) and empirical work (Schoenberger et al., 1997), one would expect the hypnosis condition to be superior to the relaxation condition. However, in the Gay study, there were no differences between relaxation and hypnosis groups on pain. Closer examination of the study reveals that the authors never refer to the hypnosis intervention as "hypnosis" with patients, and instead refer to it as "imagery." From a socio–cognitive perspective, this change in terminology may fail to activate positive expectancies and beliefs associated with hypnosis and thereby reduce its effectiveness. It is possible that their hypnosis intervention would have been more effective had they been open with patients and referred to their intervention in a way consistent with their own conceptualization and hypotheses. Overall, authors need to be clear about the methods used in delivering their hypnosis intervention to patients.

In summary, the empirical data strongly support the use of hypnotic suggestion for pain control in clinical populations. The beneficial effects of hypnosis have been demonstrated in a wide variety of patients and may have long lasting beneficial effects (Gonsalkorale, Miller, Afzal, & Whorwell, 2003); there is every reason to believe that this technique can and should be applied even more widely in the future. To ensure that this more widespread application takes place, further randomized clinical trials with larger sample sizes may be needed to provide incontrovertible evidence for such organizations as third party payers. Data on the cost-effectiveness of these interventions will also be critical in this regard. Unfortunately, pain is a part of life for a great many patients, and pain is the primary reason Americans seek medical treatment (Abbott & Fraser, 1998). In addition, pain is nearly ubiquitous for patients undergoing aversive medical treatments. It is the duty of researchers to help individuals in pain by devising and testing interventions that can reliably ameliorate their suffering.

CONCLUSION

Pain control is one of the most promising applications of hypnosis, and developments in this area have played a large part in the recent increase in enthusiasm for this modality of treatment. The evidence for the impact of hypnosis on clinical pain is strong both in meta-analyses and narrative reviews of randomized controlled studies. When applying hypnosis to pain, it is important for the clinician to understand whether the pain is acute or chronic, to assess the emotional state of the patient, and to investigate the presence of a number of potential complicating factors that might exist based on the nature of pain. There are a variety of suggestions that can be provided to patients in pain; deciding which ones to be used can be based on the theoretical orientation of the clinician as well as the nature of the presenting problem.

REFERENCES

Abbott, F. V., & Fraser, M. I. (1998). Use and abuse of over-the-counter analgesic agents. *Journal of Psychiatry and Neuroscience, 23*(1), 13–34.

Auret, K., & Schug, S. A. (2005). Underutilisation of opioids in elderly patients with chronic pain: Approaches to correcting the problem. *Drugs & Aging, 22,* 641–654.

Barabasz, A., & Watkins, J. G. (2005). *Hypnotherapeutic techniques* (2nd ed.). New York: Brunner/Routledge.

Barsky, A. J., Goodson, D. K., & Lane, R. S. (1988). The amplification of somatic symptoms. *Psychosomatic Medicine, 50,* 510–519.

Bone, R. C., Hayden, W. R., Levine, R. L., McCartney, J. R., Barkin, R. L., Clark, S., et al. (1995). Recognition, assessment, and treatment of anxiety in the critical care patient: Consensus guidelines from a working party. *Disease-a-Month, 41,* 293–360.

Bruera, E., & Pereira, J. (1997). Acute neuropsychiatric findings in a patient receiving fentanyl for cancer pain. *Pain, 69,* 199–201.

Butler, L. D., Symons, B. K., Henderson, S. L., Shortliffe, L. D., & Spiegel, D. (2005). Hypnosis reduces distress and duration of an invasive medical procedure for children. *Pediatrics, 115,* e77–e85.

Chapman, C. R. (1985). Psychological factors in postoperative pain and their treatment. In G. Smith & B. G. Covino (Eds.), *Acute Pain* (pp. 22–41). London: Butterworths.

Chapman, C. R., & Bonica, J. J. (1983). *Current Concepts: Acute pain*. Kalamazoo, MI: The Upjohn Company.

Chibnall, J. T., & Duckro, P. N. (1994). Posttraumatic stress disorder in chronic post-traumatic headache patients. *Headache, 34,* 357–361.

Chien, S. (1967). Role of the sympathetic nervous system in hemorrhage. *Physiological Review, 47,* 214–288.

Crasilneck, H. B., Stirman, J. A., & Wilson, B. J. (1955). Use of hypnosis in the management of patients with burns. *JAMA, 158,* 103–106.

Eisenberg, D. M., Kessler, R. C., Foster, C., Norlock, F. E., Calkins, D. R., & Delbanco, T. L. (1993). Unconvetional medicine in the United States: Prevalence, costs, and patterns of use. *New England Journal of Medicine, 328*(4), 246–252.

Erickson, M. (1980). *Innovative hypnotherapy* (Vol. 4). New York: Irvington Publishers.

Erickson, M., & Rossi, E. (1981). *Experiencing hypnosis: Therapeutic approaches to altered states*. New York: Irvington Publishers.

Erickson, M., Rossi, E., & Rossi, S. (1976). *Hypnotic realities: The induction of clinical hypnosis and forms of indirect suggestion*. New York: Irvington.

Erickson, M. H., & Rossi, E. L. (1980). Autohypnotic experiences of Milton Erickson. In E. L. Rossi (Ed.), *The nature of hypnosis and suggestion by Milton Erickson: The collected papers of Milton H. Erickson on hypnosis* (Vol. 1, pp. 108–132). New York: Irvington.

Esdaile, J. (1957). *Hypnosis in medicine and surgery*. New York: Julian Press.

Fordyce, W. E. (1976). *Behavioral methods for chronic pain and illness*. St. Louis, MO: Mosby.

Fordyce, W. E. (1988). Pain and suffering. *American Psychologist, 43,* 276–283.

Fromm, E., & Nash, M. R. (1997). *Psychoanalysis and hypnosis*. Madison, CT: International Universities Press.

Gay, M. C., Philippot, P., & Luminet, O. (2002). Differential effectiveness of psychological interventions for reducing osteoarthritis pain: A comparison of Erikson hypnosis and Jacobson relaxation. *European Journal of Pain, 6,* 1–16.

Geisser, M. E., Roth, R. S., Bachman, J. E., & Eckert, T. A. (1996). The relationship between symptoms of posttraumatic stress disorder and pain, affective disturbance, and disability among patients with accident and non-accident related pain. *Pain, 66,* 207–214.

Gonsalkorale, W. M., Miller, V., Afzal, A., & Whorwell, P. J. (2003). Long-term benefits of hypnotherapy for irritable bowel syndrome. *Gut, 52,* 1623–1629.

Gureje, O., Von Korff, M., Simon, G. E., & Gater, R. (1998). Persistent pain and well-being: A World Health Organization study in primary care. *JAMA, 280,* 147–151.

Haanen, H. C., Hoenderdos, H. T., van Romunde, L. K., Hop, W. C., Mallee, C., Terwiel, J. P., et al. (1991). Controlled trial of hypnotherapy in the treatment of refractory fibromyalgia. *Journal of Rheumatology, 18,* 72–75.

Hajek, P., Radil, T., & Jakoubek, B. (1991). Hypnotic skin analgesia in healthy individuals and patients with atopic eczema. *Homeostasis in Health and Disease, 33,* 156–157.

Haley, J. (1973). *Uncommon therapy: The psychiatric techniques of Milton H. Erickson, M.D.* New York: Norton.

Harandi, A. A., Esfandani, A., & Shakibaei, F. (2004). The effect of hypnotherapy on procedural pain and state anxiety related to physiotherapy in women hospitalized in a burn unit. *Contemporary Hypnosis, 21,* 28–34.

Hilgard, E. R., & Hilgard, J. R. (1975). *Hypnosis in the relief of pain.* Los Altos, CA: William Kaufmann, Inc.

Horton, J. R., & Mitzdorf, U. (1994). Clinical hypnosis in the treatment of rheumatoid arthritis. *Psychologische Beitraege, 36,* 205–212.

Hunter, J. E., & Schmidt, F. L. (1990). *Methods of meta-anlaysis: Correcting error and bias in research findings.* Newbury Park, CA: Sage.

Jacobson, L., & Mariano, A. J. (2001). General considerations of chronic pain. In J. D. Loeser, S. H. Butler, C. R. Chapman & D. C. Turk (Eds.), *Bonica's management of pain* (pp. 241–254). Philadelphia: Lippincott Williams & Wilkins.

Jaffe, S. E., & Patterson, D. R. (2004). Treating sleep problems in patients with burn injuries: Practical considerations. *Journal of Burn Care & Rehabilitation, 25,* 294–305.

Jensen, M. P., & Patterson, D. R. (2008). Hypnosis and the relief of pain and disorders. In M. Nash & A. Barnier (Eds.), *The Oxford Handbook of Hypnosis* (pp. 503–533). New York: Oxford University Press.

Jensen, M. P., Turner, J. A., Romano, J. M., & Lawler, B. K. (1994). Relationship of pain-specific beliefs to chronic pain adjustment. *Pain, 57,* 301–309.

Katz, E. R., Kellerman, J., & Ellenberg, L. (1987). Hypnosis in the reduction of acute pain and distress in children with cancer. *Journal of Pediatric Psychology, 12,* 379–394.

Katz, N. (2002). The impact of pain management on quality of life. *Journal of Pain Symptom Management, 24*(Suppl. 1), S38–S47.

Kehlet, H., & Dahl, J. B. (2003, December 6). Anaesthesia, surgery, and challenges in postoperative recovery. *The Lancet, 362,* 1921–1928.

Kihlstrom, J. F. (1992). Hypnosis: A sesquicentennial essay. *International Journal of Clinical and Experimental Hypnosis, 50,* 301–314.

Kirsch, I. (1990). *Changing expectations: A key to effective psychotherapy.* Pacific Grove, CA: Brooks/Cole.

Kirsch, I., Montgomery, G., & Sapirstein, G. (1995). Hypnosis as an adjunct to cognitive–behavioral psychotherapy: A meta-analysis. *Journal of Consulting and Clinical Psychology, 63,* 214–220.

Lang, E., & Rosen, M. (2002). Cost analysis of adjunct hypnosis with sedation during outpatient interventional radiologic procedures. *Radiology, 222,* 375–382.

Lang, E. V., Benotsch, E. G., Fick, L. J., Lutgendorf, S., Berbaum, M. L., Berbaum, K. S., et al. (2000, April 29). Adjunctive non-pharmacological analgesia for invasive medical procedures: A randomised trial. *The Lancet, 355,* 1486–1490.

Liossi, C., & Hatira, P. (2003). Clinical hypnosis in the alleviation of procedure-related pain in pediatric oncology patients. *International Journal of Clinical and Experimental Hypnosis, 51,* 4–28.

Loeser, J. D. (1999). Economic implications of pain management. *Acta Anaesthesioligica Scandinavica, 43,* 957–959.

Loeser, J. D. (Ed.). (2001). *Bonica's management of pain* (3rd ed.). Philadelphia: Lippincot, Williams, & Wilkins.

Lynn, S. J., & Rhue, J. W. (1991). *Theories of hypnosis: Current models and perspectives.* New York: Guilford Press.

Mackersie, R. C., & Karagianes, T. G. (1990). Pain management following trauma and burns. *Anesthesiology Clinics of North America, 7,* 433–449.

Melzack, R., & Perry, C. (1975). Self-regulation of pain: The use of alpha-feedback and hypnotic training for the control of chronic pain. *Experimental Neurology, 46,* 452–469.

Melzack, R., & Wall, P. (1973). *The challenge of pain.* New York: Basic Books.

Melzack, R., & Wall, P. D. (1965, November 19). Pain mechanisms: A new theory. *Science, 150,* 971–979.

Moher, D., Schulz, K. F., & Altman, D. G. (2001). The CONSORT statement: Revised recommendations for improving the quality of reports of parallel group randomized trials. *BMC Medical Research Methodology, 1,* 2.

Montgomery, G. H. (2005). *The role of hypnosis in 21st-century medicine.* Paper presented at the meeting of the American Psychology Association, Washington, DC.

Montgomery, G. H., & Bovbjerg, D. H. (2004). Presurgery distress and specific response expectancies predict postsurgery outcomes in surgery patients confronting breast cancer. *Health Psychology, 23,* 381–387.

Montgomery, G. H., Bovbjerg, D. H., Schnur, J. B., David, D., Goldfarb, A., Weltz, C., et al. (2007). A randomized clinical trial of a hypnosis intervention to control side effects in breast cancer surgery patients. *JNCI, 99,* 1304–1312.

Montgomery, G. H., David, D., Winkel, G., Silverstein, J. H., & Bovbjerg, D. H. (2002). The effectiveness of adjunctive hypnosis with surgical patients: A meta-analysis. *Anesthesia & Analgesia, 94,* 1639–1645.

Montgomery, G. H., DuHamel, K. N., & Redd, W. H. (2000). A meta-analysis of hypnotically induced analgesia: How effective is hypnosis? *International Journal of Clinical and Experimental Hypnosis, 48,* 138–153.

Montgomery, G., & Kirsch, I. (1996). Mechanisms of placebo pain reduction: An empirical investigation. *Psychological Science, 7,* 174–176.

Montgomery, G. H., & Kirsch, I. (1997). Classical conditioning and the placebo effect. *Pain, 72,* 107–113.

Montgomery, G. H., Weltz, C. R., Seltz, M., & Bovbjerg, D. H. (2002). Brief presurgery hypnosis reduces distress and pain in excisional breast biopsy patients. *International Journal of Clinical and Experimental Hypnosis, 50,* 17–32.

Niv, D., & Kreitler, S. (2001). Pain and quality of life. *Pain Practice, 1,* 150–161.

Palsson, O. S., Turner, M. J., Johnson, D. A., Burnelt, C. K., & Whitehead, W. E. (2002). Hypnosis treatment for severe irritable bowel syndrome: Investigation of mechanism and effects on symptoms. *Digestive Diseases and Sciences, 47,* 2605–2614.

Patterson, D. R. (1995). Nonopioid based approaches to burn pain. *Journal of Burn Care and Rehabilitation, 16,* 372–376.

Patterson, D. R. (1996). Burn Pain. In J. Barber (Ed.), *Hypnosis and suggestion in the treatment of pain* (pp. 267–302). New York: Norton.

Patterson, D. R. (in press). *Clinical hypnosis for pain control.* Washington, DC: American Psychological Association.

Patterson, D. R., Adcock, R. J., & Bombardier, C. H. (1997). Factors predicting hypnotic analgesia in clinical burn pain. *International Journal of Clinical and Experimental Hypnosis, 45,* 377–395.

Patterson, D. R., Everett, J. J., Bombardier, C. H., Questad, K. A., Lee, V. K., & Marvin, J. A. (1993). Psychological effects of severe burn injuries. *Psychological Bulletin, 113,* 362–378.

Patterson, D. R., Everett, J. J., Burns, G. L., & Marvin, J. A. (1992). Hypnosis for the treatment of burn pain. *Journal of Consulting and Clinical Psychology, 60,* 713–717.

Patterson, D. R., & Jensen, M. (2003). Hypnosis and clinical pain. *Psychological Bulletin, 129,* 495–521.

Patterson, D. R., & Ptacek, J. T. (1997). Baseline pain as a moderator of hypnotic analgesia for burn injury treatment. *Journal of Consulting and Clinical Psychology, 65,* 60–67.

Patterson, D. R., & Sharar, S. (2001). Burn pain. In J. Loeser (Ed.), *Bonica's management of pain* (3rd ed., pp. 780–787). Philadelphia: Lippincott Williams & Wilkins.

Rainville, P., Duncan, G. H., Price, D. D., Carrier, B., & Bushnell, M. C. (1997, August 15). Pain affect encoded in human anterior cingulate but not somatosensory cortex. *Science, 277,* 968–971.

Rhue, J. W., Lynn, S. J., & Kirsch, I. (1993). *Handbook of clinical hypnosis.* Washington, DC: American Psychological Association.

Romano, J. M., & Turner, J. A. (1985). Chronic pain and depression: Does the evidence support a relationship? *Psychological Bulletin, 97,* 18–34.

Schoenberger, N. E., Kirsch, I., Gearan, P., Montgomery, G., & Pastyrnak, S. L. (1997). Hypnotic enhancement of a cognitive behavioral treatment for public speaking anxiety. *Behavior Therapy, 28,* 127–140.

Schulz-Stubner, S. (2000). Clinical hypnosis and anesthesia: A historical review and its clinical implications in today's practice. *Bulletin of Anesthesia History, 18,* 4–5.

Smith, M. L., Glass, G. V., & Miller, T. I. (1980). *The benefits of psychotherapy.* Baltimore, MD: Johns Hopkins University Press.

Spiegel, D. (1991). Hypnosis, dissociation and trauma: Hidden and overt observers. In J. L. Singer (Ed.), *Repression and dissociation: Implications for personality theory, psychopathology and health* (pp. 121–142). Chicago: University of Chicago Press.

Spiegel, D., & Bloom, J. R. (1983). Group therapy and hypnosis reduce metastatic breast carcinoma pain. *Psychosomatic Medicine, 45,* 333–339.

Spiegel, D., Hunt, T., & Dondershine, H. E. (1988). Dissociation and hypnotizability in posttraumatic stress disorder. *American Journal of Psychiatry, 145,* 301–305.

Spiegel, D., Koopman, C., & Classen, C. (1994). Acute stress disorder and dissociation. *Australian Journal of Clinical and Experimental Hypnosis, 22,* 11–23.

Spinhoven, P., & Linssen, A. C. (1989). Education and self-hypnosis in the management of low back pain: A component analysis. *British Journal of Clinical Psychology, 28,* 145–153.

Spinhoven, P., Linssen, A. C., Van Dyck, R., & Zitman, F. G. (1992). Autogenic training and self-hypnosis in the control of tension headache. *General Hospital Psychiatry, 14,* 408–415.

Stam, H. J., McGrath, P. A., & Brooke, R. I. (1984). The effects of a cognitive–behavioral treatment program on temporomandibular pain and dysfunction syndrome. *Psychosomatic Medicine, 46,* 534–545.

Sternbach, R. A. (1986). Pain and "hassles" in the United States: Findings of the Nuprin pain report. *Pain, 27,* 69–80.

Syrjala, K. L., Cummings, C., & Donaldson, G. W. (1992). Hypnosis or cognitive behavioral training for the reduction of pain and nausea during cancer treatment: A controlled clinical trial. *Pain, 48,* 137–146.

ter Kuile, M. M., Spinhoven, P., Linssen, A. C., Zitman, F. G., Van Dyck, R., & Rooijmans, H. G. (1994). Autogenic training and cognitive self-hypnosis for the treatment of recurrent headaches in three different subject groups. *Pain, 58,* 331–340.

Thompson, S. C. (1981). Will it hurt less if I can control it? A complex answer to a simple question. *Psychological Bulletin, 90,* 89–100.

Turk, D. C., & Okifuji, A. (1998). Treatment of chronic pain patients: Clinical outcomes, cost-effectiveness, and cost-benefits of multidisciplinary pain centers. *Critical Reviews in Physical and Rehabilitation Medicine, 10,* 181–208.

Turner, J. A., & Romano, J. M. (2001). Cognitive–behavioral therapy for chronic pain. In J. D. Loeser, S. H. Butler, C. R. Chapman, & D. C. Turk (Eds.), *Bonica's management of pain* (3rd ed., pp. 1751–1758). Philadelphia: Lippincott Williams & Wilkins.

Van Dyck, R., Zitman, F. G., Linssen, A. C., & Spinhoven, P. (1991). Autogenic training and future oriented hypnotic imagery in the treatment of tension headache: Outcome and process. *International Journal of Clinical and Experimental Hypnosis, 39,* 6–23.

Wakeman, J. R., & Kaplan, J. Z. (1978). An experimental study of hypnosis in painful burns. *American Journal of Clinical Hypnosis, 21*, 3–12.

Wall, V. J., & Womack, W. (1989). Hypnotic versus active cognitive strategies for alleviation of procedural distress in pediatric oncology patients. *American Journal of Clinical Hypnosis, 31*, 181–191.

Weinstein, E. J., & Au, P. K. (1991). Use of hypnosis before and during angioplasty. *American Journal of Clinical Hypnosis, 34*, 29–37.

Weitzenhoffer, A. M., & Hilgard, E. R. (1959). *Stanford Hypnotic Susceptibility Scale Forms A & B.* Palo Alto, CA: Consulting Psychologists Press.

Wilson, L., Dworkin, S. F., Whitney, C., & LeResche, L. (1994). Somatization and pain dispersion in chronic temporomandibular disorder pain. *Pain, 57*, 55–61.

22

HYPNOSIS AND MEDICINE

NICHOLAS A. COVINO AND CORNELIA M. PINNELL

Only a small percentage of any population will approach traditional mental health services for psychological care, but the vast majority of us will become patients in a medical setting at several points in our lives. Medical illnesses, conditions, procedures, and treatments are influenced by psychological factors and, commonly, influence them. Depression, anxiety, and anger are frequent sequelae to medical illness and have been implicated as important variables in illness onset.

In recent years, medical practitioners have increased their diagnostic acumen with regard to the psychological dimensions of their patients' care. Primary care providers are likely to recognize symptoms of depression or anxiety in the patients who visit their office, diagnose them with a mood or an anxiety disorder, and prescribe antidepressant or antianxiety medications. Consequently, some of the traditional mental health services, such as psychiatric diagnosis, may be delivered by primary care physicians rather than psychiatrists, psychologists, and other psychotherapists (Pincus, Tanielian, & Marcus, 1998). Medical settings are excellent places to identify those in need of mental health care.

All clinical material has been disguised to protect patient confidentiality.

Problems of psychophysiological arousal, behavior, affect, and the patient's intrapsychic and interpersonal world (i.e., *psychodynamics*) contribute, independently and interactively, to amplify autonomic nervous system activity and intensify medical symptoms. Not only can psychological factors adversely affect physiological functioning, but they also undermine otherwise appropriate medical care. Historically, the multiple dimensions of a patient's experience of illness have been neglected by investigators championing the primacy of one psychological theory, one explanatory account for illness behavior, and one intervention, to the relative neglect of others. As Cassileth et al. (1984) noted, psychosomatic researchers tend to work parochially, failing to integrate the influential psychological variables of one illness area (e.g., Type A behavior pattern in heart disease) into another (e.g., asthma) or concentrating on the role that certain psychological factors play in the inception of an illness while ignoring their potential for symptom management.

The results of experimental investigations in behavioral medicine support the use of a variety of psychological techniques for the care of medical patients (Chiles, Lambert, & Arlen, 1999). Pertinent to our discussion, hypnosis interventions can benefit patients with a variety of medical conditions and disorders ranging from functional gastrointestinal disorders to asthma, pain, and anticipatory emesis (Covino, 2008; Montgomery, DuHamel, & Redd, 2000; Patterson & Jensen, 2003; Pinnell & Covino, 2000). Because this literature has been previously reviewed and the problems of pain, surgical anxiety, and psychosomatic disorders are presented elsewhere in this volume, we devote our attention to presenting a model for clinical intervention with medical patients and explicating the application of hypnosis to a diversity of medical disorders and conditions in this context.

CLINICAL APPLICATIONS

We adopt a biopsychosocial perspective (Engel, 1977), which proposes that most medical conditions are neither all physical nor all psychological. Numerous physical illnesses depend on the interplay of biological, social, cognitive (i.e., self-perceptions, psychodynamics), and cultural factors (Turk, 1996). For example, patients' perceptions of danger and threat and the apprehensiveness and helplessness that ensue may amplify autonomic nervous system (ANS) activity, which leads to predictable alterations of heart rate, respiratory functioning, muscle tension, adrenal activity, gastrointestinal motility, and other physiological responses. A hyperreactive cognitive style that consistently stimulates ANS activity through sympathetic arousal can not only exacerbate physiological conditions such as asthma (Hasler et al., 2005), hemorrhagic disorders (Enqvist, von Konow, & Bystedt, 1995), irritable bowel syndrome (Blanchard, 2001; Casati & Toner, 2002; see also chap. 25, this volume), and insomnia (Bonnet & Arand, 1995, 2003) but also affect invasive diagnostic and interventional procedures (Butler, Symons, Henderson, Shortliffe, & Spiegel, 2005; Lang et al., 2000; Zeltzer & LeBaron, 1982; see also chap. 23, this volume). Accordingly, relaxation training and hypnotic intervention, with suggestions to alter apprehensive thoughts, can potentially reduce sympathetic arousal and, as a consequence, physical symptoms.

Relaxation and hypnosis can also alter a variety of repetitive, avoidant, and conditioned behaviors in health settings. For example, behaviors such as scratching, rubbing, and picking at lesions and abrasions occur in repetitious cycles that reinjure the skin and prevent healing. Avoidance behaviors such as needle phobias prevent patients from keeping appointments and adhering to medical directives. Operant and classical conditioning principles may explain the intractability of certain medical problems such as bulimia (Bulik, 2005; Wilson, 2005), cigarette smoking (Covino & Bottari, 2001; Law & Tang, 1995), and anticipatory nausea and vomiting (ANV; Redd, Montgomery, & DuHamel, 2001). For example, many bulimics learn to attenuate painful affects by binging and purging, which constitute negative reinforcement (Hohlstein, Smith, & Atlast, 1998). Cigarette smoking may be reinforced by positive associations with pleasant outcomes created by media-promoted images of an exciting lifestyle. Anticipatory emesis may arise from negative associations with the emetic properties of chemotherapy and the hospital's smells, sights, and personnel, leading any of the latter to become stimuli for ANV. Hypnosis interventions can inhibit excoriating behaviors through the combination of relaxation and behavioral rehearsal, with response prevention added to relaxation and distraction strategies proving useful to patients with acne and other skin disorders (Shenefelt, 2004; Zachariae, Oster, Bjerring, & Kragballe, 1996).

Affective and medical disorders are commonly comorbid. A recent longitudinal study determined that anxiety and panic predispose adults to develop bronchial asthma with the reverse also true. Hasler et al. (2005) observed a six-fold likelihood of developing asthma over 20 years for people with panic disorder and a 4.5-fold likelihood of asthmatics developing panic and anxiety. As many as one quarter of those who present to emergency units, primary care, gastroenterology, and cardiology units with complaints of chest pain have a primary diagnosis of panic disorder (Fleet & Beitman, 1997). Indeed, the common co-occurrence of pain and affective disorder calls for multimodal interventions, which can include hypnosis as well as pharmacotherapy (Fernandez, 2002).

Adherence to medical and psychological treatment protocols can be influenced by *psychodynamics*, a term that encompasses individuals' beliefs, attitudes, emotions, and expectations, including self and body image, conflicts, and defenses. Adaptive psychodynamics and social support (e.g., social and family relationships) can prolong life (Anderson, 2004; Cohen & Willis,

1985); however, empirically supported treatment protocols may be compromised by conflicts about trust, forming a relationship, or becoming well. Accordingly, prior to implementing traditional and hypnotic interventions, practitioners should assess and adapt treatment protocols to conform to both individual and social dynamics.

As the model in Table 22.1 indicates, there are substantial opportunities for mental health and medical practitioners to use psychological techniques to assist medical patients. The figured dimensions can be described in terms of a Venn diagram, with overlapping influences rather than discrete problem areas. A simple medical procedure, for example, that would prove worrisome but manageable for one individual can be the source of profound anxiety for another with a history of psychological trauma. A person with a problem of hyperarousal (e.g., irritable bowel syndrome) might have comorbid panic disorder and be so frightened of others or rewarded by illness that undertaking medical care is difficult if not impossible.

Although the realities of managed care place constraints on the practitioner's time, all interventions should ideally begin with a proper diagnosis and formulation that includes the biological, cognitive, affective, behavioral, relational, and cultural influences on the presenting complaint. The physician or service provider must introduce discussion of the role of psychological factors in illness with sensitivity so as not to appear to blame the patient or convey the impression that the patient is fabricating symptoms. Following a brief explanation of the role of psychophysiologic arousal in illness, the health provider should explain how hypnosis, a relaxation-based technique, could facilitate ANS control to achieve symptomatic relief. It is imperative to debunk myths

TABLE 22.1
Medical Hypnosis Interventions

Problem	Hypnosis strategy	Illustrative technique
Arousal	Distract, dispute, dissociate	Breathing, watch; restructure cognition; relaxation, absorbing imagery
Behavior	Recondition, rehearse, reward	Desensitization, exposure; new associations and contingencies; practice
Affect	Medication, mastery (exposure, desensitization)	Regression, affect bridge, exposure; coping
Dynamics	Mental representations (identify, recruit, replace)	Contact comforters, become comforter
	Memory (alter)	Reframe traumatic experience, amnesia
	Meaning (associate, negotiate)	Affect bridge, theater, board room
	Motivate (enlist, avoid, advise)	Engage issue, defer, direct suggestion

and provide scientific information to mitigate fears about hypnosis and provide a rationale for why hypnosis is useful in treating the psychological aspects of the medical condition. In short, the practitioner should present a compelling theoretical and scientific rationale for the use of hypnosis as an adjunctive treatment along with the specific strategies contemplated.

Problems of Arousal

Practitioners often target excessive autonomic arousal with medication and psychological interventions at the inception of treatment insofar as ANS arousal adversely affects multiple organ systems. Relaxation interventions can not only impact muscular tension but also ameliorate dysfunctional cognitions (e.g., catastrophizing, hypervigilance to interoceptive cues) that amplify the perception of symptoms. Hypnotic suggestions that focus attention on a neutral or pleasant event (and away from worrisome thoughts) can be used to decrease autonomic arousal. Many so-called deepening techniques, such as (a) attending to breathing with its rhythmic muscle and temperature changes, (b) imagining a ride on a down elevator while releasing muscle tension, (c) picturing oneself on a staircase and imagining a walk down 20 steps, and (d) relaxing muscles or altering body temperature can be effective *distraction techniques*. These not only calm the patient but they also direct attention away from negatively arousing thoughts, thereby evoking a more relaxed state.

In the first case study we describe, we present a favorite technique in which the practitioner invites the patient, during hypnosis, to concentrate on the shape, pressure, temperature, and sensations associated with his wristwatch. The practitioner then asks him to concentrate on the way his shoe surrounds his foot with the same pressures, temperature, and attendant sensations. The practitioner can elaborate this technique by including other objects. The method distracts the patient from arousing thoughts and provides experiential confirmation of the suggestion that "feelings and sensations follow perception, and the latter can be manipulated and managed." This exercise helps to convince the patient that perception is intimately tied to distressing thoughts and sensations, which can be altered with hypnosis to achieve symptom relief.

Some patients experience difficulty abandoning a vigilant stance and require help to reframe dysfunctional thoughts or to allay their irrational concerns. For these patients, cognitive–behavioral techniques (Beck, 1995) that include identifying automatic thoughts and core beliefs followed by cognitive restructuring strategies such as reframing, decatastrophizing, or disputation, are required. In hypnosis, maladaptive cognitions can be disputed and reframed and new ideas presented. The surgical candidate, afraid that the procedure will be too painful, will be encouraged to concentrate on more constructive thoughts such as, "There are ample medicines available to keep me comfortable" and

"The surgical team is expertly trained and I will be in excellent hands." Mantras such as, "What the mind thinks about, the body feels" can be even more compelling following a distraction exercise such as the one we described previously.

Some people demonstrate a capacity to become absorbed in pleasant fantasy to the extent that disturbing ideas lose their evocative influence. Well-known hypnotic approaches such as visualizing a favorite place, experiencing warm and loose muscles, and imagining cool air elevating the diaphragm and warm air leaving the mouth are useful relaxation methods for these patients. Patients with a significant capacity to experience absorption or meditative states will require less direction for their imaginings, and the suggestion to experience the relaxing image "as if they are there in the moment" may prove sufficient.

Problems of Behavior

Many so-called habit disorders are behavioral manifestations of tension reduction. For patients with bulimia, tobacco dependence, and dermatologic problems, for example, hypnotic training to reduce psychophysiologic arousal is often an important beginning step in treatment. For patients who are anxious and who fail to profit sufficiently from distraction, disputation, and dissociation techniques, therapists can use hypnosis to desensitize maladaptive behaviors and recondition and rehearse adaptive behaviors. The imaginative nature of hypnosis can create a "workspace" to mentally practice improved performance, virtually experience fearful situations, and recondition maladaptive behaviors. In the same fashion as athletes, public speakers, actors, and artists enhance their performances through visualization, surgical candidates and patients with unusual fears of medical procedures can use hypnosis to recognize the interoceptive cues and discriminative stimuli of anxiety and mentally rehearse adaptive responses prior to real-life exposure to the feared situation.

During hypnosis, the patient facing an upcoming surgery, for example, is first trained to experience relaxation on a reliable basis. At times, this state is *named*; that is, it is associated with taking a deep breath or is linked to a behavior such as slowly rubbing the index finger and thumb together. Next, the patient is invited to recognize thoughts pertaining to the procedure, consider them for any extraordinary meaning to be discussed later, and practice dismissing or countering them with comforting thoughts. After mastering this task, the patient is guided to imagine the trip to the hospital, registering as a patient, smelling the odors and attending to the environment's sounds, meeting staff, changing clothes, sitting in the preoperation room practicing the mastered relaxation exercises, and moving into the procedure room while entertaining comforting thoughts. Examples of such thoughts might be, "This procedure begins my recovery to health" or "These doctors do this work all day, every day. I am in good hands and can let them do their work. I will just go to my sanctuary in my imagination and wait." The same strategy is useful in treating anticipatory emesis related to chemotherapy, or with procedures such as gynecologic examinations, physical therapy, phlebotomy, and other procedures exacerbated by muscle tension.

Some patients are so fearful of necessary procedures that they avoid them for many years. When forced to confront feared dental work, magnetic resonance imaging, needles, surgery or other medical treatment, patients who are phobic may flee the situation or require sedation to complete the work. When this occurs, procedures must be rescheduled, and patients who are sedated will require extended monitoring by hospital personnel, increasing the cost of care. In many such cases, the combination of conditioning and imaginative processes maintains the problem and can potentially be enlisted in the solution.

Phobias and Panic

Systematic desensitization (Wolpe, 1958) is commonly used to ameliorate anxious avoidance by providing graded exposure to the feared object or situation. In graded exposure, patients experience their fears in a stepwise, hierarchical manner, starting with the least fear-evoking situation. Patients move from the bottom of the hierarchy to the most worrisome situation as their fear is nullified at each step by relaxation suggested during hypnosis. For patients familiar with the children's book *The Little Prince*, the instructions of the Fox to the boy who wished to befriend him (i.e., to avoid rushing up but to approach a little bit at a time, day by day, and thereby "tame" him) are sensible and inviting. This procedure may be enhanced through the use of hypnotic suggestion. Patients who are hypnotized may raise a signal finger when they experience themselves in a relaxed and safe place. This safe place or sanctuary becomes a grounding, or anchoring, point from which the lowest distressing image is presented first. As the patient experiences any anxiety (e.g., thoughts, feelings, physical sensations), the signal finger rises, and the scene is switched to the place of sanctuary for about 3 minutes. Subsequent presentations proceed until the patient can tolerate imagining the scene without distress for three administrations. After mastering the anxiety associated with one level, the next item in the hierarchy is presented and so on throughout the entire set of scenes. Our clinical experience is that patients have considerable difficulty with the extremes of the anxiety hierarchy but move rather quickly through the midrange.

A radically different treatment approach (Anthony & Barlow, 2002; Barlow, 2001; Barlow & Craske, 2000) relies on intensive interoceptive exposure to fear-related sensations. Rather than begin with the lowest item on the hierarchy, patients imaginatively experience the most anxiety-eliciting stimuli for extended periods of time, sometimes for several hours across several days, until the fear response extinguishes or habituates (Stampfl, 1961). Desensitization is eschewed as just another avoidance technique, with priority placed on mastering the cognitive, behavioral, and interoceptive cues to panic. Practitioners need to titrate patient affect and provide suggestions for mastery to counteract high levels of anxiety that may peak with intense exposure. Hypnosis is particularly useful to engage the imagination of the patient whose anxiety and panic are fed by imagery. Teaching the person to use neutral or relaxing imagery allows for a sense of control over automatic arousal. Moving from a position where imagery is reliably absorbing and relaxing to suggestions in hypnosis that attend to the neutral image then to the more minimally disturbing and then back to the neutral image provides a sense of mastery and control to the patient.

Habit Disorders

Urges are often triggers for binge eating, scratching or picking skin lesions, and smoking. So compelling is the urge to act that patients describe the sensation as physiological and irresistible. For such patients, hypnotically assisted response prevention, behavioral rehearsal, and reconditioning are keys to extinguishing maladaptive behaviors. During hypnosis, the sights, sounds, and sensations related to the urge can be attended to and intensified, while the imagined response is prevented. Over time, the link between the urge and the action is severed, as patients master their urges.

Patients with *trichotillomania*, another habit-like disorder, twist and pull their hair until they sometimes develop bald spots. These patients can be invited to use hypnosis to imagine recent situations and emotions connected to hair-pulling. After they master the ability to achieve a relaxed state during hypnosis, they imagine the target scene as if it is real and experience a flood of intense feelings and urges. Using a hand-levitation technique, they are invited to experience the automatic movement of their hand with outspread fingers in its approach to their head. As the hand nears its destination, patients picture a force field that blocks the hand and closes the fingers into a fist. The hand then falls to the side or might rub the head with a closed fist. Alternately, it can be suggested that when the hand touches the head, it will become increasingly heavy, and when it reaches the resting surface, the entire body will relax. These response-prevention exercises can be practiced repeatedly for several sessions. Patients can be positively reinforced for new behaviors and told that their hands will become "healing hands" that can rub or gently touch but not pull at or hurt sore areas, and they may be invited to practice these newly acquired behaviors. Images of past success experiences may be accessed with suggestions to apply the feelings and sensations of past accomplishments to the challenging situation at hand.

The same technique can be used to master urges associated with other habits that are controlled by strong operant cues. With smokers, the practitioner can provide the following suggestions: (a) not smoke for the day prior to the session; (b) during hypnosis, concentrate on (e.g., see, smell, anticipate) the taste of a cigarette; (c) imagine opening the pack and inhaling the aroma; (c) attend to the anticipatory saliva and increased heart rate; (d) imagine the sensations of the cigarette in the mouth; (e) hear the match being struck and smell the sulfur; (f) take a deep breath in expectation; and (g) blow out the match. After the images unfold, the practitioner suggests full-body relaxation, invoking imagery of a quiet place or sanctuary, and reinforces not only the idea that the patient experienced and mastered an urge but also the idea that the "mind controlled the body." Sequences of images relevant to binge eating, scratching or picking at skin lesions, and nausea and vomiting can likewise be developed.

Many of the behavior and habit problems we have discussed can also benefit from behavioral rehearsal and relapse prevention techniques (Marlatt & Donovan, 2005). Relapse prevention requires identifying circumstances and emotional states that increase the probability of relapse or are threats to maintaining behavior change. For example, affectively charged situations in which the target substances (e.g., cigarettes, food, alcohol) are readily available are common occasions for relapse. The attributions that patients make in such high-risk situations (e.g., "I am a hopeless addict," "I have no willpower," "This will never work for me") have a critical influence on the ability to maintain the desired behavior.

Hypnosis-assisted behavioral rehearsal techniques teach adaptive responses in high-risk situations and include conveying the idea to the patient that "slips" are an inevitable part of the recovery process and do not necessarily signify a lack of willpower. Practicing imagery such as recalling efforts to ride a bicycle or to speak a language with attendant mistakes and miscues are often presented in hypnosis to normalize abstinence failure, praise successive approximations to goals, and emphasize the educational (i.e., vs. moral or medical) nature of behavior change.

Problems of Affect

Affect disorders adversely influence many health-related conditions. A robust literature indicates that chronic problems with anger, anxiety, and depression are associated with physiologic changes that accompany coronary artery disease (Rozanski, Blumenthal, & Kaplan, 1999). Individuals with major mental illness often engage in behaviors that contribute to heart disease (e.g., poor nutrition, smoking, lack of exercise). However, affective spectrum disorders are powerful predictors of poor psychosocial outcome and poor physical health, especially in later life (i.e., ages 65 and above; Vaillant, Orav, Meyer, Vaillant, & Roston, 1996). Base-rate data indicate that 4% to 8% of medical patients experience panic disorder. However, estimates of the prevalence of panic disorder among asthmatics escalate to 8% to 24%. Research suggests that the link between panic and asthma can be accounted for in terms of a variety of moderator variables, including increased interoceptive sensitivity, catastrophic thinking that provokes airways reactivity, and sensitization of neural pathways by repetitive hyperventilation and hypoxia (Kayton, Richardson, Lozano, & McCauley, 2004).

Mastering emotions, whether anger, anxiety or depression, is a complex process that often requires recognition, experience, labeling, and coping. Practitioners may use many imaginative strategies during hypnosis (e.g., age regression, affective bridge, guided imagery) to invite patients to revisit an affect-laden experience. Attention paid to the triggers and elements of the emotional experience (e.g., sights, sounds, cognitions, feelings, physical sensations) allows patients to become better acquainted with their emotions. For example, an age regression technique can be used to invite patients to vividly remember a previous episode of heightened emotion with accompanying physiological sensations (e.g., muscles, heart rate, salivation, respiration), thoughts, contextual stimuli, and feelings. The *affective bridge* suggestion, in which patients identify a dominant aspect of a present-affective experience and associate it with similar past occurrences (i.e., "travel across the bridge"), is a useful way to both elaborate on the nuances of a particular emotion and to better identify it and understand its possible origins and associations.

A few caveats are noteworthy. Mastery of difficult emotions often requires controlled conditions. Hypnosis allows identified feelings to be practiced in the "play space" of imagination. Not uncommonly, an imaginative person will resist this type of exercise or become suddenly flooded with emotion. Our experience is that this often occurs with highly imaginative persons, individuals with a trauma history, and patients with serious personality disorders (e.g., borderline personality disorder). It may be necessary for patients to proceed in a stepwise or graded approach to highly emotional scenes, and it may be necessary for the therapist both to (a) include suggestions for titrating affect and achieving mastery of emotions and (b) provide calming imagery if emotions verge on becoming overwhelming.

Images of safe places, sanctuaries, and so forth, can be springboards for encountering anxious imagery. Finger cues (e.g., lifting one or more fingers; so-called ideomotor signaling) can be used to indicate when a person has "entered" such a place and as a means of communicating nonverbally with the therapist on a moment-to-moment basis. From this safe ground, the person can explore the physical sensations, thoughts and feelings of safety and comfort, and then imagine more aversive scenes to achieve the same level of comfort. Finger signals can also be used to indicate if emotions become intolerable.

Research suggests that cognitive–behavioral treatments (CBT) are highly effective in the treatment of depression and that hypnosis can increase the effectiveness of a variety of problems treated with CBT (Kirsch, Montgomery, & Sapirstein, 1995). Recently, research indicates that hypnosis can improve outcomes associated with treatment of depression (Alladin & Alibhai, 2007). Yapko (2001; see also chap. 15, this volume) recommends the following approach to treating depression: (a) Distinguish past from future events, (b) build the expectation of future possibilities, (c) set goals, (d) identify resources to meet goals, (e) differentiate mood and action, (f) support experimentation, and (g) generalize new learning and associations to contexts beyond the hypnotic situation. With the use of hypnosis for increasing coping skills and for relapse prevention training, patients are trained to break life-long maladaptive patterns.

Problems of Psychodynamics

Theoretical, clinical, and political controversies in the field involving therapeutic action, psychopathology, and memory have marginalized the use of hypnosis in psychodynamic treatment. Freud initiated this dismissal when he likened hypnosis to copper (Freud, 1919) and painting (Freud, 1905); placing substance where there was nothing. Freud compared hypnosis with the pure gold of psychoanalysis, which operated like sculpture, removing obstacles to the pure form beneath the rock. There is little current theoretical work in this area and less research. Nevertheless, there are many ways that hypnosis and psychoanalysis can be reunited to assist psychotherapists today.

Elgan Baker (1981, 1983), a psychoanalyst, contended that hypnosis can facilitate the impression of the therapist as a caring, constant, and protective person to assist patients with significant developmental problems. In hypnosis, Baker had patients imagine pleasant events as a touchstone with periodic open-eye checks on the presence of the therapist to reassure them of the therapist's constant presence. Patients were then invited to picture themselves in a relaxed setting; the therapist in a relaxed setting; and both patient and therapist engaged in a nurturing, safe interaction. Once such a relationship was firmly established, the work of addressing and integrating complex and problematic emotions began with the help of hypnosis and in a talking therapy. Baker's logic was that positive "mental representations" or "object relations" related to the therapist influence feelings and behavior and can be developed and rehearsed in hypnosis for individuals whose life circumstances did not facilitate secure interpersonal attachments. Further, discussions with and without the aid of hypnosis are useful ways to explore the patient's associations, integrate thoughts and feelings, and regulate emotions.

It is possible to use a similar method with surgical candidates and others about to enter anxiety-arousing situations. In the same way that children use stuffed animals and other "transitional objects" to help them to manage anxiety (Winnicott, 1971), hypnosis can be used to help patients to recall and experience comforting sensations, images, and related emotions. As these are recalled and imaginatively engaged, patients are not only able to distract themselves from troublesome thoughts and emotions but are also able to reduce their fears and psychophysiologic arousal. Alternatively, patients with traumatic memories of surgery, dentistry, or other treatments can use hypnosis to suppress highly aversive memories and reassure themselves that present or future circumstances will not echo their past ordeal. With hypnosis, memories can become dim, clouded, sequestered, forgotten, or rewritten with an improved ending that allows the patient to enter the new experience with less interference or priming from prior, adverse experiences.

Even the most empirically supported intervention is likely to fail when presented to a reluctant patient. For some therapists, failure to comply with a treatment protocol indicates that the patient is not ready for treatment, and such a person may be dismissed until ready. For others, the very presence of a patient in the consulting room is a sign of motivation, even though the person might be conflicted about pursuing treatment. Conflict of this nature can be explored with hypnosis.

Conflict can be represented during hypnosis by inviting the patient to imagine a play in a theater with actors expressing, symbolically or not, various aspects of the patient's conflicting motives about fully participating in treatment. To provide a helpful way to identify issues with a modicum of emotional distance, conflicted patients also may be asked during hypnosis to picture a meeting of a board of trustees, with individuals around the table representing disparate points of view. As the chairperson of this board, the patient solicits and weighs each point of view. Practitioner and patient can discuss these different perspectives apart from hypnosis and then revisit the meeting to encourage the group to decide on a more unified, progressive course of action. Sometimes, progress means "tabling," or deferring, an issue for discussion at a later day; sometimes, a particularly motivating issue can be expressed as a mantra to provide motivation to change. When hypnosis is used to facilitate association, exploration, and motivation, issues of veridicality (e.g., "Does the therapist agree with me?") are often less important than the fact that the power of imaginative, focused attention to facilitate change is made available to patient and therapist.

CLINICAL MATERIAL

Very simple hypnotic strategies can be of great benefit to imaginative persons whose vivid fantasies often lead to increased autonomic activity. For these, distractions and relaxation strategies take center stage in their mind so that more distressing images are able to be avoided. In keeping with more traditional psychoanalysis, imagery in hypnosis can be used as a free association technique to allow the patient to identify and work through conflicts and fears more symbolically.

Peter, a 45-year-old man, was referred by his primary care physician for help with intermittent insomnia. For weeks, Peter lay in bed, unable to sleep, ruminating about the affairs of the day, the past, and the future. His sleep was fitful, delayed, and disturbing to his partner. His insomnia was a relatively new symptom and seemed to be connected to challenges at work and impending career changes.

After the practitioner provided a brief explanation regarding the connections among perception, arousal, and sleep, Peter was invited to focus with hypnosis on the thermal, muscular, and kinesthetic experience of his shoe surrounding his foot. With a finger to signal the therapist that he could indeed differentiate the pressure, temperature, and tension of the foot within the shoe, he was then directed to become aware of the same sensations around the wrist with his watch. After he became able to easily shift his focus and attend to the presented sensations, he was told the following:

> The brain receives constant stimuli, but the mind edits what it concentrates on. You might not be able to control what comes to your attention, but you can concentrate on ideas and sensations that are interesting, calming, and quieting. Whatever might be important will keep for the morning. At night, you need only to rest, not to be bothered with sleep.

With this "lesson" mastered, he was quickly able to keep arousing thoughts at bay during the night and to restore his usual pattern of sleep.

A 68-year-old woman named Hilary came for help with hypnosis in advance of hip-replacement surgery. She carried an article from a newspaper with her that was a brief biography of the therapist. Although the report was several years old, Hilary had saved the piece "in the event that I would ever need to see someone for hypnosis." The reporter emphasized the spiritual journey of the psychologist and presented the doctor as "kind and accessible." Hilary was a spiritual person whose work with a Pentecostal church was quite important to her.

This was the first surgical experience for Hilary, whose only other medical problem was a history of hypertension, for which she was prescribed an antihypertensive medication. Although married, she felt distant from her husband, who was still a busy attorney. The couple had two grown children and a grandchild. Hilary had retired after a long career as a high school teacher of English and art. Even in retirement, she still tutored high school students and managed to spend several hours each day with creative arts (i.e., poetry, painting).

Hilary began to use hypnosis for relaxation and anxiety management. Her capacity to become actively absorbed in fantasy for prolonged periods provided her with a feeling of success. Nevertheless, she regularly found herself experiencing significant episodes of sudden panic, shortness of breath, sweating, and heart palpitations. Even after four sessions that emphasized relaxation training, imaginative visits to the hospital, and some behavioral rehearsal for anxiety management, Hilary still reported occasional breakthrough panic experiences during and apart from hypnosis.

The practitioner invited Hilary to use the panic as a bridge to some experience in her life that felt similar, which led her to think about her son. As she used hypnosis to conjure an imaginary theater, the image of two people engaged in a heated argument came to her. In short order, she saw an older woman and a younger man become so furious that they stormed off the stage. In tears, Hilary described a relatively recent conflict with her son that resulted in their estrangement. Hilary revealed her considerable fear that she would die during the upcoming surgery and leave this relationship and her family in shambles. Although she feared his anger and disapproval, Hilary reached out to her son through telephone calls and even traveled some distance to his home to leave an apologetic note, without a response.

During hypnosis, Hilary was able to imagine a department meeting at her school where she was chairperson. As she looked over the sea of faces at the meeting, she identified several individuals with strong points of view and stronger emotions about an issue that she needed to make a decision about. She spent time engaging a number of the individuals and became familiar with the range of emotions and viewpoints. Although each had a voice and something to offer to the discussion, Hilary was able to see that no one person had a purchase on truth. Even as she considered the whole group, it was clear that she felt closer to, and more in agreement with, some individuals than others. Although her "critics" had certain value, she was able to see them as department members and herself as the leader who could solicit the advice and support of the more benign and cooperative teachers.

With the use of this metaphor, Hilary was able to acknowledge her disagreement with her son and place it in a larger context. Because she could forgive herself for her part in the conflict, she was able to understand his point of view, forgive him for walking away, and accept that he was overcome with an emotion that they would both have to manage. Having done this work, she was able to imagine herself in the hospital, coping successfully with her surgery, recovering speedily, moving easily when directed by therapists and enjoying her newly earned mobility. The work during hypnosis helped Hilary prepare for and endure an event that otherwise would have evoked considerable anxiety.

RESEARCH AND APPRAISAL

When we previously reviewed the empirical support for the use of hypnosis in medicine in the 2000 special issue of the *International Journal of Clinical and Experimental Hypnosis* (Pinnell & Covino, 2000), we identified several studies that qualified as "possibly efficacious" interventions by the Chambless and Hollon (1998) criteria. At that time, we determined that there was moderate evidence that hypnosis offered to patients undergoing surgical interventions lessened their anxiety and was superior to "standard care" or supportive treatments in reducing the use of analgesic medications and pain reports (Lambert, 1996; Lang, Joyce, Spiegel, Hamilton, & Lee, 1996). Lang et al. (2000) replicated the success of hypnosis on pain and drug management among surgical patients and also found that patients in the hypnosis group were treated by surgeons in a significantly shorter period of time (see chap. 23, this volume).

In another study, young children who were scheduled for a painful, and usually frightening, radiologic procedure (i.e., voiding cystourethrography) were randomly assigned to routine care and to receive hypnosis training for use during the procedure (Butler et al., 2005). Not only did parents, children, and medical staff report less distress for the intervention group, but also the time the children were subjected to the painful procedure averaged 14 minutes less with hypnosis.

Flory, Salazar, and Lang (2007; see also chap. 23, this volume) reviewed several methodologically sound studies (i.e., prospective randomized controlled trials) and concluded the following:

> There is overwhelming evidence for the effectiveness of hypnosis to reduce acute distress and pain during procedures. There is also support that hypnotic techniques can ameliorate the effects of analgesia and anesthesia, stabilize vital signs, reduce complications, facilitate healing and recovery, and overall reduce health care costs. (p. 310)

Moreover, the benefits of hypnosis were experienced by adult and pediatric patients alike. The authors noted, "there is evidence that adjunctive hypnosis is superior to standard medical care both in terms of quality of care and costs" (p. 311). Brown and Hammond (2007) reviewed the extant literature on the use of hypnosis in prenatal obstetrics and for pain management during labor and delivery. They found that a large percentage of women who used hypnosis during delivery were able to deliver without the use of medication. It is worth mentioning that hypnotic interventions may result in rare, relatively few, and transient adverse effects.

Since the 2000 review, a number of studies examining the effect of hypnosis on irritable bowel syndrome have added to the considerable support for CBT in this illness area (Blanchard, 2001; see also chap. 25, this volume). Gastrointestinal symptoms were improved in a randomized trial with six sessions of "gut-focused" hypnotherapy versus an intervention package of patient education, suggestions, and coping-skills training (Forbes, MacAuley, & Chiotakakou-Faliakou, 2000). In a wait list controlled study, hypnosis interventions facilitated an 87% reduction in symptoms along with a significant reduction in anxiety (Palsson, Turner, Johnson, Burnett, & Whitehead, 2002). Although the two studies did not include a control group, significant improvement in quality of life and patient reports of bowel symptoms were found for a large number ($N = 250$) of consecutively admitted patients who were treated with hypnosis (Gonsalkorale, Houghton, & Whorwell, 2002), and symptom improvement remained for 204 of those treated with hypnosis who were followed-up at 5 or more years (Gonsalkorale, Miller, Afzal, & Whorwell, 2003). Many of the studies in this area lack methodological soundness, especially with regard to randomization, sample size and intervention standardization. However, reviewers have noted that the impact of hypnosis training on patients who failed to profit from otherwise appropriate medical treatments is substantial and deserves much closer attention (Palsson, 2006; Whitehead, 2006).

There is some good evidence supporting the use of hypnosis in reducing psychophysiological arousal. Among surgical patients, this can translate to improved patient comfort and compliance as well as to reduced health care costs. For those with IBS, it can mean relief from pain and improved quality of life. The extant empirical evidence regarding the effectiveness of hypnosis and relaxation strategies in the treatment of hyperemesis (i.e., nausea, vomiting) is inconsistent, yet promising. Randomized controlled trials involving children with cancer (Jacknow, Tschann, Link, & Boyce, 1994; Zeltzer, Dolgin, LeBaron, & LeBaron, 1991) found that those who used hypnosis reduced anticipatory nausea better than others who used distraction techniques or group support. The more challenging problem of postoperative nausea and vomiting was also managed with significantly fewer symptoms and medication requests by surgical patients who were trained to use hypnosis for symptom management than those who had "usual care" (Enqvist, Bjorklund, Engman, & Jakobson, 1997). Néron and Stephenson (2007) conducted a systematic critical review of the evidence accumulated from 1999 to 2006 for the effectiveness of hypnotherapy for anxiolysis, analgesia, and emesis in the treatment of patients with cancer. They concluded that more recent studies have failed to provide empirical support for the effectiveness of hypnotherapy in the treatment of nausea and emesis. There is a clear need for well-designed and methodologically sound studies to further explore the potential use of hypnotherapy for reducing nausea and emesis.

Graci and Hardie (2007) discussed the inconsistent findings regarding the effectiveness of clinical hypnosis in treating insomnia disorders. The authors underscored the pressing need for well-designed studies to demonstrate that hypnosis could be effective in the treatment of sleep disorders. Furthermore, they emphasized that hypnosis should be used in conjunction with CBT interventions, as part of a comprehensive multitreatment approach.

A review of 18 studies using cognitive–behavioral interventions for pain, insomnia, weight control, and anxiety found a significant advantage for patients when hypnosis is added to CBT (Kirsch et al., 1995). A subsequent meta-analysis of the most frequent (i.e., weight control) studies found that the clinical impact of adding hypnosis was mainly evident at evaluations several months posttreatment. This suggests a skill acquisition process that increases and improves with time (Kirsch, 1996).

Debate remains regarding the mind–body interface at the level of immune function and the role of hypnosis. Skin diseases, such as urticaria, psoriasis, and atopic dermatitis, which are characterized by lesions caused by an "upregulation" of the immune function and by inflammatory reactions have been hypothesized to be psychogenic in nature (Zachariae, 2001). In a series of case studies, Ewin (1986) demonstrated an important role for hypnosis in the healing process for burns. Moderate improvement in patients with stable psoriasis was observed following hypnosis and direct suggestions for stress management, analgesia, and symptom control but without any association with hypnotizability (Zachariae et al., 1996). Several reports on the treatment of warts (Ewin, 1992; Spanos, Stenstrom, & Johnston, 1988; Spanos, Williams, & Gynn, 1990) found support for the use of hypnosis, although it was limited perhaps to its suggestive component. However, two well-controlled studies failed to alter delayed-type hypersensitivity response in participants who were highly hypnotizable (Locke et al., 1994). Future studies with longer interventions and extended follow-up will be necessary to clarify the limited findings in this area (Kiecolt-Glaser, McGuire, Robles, & Glaser, 2002).

Flammer and Alladin (2007) examined the effectiveness of hypnosis in the treatment of psychosomatic illnesses by carefully selecting and critically evaluating 22 randomized controlled clinical studies that met their inclusion criteria. They also conducted a meta-analysis to determine the size of the treatment effect. The disorders treated included tinnitus, insomnia, enuresis, asthma, hay fever, irritable bowel syndrome, chronic pain, chronic headache, duodenal ulcer, atopic dermatitis, and so forth. Flammer and Alladin categorized the types of hypnotic interventions used by various researchers as "classical hypnosis, modern hypnosis, and mixed form of hypnosis" (p. 255), because they were interested in the differential effects of different types of suggestions. The majority of the studies included hypnotic suggestions aimed at symptomatic treatment. Overall, they found hypnosis to have a medium effectiveness ($d = .61$) for psychosomatic disorders. The examination of the differential effectiveness of types of hypnosis interventions used across studies revealed the superiority of modern hypnosis interventions (i.e., metaphors, age regression, indirect suggestions) over classical hypnosis interventions (i.e., visualization, imagery, direct suggestions). Flammer and Alladin concluded that hypnosis is an effective adjunctive treatment for psychosomatic disorders. On the basis of their analysis, they suggested possible avenues to further increase the effectiveness of hypnotherapy by expanding the scope of interventions beyond suggestions aimed at symptom relief.

In general, the usual methodological problems of sample size, subject heterogeneity, inadequately described interventions, and absent follow-up limit the support for hypnosis in this area. Research with medical patients is further complicated by the variability that often exists with regard to illness onset, symptom severity, comorbidity, medications prescribed, and treatment history. However, the most limiting factor is the absence of current research in illness areas that may well respond to hypnosis interventions (e.g., asthma, bulimia, diabetes, insomnia). As researchers in this area are able to distance themselves from early Freudian topographical models that emphasize memory retrieval and initiate investigations on the use of hypnosis to foster affect management, emotional development, and psychological functioning, new opportunities will become available to use hypnosis in psychodynamic and other types of psychotherapy.

CONCLUSION

With the current emphasis on "evidence-based treatments," physicians, insurers, and patients look for research support prior to undertaking an "alternative medical treatment." This review revealed a number of ways that hypnosis can be of considerable benefit to medical patients. Experienced practitioners, no matter how devoted they are to a particular orientation, understand the importance of drawing from many theoretical perspectives in their work with patients, especially the medically ill. The usual need for dialogue between clinicians and researchers is particularly acute in this area and at this time when helpful hypnotic interventions battle for limited health care dollars and the public willingly embraces additions to traditional medical care.

REFERENCES

Alladin, A., & Alibhai, A. (2007). Cognitive hypnotherapy for depression: An empirical investigation. *International Journal of Clinical and Experimental Hypnosis, 55,* 147–163.

Anderson, N. (2004). *Emotional longevity: What really determines how long you live.* New York: Viking Penguin.

Anthony, M. M., & Barlow, D. H. (Eds.). (2002). *Handbook of assessment and treatment planning for psychological disorders.* New York: Guilford Press.

Baker, E. L. (1981). A hypnotherapeutic approach to enhance object relatedness in psychotic patients. *International Journal of Clinical and Experimental Hypnosis, 29,* 136–147.

Baker, E. L. (1983). The use of hypnotic techniques with psychotics. *American Journal of Clinical Hypnosis, 25,* 283–288.

Barlow, D. H. (2001). *Anxiety and its disorders: The nature and treatment of anxiety and panic* (2nd ed.). New York: Guilford Press.

Barlow, D. H., & Craske, M. G. (2000). *Mastery of your anxiety and panic (MAP–3).* San Antonio, TX: Psychological Corporation.

Beck, J. S. (1995). *Cognitive therapy: Basics and beyond.* New York: Guilford Press.

Blanchard, E. B. (2001). *Irritable bowel syndrome: Psychosocial assessment and treatment.* Washington, DC: American Psychological Association.

Bonnet, M. H., & Arand, D. L. (1995). 24-Hour metabolic rate in insomniacs and matched normal sleepers. *Sleep: Journal of Sleep and Sleep Disorders Research, 18,* 581–588.

Bonnet, M. H., & Arand, D. L. (2003). Situational insomnia: Consistency, predictors, and outcomes. *Sleep: Journal of Sleep and Sleep Disorders Research, 26,* 1029–1036.

Brown, D. C., & Hammond, D. C. (2007). Evidence-based clinical hypnosis for obstetrics, labor, and delivery, and preterm labor. *International Journal of Clinical and Experimental Hypnosis, 55,* 355–371.

Bulik, C. M. (2005). Exploring the gene–environment nexus in eating disorders. *Journal of Psychiatry and Neuroscience, 30,* 335–339.

Butler, L., Symons, B., Henderson, S., Shortliffe, L., & Spiegel, D. (2005). Hypnosis reduces distress and duration of an invasive medical procedure for children. *Pediatrics, 115,* 77–85.

Casati J., & Toner, B. (2002). Diseases of the digestive system. In T. Boll (Editor-in-Chief), S. B. Johnson, N. W. Perry, & R. H. Rozensky (Vol. Eds.), *Handbook of clinical health psychology: Vol. 1. Medical disorders and behavioral applications* (pp. 283–305). Washington DC: American Psychological Association.

Cassileth, B. R., Lusk, E. J., Strouse, T. B., Miller, D. S., Brown, L. L., Cross, P. A., & Tenaglia, A. N. (1984). Psychosocial status in chronic illness: A comparative analysis of six diagnostic groups. *The New England Journal of Medicine, 311,* 506–511.

Chambless, D. L., & Hollon, S. D. (1998). Defining empirically supported therapies. *Journal of Consulting and Clinical Psychology, 66*, 7–18.

Chiles, J. A., Lambert, M. J., & Arlin, A. L. (1999). The impact of psychological interventions on medical cost offset: A meta-analytic review. *Clinical Psychology: Science and Practice, 6*, 204–220.

Cohen, S., & Willis, T. (1985). Stress, social support, and the buffering hypothesis. *Psychological Bulletin, 98*, 310–357.

Covino, N. A. (2008). Medical illnesses, conditions, and procedures. In M. Nash & A. Barnier (Eds.), *The Oxford handbook of hypnosis* (pp. 611–624). Oxford, England: Oxford University Press.

Covino, N. A., & Bottari, M. (2001). Hypnosis, behavioral theory, and smoking cessation. *Journal of Dental Education, 65*, 340–347.

Engle, G. (1977, April 8). The need for a new medical model: A challenge for biomedicine. *Science, 196*, 129–136.

Enqvist, B., Bjorklund, C., Engman, M., & Jakobsson, J. (1997). Preoperative hypnosis reduces postoperative vomiting after surgery of the breasts: A prospective, randomized and blinded study. *Acta Anaesthiologica Scandinavica, 41*, 1028–1032.

Enqvist, B., von Konow, L., & Bystedt, H. (1995). Pre- and perioperative suggestion in maxillofacial surgery: Effects on blood loss and recovery. *International Journal of Clinical and Experimental Hypnosis, 43*, 284–294.

Ewin, D. (1986). The effect of hypnosis and mind set on burns. *Psychiatric Annals, 16*, 115–118.

Ewin, D. (1992). Hypnotherapy for warts (Verruca Vulgaris): 41 consecutive cases with 33 cures. *American Journal of Clinical Hypnosis, 35*, 1–10.

Fernandez, E. (2002). *Anxiety, depression, and anger in pain: Research findings and clinical options.* Dallas, TX: Advanced Psychological Resources.

Flammer, E., & Alladin, A. (2007). The efficacy of hypnotherapy in the treatment of psychosomatic disorders: Meta-analytical evidence. *International Journal of Clinical and Experimental Hypnosis, 55*, 251–274.

Fleet, R. P., & Beitman, B. D. (1997). Unexplained chest pain: When is it panic disorder? *Clinical Cardiology, 20*, 187–194.

Flory, N., Salazar, G. M. M., & Lang, E. V. (2007). Hypnosis for acute distress management during medical procedures. *International Journal of Clinical and Experimental Hypnosis, 55*, 303–317.

Forbes, A., MacAuley, S., & Chiotakakou-Faliakou, E. (2000). Hypnotherapy and therapeutic audiotape: Effective in previously unsuccessfully treated irritable bowel syndrome? *International Journal of Colorectal Disease, 15*, 328–334.

Freud, S. (1905). On psychotherapy. *The standard edition of the complete psychological works of Sigmund Freud, Volume VII (1901–1905): A Case of Hysteria. Three essays on sexuality and other works* (pp. 255–268). New York: W. W. Norton & Co.

Freud, S. (1919). Lines of advance in psychoanalytic therapy. *The standard edition of the complete psychological works of Sigmund Freud, Volume XVII (1917–1919):*

An infantile neurosis and other works (pp. 157–168). New York: W. W. Norton & Co.

Gonsalkorale, W. M., Houghton, L. A., & Whorwell, P. J. (2002). Hypnotherapy in irritable bowel syndrome: A large-scale audit of a clinical service with examination of factors influencing responsiveness. *American Journal of Gastroenterology, 97*, 954–961.

Gonsalkorale, W. M., Miller, V., Afzal, A., & Whorwell, P. J. (2003). Long-term benefits of hypnotherapy for irritable bowel syndrome. *Gut, 52*, 1623–1629.

Graci, G. M., & Hardie, J. C. (2007). Evidence-based hypnotherapy for the management of sleep disorders. *International Journal of Clinical and Experimental Hypnosis, 55*, 288–302.

Hasler, G., Gergen, P. J., Kleinbaum, D. G., Ajdacic, V., Gamma, A., Eich, D., et al. (2005). Asthma and panic in young adults: A 20-year prospective community study. *American Journal of Respiratory and Critical Care Medicine, 171*, 1224–1230.

Hohlstein, L. A., Smith, G. T., & Atlast, J. G. (1998). An application of expectancy theory to eating disorders: Development and validation of measures of eating and dieting expectancies. *Psychological Assessment, 10*, 49–58.

Jacknow, D. S., Tschann, J. M., Link, M. P., & Boyce, W. T. (1994). Hypnosis in the prevention of chemotherapy-related nausea and vomiting in children: A prospective study. *Journal of Developmental and Behavioral Pediatrics, 15*, 258–264.

Kayton, W. J., Richardson, L., Lozano, P., & McCauley, E. (2004). The relationship of asthma and anxiety disorders. *Psychosomatic Medicine, 66*, 349–355.

Kiecolt-Glaser, J. K., McGuire, L., Robles, T. F., & Glaser, R. (2002). Psychoneuroimmunology: Psychological influences on immune function and health. *Journal of Consulting and Clinical Psychology, 70*, 537–547.

Kirsch, I. (1996). Hypnotic enhancement of cognitive–behavioral weight loss treatments: Another meta-reanalysis. *Journal of Consulting and Clinical Psychology, 64*, 517–519.

Kirsch, I., Montgomery, G., & Sapirstein, G. (1995). Hypnosis as an adjunct to cognitive–behavioral psychotherapy: A meta-analysis. *Journal of Consulting and Clinical Psychology, 63*, 214–220.

Lambert, S. A. (1996). The effects of hypnosis/guided imagery on the postoperative course of children. *Developmental and Behavioral Pediatrics, 17*, 307–310.

Lang, E. V., Benotsch, E. G., Fick, L. J., Lutgendorf, S., Berbaum, M. L., Berbaum, K. S., et al. (2000, April 29). Adjunctive nonpharmacological analgesia for invasive medical procedures: A randomized trial. *The Lancet, 355*, 1486–1490.

Lang, E. V., Joyce, J. S., Spiegel, D., Hamilton, D., & Lee, K. K. (1996). Self-hypnotic relaxation during interventional radiological procedures: Effects on pain perception and intravenous drug use. *International Journal of Clinical and Experimental Hypnosis, 44*, 106–119.

Law, M., & Tang, J. L. (1995). An analysis of the effectiveness of interventions intended to help people stop smoking. *Archives of Internal Medicine, 155*, 1933–1941.

Locke, S. E., Ransil, B. J., Covino, N. A., Toczydolwski, J., Lohse, C. M., Dvorak, H. E., et al. (1987). Failure of hypnotic suggestion to alter immune response to delayed-type hypersensitivity antigens. *Annuals of the New York Academy of Science, 496*, 745–749.

Locke, S. E., Ransil, B. J., Zachariae, R., Molay, F., Tollins, K., Covino, N. A., & Danforth, D. (1994). Effect of hypnotic suggestion on the delayed-type hypersensitivity response. *JAMA, 272*, 47–52.

Marlatt, G. A., & Donovan, D. M. (2005). *Relapse prevention: Maintenance strategies in the treatment of addictive behaviors.* New York: Guilford Press.

Montgomery, G. H., DuHamel, K. N., & Redd, W. H. (2000). A meta-analysis of hypnotically induced analgesia: How effective is hypnosis? *International Journal of Clinical and Experimental Hypnosis, 48*, 138–153.

Néron, S., & Stephenson, R. (2007). Effectiveness of hypnotherapy with cancer patients' trajectory: Emesis, acute pain, and analgesia and anxiolysis in procedures. *International Journal of Clinical and Experimental Hypnosis, 55*, 336–354.

Palsson, O. S. (2006). The nature of IBS and the need for a psychological approach. *International Journal of Clinical and Experimental Hypnosis, 54*, 1–6.

Palsson, O. S., Turner, M. J., Johnson, D. A., Burnett, C. K., & Whitehead, W. E. (2002). Hypnosis treatment for severe irritable bowel syndrome: Investigation of mechanism and effects on symptoms. *Digestive Diseases and Science, 47*, 2605–2614.

Patterson, D. R., & Jensen, M. P. (2003). Hypnosis and clinical pain. *Psychological Bulletin, 129*, 495–521.

Pincus, H. A., Tanielian, T. L., & Marcus, S. C. (1998). Prescribing trends in psychotropic medications. *JAMA, 279*, 526–531.

Pinnell, C. M., & Covino, N. A. (2000). Empirical findings on the use of hypnosis in medicine: A critical review. *International Journal of Clinical and Experimental Hypnosis, 48*, 174–194.

Redd, W. H., Montgomery, G. H., & DuHamel K. N. (2001). Behavioral intervention for cancer treatment side effects. *Journal of the National Cancer Institute, 93*, 810–823.

Rozanski, A., Blumenthal, J. A., & Kaplan, J. (1999). Impact of psychological factors on the pathogenesis of cardiovascular disease and implications for therapy. *Circulation, 99*, 2192–2217.

Shenefelt, P. D. (2004). Using hypnosis to facilitate resolution of psychogenic excoriations in acne excoriée. *American Journal of Clinical Hypnosis, 46*, 239–245.

Spanos, N. P., Stenstrom, R. J., & Johnston, J. C. (1988). Hypnosis, placebo, and suggestion in the treatment of warts. *Psychosomatic Medicine, 50*, 245–260.

Spanos, N. P., Williams, V., & Gynn, M. (1990). Effects of hypnotic, placebo, and salicylic acid treatments on wart regression. *Psychosomatic Medicine, 52*, 109–114.

Stampfl, T. G. (1961). The implosive therapy: A learning theory derived psychodynamic therapeutic technique. In A. E. Lebarba & C. E. Dent (Eds.), *Critical issues in clinical psychology* (496–503). New York: Academic Press.

Turk, D. (1996). Psychological aspects of pain and disability. *Journal of Musculo-skeletal Pain, 4*, 145–154.

Vaillant, G. E., Orav, J., Meyer, S. E., Vaillant, L. M., & Roston, D. (1996). Late-life consequences of affective spectrum disorder. *International Psychogeriatrics, 8*, 13–32.

Whitehead, W. E. (2006). Hypnosis for irritable bowel syndrome: The empirical evidence of therapeutic effects. *International Journal of Clinical and Experimental Hypnosis, 54*, 7–20.

Wilson, G. T. (2005). Psychological treatment of eating disorders. *Annual Review of Clinical Psychology, 1*, 439–465.

Winnicott, D. W. (1971). *Playing and reality*. London: Routledge.

Wolpe, J. (1958). *Psychotherapy by reciprocal inhibition*. Stanford, CA: Stanford University Press.

Yapko, M. (2001). *Treating depression with hypnosis: Integrating cognitive–behavioral and strategic approaches*. Philadelphia: Brunner-Routledge.

Zachariae, R. (2001). Hypnosis and immunity. *Psychoneuroimmunology, 2*, 133–160.

Zachariae, R., Oster, H., Bjerring, P., & Kragballe, K. (1996). Effects of psychologic intervention on psoriasis: A preliminary report. *Journal of the American Academic of Dermatology, 34*, 1008–1015.

Zeltzer, L. K., Dolgin, M. J., LeBaron, S., & LeBaron, C. (1991). A randomized, controlled study of behavioral intervention for chemotherapy distress in children with cancer. *Pediatrics, 88*, 34–42.

Zeltzer, L. K., & LeBaron, S. (1982). Hypnosis and nonhypnotic techniques for reduction of pain and anxiety during painful procedures in children and adolescents with cancer. *Journal of Pediatrics, 101*, 1032–1035.

23

HYPNOSIS DURING INVASIVE MEDICAL AND SURGICAL PROCEDURES

GLORIA MARIA MARTINEZ SALAZAR, SALOMAO FAINTUCH,
ELEANOR LASER, AND ELVIRA LANG

Surgery has greatly evolved from the traditional large-incision approach to less- and minimally invasive techniques that often no longer require general anesthesia. Within this trend, the field of interventional radiology has blossomed. Currently, specially trained physicians advance instruments under image-guidance (i.e., X-ray, ultrasound, magnetic resonance imaging) through tiny skin openings to perform, for example, angioplasties; remove pus, kidney stones, or gallstones; open up blocked veins or bile ducts; occlude varicose veins with laser; and occlude tumor vessels. Similarly, interventional pulmonology, gastroenterology, and cardiology have expanded using comparable techniques. Technical refinements have greatly reduced the mechanical risks of these procedures, but despite these advances in procedures and anesthetic techniques, even minimally invasive surgical interventions still involve some physical and emotional cost to patients (Hatsiopoulou, Cohen, & Lang, 2003; Johnston, 2001; Martin & Lennox, 2003). Patients' tolerance to being awake but immobilized on a procedure table, often in a darkened room, conscious of potential complications, and captive to the surrounding

---

Clinical material has been disguised to protect patient confidentiality.

health care providers can become a safety-limiting scenario. Herein lays a tremendous opportunity for those willing to improve the patients' emotional experience. Hypnotic techniques, which have been used with some success to alleviate pain during major surgery before introduction of general anesthesia (Esdaile, 1846/1957), are ideally suited as an adjunct to modest medication for minimally invasive medical procedures. Furthermore, adjunct hypnosis should not be merely utilized by a select group of practitioners for a select group of patients, but should rather be broadly introduced into medical practice.

Research has shown sufficient evidence that hypnotic techniques can be safely and effectively integrated into the modern medical environment for better health and cost savings. Such a movement will likely be consumer-driven; patients who have experienced hypnosis once on the procedure table will request it again, tell their neighbors, make it public, and select their health care facilities accordingly. Consequently, these services and training should be provided to the next generation of medical personnel on site. This vision recognizes that in a busy and often hectic clinical setting, there may be no extra time for psychological preparation of patients during a separate office or hospital visit. Our work has therefore focused on nonpharmacologic techniques that can be applied on the procedure table to hypnosis-naive patients without disturbing or prolonging the ongoing procedure. Because hypnotic techniques are relatively generic and well-explained in other chapters of this volume, we focus in this chapter on the unique task of assisting patients in a noisy, sabotage-prone environment distinct from the tranquil office setting. We also present a review of the use of hypnosis in different medical settings.

CLINICAL APPLICATIONS

Pharmacological therapy has been the main approach for addressing pain and anxiety during and after invasive procedures, mostly in combinations of analgesics and sedatives (Martin & Lennox, 2003). These medications, however, can induce cardiovascular depression, hypoxia, apnea, unconsciousness, and, rarely, death, even in dosages usually well-tolerated (Greenberg, Faerber, Aspinall, & Adams, 1993; Ronchera-Oms et al., 1994; Yaster & Cravero, 2004). Therefore, an application that provides comfort while reducing or eliminating the need for drugs is highly desirable.

The clinical practice guidelines for acute pain management published by the Public Health Service, mentions relaxation exercises and cognitive approaches but do not provide specifics or outcome data (Acute Pain Management Guideline Panel, 1992). Some patients, when confronted with distress, resort to their own cognitive nonpharmacologic means of coping, such as imagination of pleasant scenes, distraction, relaxation, hypnosis, or meditation (Hilgard, 1977; Quirk, Letendre, Ciottone, & Lingley, 1989; Spanos, Radtke-Bodorik, Ferguson, & Jones, 1979). Whereas hypnosis as the sole means of analgesia during open surgery (Bernstein, 1965; Blankfield, 1991; Bowen, 1973; Crasilneck, McCranie, & Jenkins, 1956; Esdaile, 1957; Kroger & DeLee, 1957; Levitan & Harbaugh, 1989, 1992; Marmer, 1959; Mason, 1955; Ruiz & Fernandez, 1960; Schwarcz, 1965; Tinterow, 1960) can be used in select patients only, hypnosis and suggestion as adjuncts to or replacement of pharmacologic analgesia are becoming attractive options and are relatively independent of the patients' hypnotizability to be effective (Blankfield, 1991; Bonilla, Quigley, & Bowers, 1961; Fredericks, 1978; Lang et al., 2000; Lang, Joyce, Spiegel, Hamilton, & Lee, 1996).

A wide range of procedures can be effectively managed with medications and adjunct hypnosis (Stewart, 2005). Despite substantial variation in hypnotic techniques among numerous reports and randomized trials, patients treated with hypnosis experience substantial benefits for different medical purposes, indicating an expanded role for its use. In the largest prospective randomized trial of its kind, adjunct hypnosis reduced pain, anxiety, drug use, and complications during invasive procedures in the vasculature and the kidneys (Lang et al., 2000). Brief hypnosis has also been documented to be beneficial before excisional breast biopsies, as shown in a study designed to determine the impact of that method on patients' postsurgical pain and distress by analyzing 20 cases that were randomly assigned to a hypnosis or control group (i.e., standard care). In this setting, hypnosis significantly reduced postsurgical pain and distress (Montgomery, Weltz, Seltz, & Bovbjerg, 2002). A 1999 review of more than 1,650 surgical cases using hypnosis as an adjunct to conscious sedation favored the safety and patient comfort provided by hypnosis (Faymonville, Meurisse, & Fissette, 1999). This form of anesthesia was applied as an alternative to general anesthesia for a wide range of surgical procedures, including neck lift, thyroidectomy, cervicotomy for hyperparathyroidism, correction of mammary ptosis, breast augmentation, tubal ligation, nasal septorhinoplasty, debridement with skin grafting, and calvarial bone graft (i.e., maxillofacial reconstruction), as well as some minor surgical procedures (e.g., turbinoplasty, wisdom teeth). The authors proposed the use of this technique as a safe alternative to standard anesthetic protocols and also indicated that the major benefit for its use is the capability of patients' participation during their procedure, ensuing a faster recovery and shorter hospital stay.

The contribution of hypnosis to surgery and anesthesiology and its effects on physiologic response are being investigated in studies with percutaneous transluminal coronary angioplasty (PTCA). The selective influence of hypnosis on cardiac vegetative tone is well known (Hippel, Hole, & Kaschka, 2001). In a report published in 2004, results showed a selective influence of hypnosis on the mechanisms that regulate the sympathetic drive during PTCA, in particular, a selective inhibition on central autonomic nervous pathways (Baglini et al., 2004). This may account for the greater hemodynamic stability achieved with adjunct hypnosis during interventional radiological procedures (Lang et al., 2000).

Moreover, the clinical benefits of hypnosis can be extended to a higher cost effectiveness as compared with the usual standard treatment. Recent studies (Faintuch, Lang, & Rosen, 2004; Lang & Rosen, 2002) assessed this by using decision analysis model software. The decision analysis model postulated the following possible outcomes with the use of hypnosis and standard treatment: (a) uncomplicated sedation, (b) oversedation, and (c) undersedation. Uncomplicated sedation was assumed to have no additional cost. Oversedation or undersedation could result either in (a) no additional cost, (b) cost associated with intense observation, or (c) cost associated with admission. Probabilities of occurrence and associated cost for each of these scenarios resulted in the overall cost assessment of both treatments. The cost associated with standard sedation was $638, compared with $300 for cases performed with adjunct hypnosis (i.e., resulting in a saving of $338/case with hypnosis). Using our base case rates, we found the use of hypnosis reduced room time; however, hypnosis would still remain more cost effective even if it added an additional 58.2 minutes to the room time. The cost advantage of adjunct hypnosis persisted even if a health care provider dedicated to only performing hypnosis were added to the team, unless this person's hourly wage exceeded $330/hour.

Techniques and Procedures

Many reports in the literature are based on either the use of audiotapes or live hypnotherapy providers outside the procedure room (Bennett, Benson, & Kuiken, 1986; Blankfield, 1991; Enqvist, von Konow, & Bystedt, 1995; Montgomery, Weltz, et al., 2002). Tapes promoting relaxation have also been used to reduce drug use during dental surgery (Corah, Gale, & Illig, 1979; Ghoneim, Block, Sarasin, Davis, & Marchman, 2000), gastrointestinal endoscopy (Wilson, Moore, Randolph, & Hanson, 1982), and femoral angiography (Mandle et al., 1990). Tapes were rejected by 13% of the patients who received such to practice relaxation and imagery to increase breast milk production (Feher, Berger, Johnson, & Wilde, 1989). Also, because of the lack of a therapist–patient relationship, tapes might not be as powerful in preventing adverse effects such as vomiting (Ghoneim et al., 2000). In general, the presence of a live therapist is felt to be superior (Blankfield, 1991). Very anxious patients may also need a process that addresses their worries specifically before they will be able to relax and engage in hypnosis. This opportunity would be lost if only a standard electronic medium were used. We also found that patients' preferences for pleasant imagery during self-hypnotic relaxation were highly individual and quite variable (i.e., not necessarily predictable; Fick, Lang, Benotsch, Lutgendorf, & Logan, 1999). Patients chose as their pleasant and safe place scenarios ranging from gambling in Las Vegas to building birdhouses, canning vegetables, or floating over the clouds with deceased loved ones.

Despite ongoing theoretical discussion of what hypnosis is, leaders in the field surmise that all hypnosis is self-hypnosis (Hammond, 1998). A semantic focus on self-hypnosis (i.e., which emphasizes the patient's contribution) rather than hypnosis (i.e., which focuses on the power of the provider) has practical implications in the modern medical environment, which often leaves the patient feeling devoid of control. It gives the patient a sense of control and reduces feelings of guilt or failure on the side of the therapist, particularly in a setting in which no pretesting for hypnotizability is done and where patients did not come actively seeking hypnosis. We teach our hypnosis providers that all they do is help patients help themselves; if a patient does not enter a deep state of hypnosis, providers should not blame themselves. However, if a patient has an excellent experience, providers should not take credit but acknowledge the patient's contribution. In our clinical practice, we find that this approach provides patients with a tremendous sense of pride and fulfillment at having been able to help themselves.

Typically, patients who come for a doctor's visit or a medical procedure are highly suggestible (H. Spiegel, 1997). Unfortunately, there are strong belief systems in the medical community that alerting patients with the use of negative suggestions about upcoming pain and distressing feelings during procedures expresses sympathy (Lang et al., 2005). Therefore, therapists who prepare patients prior to procedures and are not in the procedure room with them may want to be particularly conscious of these negative suggestions (e.g., telling patients that the local anesthetic injection will "sting and burn") and include measures of immunization against such comments. However, it is important to recognize the emotional investment of the members of the procedure team in the patient's pain management, and it is crucial to acknowledge their experience and enlist their contribution and collaboration when designing hypnosis programs in medical settings.

Hypnotizability

The procedure room does not permit for feasible assessment of a patient's hypnotizability. Furthermore, testing for hypnotizability before the procedure could affect expectancy of patients and personnel and thereby alter outcome (Chaves & Barber, 1974; Jacobs, Kurtz, & Strube, 1995; H. Spiegel & Spiegel, 1978; Stam & Spanos, 1980). In a previous study (Lang, Joyce, et al., 1996) we used the Hypnotic Induction Profile test (HIP; H. Spiegel & Spiegel) as a measure of hypnotizability after patients' procedures. The HIP possesses outcome validity and is relatively unaffected by prior hypnotic experiences (H. Spiegel & Spiegel). Our results showed that patients in both our standard care and hypnosis groups had nearly identical average HIP scores after the procedure, as expected for a successful randomization. Benefit from hypnosis was also relatively independent of hypnotizability.

Hypnotic Analgesia Method

Nonpharmacologic analgesia aims at inducing a state of attentive, receptive concentration that allows patients to explore their own capacity to interact with a painful or uncomfortable situation (D. Spiegel, 1989). Treatment includes establishment of rapport, correct use of language and suggestions, relaxation training, hypnosis, patient-initiated imagery, and provisions for addressing patients' worries and fears, if necessary.

We prefer an approach validated in the interventional radiology setting, which has been proven safe for patient and therapist in prior studies (Lang & Berbaum, 1997; Lang et al., 2000; Lang, Spiegel, Lutgendorf, & Logan, 1996). Typically, we perform all hypnotic treatment in the procedure room, while the patient is lying on the procedure table. In our clinical practice, this is often the first time that patients are exposed to the idea of having medical hypnosis during their procedure, and therefore, patient hypnotizability is not assessed prior to hypnosis. The main reason for this is the lack of time and structure for a preparatory visit in the busy clinical interventional radiology setting. Emphasis is placed on rapid (i.e., "instant") rapport techniques in the form of structured attentive behavior to establish the patient–provider relationship. Detailed descriptions of the standardized interventions of structure attentive behavior have been published (Lang et al., 1999).

Structured attentive behaviors include the following components: (a) matching the patients' verbal communication pattern, (b) matching the patients' nonverbal communication pattern, (c) listening attentively, (d) providing the perception of control (e.g., "Let us know at any time what we can do for you"), (e) swiftly responding to patients' requests, (f) encouraging the patient, (g) using emotionally neutral descriptors when painful stimuli are imminent (e.g., "What are you experiencing?", "Focus on a sensation of fullness, numbness, coolness, or warmth"), and (h) avoiding negatively loaded suggestions (e.g., "How bad is your pain?", "You will feel a sting and burn now").

For guidance to self-hypnotic relaxation, we typically use scripts, in part because much of our work occurs in a research context. Scripts assure reproducibility and also help the hypnosis providers, many of whom were trained de novo, to internalize hypnotic language. Seeing a hypnosis provider sit down, put on glasses, and start reading a script also has some comforting aspects in the procedure suite for patients and personnel: It removes notions of mind-control as asserted in popular culture depictions (i.e., movies, books, TV). It also conveys to the procedure team that hypnosis is something they could learn with the support of a script and that language is important.

The script in our first pilot study (Lang et al., 1996) used progressive muscle relaxation from the head and moving down the entire body, use of a signal breath to release tension and discomfort, and guidance to a pleasant scene in nature or other location. When feelings of discomfort, anxiety, or pain were expressed, the patients were asked to think of an image that best represented the experience and were guided to transform this image into something emotionally more manageable. With subsequent clinical use, we realized that progressive muscle relaxation took too long for a busy interventional suite and that underlying fears, if left unaddressed early on, prevented patients from relaxing. We then experimented with an approach that started by asking patients what they were experiencing. When fears and anxieties were mentioned, which was not uncommon, we immediately started the process of converting those distressing feelings using a guided imagery process and used the resultant imagery to further structure self-hypnotic relaxation. For example, if a patient described feeling as if vultures were coming down to get him, we would suggest that the birds would fly away and leave behind beautiful, soft feathers, becoming a wonderful, cozy down blanket of protection into which the patient could sink deeper and deeper. Some patients, however, would not generate or share imagery and additional interventions made the process less reproducible and "weird" in the eyes of the procedure team.

We then experimented with inductions that used walking down stairs or counting numbers back from 100. However, interruptions to which patients are subjected on the operating table made these approaches cumbersome. For example, one of the authors guided a patient to walk down from stairs 10 to 9 and then to 8, but a relief nurse walked into the room, went straight to the patient, and introduced herself loudly. Starting again from stair 10 downward—this time to stair 5—the patient's concentration was broken again when the operator yelled a command. Disenchantment with walking up and down the stairs on the part of the provider ended usage of this induction script. It became clear that the next script must be immune to interruptions, be quick to apply, address fears early in a way that would be easily manageable, and release the patient's imagery without resistance. David Spiegel kindly developed the hypnosis script for us that we modified slightly over time to include elements unique to the environment. This script resulted in rapid induction and was used successfully in our study published in *The Lancet* (Lang et al., 2000) and in subsequent prospective randomized trials. For a free download of the hypnosis scripts we use for analgesia during medical procedures, please refer to our Web site: http://www.hypnalgesics.com.

In our clinical practice, we introduce the nature of hypnosis by asking the patients whether they have ever experienced getting caught up in a movie or book. For skeptics we add that this experience shows that one cannot be hypnotized against one's will, because getting involved in a movie or book will not happen with a movie or book one does not like. Also, one can always close a book or turn off the movie. This introduction may often be the only explanation we give patients about the mechanisms of hypnosis. Also, we explain to the patients that there may be distracting noises in the procedure room and that health care workers may make negative suggestions (e.g., "This won't hurt that much," "You will feel a sting and a burn"), and we provide suggestions to immunize them against such negative comments.

The induction of hypnosis begins with an eye-roll induction, which is useful in this hospital setting because whenever there is an interruption, it is easy to repeat the eye roll. Once the patients learn the induction, we may also tell them that it is something they can use now and also later, when they return to the ward, their home, or whenever they wish to relax deeply.

CLINICAL MATERIAL

Rather than present a single case of a person who undergoes our procedures, we describe the experiences of a group of patients who participated in a prospective randomized trial that was published in *The Lancet* (Lang, 2000). In this study, 241 patients undergoing peripheral vascular and percutaneous renal interventions were randomized to receive intraoperatively standard care treatment ($n = 79$), structured attention ($n = 80$), or self-hypnotic relaxation ($n = 82$). As we described before, we used the eight key elements of structured empathic attention; to the hypnosis group, we added the reading of a self-hypnotic relaxation script. An additional provider (i.e., a live therapist) supplied both hypnosis and structured attentive behavior in the procedure room. During the research period, all four providers were trained anew to reflect what an average competent health care worker could do with specific training. This training consisted of 24 hours of classroom instruction and role-play in hypnosis and structured attention, with an additional 8 hours of workshop training.

All patients had free access to an intravenous sedative or narcotic that was controlled by the patient. Pain and anxiety levels were assessed through verbal scores reported on scales from 0 to 10 (i.e., where 0 = *no pain and no anxiety at all* and 10 = *worst pain possible or terror*). Scores were obtained before and every 15 minutes during the procedure. Use of moderate sedation was recorded as 1 unit, corresponding to either 50 μg of fentanyl or 1 mg of mida-zolam (i.e., the amount of drugs required and received). Possible adverse effects were also recorded through monitoring of physiologic parameters (e.g., heart rate, blood pressure, oxygen saturation).

The results showed that pain increased linearly with procedure time in the standard care group and in the attention control group but not in the hyp-nosis group. Anxiety decreased linearly with procedure duration in all three groups. The difference in slopes was significant for the hypnosis group as com-pared with the standard care group. Analysis of drug administration during the procedure showed that patients in the standard care group had significantly higher drug use than those in the attention group and in the hypnosis group.

It is interesting that adverse effects were also less frequent in the hypno-sis group. Whereas one could have expected a given improvement of hemo-dynamic stability in the empathy and hypnosis group merely based on a reduction of drug use, the significant reduction of hemodynamic instability in the hypnosis group suggests that hypnosis-specific effects are responsible for this clinically important outcome. Also, average procedure duration was sig-nificantly shorter in the hypnosis group than in the standard group (i.e., 61 vs. 78 minutes). Procedure duration for the attention group was between, but not significantly different from, that of the other two groups (M = 67 minutes).

RESEARCH AND APPRAISAL

Many reports about the effectiveness of adjunct hypnosis are either anecdotal, based on case series, or retrospective in nature. The researchers involved believed in their methodology—the effect of hypnosis is obvious to anyone who has ever worked with it—but widespread introduction into the operating room will require evidence-based justification. Safety and efficacy of acute pain management are still a challenge to doctors, particularly in the pediatric population (Yaster & Cravero, 2004). The observation that chil-dren have an increased susceptibility for hypnosis (Morgan & Hilgard, 1972) makes its use attractive for this setting.

As such, the benefits for the use of hypnosis were assessed in a random-ized study with 44 children undergoing voiding cystourethrography, one of the most common radiologic procedures performed to evaluate vesicoureteral reflux in children (Butler, Symons, Henderson, Shortliffe, & Spiegel, 2005). Children assigned to the hypnosis group demonstrated significantly lower dis-tress levels during the procedure as compared with the control group, and par-ents of the children also reported that the procedure was significantly less traumatic for their children as compared with their previous procedures. Moreover, the medical staff reported less difficulty in performing the procedure in the hypnosis group; they also reported shorter procedure times as compared with the control condition.

The effect of hypnosis on postoperative pain was assessed in another randomized study (Huth, Broome, & Good, 2004) in which 75 children undergoing tonsillectomy with or without adenoidectomy were assigned to either a hypnosis treatment group or to a control group. In the treatment group, parents and children were given professionally developed imagery booklets, a videotape presentation (with deep breathing and imagery techniques) and an audiotape for school-age children (with deep breathing, muscle relaxation, music, and suggestions for picturing a park) 2 to 22 days prior to the scheduled surgery in order to teach the child imagery skills for postoperative pain management. This material was also provided postoperatively in ambulatory surgery, 1 to 4 hours after the procedure (Time 2) and 22 to 27 hours after discharge at home (Time 3). Measurements of sensory and affective pain, as well as the anxiety were performed at Time 2 and Time 3. The results showed that in the treatment group, less pain and anxiety was reported at Time 2 as compared with the control group, although no differences were observed in Time 3 between the groups.

Montgomery, David, Winkel, Silverstein, and Bovberg (2002) presented a meta-analysis that documented the beneficial impact of the use of adjunct hypnosis in surgical patients by calculating 22 effect sizes of 20 controlled published studies. Clinical outcomes were categorized and a secondary analysis of the differences was performed. The categories included (a) negative affect (e.g., anxiety, depression), which was measured by both self-report and observations by others (e.g., nurses); (b) pain (i.e., both self-report and observations by others); (c) pain medication (e.g., analgesics, anesthetics); (d) physiological indicators (e.g., blood pressure, heart rate, catecholamine levels); (e) recovery (e.g., return of muscular strength, postoperative vomiting, fatigue); and (f) treatment time (e.g., length of the procedure, inpatient stay). The results indicated that, on average, 89% of surgical patients in the studies investigated benefited from adjunctive hypnosis techniques relative to patients in control conditions. Likewise, the beneficial effects were apparent in each of the six clinical outcome categories selected for the study.

Another application in pain management is the use of hypnosis in the burn care unit. Pain related to daily dressing changes and wound debridements produce significant nociception (Patterson et al., 1993). Numerous case reports demonstrate the benefits of the use of hypnosis for this purpose (Patterson, Questad, & Boltwood, 1987); however, Patterson and his colleagues conducted the first controlled trial in 1992 (Patterson, Everett, Burns, & Marvin, 1992). In this study, 30 patients undergoing dressing changes in a major regional burn unit were randomly assigned to one of the three following conditions: hypnosis, attention and information control condition, and no-treatment control condition. The hypnosis condition was based on a rapid induction analgesia model modified for burn wound debridement (Patterson, Questad, & deLateour, 1989). The attention and information control condition included interaction with psychologists; participants and nurses were led to believe that participants were hypnotized. Patients in the no-treatment control condition received only opioid medication.

The patients were seen on two different occasions during the dressing changes: on the 1st day (i.e., pretreatment), in which patients were given only the pain medication in all three groups, and on the 2nd day (i.e., posttreatment), in which one of the three conditions described previously was provided to each group in addition to pain medication. For pain assessment, investigators used a visual analog scale anchored on one end with the words, "worst pain possible" and on the other end with, "no pain." The patients were asked to describe the pain during the wound care using the visual analog scale within 3 hours after the procedure on the 1st day (i.e., pretreatment) and 2nd day (i.e., posttreatment) of dressing changes. The authors compared the patients' self-ratings of pain in the 1st and the 2nd day of wound care for each group. The researchers found that hypnotized patients experienced superior pain relief as compared with a control condition and reported decreased pain relative to the group that believed they had hypnosis treatment.

Subsequently, in a prospective randomized study comparing hypnosis with a stress-reducing strategy (Frenay, Faymonville, Devlieger, Albert, & Vanderkelen, 2001), 30 patients with a total burned surface area of 10% to 25% were randomly assigned to hypnosis or a nonhypnotic stress-reducing strategy group. Measurements of patients' anxiety, pain, pain control, and satisfaction were collected on Days 1, 3, 5, 7, 8, 10, 12, and 14 by means of a visual analog scale before, during, and after each dressing change while in the hospital. In the hypnosis condition, a psychologist was present during the wound changes and invited the patient to choose a pleasant life experience to recollect. The psychologist provided the patient with positive suggestions to transform sensations and to dissociate the patient from his or her pain. The following stress-reducing strategies were applied in the same setting: (a) instruction in behaviors (i.e., deep breathing, relaxation procedures) to buffer responses to pain and stressful stimuli and (b) positive evocation to focus the patient on recreating a pleasant memory and to create a positive emotional state to offset the effects of negative life events. The results showed that the hypnosis group presented with lower anxiety scores, but no difference was observed between the two groups regarding pain scores and satisfaction.

Psychological approaches for pain control in the surgical setting were also evaluated during more invasive procedures (Faymonville et al., 1997) by studying 60 patients scheduled for elective plastic surgery under local anesthesia and intravenous sedation, randomly assigned to a stress-reducing strategy (i.e., control) or hypnosis group. Before randomization and surgery, all patients used visual analog scales (VAS) to assess their level of anxiety and predicted level of control during surgery. In the hypnosis group, patients were invited to choose a pleasant life experience to relive during surgery, followed by induction of hypnotic state using eye fixation, muscle relaxation, and permissive and indirect suggestions. In the control group, stress-reducing strategies were provided to the participants by suggesting behaviors (i.e., deep breathing, relaxation procedures) to buffer responses to pain and stressful stimuli. Positive evocation was provided to focus the patient on recreating a pleasant memory and to create a positive emotional state to offset the effects of negative life events. For each case, intraoperative occurrence of verbal and nonverbal discomfort and pain complaints detected by a psychologist observer, requirements for midazolam and alfentanil, and operative surgical conditions were rated by the surgeon on a VAS scale. Postoperatively, pain and anxiety were assessed before discharge from the hospital, as was satisfaction with the anesthetic procedure and the level of control perceived during surgery. The researchers reported that peri- and postoperative anxiety and pain were significantly lower in the hypnosis group, despite the fewer requirements for drugs as compared with the other group. The hypnosis group also presented with more stable vital signs and reported greater satisfaction and better surgical conditions compared with the stress-reducing strategies group.

One of the major concerns in hypnosis clinical trials is to examine the effects of hypnosis in conjunction with a control group adequate to make inferences regarding the variables responsible for treatment outcomes. Such controls are particularly important in studies of the management of chronic pain (Jensen & Patterson, 2005). Ideally, research designs should include standard care and attention control groups, although identifying the "active ingredient" in the outcome can still remain challenging. Patients who are aided by an external focus intraoperatively (e.g., by a provider displaying empathic structured attention only) can postoperatively be less able or willing to follow suggestions measuring hypnotizability than patients who experience self-hypnotic relaxation (Koch, Lang, Hatsiopoulou, Berbaum, & Anderson, 2003). Such a short-term adverse effect of attention control treatment can represent a further conundrum in designing controlled hypnosis trials, particularly those in which the researchers wish to measure hypnotizability.

Our current research focuses on examining the generalizability of the treatment effects we obtained in the research described earlier to different medical scenarios and patient populations. Our earlier positive findings (Lang et al., 1999, 2000) of faster and safer interventional radiology procedures were based mostly on patients undergoing procedures such as balloon angioplasty or percutaneous kidney drainage. In contrast, our current randomized clinical trial aims to assess the effects of hypnosis on patients undergoing some of the more (or most) aggressive procedures performed in the interventional radiology setting, namely, image-guided tumor therapies. Examples of image-guided tumor interventions include uterine artery embolization (i.e., to treat uterine fibroids) or transarterial liver chemo-embolization or percutaneous radiofrequency ablation (i.e., to treat malignant liver tumors, primary or metastases). These treatment modalities are associated with massive tissue necrosis immediately following the intervention and can potentially be more painful and uncomfortable compared with angioplasty or kidney procedures. Also, they encompass patient populations with specific and interesting psychological profiles, for example, patients with fibroids (i.e., women, usually anxious after experiencing menorrhagia and cramps for a long time) and patients with liver cancer (i.e., frequently older patients, who have a malignant cancer so advanced that cannot be surgically removed). This clinical trial also aims to investigate the effect of a single self-hypnotic intervention during a procedure on subsequent procedures of the same kind, insofar as patients frequently present for multiple treatment sessions.

We currently are conducting another study in a completely different setting in the area of breast imaging for women undergoing large core breast biopsy for suspicious lesions seen on screening mammogram or breast ultrasound. Image-guided breast biopsies are performed in a purely outpatient context for women with heightened baseline anxiety, fearful that their biopsy will reveal breast cancer. As opposed to the other interventional radiology procedures we have described, this procedure is performed solely under local anesthesia. Intravenous moderate sedation or oral sedatives are not desirable for this patient population who will likely drive home following the biopsy. This randomized trial of self-hypnosis promises to yield unique insights in an interventional scenario in which patients experience heightened fear and anxiety and in which few options of pharmacologic analgesia or anxiolysis are available.

CONCLUSION

Hypnotic relaxation has the potential to benefit millions of patients by reducing cognitive and physiologic distress associated with invasive medical procedures. The possibilities for improved patient safety and comfort are significant. There is currently a significant amount of evidence in the medical literature to support widespread clinical application of hypnosis for invasive medical procedures. It is important that cost analyses have demonstrated that the introduction of hypnosis in the currently expensive and high tech medical environment can lead to significant savings for the health care system.

REFERENCES

Acute Pain Management Guideline Panel. (1992). *Acute pain management: Operative or medical procedures and trauma: Clinical practice guideline* (AHCPR Publication No. 92–0032). Rockville, MD: U.S. Department of Health and Human Services.

Baglini, R., Sesana, M., Capuano, C., Gnecchi-Ruscone, T., Ugo, L., & Danzi, G. (2004). Effect of hypnotic sedation during percutaneous transluminal coronary angioplasty on myocardial ischemia and cardiac sympathetic drive. *American Journal of Cardiology, 93,* 1035–1038.

Bennett, H. L., Benson, D. R., & Kuiken, D. A. (1986). Preoperative instructions for decreased bleeding during spine surgery [Abstract]. *Anesthesiology, 65,* A245.

Bernstein, M. R. (1965). Significant value of hypnoanaesthesia: Three clinical examples. *American Journal of Clinical Hypnosis, 7,* 259–260.

Blankfield, R. P. (1991). Suggestion, relaxation, and hypnosis as adjuncts in the care of surgery patients: A review of the literature. *American Journal of Clinical Hypnosis, 33,* 172–186.

Bonilla, K. B., Quigley, W. F., & Bowers, W. F. (1961). Experiences with hypnosis on a surgical service. *Military Medicine, 126,* 364–370.

Bowen, D. E. (1973). Transurethral resection under self-hypnosis. *American Journal of Clinical Hypnosis, 16,* 132–134.

Butler, L. D., Symons, B. K., Henderson, S. L., Shortliffe, L. D., & Spiegel, D. (2005). Hypnosis reduces distress and duration of an invasive medical procedure for children. *Journal of Pediatrics, 115,* 77–85.

Chaves, J. F., & Barber, T. X. (1974). Cognitive strategies, experimenter modeling, and expectation in the attentuation of pain. *Journal of Abnormal Psychology, 83,* 356–363.

Corah, N. L., Gale, E. N., & Illig, S. J. (1979). The use of relaxation and distraction during dental procedures. *Journal of the American Dental Association, 98,* 390–394.

Crasilneck, H. B., McCranie, E. J., & Jenkins, M. T. (1956). Special indications for hypnosis as method of anesthesia. *JAMA, 126,* 1606–1608.

Enqvist, B., von Konow, L., & Bystedt, H. (1995). Pre- and perioperative suggestion in maxillofacial surgery: Effects on blood loss and recovery. *International Journal of Clinical and Experimental Hypnosis, 63,* 284–294.

Esdaile, J. (1957). *Hypnosis in medicine and surgery.* New York: Julian Press. (Reprinted from *Mesmerism in India and its practical application in surgery and medicine,* 1846, London: Longman, Brown, Green, & Longmans)

Faintuch, S., Lang, E. V., & Rosen, M. P. (2004). Cost-effectiveness of self-hypnosis during outpatient interventional radiologic procedures: Update and impact. *Sociedad Iberoamericana de Informacion Cientifica.* Retrieved from htp://www.trabajosdistinguidos.com

Faymonville, M. E., Mambourg, P. H., Joris, J., Vrijens, B., Fissette, J., Albert, A., et al. (1997). Psychological approaches during conscious sedation: Hypnosis versus stress reducing strategies: A prospective randomized study. *Journal of Pain, 73*, 361–367.

Faymonville, M. E., Meurisse, M., & Fissette, J. (1999). Hypnosedation: A valuable alternative to traditional anaesthetic techniques. *Acta Chirurgica Belgica, 99*, 141–146.

Feher, S. D. K., Berger, L. R., Johnson, J. D., & Wilde, J. B. (1989). Increasing breast milk production for premature infants with relaxation/imagery audiotape. *Pediatrics, 83*, 57–60.

Fick, L. J., Lang, E. V., Benotsch, E. G., Lutgendorf, S., & Logan, H. L. (1999). Imagery content during nonpharmacologic analgesia in the procedure suite: Where your patients would rather be. *Academic Radiology, 6*, 457–463.

Fredericks, L. E. (1978). Teaching of hypnosis in the overall approach to the surgical patient. *American Journal of Clinical Hypnosis, 22*, 175–183.

Frenay, M. C., Faymonville, M. E., Devlieger, S., Albert, A., & Vanderkelen, A. (2001). Psychological approaches during dressing changes of burned patients: A prospective randomised study comparing hypnosis against stress reducing strategy. *Journal of the International Society For Burn Injuries, 27*, 793–799.

Ghoneim, M. M., Block, R. I., Sarasin, D. S., Davis, C. S., & Marchman, J. N. (2000). Tape-recorded hypnosis instructions as adjuvant in the care of patients scheduled for third molar surgery. *Anesthesia and Analgesia, 90*, 64–68.

Greenberg, S. B., Faerber, E. N., Aspinall, C. L., & Adams, R. C. (1993). High-dose chloral hydrate sedation for children undergoing MR imaging: Safety and efficacy in relation to age. *American Journal of Roentgenology, 161*, 639–641.

Hammond, D. C. (1998). *Hypnotic induction & suggestion*. Chicago: American Society of Clinical Hypnosis.

Hatsiopoulou, O., Cohen, R. I., & Lang, E. (2003). Postprocedure pain management of interventional radiology patients. *Journal of Vascular and Interventional Radiology, 14*, 1373–1385.

Hilgard, E. R. (1977). *Divided consciousness: Multiple controls in human thought and action*. New York: Wiley.

Hippel, C. V., Hole, G., & Kaschka, W. P. (2001). Autonomic profile under hypnosis as assessed by heart rate variability and spectral analysis. *Pharmacopsychiatry, 34*, 11–113.

Huth, M. M., Broome, M. E., & Good, M. (2004). Imagery reduces children's postoperative pain. *Journal of Pain, 110*, 439–448.

Jacobs, A. L., Kurtz, R. M., & Strube, M. J. (1995). Hypnotic analgesia, expectancy effects, and choice of design: A reexamination. *International Journal of Clinical and Experimental Hypnosis, 43*, 55–61.

Jensen, M. P., & Patterson, D. R. (2005). Control conditions in hypnotic–analgesia clinical trials: Challenges and recommendations. *International Journal of Clinical and Experimental Hypnosis, 53*, 170–197.

Johnston, M. (2001). Impending surgery. In S. Fisher & J. Reason (Eds.), *Handbook of life stress, cognition, and health* (pp. 79–100). New York: Wiley.

Koch, T., Lang, E. V., Hatsiopoulou, O., Berbaum, K., & Anderson, B. (2003). Adverse short-term effects of attention control on treatment of hypnotizability: A challenge in designing controlled hypnosis trials. *International Journal of Clinical and Experimental Hypnosis, 51*, 357–368.

Kroger, W. S., & DeLee, S. T. (1957). Hypnoanesthesia for Cesarean section and hysterectomy. *JAMA, 163*, 442–444.

Lang, E. V., Benotsch, E. G., Fick, L. J., Lutgendorf, S., Berbaum, M. L., Berbaum, K. S., et al. (2000, April 29). Adjunctive nonpharmacologic analgesia for invasive medical procedures: A randomized trial. *The Lancet, 355*, 1486–1490.

Lang, E. V., & Berbaum, K. S. (1997). Educating interventional radiology personnel in nonpharmacologic analgesia: Effect on patients' pain perception. *Academic Radiology, 4*, 753–757.

Lang, E. V., Hatsiopoulou, O., Koch, T., Berbaum, K., Lutgendorf, S., Kettenmann, E., et al. (2005). Can words hurt? Patient–provider interactions during invasive medical procedures. *Journal of Pain, 114*, 303–309.

Lang, E. V., Joyce, J. S., Spiegel, D., Hamilton, D., & Lee, K. (1996). Self-hypnotic relaxation during interventional radiological procedures: Effects on pain perception and intravenous drug use. *International Journal of Clinical and Experimental Hypnosis, 44*, 106–119.

Lang, E. V., Lutgendorf, S., Logan, H., Benotsch, E., Laser, E., & Spiegel, D. (1999). Nonpharmacologic analgesia and anxiolysis for interventional radiological procedures. *Seminars in Interventional Radiology, 16*, 113–123.

Lang, E. V., & Rosen, M. (2002). Cost analysis of adjunct hypnosis for sedation during outpatient interventional procedures. *Radiology, 222*, 375–382.

Lang, E. V., Spiegel, D., Lutgendorf, S., & Logan, H. (1996). *Empathic attention and self-hypnotic relaxation for interventional radiological procedures.* Iowa City, IA: The University of Iowa.

Levitan, A. A., & Harbaugh. T. E. (1989). Hypnoanalgesia and hypnotizability. *Hypnosis, 16*, 140–148.

Levitan, A. A., & Harbaugh, T. E. (1992). Hypnotizability and hypnoanalgesia: Hypnotizability of patients using hypnoanalgesia during surgery. *American Journal of Clinical Hypnosis, 34*, 223–226.

Mandle, C. L., Domar, A. D., Harrington, D. P., Leserman, J., Bozadjian, E. M., Friedman, R., et al. (1990). Relaxation response in femoral angiography. *Radiology, 174*, 737–739.

Marmer, M. J. (1959). Hypnoanalgesia and hypnoanesthesia for cardiac surgery. *JAMA, 171*, 512–517.

Martin, M. L., & Lennox, P. H. (2003). Sedation and analgesia in the interventional radiology department. *Journal of Vascular and Interventional Radiology, 14*, 1119–1128.

Mason, A. A. (1955). Surgery under hypnosis. *Anaesthesia, 10,* 295–299.

Montgomery, G. H., David, D., Winkel, G., Silverstein, J. H., & Bovbjerg, D. H. (2002). The effectiveness of adjunctive hypnosis with surgical patients: A meta-analysis. *Anesthesia and Analgesia, 94,* 1639–1645.

Montgomery, G. H., Weltz, C. R., Seltz, M., & Bovbjerg, D. H. (2002). Brief presurgery hypnosis reduces stress and pain in excisional breast biopsy patients. *International Journal of Clinical and Experimental Hypnosis, 50,* 17–32.

Morgan, A. H., & Hilgard, E. R. (1972). Age differences in susceptibility to hypnosis. *International Journal of Clinical and Experimental Hypnosis, 21,* 78–85.

Patterson, D. R., Everett, J. J., Bombardier, C. H., Questad, K. A., Lee, V. K., & Marvin, J. A. (1993). Psychological effects of severe burn injuries. *Psychological Bulletin, 113,* 362–378.

Patterson, D. R., Everett, J. J., Burns, G. L., & Marvin, J. A. (1992). Hypnosis for the treatment of burn pain. *Journal of Consulting and Clinical Psychology, 5,* 713–717.

Patterson, D. R., Questad, K. A., & Boltwood, M. D. (1987). Hypnotherapy as a treatment for pain in patients with burns: Research and clinical considerations. *Journal of Burn Care and Rehabilitation, 8,* 263–268.

Patterson, D. R., Questad, K. A., & deLateour, B. J. (1989). Hypnotherapy as an adjunct to narcotic analgesia for the treatment of pain for burn debridement. *American Journal of Clinical Hypnosis, 31,* 156–163.

Quirk, M. E., Letendre, A. J., Ciottone, R. A., & Lingley, J. F. (1989). Anxiety of patients undergoing MRI imaging. *Radiology, 170,* 463–466.

Ronchera-Oms, C. L., Casillas, C., Martí-Bonmati, L., Poyatos, C., Tomás, J., & Sobejano, A., et al. (1994). Oral chloral hydrate provides effective and safe sedation in pediatric magnetic resonance imaging. *Journal of Clinical Pharmacy and Therapeutics, 19,* 239–243.

Ruiz, O. R. G., & Fernandez, A. (1960). Hypnosis as an anesthetic in ophthalmology. *American Journal of Ophthalmology, 50,* 163.

Schwarcz, B. E. (1965). Hypnoanalgesia and hypnoanesthesia in urology. *Surgical Clinics of North America, 45,* 1547–1555.

Spanos, N. P., Radtke-Bodorik, H. L., Ferguson, J., & Jones, B. (1979). The effects of hypnotic susceptibility suggestions for analgesia and the utilization of cognitive strategies on the reduction of pain. *Journal of Abnormal Psychology, 88,* 282–292.

Spiegel, D. (1989). Uses and abuses of hypnosis. *Integrative Psychiatry, 6,* 211–222.

Spiegel, H. (1997). Nocebo: The power of suggestibility. *American Journal of Preventative Medicine, 26,* 616–621.

Spiegel, H., & Spiegel, D. (1978). *Trance and treatment: Clinical uses of hypnosis.* New York: Basic Books.

Stam, H. J., & Spanos, N. P. (1980). Experimental designs, expectancy effects, and hypnotic analgesia. *Journal of Abnormal Psychology, 89,* 751–762.

Stewart, J. H. (2005). Hypnosis in contemporary medicine. *Mayo Clinic Proceedings*, 80, 511–524.

Tinterow, M. T. (1960). Hypnotic anesthesia for major surgical procedures. *American Surgeon, 26*, 732–737.

Wilson, J. F., Moore, R. W., Randolph, S., & Hanson, B. J. (1982). Behavioral preparation of patients for gastrointestinal endoscopy: Information, relaxation, and coping style. *Journal of Human Stress, 8*, 13–23.

Yaster, M., & Cravero, J. P. (2004). The continuing conundrum of sedation for painful and nonpainful procedures. *Journal of Pediatrics, 14*, 10–12.

24

HYPNOSIS AND SMOKING CESSATION: RESEARCH AND APPLICATION

JOSEPH P. GREEN

According to the U.S. Department of Health and Human Services (USDHHS; 2004), smoking is the leading cause of preventable morbidity and mortality. In the executive summary of a recent surgeon general's report, the following conclusions were drawn:

1. Smoking harms nearly every organ of the body, causing many diseases and reducing the health of smokers in general.
2. Quitting smoking has immediate as well as long-term benefits, reducing the risks for diseases caused by smoking and improving health in general.
3. Smoking cigarettes with lower machine-measured yields of tar and nicotine provides no clear benefit to health.
4. The list of diseases caused by smoking has been expanded to include abdominal aortic aneurysm, acute myeloid leukemia,

As I note in the chapter, Steven Jay Lynn and his colleagues were the original developers of the smoking cessation program. Although I was not one of the original authors, I have worked closely with Lynn over the past 2 decades improving the program. The reader should be informed that it is within this capacity that I use the terms *we* and *our* to describe the program. I am grateful to Lynn for his helpful comments and editorial assistance with earlier drafts of this chapter.
All clinical material has been disguised to protect patient confidentiality.

cataracts, cervical cancer, kidney cancer, pancreatic cancer, pneumonia, periodontitis, and stomach cancer. (p. 8)

Since the initial 1964 surgeon general's report, the USDHHS has issued no less than 27 reports on the adverse health effects associated with smoking and secondhand smoke. In spite of the widespread knowledge about the dangers associated with smoking and secondhand smoke, nearly a quarter of Americans (22.5%) continue to smoke (Centers for Disease Control [CDC], 2004). According to a 2002 survey, a higher percentage of males (25.2%) than females (20.0%) smoked on a daily basis or at least on "some days" (CDC, 2004). Extrapolating from the results of the survey, about 45.8 million U.S. adults smoke cigarettes. The good news is that for the first time in nearly 50 years, more U.S. adults have quit smoking than are current smokers: According to CDC statistics, 50.1% of those who had ever smoked had quit. There are a number of treatment options available to smokers who want to become non-smokers. Hypnosis continues to be one the most popular methods for achieving smoking abstinence (Lynn & Kirsch, 2006). In the Clinical Applications section of this chapter, I will describe in detail our two-session, cognitive behavioral program using hypnotic suggestions for smoking cessation. To supplement previous descriptions of the program (see Lynn, Neufeld, Rhue, & Matorin, 1993; Green, 1996, 2000), I update our original approach and present an expanded rationale for various components of the program. The clinical efficacy of other suggestion-based treatments for smoking cessation will be reviewed in the Research and Appraisal section of this chapter.

CLINICAL APPLICATIONS

In 1988, Neufeld and Lynn (1988) developed a single session hypnosis-based treatment for smoking. The program was developed in conjunction with the American Lung Association of Ohio. Lynn, Neufeld, and Rhue (1992) expanded the protocol into a two-session approach culling various cognitive, behavioral, and hypnotic strategies together (see also Lynn, et al., 1993). In a series of book chapters, I (Green, 1996, 1998, 2000) illustrated the specifics of the Lynn et al. (1993) program in both individual and group formats. Over the years, we have made several modifications to the original protocol (see Lynn & Kirsch, 2006). What follows is the latest refinement of the smoking cessation approach that we currently use.

Our program can be used to treat a single individual or a fairly large group (e.g., about 50 people). The protocol involves two sessions, spaced a week apart. The first session (approximately 90 minutes) educates the client about the dangers of smoking and secondhand smoke and describes cognitive, behavioral, and hypnotic strategies to help him or her become a nonsmoker.

As originally designed, the therapist personally meets with an individual client or a group of clients to discuss the information and strategies comprising our first session. In an effort to provide this information in a more expedient manner, I have recently created a 1-hour DVD (with approximately 60 slides and a running narrative) and corresponding handouts detailing the informational and educational components of our first session. Clients can now review the DVD and related written materials prior to coming to therapy. We are currently testing whether outcome rates differ as a function of these two different delivery methods. The second session (approximately 60 minutes) presents a variety of hypnotic suggestions to achieve smoking abstinence. The hypnosis scripts have also been recorded on CD, and we are currently investigating the impact of delivering our entire program in a home-study format. If a home-study program can be shown to be effective, it could enable a large number of individuals to undergo this type of smoking cessation treatment.

Cognitive and Behavioral Skills

The treatment protocol and the self-hypnosis script contain cognitive and behavioral strategies to instill confidence, enhance self-efficacy, substitute adaptive behaviors for smoking, improve self-image, and manage stress and negative affect. Techniques such as minimizing negative self-talk, identifying triggers and stimulus control, self-monitoring and self-reward, contingency management, and cue-controlled relaxation (i.e., anchoring) are all key components of the smoking cessation protocol.

Education

The health risks associated with smoking are well established. In fact, most of our clients do not need to be convinced that smoking is harmful to their health. In addition to reviewing the information about the risks associated with smoking, we point out the dangers of secondhand smoke, including the link between secondhand smoke and lung cancer in nonsmoking adults and its association with children's vulnerability to respiratory infections, middle ear infections, and asthma. A periodic review of the Web sites of the CDC or the American Lung Association can keep the clinician informed about the risks associated with smoking and provide the necessary information to respond to individual questions and needs of particular clients.

Smoking as a Learned Behavior

Smoking is a habit that is reinforced many times. Nicotine is positively reinforcing because it decreases anxiety and increases arousal (Pomerleau &

Pomerleau, 1994). Appreciating the reinforcing pharmacological effects of nicotine helps clients understand the difficulty of trying to quit. Recognizing that these effects dissipate within days of stopping encourages clients to stick with the program. To help clients to understand the strength of their habit, and appreciate the effort required to stop smoking, we ask them to estimate of the number of times they have smoked. To estimate this number, clients multiply the number of cigarettes smoked per day by an average of 10 inhalations per cigarette multiplied by 365 days a year multiplied by the number of years smoked.

Self-Monitoring

Between the first and second sessions, clients record the number of cigarettes that they smoke, the location and circumstances of smoking, their mood, and their level of craving for each cigarette. This process aids in identifying environmental conditions and situations associated with smoking. Research (e.g., Abrams & Wilson, 1977) has shown that the process of self-monitoring itself can result in a reduction of smoking behavior as clients become more cognizant of the circumstances associated with smoking.

Identifying Triggers and Stimulus Control

To increase awareness of smoking triggers, participants make an inventory of when, where, and why they smoke. Common triggers include driving, after eating meals, after drinking their morning cup of coffee, watching TV, while drinking in bars, and in response to negative feelings. Stimulus control refers to manipulating the environment to reduce exposure to stimulus cues that are associated with smoking. Altering morning routines, listening to a different radio station while driving, avoiding smoking sections of restaurants and buildings, rearranging furniture in the TV room, removing ash trays within the home and office, and making other changes to the environment or daily routine can help reduce visual cues that, in the past, might have been associated with smoking. Such changes also alert and remind the client about their desire to achieve smoking abstinence. During the first couple of weeks of treatment, it is especially important for the client to avoid situations and environments (and sometimes certain individuals) typically associated with smoking in the past.

Enhancing Self-Efficacy

Strong motivation is key to successfully achieving smoking cessation (see Perry, Gelfand, & Marcovitch, 1979; Perry & Mullin, 1975). Accordingly, our program emphasizes positive self-predictions and self-efficacy (Bandura, 1982). During hypnosis, we encourage clients to see themselves successfully changing their lives and resisting the urge to smoke. They are also given suggestions to strengthen their resolve to become a nonsmoker. Clients rate their motivation on a scale from 1, *not at all motivated*, to 5, *extremely motivated*. Previous research indicates that ratings of 3 or higher are associated with successful treatment (see Lynn et al., 1993).

Reviewing Reasons-to-Quit Cards

As an assignment, participants write out all of their reasons to quit smoking. During the first session, clients write their top three to five reasons to stop smoking on several wallet-size cards. These cards serve as reminders and can be placed throughout the client's home, car, or office and, during the monitoring phase of the program, inside the plastic cover of their cigarette box. We instruct clients to regularly review their reasons for being a nonsmoker. We instruct participants during hypnosis to imagine themselves writing out all of their reasons to stop smoking on a mental chalkboard.

Anchoring Feelings of Mastery

During hypnosis, clients are encouraged to anchor feelings of calm, comfort, and confidence by bringing a finger and thumb together to create a circle. They are told that they can use their anchor anytime, anywhere, pairing it with slow deep breaths, to discretely remind themselves of their commitment to health. The repeated pairing of a physical anchor with subjective feelings of well-being, confidence, and relaxation can lead to a conditioned calming effect that reduces stress and helps manage the urge to smoke.

Self-Reinforcement (Contingency Management)

Contingency management and the use of rewards to sustain new or desired behavior are significant components of behavior modification protocols (Masters, Burish, Hollon, & Rimm, 1987). Determining what stimuli are reinforcing is key (Becker, 1971; Skinner, 1966). Clients often suggest that they can reinforce nonsmoking by paying themselves money, perhaps the money they would have spent on cigarettes. If money is used as a reward for not smoking, we encourage clients to develop a detailed plan regarding how much they will earn, when they will reward themselves, and how they will spend the money. For example, if a client's reward is to purchase a new television or iPod, we encourage them to place pictures of these products throughout their home or workplace to remind them of their incentive. Of course, stimuli other than money can be used as self-rewards too (see Green, 1998). Clinicians should work with their clients to determine the most effective rewards.

Visualizing Oneself as a Nonsmoker

An essential part of the hypnosis script involves clients visualizing themselves as nonsmoking persons. Clients imagine themselves successfully resisting the urge to smoke in situations in which they smoked in the past. They mentally rehearse requesting the nonsmoking section of a restaurant. Clients imagine themselves being congratulated and publicly applauded for not smoking. During hypnosis, clients are encouraged to proudly say to themselves, "I am a nonsmoker!" to embolden their newfound identity as a nonsmoking individual. Research suggests that the extent to which people can visualize themselves as a nonsmoker predicts long-term abstinence (Tobin, Reynolds, Holroyd, & Creer, 1986).

Social Support

To encourage social support, clients are encouraged to inform their spouses, coworkers, family, neighbors, and friends about their desire to stop smoking. When treating groups, we assign two or three people to a team and ask that members call or e-mail one another to offer support and encouragement (obtaining a commitment to contract with a friend for regular support can be used with individual cases). Such a buddy system can be helpful. For individuals reluctant to participate, there are online (e.g., supportive chat rooms) and telephone-based resources (e.g., The Ohio Tobacco Quitline) available. We instruct clients to complete a behavioral contract that clearly states their goal. As a way to enlist the support of others, clients and cosigners sign the contract. Imagining positive feedback from others as well as actually receiving support and encouragement from others positively reinforces their nonsmoking behavior.

Relapse Prevention and Gain Maintenance

Identifying trigger situations and developing specific plans to constructively respond to these situations are key ingredients of relapse prevention. Because the belief in one's ability to cope in high-risk smoking situations is a predictor of long-term abstinence (see Collettii, Supnick, & Payne, 1985), our clients identify trigger situations, develop coping responses, and mentally rehearse their plans. We discuss the importance of monitoring emotions and managing stress. Although complete smoking abstinence is the ostensible goal of treatment, we recognize that clients do, on occasion, lapse. When this occurs, we encourage clients to redouble their efforts, seek social support, and recommit to living a smoke-free life. In an attempt to dissuade clients from interpreting a smoking lapse as evidence that they have failed and lost all treatment gains, we discuss the maxim, "A lapse does not mean a relapse!"

Nicotine Fading

Between the first and second sessions, participants are encouraged to decrease their smoking by 10% to 15% each day so that they are not smoking at all on the day of the second session. Also, participants may switch brands during this week in an attempt to both reduce the amount of nicotine and tar contained within each cigarette and also to alter the taste and physical cues associated with their preferred brand. Although participants are told that the official quit day is the day of our second session, some clients are motivated to quit on the 1st day of treatment. When a client announces at our first session that they have already stopped smoking (at least for that day), we often try to capitalize on this motivation. We still review all of the first-session materials and use the initial CD; however, we would likely instruct them to begin the second CD the next day.

Reframing and Managing Withdrawal Symptoms (The Winning Edge)

The client's knowledge about the dangers of smoking, the newfound confidence and determination to succeed, the newly developed self-hypnosis skill, the development and use of an anchor, and all of the other strategies, coping skills, and supportive constructs of the program are collectively referred to as *The Winning Edge*. By gradually reducing the amount of nicotine in the body through nicotine fading, withdrawal symptoms are minimized. We discuss the time-limited nature of withdrawal symptoms. Intense cravings to smoke typically dissipate after only a couple of weeks of smoking abstinence. Furthermore, after a couple of months of not smoking, ex-smokers usually report less anxiety and depression compared with when they were smoking. Rehearsing a detailed plan to cope with withdrawal symptoms (e.g., taking a walk, drinking a glass of water, talking with someone, listening to music or their hypnosis CD) and reminding oneself of the time-limited nature of withdrawal symptoms can take the edge off withdrawal symptoms.

Concerns About Weight Gain

Approximately 80% of individuals trying to quit smoking will gain weight (USDHHS, 1990). Results from nonhypnosis studies suggest that women gain more weight following successful smoking cessation than men (see Hall,

Ginsberg, & Jones, 1986; Williamson et al., 1991). Williamson et al. (1991) reported an average weight gain of approximately 9 pounds for women and 6 pounds for men. Only a small percentage of individuals (i.e., less than 5% of those who successfully abstain from smoking) gain more than 20 pounds (USDHHS, 1990). A handful of studies reported an association between gaining weight and successfully quitting smoking following hypnosis-based treatments (e.g., Baer, Carey, & Meminger, 1986; Barabasz, Baer, Sheehan, & Barabasz, 1986; Javel, 1980; Sheehan & Surman, 1982).

Given the similarity of findings across nonhypnosis and hypnosis approaches, mild weight gain should be an anticipated outcome of successful treatment. It is also worth noting, however, that many clients succeed in treatment without gaining an appreciable amount of weight. Because weight gain is associated with relapse risk (see Perkins, Epstein, & Pastor, 1990), a thorough discussion of the possibility that mild weight gain may be a trade-off for successful treatment is warranted. The addition of a novel weight management program or the initiation of a new and time-consuming exercise program can complicate treatment and undermine the chances of achieving smoking cessation (see Green, 2000). Our program, using a minimal strategy on the basis of the recommendations by Black, Coe, Friesen, and Wurzmann (1984), encourages a well-balanced diet, consuming foods slowly, drinking plenty of water, and engaging in nonstrenuous exercise, such as walking, to improve mood, enhance self-esteem, and to minimize weight gain posttreatment. Embedded within the script to stop smoking are suggestions to "take care of your body," "eat in moderation," and "enjoy exercising to keep the body strong and healthy."

Learning Self-Hypnosis

We introduce hypnosis as *self-hypnosis*, a skill that can be learned and mastered through daily practice. We dispel myths commonly associated with hypnosis (e.g., that one can get "stuck" in hypnosis; that hypnosis involves a loss of will; that hypnotized persons are under the spell of the hypnotist) and inform clients that hypnosis can empower them to accomplish their goals, strengthen their resolve to stop smoking, and enhance their motivation to succeed. We inform clients that there is nothing magical about hypnosis and that hard work is required to achieve smoking abstinence. We stress that the clinician will act as a guide or coach; however, the client's own motivation and effort will ultimately determine success.

During the first session, clients gain valuable experience with hypnosis. They receive suggestions for (a) calmness and releasing tension, along with deepening suggestions; (b) imagining a special place of comfort and safety; (c) visualizing a future (nonsmoking) self; and (d) anchoring feelings of empowerment and confidence. The first script (approximately 15 minutes in length) contains references to successfully resisting urges to smoke, becoming stronger and healthier, and living a smoke-free life. The bulk of the script, however, focuses on relaxation, feeling calm and secure, and visualization exercises to give clients experience with hypnosis and practice in using their imaginative abilities. At the conclusion of the first session, clients receive a copy of the CD for home practice. During the second session, the hypnosis script (approximately 30 minutes long) specifically targets the smoking habit, including urge management and acquiring adaptive behaviors that substitute for smoking. As before, clients are given a copy of the CD and are encouraged to listen to it twice daily.

Description of Second Session

The second session begins with a review of the previous week and a discussion of any difficulties experienced by clients. Regardless of whether participants were successful in completely reducing their smoking consumption to zero, all are invited to participate in the second hypnosis session. With clients who express pessimism about stopping entirely, we inform the group that it often takes more than one attempt to quit smoking forever. Although the stated goal is for everyone in the group to never smoke again, we share the fact that not everyone succeeds at the same rate and time. All participants are invited to crumple up their remaining cigarettes and to throw them (along with other smoking paraphernalia) into a large trashcan. The group claps while each individual completes this ceremony and declares that he or she is a nonsmoker. The following script, used in the second session, is presented to clients as a hypnosis-based intervention to help them achieve their goal of being a nonsmoker the rest of their life.

> Let's begin our work together by having you close your eyes and just relax. That's it, eyes closed and relax. I wonder if you can let yourself relax even more, calm and at ease, relaxed and secure, your mind and body working together, your conscious and your unconscious mind working together for your best good . . . partners . . . partners to protect your health, your well-being, your life, your breath. With each breath, let go of more and more tension, let go of whatever tension you don't need. You don't need it . . . you don't want it . . . you don't have to have it. Let any tension you don't need move out of your body, flow away from you. You don't need it, you can let go of it to feel even more comfortable. Even if your attention wanders, it's alright, but keep coming back to my voice, as I give you helpful suggestions . . . suggestions you can use.
>
> Calm . . . peace . . . at ease . . . serene . . . nothing to bother, nothing to disturb . . . calm . . . relaxed and secure . . . centered . . . feel the strength that is within you, as you let any remaining tension that you don't need,

don't want . . . drain out of you . . . leave you with each breath . . . feel the tension you don't need . . . flow out of your fingertips, out of your toes . . . with you feeling calmer and calmer . . . more and more open to suggestions . . . more and more tuned into your best interests . . . wouldn't it feel good to move even deeper into a wonderful state of mind, of being, imagine a favorite scene, a scene of a special place, your spot, your place, where you feel just right, so centered, so secure.

Don't fall over the edge of sleep, remain awake, yet so deeply relaxed, just on the edge, with me communicating with the deepest levels of your understanding . . . all the while knowing you can tap the strength that you need from inside yourself . . . strength you will discover . . . strength that is within . . . wisdom that is there for you . . . courage that is a part of you . . . strength and courage to be what you can be . . . to do what you need to do . . . to be a nonsmoker as you were for so many years before you first smoked.

Just like you let go of the tension you don't need, you can let go of any and all urges to smoke . . . just let them go . . . if they come back . . . you can just let them go . . . they will pass . . . but you don't even have to think about that now . . . as you are aware of a deepening sense . . . a sense of the strength that is within . . . deep within you . . . discover it . . . it's there . . . now move toward this place in your mind . . . in your imagination . . . in your being . . . this place where you are centered and secure . . . a place where you can return to anytime you wish . . . anytime you want . . . moving and moving and moving . . . flowing and flowing and flowing.

You can change your position anytime you want to make yourself comfortable . . . to go even deeper, go even deeper into your desire to preserve your health to be a nonsmoker . . . your need to free yourself from this habit . . . nothing to bother now . . . nothing to disturb . . . you can do this . . . you can be smoke free . . . you can do this . . . yes . . . learning to do this . . . more and more . . . more and more . . . on so many levels . . . your mind more calm and clear . . . different muscle groups relaxing . . . wouldn't it be nice to relax even more? I wonder which muscles are more relaxed . . . your neck or your eyelids . . . your legs or your arms . . . it doesn't matter for now . . . does it? . . . it really doesn't matter . . . as you approach this place . . . or are you there now . . . I don't really know . . . and is your breathing becoming slower . . . as you relax . . . as you let go . . . or are you feeling heavy or light, floating or heavy . . . or perhaps a relaxed, heavy floating feeling all in one . . . can you feel comfort and security wrapping around you like a blanket that is so comfortable?

Or is your conscious mind wandering while your unconscious mind tunes into the deepest meanings, your deepest desires to be a nonsmoker . . . or are you ready to relax even more. Go deeper now if you like . . . so comfortable and at ease . . . strength is within . . . move toward that place or maybe you are there . . . taking the steps you need . . . learning . . .

to get where you are going . . . to where you want to go . . . notice the words and images that are coming easily and naturally to you . . . healing words and images . . . cleansing words and images . . . freeing words and images . . . perhaps a key phrase is coming to you . . . something you can say any time you want . . . any time you wish . . . a phrase that touches the deepest core of your being . . . a phrase that cushions you . . . supports you. Or, maybe it's an image . . . I don't know . . . you can say this phrase or visualize your image any time you want . . . say it now . . . take a deep breath and say your key phrase to yourself right now. And again . . . breathe in . . . say your key phrase and release. You can use relaxation and your key phrase to anchor your resolve to be a nonsmoker forever.

As you do this, think of all the many reasons you have to stop smoking forever. Imagine a writing board . . . a chalkboard perhaps, or maybe a writing tablet. See it clearly in your mind. Now write down your reasons for quitting . . . list them on the writing board or tablet. And hear your words reading your reasons as you imagine writing them down . . . write why you will stop smoking . . . listen to your voice saying to yourself . . . talking to yourself . . . about why you will stop smoking . . . think of all the benefits . . . all you have to gain . . . health . . . money saved . . . loved ones . . . so many benefits . . . think of even more reasons . . . let them move you deeper and deeper . . . swell your confidence . . . help you as you move toward your goal, your life can mean so much to you . . . so much you have to look forward to. Take a moment and list your reasons to be a nonsmoker for life! [*Pause 30 seconds.*]

Good. And continue to relax. Perhaps your hands feel more relaxed than your feet . . . your breathing so easy . . . perhaps, if you like, you can feel your head moving ever so slightly . . . just a nod to signify a "yes" to your intention to stop smoking, just a little nod, feel your head nod, move up and down ever so slightly, a slight nod to signify yes, yes . . . yes to your intention to stop smoking. Go ahead and gently let your head nod yes. Your unconscious mind communicating with your conscious mind your desire to be free of smoking . . . yes . . . yes . . . yes. Even if you did not feel your head move, just say yes, say yes to yourself, yes to your intention to stop smoking. Now just let your head and body settle into a comfortable resting position and begin to create a sense of yourself, perhaps an image of yourself as a nonsmoker . . . perhaps you see yourself with others . . . or perhaps are you alone . . . feeling a sense that you can say yes, yes to your health . . . say yes to yourself . . . yes . . . take a moment to see yourself as a nonsmoker . . . create this image . . . see it, feel it becoming more and more real to you . . . feel a sense of the strength that is within . . . can you feel it . . . or is it becoming so much a part of you that you do not notice it? See your future self . . . the self you want to be . . . the self that is within you. Take a moment and do this now. [*Pause 30 seconds.*]

So comfortable now . . . your need to smoke . . . any urges to smoke once a part of you are fading . . . they are dissolving . . . detaching from you . . . breaking up . . . like clouds in the wind . . . like clouds on a day that the sun begins to shine through . . . the light . . . the diffuse light . . . the breeze . . . the wind . . . the gentle calm . . . it all helps you to believe that you can be a nonsmoker for life . . . see yourself doing something else in situations in which you smoked in the past . . . now in your past . . . you can resist smoking . . . any urges that come up . . . you can watch them fade . . . fade . . . like clouds in the wind . . . use your key phrase now . . . you know your strength is within . . . see yourself as a nonsmoker . . . it is coming clearer to you . . . the light is illuminating you, your reasons to stop smoking . . . your will . . . your resolve . . . the power is within you . . . you know that smoking is a poison . . . you respect yourself . . . you will protect your body . . . you need your body . . . it needs you . . . your strength . . . your willpower, watch the urge fade should it arise after our session today . . . let it come and feel it go.

Think about what you can do besides smoking . . . so many things . . . your conscious working with your unconscious mind . . . help you to decide what to do . . . you know that you are capable of taking care . . . taking good care . . . of others . . . of yourself . . . get in touch with your kindness . . . your caring . . . direct this toward yourself . . . learn the art of flowing with an urge . . . riding it out . . . observe it . . . breathe it out . . . it leaves your body with each breath . . . let the tension go . . . let the urge go . . . it will pass . . . ride it like a wave . . . it passes . . . go on with your life . . . don't smoke . . . go on with your life . . . don't smoke . . . breathe any urge out . . . observe it, and let it go . . . it will be replaced by something else . . . trust that it will pass . . . remember your commitment to respect your body . . . take care of yourself . . . trust that the urge will pass . . . you are your body's keeper . . . you can do so many things beside smoking . . . any urge passes . . . ride it like a wave . . . a wave that flows into the water and exists no more as it once was . . . let it flow away . . . fade away . . . you ride it out . . . you choose not to smoke . . . you get to know the person you can be as a nonsmoker . . . you do it . . . do it today . . . it is important . . . you do it.

See yourself in social situations . . . notice others supporting you . . . noticing you are not smoking anymore . . . feel their respect for you . . . you are in control . . . you can avoid situations in which you would be likely to smoke . . . you care about yourself . . . you take care of yourself . . . you know what you have to do . . . say yes to this.

Reward yourself for not smoking . . . you are saving money . . . you are preserving your health . . . you are letting urges pass . . . exercise . . . eat in moderation . . . take care of yourself . . . feel pride . . . reward yourself . . . you deserve it . . . how can you do this? Show yourself you can be good to yourself . . . yes . . . see yourself as the person you want to be . . . move toward strength . . . be that person . . . be that person. Take a brief moment and feel the pride, the sense of accomplishment, for achieving your goal. [*Pause 10 seconds.*]

Wouldn't it be nice to feel your senses awakening? As a nonsmoker, your senses will come alive . . . touch . . . smell . . . as a nonsmoker . . .

you begin to taste . . . really taste . . . you smell fresh . . . free of the stench of cigarettes . . . free of their clinging odor . . . fresh . . . beginning to regain your senses . . . becoming aware . . . like a newborn baby . . . before your senses were dulled . . . your body is healing . . . healing . . . able to taste your foods . . . as you chew them slowly . . . with enjoyment . . . eat in moderation . . . not too much . . . exercise . . . if you wish . . . you are a nonsmoker today . . . from this moment on . . . say this to yourself . . . "I am a nonsmoker from this moment on" . . . yes . . . say yes to it . . . yes . . .

Discover this strength that is within you . . . realize what you can do . . . yes . . . capable of so much . . . perhaps now you can absorb this fact— every day of your life you are a nonsmoker . . . you do not smoke when you sleep . . . perhaps for 8 hours a day you did not smoke . . . perhaps more . . . perhaps less . . . you do not feel deprived yet you are not smoking when you sleep . . . your conscious and unconscious mind working together . . . your body relaxed . . . your body healing . . . now when you do not smoke during the day . . . you will heal your body even more . . . you can relax too . . . with what you have learned . . . with what you have learned.

Wouldn't it be so good to feel good . . . really good . . . peace . . . peace and serenity . . . comfort and ease . . . relaxed and healthy . . . even more secure in yourself . . . a sense of feeling worthwhile . . . now, as you experience these feelings, please bring your thumb and forefinger together. Or, if you wish, you may bring your ring finger and thumb together. Use any hand you want. Whatever feels good. Just lightly touch a finger and thumb together . . . make your anchor and feel so good and relax . . . more and more . . . more and more . . . even more confident . . . even better . . . gentle relaxation . . . gentle waves of relaxation . . . flow with a sense of ease . . . secure . . . deep . . . deep . . . relaxed . . . so good . . . so calm . . . at ease . . . yes . . . feel this in your entire body . . . relax even deeper, if you like . . . it is you who creates the feelings . . . so deep . . . you create the feeling . . . your strength . . . your security . . . is within . . . create these feelings . . . make the feelings move and flow together with your need to be a nonsmoker . . . relaxing . . . coping effectively . . . that anchor . . . a symbol of your conscious and unconscious mind working together . . . flowing together to create a new you . . . the you you want to be . . . your mind and body working together . . . to help you control your thoughts and feelings in ways that are productive . . . good for you . . . for your health . . . for your self-respect. Use your anchor anytime you wish. Use your anchor as you practice self- hypnosis, and to relax your body throughout your day. Your anchor is a powerful symbol of peace and serenity, your resolve to be healthy, and your commitment to life.

Go deep into your comfort . . . deep . . . deeper and deeper . . . learning, firming your resolve . . . at ease . . . nothing to bother, nothing to disturb . . . as you go deeper and deeper and deeper, you become more aware of what you are and what you can be . . . how you can use what you have learned . . . how you will help yourself to be a nonsmoker for life . . . a new you . . . see yourself not smoking in situations in the past in which you were tempted to smoke, see yourself substituting healthy behaviors for smoking . . . choosing health and well-being . . . your senses alive . . . proud, in control . . . you can do it . . . you will do it . . . use your key phrase . . . use your anchor . . . find ways to reinforce your sense of accomplishment . . . control what you do and what you do not do . . . you are no longer a slave to smoking . . . yes . . . more in charge of your life . . . say this firmly to yourself. . . . Say to yourself right now, "I am in charge" . . . "I am in control" . . . "my strength is within" . . . "I am a nonsmoker."

The more you practice . . . the more you develop your skills, the better you feel . . . practice early in the morning . . . practice during the day . . . as you do the things you do in your life . . . as you live and learn . . . more and more and more . . . more and more . . . you can program your own mind . . . to be a nonsmoker . . . tune yourself . . . tune your feelings . . . like you would tune a precision instrument . . . use your anchor . . . say your key phrase . . . review your reasons for not smoking . . . if you experience any urges . . . use your lifetime of learnings to focus on your health and well-being and just let the urge fade away . . . it will fade away . . . it will move past you, it will drift away from you, it will dissipate, like clouds in the wind . . . like a ripple of water fading away . . . use your anchor.

Now, as we near the close of today's session, take a deep breath and hold it in for four counts, and then as you slowly exhale, say your key phrase. And, again. As you exhale, use your anchor and say your key phrase. [*Pause 5 seconds*.] And, once again.

Take a moment and enjoy the relaxation of your body. Your conscious and unconscious mind working together. Review all that you have learned. Center your mind on your goal to never smoke again. You can do this. You are a nonsmoker. Take a moment right now . . . use your anchor, and your key phrase. [*Pause 30 seconds*.]

Wonderful. Remember to practice your self-hypnosis on a daily basis. Use everything you have learned, and will continue to learn, to live a happy and healthy life.

I will now count backward from 10 to 1 and you will gradually wake up. You will open your eyes at 2, and you will feel refreshed, alert, and ready for life. 10 . . . 9 . . . 8 . . . 7 . . . 6 . . . 5 . . . 4 . . . 3 . . . 2 . . . 1 (open your eyes, wide awake).[1]

---

[1] From *Essentials of clinical hypnosis: An evidenced-based approach* (pp. 90–95), by S. J. Lynn and I. Kirsch, 2006, Washington, DC: American Psychological Association. Copyright 2006 by the American Psychological Association.

CLINICAL MATERIAL

The following case describes the successful treatment of Oliver with the smoking cessation program.

Oliver is a 34-year-old Caucasian male computer programmer who requested help to stop smoking. He reported smoking for just over a dozen years, averaging about a pack a day. Oliver also chewed tobacco for nearly 4 years prior to commencing his smoking habit. Oliver was well aware of the health risks associated with smoking, and he had tried to stop smoking on at least 10 previous occasions. He reported that his previous cessation attempts were unsuccessful and short-lived with the exception of not smoking for 3 months during military boot camp where smoking was prohibited. When we met for our first session, Oliver stated that he had never been hypnotized before and that he was a "bit skeptical about hypnosis." However, given the lack of lasting results from trying to quit on his own, he was "willing to try anything."

Oliver reported that the birth of his second child served as a clarion call for him to take better care of himself. "What am I doing smoking these things?" he asked himself with increased frequency. Oliver reported that he wanted to stop smoking so that he could live a longer and healthier life with his wife and children. In addition, it was clear from our conversation that Oliver was disappointed that he had not been able to quit on his own. He seemed personally challenged, wanting to prove that he could exert the self-control needed to successfully stop smoking. In spite of his uncertainty about whether hypnosis might be helpful, he presented a highly motivated attitude to succeed.

When we met for the second session, Oliver seemed more optimistic that this attempt to stop smoking would, in fact, be his last. He announced that he was "ready to quit smoking for good." Following the hypnosis session, Oliver reported experiencing "a great deal of relaxation" and that he was able to "see himself clearly" in various settings successfully resisting the urge to smoke. He also stated that he enjoyed the hypnosis session, and he wondered out loud about whether "this hypnosis thing" might help him deal with stress at work. Another positive sign was the fact that Oliver had publicly announced his plan to stop smoking and actively sought the help and encouragement of his family and friends.

At the 3-month follow-up, Oliver reported that he was completely smoke-free and that he had not lapsed since our last session. He recalled having moderately strong urges to smoke during the first 2 months of treatment but was able to resist them by using his anchor, "slowing himself down," and substituting alternative behaviors. "About 2 months into it," he reported, "I didn't experience strong urges anymore." Oliver maintained his success over time. During a recent conversation nearly 5 years after our work together, Oliver reported that he continued to be smoke-free. He was pleased with his success and reported feeling stronger, both physically and mentally. Reflecting on our protocol, Oliver said, "I liked your program because it was easy to complete and effective."

RESEARCH AND APPRAISAL

Using hypnosis for smoking cessation has generated widely disparate success rates. Early anecdotal reports claimed success rates as high as 94% (Von Dedenroth, 1964). After reviewing 17 mostly clinical studies, Holroyd (1980) reported that more than half of those treated with multiple, individualized sessions consisting of hypnosis, counseling, and supportive therapy were not smoking at 6 months follow-up. In contrast, the success rates from controlled investigations (Barkley, Hastings, & Jackson, 1977; MacHovec & Man, 1978; Pederson, Scrimgeour, & Lefcoe, 1975) yielded considerably lower success rates, in the 0% to 50% range (Holroyd, 1980).

Viswesvaran and Schmidt (1992) meta-analyzed 633 smoking cessation studies, including 48 trials involving hypnosis. Hypnosis fared better than comparison treatments (e.g., nicotine chewing gum, smoke aversion, 5-day plans) and secured an overall success rate of 36%. Requiring randomized controlled trials and follow-up periods of at least 6 months duration, Law and Tang's (1995) analysis of 10 studies found that hypnosis was effective with 23% of participants. Law and Tang concluded that the effect for hypnosis is unproved, however, because the trials relied solely on verbal report without biochemical confirmation. A recent study (Abbot, Stead, White, & Barnes, 2008) echoed the same criticism, citing the paucity of experimentally sound investigations.

Green and Lynn (2000) examined 59 smoking cessation studies and concluded that, as judged against Chambless and Hollon's (1998) criteria for evaluating the empirical support of diverse psychotherapies, hypnosis was a "possibly efficacious" treatment. More specifically, hypnotic interventions were more effective than no-treatment or wait-list control conditions. However, hypnosis was not necessarily superior to alternative treatments (e.g., rapid smoking), and the evidence concerning whether hypnosis was superior to a placebo was mixed (Green & Lynn, 2000). Unfortunately, the evidence to date presents an ambiguous picture. It is unclear, for example, whether hypnosis per se is responsible for the treatment gains or whether hypnosis is superior to other treatments. The lack of experimental controls and the failure to obtain biochemical confirmation of verbal reports continue to provide fodder for critics. Nevertheless, hypnosis procedures are brief, safe, cost-effective, and appear to be a viable entry-level treatment for smoking.

Researchers are beginning to address some of the limitations of earlier studies. For example, Gary Elkins and colleagues recently reported the results of a prospective study comparing hypnotherapy and supportive counseling with wait-list controls (Elkins, Marcus, Bates, & Rajab, 2006). Participants were randomly assigned to a condition and smoking status was confirmed by means of a respiratory-based measure of carbon monoxide. Whereas the authors used a standardized treatment script, they included a couple of individually tailored suggestions (e.g., to imagine being in a favorite place, to foresee the personal benefits of not smoking). At 6 months follow-up, 40% of the treated patients were still not smoking. This result is encouraging and warrants a larger scale investigation across multiple treatment sites.

Research suggests that there is a need to tailor smoking cessation treatments to specific populations. According to the 1998 National Health Institute Survey of U.S. adults, 50.9% of men and 46.1% of women who had ever smoked had quit (USDHHS, 2001). Within the nonhypnosis literature, there is evidence that women may have a more difficult time stopping smoking relative to men (Escobedo & Peddicord, 1996; Fiore et al., 1994; Perkins, 1999; Wetter et al., 1994), although the magnitude of this difference has been debated (see USDHHS, 1980).

To examine whether gender influences smoking cessation outcome across hypnosis-based treatments, Green, Lynn, and Montgomery (2006, 2008) performed two meta-analyses with overlapping data sets. Across both analyses, we found an average success rate of 31% for males and 23% for females. Meta-analyses of the larger data set, consisting of 24 reports, obtained a small but significant mean effect size of .25, indicating that the odds for successful treatment were 1.29 times greater for males than females (Green, Lynn, & Montgomery, 2008). These results suggest that there may be a link between gender and outcome across hypnosis-based treatments for smoking cessation. Although the magnitude of this potential gender-based effect should not dissuade women from seeking hypnosis-based treatments for smoking cessation, our findings should alert clinicians to carefully consider gender-related variables and concerns that might impact outcome.

Clinicians should attend to a number of findings from the nonhypnosis literature on smoking cessation. For example, smokers are 4 times as likely to experience depression as nonsmokers (Glassman et al., 1988), women are twice as likely to be depressed than are men (Blazer, Kessler, McGonagle, & Swartz, 1994), being female is a risk factor for depression during nicotine withdrawal (Brandon & Baker, 1991), and acute menstrual distress negatively predicts smoking cessation outcome (Pomerleau, 1996). In addition to working with clients to help them manage their negative affect, clinicians should carefully consider the benefits of using antidepressant medication with patients who are vulnerable to negative mood states (see Green, 2000).

Within the hypnosis literature on smoking cessation, gender differences have been reported across a few important variables. For example, women tend to be more fearful of gaining weight (Johnson & Karkut, 1994), and women actually gain more weight than men during cessation attempts (Barabasz et al., 1986). Clinicians should assess their clients' concerns about weight gain and be willing to tailor their approach when working with individuals who are especially fearful of gaining weight or who are particularly sensitive about gaining a few pounds.

CONCLUSION

Hypnosis continues to be a widely popular and effective means of stopping smoking. Examining the current state of evidence, hypnosis-based interventions appear to fare as well as most other nonhypnotic interventions. However, hypnosis as a treatment modality historically has been, and will continue to be, criticized because of the general absence of experimental controls, randomized trials, and biochemical verification of reports of abstinence. These limitations notwithstanding, hypnosis holds much promise as a cost-effective and viable treatment for smoking cessation. Although researchers struggle to isolate and examine the plethora of treatment variables and individual characteristics that can impact outcome, clinicians enthusiastically navigate through this morass of uncertainty and report great success. In this chapter, I illustrated the successful application of our two-session, hypnosis-based treatment for smoking cessation. It is hoped that in the near future, well-designed and well-controlled studies on the effectiveness of hypnosis-based treatments will compliment these encouraging anecdotal reports.

REFERENCES

Abbot, N. C., Stead, L. F., White, A. R., & Barnes, J. (2008). Hypnotherapy for smoking cessation (Article Number CD001008. DOI: 10.1002/14651858). *Cochrane Database of Systematic Reviews, 2*. Retrieved March 6, 2008 from http://www.Cochrane.org/reviews/ /es/ab001008.html

Abrams, D. B., & Wilson, G. T. (1977). Self-monitoring and reactivity in the modification of cigarette smoking. *Journal of Consulting and Clinical Psychology, 47*, 243–251.

Baer, L., Carey, R. J., & Meminger, S. R. (1986). Hypnosis for smoking cessation: A clinical follow-up. *International Journal of Psychosomatics, 33*, 13–16.

Bandura, A. (1982). Self-efficacy: Toward a unifying theory of behavioral change. *Psychological Review, 84*, 191–255.

Barabasz, A. F., Baer, L., Sheehan, D., & Barabasz, M. (1986). A 3-year follow-up of hypnosis and restricted environmental stimulation therapy for smoking. *International Journal of Clinical and Experimental Hypnosis, 34*, 169–181.

Barkley, R. A., Hastings, J. E., and Jackson, T. L. (1977). The effects of rapid smoking and hypnosis in the treatment of smoking behavior. *International Journal of Clinical and Experimental Hypnosis, 25*, 7–17.

Becker, W.C. (1971). *Parents are teachers*. Champaign, IL: Research Press.

Black, D. R., Coe, W. C., Friesen, J. G., & Wurzmann, A. G. (1984). Minimal interventions for weight control: A cost-effective alternative. *Journal of Addictive Behaviors, 9*, 279–285.

Blazer, D., Kessler, R., McGonagle, K., & Swartz, M. S. (1994). The prevalence and distribution of major depression in a national community sample: The National Comorbidity Survey. *American Journal of Psychiatry, 151*, 979–986.

Brandon, T. H., & Baker, T. B. (1991). The Smoking Consequences Questionnaire: The subjective expected utility of smoking in college students. *Psychological Assessment, 3*, 484–491.

Centers for Disease Control and Prevention. (2004, May 28). Cigarette smoking among adults—United States 2002. *Morbidity and Mortality Weekly, 53*, 427–431.

Chambless, D. L., & Hollon, S. D. (1998). Defining empirically supported therapies. *Journal of Consulting and Clinical Psychology, 66*, 7–18.

Collettii, G., Supnick, J. A., & Payne, T. (1985). The Smoking Self-Efficacy Questionnaire (SSEQ): Preliminary scale development and validation. *Behavioral Assessment, 7*, 249–260.

Elkins, G., Marcus, J., Bates, J., & Rajab, M. H. (2006). Intensive hypnotherapy for smoking cessation: A prospective study. *International Journal of Clinical and Experimental Hypnosis, 54*, 303–315.

Escobedo, L. G., & Peddicord, J. P. (1996). Smoking prevalence in U.S. birth cohorts: The influence of gender and education. *American Journal of Public Health, 86*, 231–236.

Fiore, M. C., Kenford, S. L., Jorenby, D. E., Wetter, D. W., Smith, S. S., & Baker, T. B. (1994). Two studies of the clinical effectiveness of the nicotine patch with different counseling treatments. *Chest, 105*, 524–533.

Glassman, A., Stetner, F., Walsh, B., Raizman, P. S., Fleiss, J. L., Cooper, T. B., et al. (1988). Heavy smokers, smoking cessation, and clonidine: Results of a double-blind randomized trial. *JAMA, 259*, 2863–2866.

Green, J. P. (1996). Cognitive–behavioral hypnotherapy for smoking cessation: A case study in a group setting. In S. J. Lynn, I. Kirsch, & J. W. Rhue (Eds.),

Casebook of clinical hypnosis (pp. 223–248). Washington, DC: American Psychological Association.

Green, J. P. (1998). Hypnosis and the treatment of smoking cessation and weight loss. In I. Kirsch, A. Capafons, E. Cardeña-Buelna, & S. Amigó (Eds.), *Clinical hypnosis and self-regulation: Cognitive–behavioral perspectives* (pp. 249–276). Washington, DC: American Psychological Association.

Green, J. P. (2000). Treating women who smoke: The benefits of using hypnosis. In L. M. Hornyak & J. P. Green (Eds.), *Healing from within: The use of hypnosis in women's health care* (pp. 91–117). Washington, DC: American Psychological Association.

Green, J. P., & Lynn, S. J. (2000). Hypnosis and suggestion-based approaches to smoking cessation: An examination of the evidence. *International Journal of Clinical and Experimental Hypnosis, 48,* 195–224.

Green, J. P., Lynn, S. J., & Montgomery, G. H. (2006). A meta-analysis of gender, smoking cessation, and hypnosis: A brief communication. *International Journal of Clinical and Experimental Hypnosis, 54,* 224–233.

Green, J. P., Lynn, S. J., & Montgomery, G. H. (2008). Gender-related differences in hypnosis-based treatments for smoking: A follow-up meta-analysis. *American Journal of Clinical Hypnosis, 50,* 259–271.

Hall, S., Ginsberg, D., & Jones, R. (1986). Smoking cessation and weight gain. *Journal of Consulting and Clinical Psychology, 54,* 342–346.

Holroyd, J. (1980). Hypnosis treatment for smoking: An evaluative review. *International Journal of Clinical and Experimental Hypnosis, 28,* 341–357.

Javel, A. F. (1980). One-session hypnotherapy for smoking: A controlled study. *Psychological Reports, 46,* 895–899.

Johnson, D. L., & Karkut, R. T. (1994). Performance by gender in a stop-smoking program combining hypnosis and aversion. *Psychological Reports, 75,* 851–857.

Law, M., & Tang, J. L. (1995). An analysis of the effectiveness of interventions intended to help people stop smoking. *Archives of Internal Medicine, 155,* 1933–1941.

Lynn, S. J., & Kirsch, I. (2006). *Essentials of clinical hypnosis: An evidenced-based approach.* Washington, DC: American Psychological Association.

Lynn, S. J., Neufeld, V., & Rhue, J. W. (1992). *A cognitive–behavioral hypnosis smoking cessation program: Treatment manual and procedures.* Unpublished manuscript, Ohio University, Athens.

Lynn, S. J., Neufeld, V., Rhue, J. W., & Matorin, A. (1993). Hypnosis and smoking cessation: A cognitive behavioral treatment. In J. W. Rhue, S. J. Lynn, & I. Kirsch (Eds.), *Handbook of clinical hypnosis* (pp. 555–585). Washington, DC: American Psychological Association.

MacHovec, F. J., & Man, S. C. (1978). Acupuncture and hypnosis compared: Fifty-eight cases. *The American Journal of Clinical Hypnosis, 21,* 45–47.

Masters, J. C., Burish, T. G., Hollon, S. D., & Rimm, D. C. (1987). *Behavior therapy: Techniques and empirical findings* (3rd ed.). San Diego, CA: Harcourt Brace Jovanovich.

Neufeld, V., & Lynn, S. J. (1988). A single-session group self-hypnosis smoking cessation: A brief communication. *International Journal of Clinical and Experimental Hypnosis, 36,* 75–79.

Pederson, L. L., Scrimgeour, W. G., & Lefcoe, N. M. (1975). Comparison of hypnosis plus counseling, counseling alone, and hypnosis alone in a community service smoking withdrawal program. *Journal of Consulting and Clinical Psychology, 43,* 920.

Perkins, K. A. (1999). Nicotine discrimination in men and women. *Pharmacology Biochemistry and Behavior, 64,* 295–299.

Perkins, K. A., Epstein, L. H., & Pastor, S. (1990). Changes in energy balance following smoking cessation and resumption of smoking in women. *Journal of Consulting and Clinical Psychology, 58,* 121–125.

Perry, C., Gelfand, R., & Marcovitch, P. (1979). The relevance of hypnotic susceptibility in the clinical context. *Journal of Abnormal Psychology, 88,* 592–603.

Perry, C., & Mullen, G. (1975). The effects of hypnotic susceptibility on reducing smoking behavior treated by a hypnotic technique. *Journal of Clinical Psychology, 31,* 498–505.

Pomerleau, C. S. (1996). Smoking and nicotine replacement treatment issues specific to women. *American Journal of Health Behavior, 20,* 291–299.

Pomerleau, C. S., & Pomerleau, O. F. (1994). Gender differences in frequency of smoking withdrawal symptoms. *Annals of Behavioral Medicine, 16*(Suppl.), S118.

Sheehan, D. V., & Surman, O. S. (1982). Follow-up study of hypnotherapy for smoking. *Journal of the American Society of Psychosomatic Dentistry and Medicine, 29,* 6–16.

Skinner, B. F. (1966). Operant behavior. In W. K. Honig (Ed.), *Operant behavior: Areas of research and application* (pp. 12–32). New York: Appleton-Century-Crofts.

Tobin, D. L., Reynolds, R. V. C., Holroyd, K. A., & Creer, T. L. (1986). Self-management and social learning theory. In K. A. Holroyd & T. L. Creer (Eds.), *Self-management of chronic disease: Handbook of clinical interventions and research.* Orlando, FL: Academic Press.

U.S. Department of Health and Human Services. (1980). *The health consequences of smoking for women: A report of the surgeon general.* Washington, DC: U.S. Government Printing Office.

U.S. Department of Health and Human Services. (1990). *The health benefits of smoking cessation: A report of the surgeon general* (DHHS Publication No. [CDC] 90–8416). Atlanta, GA: U.S. Department of Health and Human Services.

U.S. Department of Health and Human Services. (2001). *Women and smoking: A report of the surgeon general.* Rockville, MD: U.S. Department of Health and Human Services.

U.S. Department of Health and Human Services. (2004). *The health consequences of smoking: A report of the surgeon general.* Atlanta, GA: Department of Health and Human Services.

Viswesvaran, C., & Schmidt, F. (1992). A meta-analytic comparison of the effectiveness of smoking cessation methods. *Journal of Applied Psychology, 77,* 554–561.

Von Dedenroth, T. E. A. (1964). The use of hypnosis with "tobaccomaniacs." *American Journal of Clinical Hypnosis, 12,* 230–238.

Wetter, D. W., Smith, S. S., Kenford, S. L., Jorenby, D. E., Fiore, M. C., Hurt, R. D., et al. (1994). Smoking outcome expectancies: Factor structure, predictive validity, and discriminant validity. *Journal of Abnormal Psychology, 103,* 801–811.

Williamson, D. F., Madans, J., Anda, R. F., Kleinman, J. C., Giovino, G. A., & Byers, T. (1991). Smoking cessation and severity of weight gain in a national cohort. *The New England Journal of Medicine, 324,* 739–745.

25

HYPNOSIS FOR MEDICALLY UNEXPLAINED SYMPTOMS AND SOMATOFORM DISORDERS

MICHAEL N. HALLQUIST, AMANDA DEMING, ABIGAIL MATTHEWS, AND JOHN F. CHAVES

Approximately one third of patients in primary care settings present with physical symptoms that cannot be attributed to an identifiable medical cause (Barsky & Borus, 1995; Faravelli et al., 1997; Kroenke & Mangelsdorff, 1989). When severe, such medically unexplained symptoms may be sufficient to qualify for a *somatoform disorder* diagnosis, a class of psychiatric disorders that describes patients with long-standing and impairing physical symptoms that defy medical explanation and are assumed to be due to psychological factors. Several studies have estimated the prevalence of somatoform disorders among primary care patients in the range of 15% to 25% (Arnold, de Waal, Eekhof, & van Hemert, 2006; Faravelli et al., 1997; Toft et al., 2005). Medically unexplained symptoms and somatoform disorders have often been presumed to be related to *somatization*, which describes "a tendency to experience and communicate somatic distress and symptoms unaccounted for by pathological findings, to attribute them to physical illness, and to seek medical help for them" (Lipowski, 1988, p. 1359). As described in more detail later, however, recent conceptualizations make more explicit assertions about

---

All clinical material has been disguised to protect patient confidentiality.

the conversion of psychological difficulties into physical symptoms (e.g., Brown, 2004).

In this chapter, we review the different types of somatoform disorders, describe challenges in diagnosing and treating somatoform disorders, and provide a historical overview and theoretical rationale for using hypnosis to treat such disorders. The case we present illustrates how hypnosis can be used as an adjunct to cognitive–behavioral treatment of a woman who presented with multiple physical complaints, some of which defied medical explanation. The research we review suggests that hypnosis can be a cost-effective ancillary treatment for somatoform disorders.

DESCRIBING SOMATOFORM DISORDERS

The *Diagnostic and Statistical Manual of Mental Disorders* (4th ed.; American Psychiatric Association, 1994) describes six somatoform disorders that reflect the severity and breadth of medically unexplained symptoms. *Somatization disorder* is characterized by long-standing polysymptomatic somatic complaints, including pain, gastrointestinal, sexual, and pseudoneurological symptoms. *Undifferentiated somatoform disorder* represents a less severe form of somatization disorder and is defined by at least one physical complaint (e.g., numbness) that defies adequate medical explanation and is present for at least 6 months. *Pain disorder* is defined by the presence of clinically significant pain that cannot be attributed to medical causes. Unexplained neurological symptoms, such as paralysis, impaired balance, double vision, blindness, and seizures, are the hallmark of *conversion disorder*. *Hypochondriasis* is characterized by a preoccupation with fears of having an undiagnosed disease or conviction that one has a serious disease, based on the misinterpretation of bodily symptoms. Last, *somatoform disorder not otherwise specified* is a diagnostic catchall entity that is used when clinically significant medically unexplained symptoms are present, but criteria are not met for another somatoform disorder.

The diagnostic validity of somatoform disorders has been called into question because of the lack of clear, observable criteria used to identify these disorders (Looper & Kirmayer, 2002). Rather, somatoform disorders are typically diagnosed after medical assessment fails to identify an organic condition that adequately accounts for somatic symptoms. Thus, the presumed causal effect of psychological processes on medically unexplained symptoms is inferred rather than observed (Looper & Kirmayer, 2002). In cases in which psychological processes play a central role in the manifestation of physical symptoms though the patient remains convinced of a medical disorder, several medical diagnostic procedures are often conducted with equivocal results (Benjamin & Eminson, 1992). Nevertheless, it is certainly important to complete a thorough medical diagnostic assessment, as additional testing may help to identify the pathophysiology of the symptoms and to inform treatment. For example, patients with hypothyroidism often present with many symptoms of depression, but supplemental thyroid hormone therapy typically alleviates such symptoms (Rack & Makela, 2000).

HYPNOTIC INTERVENTIONS FOR MEDICALLY UNEXPLAINED SYMPTOMS

Despite the frequency with which patients report medically unexplained symptoms, referrals for psychosocial treatment are often met with resistance because many patients view psychological explanations for physical symptoms as invalidating and stigmatizing (Kirmayer, 1988). Many patients prefer not to seek psychological services and are more likely to remain in the medical service system, seeking further medical consultation and even exploratory surgeries, creating a costly burden on the health care system (Brown, 2004; Smith, Monson, & Ray, 1986). As we describe in greater detail later, hypnotic interventions may be useful in the treatment of somatoform disorders and medically unexplained symptoms.

The history of the study of hypnosis, hysteria, and somatoform disorders are closely entwined. The Egyptians were the first to describe the phenomenon of *hysteria*, defining it as a wandering of the uterus to the part of the body afflicted with pain or discomfort. Hysteria was defined by unexplained medical symptoms, such as a feeling of suffocation, paralysis of the limbs, fainting spells, a sudden inability to speak, loss of hearing, and epileptic fits. Paul Briquet (1859) described and classified somatic symptoms, which were increasingly understood as reflecting the dynamic interplay between the mind and the body. This emerging conceptualization was abetted by the work of Jean Charcot (1825–1893), the famous French neurologist, who explored the origins of hysteria in hopes of identifying the long-term course of the disorder. Charcot experimented with hypnosis to treat individuals with hysteria and argued that hypnosis was a type of pathology or illness specific to hysterics (see chap. 2, this volume).

Hypnosis is no longer considered a pathological condition. However, Charcot's efforts were significant insofar as they highlighted the link between mental processes and somatic symptoms, which attracted the attention of Sigmund Freud, who observed Charcot's methods. Breuer and Freud's *Studies in Hysteria* (1895/1974) elucidated the influential concept of *conversion*, the process by which intrapsychic activity, especially repression of psychological conflict, generates symptoms of hysteria as a psychological defense against anxiety.

This perspective, along with Pierre Janet's (1889) dissociation-based account of somatization, paved the groundwork for an early understanding of the psychogenic nature of medically unexplained symptoms (Woolfolk & Allen, 2007). Janet's work was significant because he underscored the automatic, spontaneous nature of hysterical symptoms, rather than viewing them as a deliberate attempt to receive medical attention. He also noted that many hysterical reactions were typified by a narrowing of attention on the body and a failure to integrate unconscious aspects of emotional experience into the larger personality structure (Lynn & Rhue, 1994).

The imprint of Janet's views of dissociation can be seen in Hilgard's (1977, 1986) *neodissociation theory*, which posits that information processing occurs along multiple autonomous yet potentially interconnected paths. A corollary of this perspective is that the psychological determinants of psychogenic symptoms can be dissociated from conscious awareness. Hilgard drew important parallels between hypnosis and dissociative states and noted that hypnotic phenomena, including analgesia, numbness, and paralysis, closely trace symptoms of conversion disorders and hysterical responses. Hilgard argued that because hypnosis itself is a dissociative process, it can be particularly useful in the treatment of hysterical and somatoform conditions.

In a related manner, contemporary biopsychosocial models emphasize the automatic processing of information and dissociations between physical sensations and mental schema, potentially bolstering the rationale for the use of hypnosis. According to Brown (2004), unexplained medical symptoms arise when people misinterpret innocuous bodily sensations as symptoms of medical illness. Brown emphasizes the role of two dissociable attentional systems responsible for the experience of volition and the control of cognitions and behaviors: the *supervisory attentional system* (i.e., a coordinated attention system for planning and willed actions) and the *primary attentional system*, respectively. In essence, medically unexplained symptoms arise when the primary attentional system, which is responsible for (automatically) selecting the focus of attention and constructing a representation of current experience, inappropriately selects sensory information on the basis of bodily representations stored in memory, rather than accurately perceiving the current bodily state. For example, on the basis of past experiences, people may mistakenly conclude that harmless minor aches and pains and ambiguous physical sensations are symptoms of tissue damage or disease.

Such misinterpretations are influenced by numerous sources, including (a) an actual history of illness; (b) prolonged exposure to the illnesses of others (e.g., as in the case of medical students); (c) sociocultural influences, such as media representations of specific illnesses (e.g., excessive thrashing about during a nonepileptic seizure); (d) an attentional bias to focus on bodily sensations that may be a byproduct of physical or sexual trauma; (e) excessive parental concerns about physical health during childhood; and (f) rumination about physical problems (Deary, Chalder, & Sharpe, 2007; Robbins & Kirmayer, 1991). In turn, catastrophic beliefs about illness (e.g., the idea that minor pains are symptoms of serious illness or tissue damage) amplify perceived symptoms and anxiety (Barsky, 1992) and inhibit adequate coping in the face of stressful life circumstances, which perpetuates and potentially exacerbates a maladaptive focus on physical sensations (Deary et al., 2007). Because the faulty constructions of bodily awareness and mistaken interpretations regarding physical symptoms often arise automatically and are dissociated from conscious deliberation or forethought, they are rarely questioned in light of more objective evidence of disease and often resist reassurance by medical professionals.

Brown's theory, and dissociation theory more generally, suggest that hypnosis might be useful in creating more adaptive interpretations related to physical sensations and experiences (e.g., sensations do not indicate illness), helping individuals to consciously understand their catastrophic associations to physical symptoms and sensations. In addition, hypnotic suggestions may help to quell the unconscious generation of symptoms attributable to faulty attentional selection by deconstructing and altering the sensations underlying the symptoms.

CLINICAL APPLICATIONS

Hypnosis can be useful in many aspects of the treatment of patients with medically unexplained symptoms. In addition to using the hypnotic suggestions for symptom remission, hypnosis may be helpful for enhancing the therapeutic alliance and increasing patients' insight into psychological components of their physical symptoms. Five clinical applications are considered below: (a) using hypnosis to build rapport and diffuse stigma, (b) using direct hypnotic suggestions for symptom alleviation, (c) using symptom induction as a means to symptom remission, (d) deconstructing symptoms using hypnosis, and (e) using hypnotic age regression to explore the origin of somatic symptoms.

Using Hypnosis to Build Rapport and to Defuse Stigma

Many patients with medically unexplained symptoms or functional somatic syndromes have repeatedly heard a version of the old adage, "It's all in your head," whether from medical professionals, family, or friends. Such stigmatization of patients experiencing chronic fatigue, debilitating pain, paralysis, or nonepileptic seizures, for example, can be profoundly discouraging (Looper & Kirmayer, 2004). If patients with medically unexplained somatic symptoms could will away their problems, many of them probably would choose to do so. Nevertheless, some patients may report pain-related symptoms in order to receive financial compensation, particularly as related to worker's compensation litigation (Rohling, Binder, & Langhinrichsen-Rohling, 1995). As a result of having their medically unexplained symptoms described as psychological, many patients enter mental health treatment with a grudge toward their physician and with a negative attitude about psychotherapy. Indeed, patients may feel that to demonstrate the validity of their medical symptoms, they must not respond to psychotherapy for fear that remission would indicate a psychological cause.

Similar to Erickson's (1983) utilization approach, which emphasized that the patient's perspective must be accepted and used as the starting point for intervention, hypnosis can be used to ally oneself with patients with medically unexplained symptoms. Hypnosis can facilitate the development of a therapeutic alliance because it emphasizes changing perception and experience without having to "think differently" (e.g., cognitive restructuring), which could threaten perceived symptom validity. Although challenging and reframing catastrophic cognitions about pain are likely important treatment techniques, such techniques may not lend themselves well to early psychotherapy sessions. Rather, initial work with clients with functional somatic syndromes or medically unexplained symptoms should focus closely on developing a therapeutic alliance, which is both a predictor of treatment efficacy and therapy duration (Horvath & Bedi, 2002). Indeed, by steering clear of cognitive restructuring techniques early in therapy (which may be perceived as trying to talk the patient out of her symptoms), therapists can circumvent a polarized discussion in which the patient attempts to convince the therapist that his or her symptoms are entirely medical and the therapist tries to point out possible psychological mechanisms of physical symptoms.

The following is an abridged example of an actual patient treated by Hallquist, which illustrates how hypnosis can be leveraged early in therapy as a technique to help build a therapeutic alliance with this population.

> *Patient:* I really didn't want to come here today. My doctor told me I need to see a psychologist, but he is obviously an idiot. My back hurts because I injured it, not because I am depressed. It has been hurting for 6 months now, ever since I slipped on the ice coming out of the supermarket and whacked my tailbone. My doctor said that the pain should have gone away by now and that there is nothing wrong with my back. He's given me all sorts of tests, like an MRI and a CAT scan, and he says there's no problem, and he said I shouldn't take muscle relaxants or pain killers anymore. But it still hurts, and I have a hard time going to work or playing with my kids sometimes!

Therapist: Help me to understand. It sounds like you injured your back 6 months ago, and you have had a lot of pain since then, the sort of pain that keeps you from living the life you want to live. But what is your understanding of why he wanted you to consult a psychologist?

Patient: He said that psychological problems can cause pain, and he thought that my sadness could be causing my back pain. But I am sad because of the pain, not the other way around! He doesn't believe me. Do you?

Therapist: Well, I certainly believe that you've been in a lot of pain since your injury and that it's getting in the way of your life. I am certainly not here to try to talk you out of your experience. If you say you're in pain, then you're in pain. So, sadness aside for the moment, what if we could work in here on reducing your pain? What if we could help you to get back to playing with your kids?

Patient: Well, of course that would be ideal, but how are you going to help me to do that? I need medical attention—surgery perhaps—to get rid of my pain.

Therapist: I would like to suggest that we focus initially on using hypnosis to help you manage your pain. Hypnosis is a skill that I can teach you that uses guided imagery and suggestions for comfort and relaxation to help you keep your pain at bay. There is a large amount of research behind using hypnosis for pain management. Hypnosis can really help people to use their mind to control pain that's felt in the body.

Patient: How does hypnosis work? I mean, how will this help?

Therapist: Hypnosis works because people find that by focusing in on suggestions for relaxation, by really allowing themselves to focus their attention on deep comfort, they actually begin to experience comfort. See, hypnosis is just a state of deeply focused attention, where you are listening very closely to suggestions I am offering, and listening to those suggestions helps you to feel them. But you always have the option not to listen to any suggestion I make: The choice is yours.

Patient: So, you really think that hypnosis can help me to manage my pain?

Therapist: I definitely do. Many people have had great success using hypnosis to reduce pain. As I said, you're in a lot of pain right now, and I want to be helpful to you. I think that hypnosis can really be a useful skill for you to manage your pain.

Using Direct Hypnotic Suggestions for Symptom Alleviation

Perhaps the most direct hypnotic intervention for medically unexplained symptoms is to use imagery and ideomotor suggestions to reduce the frequency or severity of such symptoms. For example, for patients with symptoms of irritable bowel syndrome (IBS), hypnotic suggestions could be used to suggest relaxation of the abdominal area and cooling of the intestines. Patients with medically unexplained paralysis might benefit from hypnotic suggestions for small muscular twitches or increased sensation in the affected area (Moene, Spinhoven, Hoogduin, & van Dyck, 2003). Using this approach, it is important to develop suggestions that creatively target the particular symptoms presented by the patient. Consider the following example of symptom alleviation suggestions (following a hypnotic induction) for medically unexplained tension headaches related to somatization disorder.

Therapist:	You mentioned earlier, Susan, that you have a nasty headache right now that has been bothering you all day. Now that you are in a comfortable state of hypnosis, I would like you to pay attention to the sensations in your head so that we can bring a greater sense of relaxation and comfort to this area. Please nod your head now if you can still feel the headache, or shake your head if it has gone away. [*Patient nods head.*] Good, so you are in contact with feelings of head ache. Now, while staying completely hypnotized, please tell me just a few words that describe your headache.
Patient:	Pounding, tense, aching; I can feel it right in the front of my forehead.
Therapist:	I would like to offer some suggestions for greater comfort that you can use in the future if you have other headaches. Allow yourself to imagine that your head is a balloon that has been blown up too much and is almost ready to pop. The balloon is too full of air, and there is a lot of tension in that balloon. Feel that tension in your head right now, that throbbing; you may even be able to feel your pulse in your skull. And imagine that you are letting out some air from the balloon so that it's not so tight. With each time you exhale your breath, feel the balloon deflate just a little bit. I wonder how you will notice the tension decreasing ever so slightly right now. It may be barely perceptible at first, but just focus on your breathing and imagine the air being let out of that balloon. Allow yourself to experience as much comfort as you can in your head and neck; notice whether you can release some tension in your shoulders with each breath, even if just a little bit at first.

Using Symptom Induction as a Means to Symptom Remission

For medically unexplained symptoms, particularly those in the conversion disorder realm (e.g., paralysis, numbness), the voluntary induction of similar symptoms may help the patient to control involuntary symptoms (i.e., those perceived as not being under the patient's control). As noted elsewhere in this volume, the similarities between conversion symptoms and hypnotic phenomena have been discussed since the 19th century (Moene et al., 2003). For example, classic hypnotic phenomena include glove anesthesia, suggested limb paralysis, and hypnotic deafness, all of which occur among patients with conversion disorder. One important difference between patients with conversion disorder and hypnotized participants, however, is that the latter view the pseudoneurological symptoms as resulting from the hypnotist's suggestions, and typically, hypnotic participants are not concerned that the symptoms will remain after hypnosis. Conversely, patients with conversion disorder see their symptoms as interminable and outside of their control.

Thus, although the phenomenology of conversion symptoms is often similar for these two groups, there is a fundamental difference in attribution of cause. Although perhaps initially counterintuitive to patients with medically unexplained symptoms, hypnotic suggestions that induce somatic symptoms may help to bring symptoms under patients' control by helping them to discover their capacity to alter sensation through suggestion. Clinically, such an approach may require a bit of salesmanship with patients, particularly when they express concern that the therapist is trying to convince them that their symptoms are all in their head. One way of presenting such an intervention is to tell the patient that you are interested in exploring the details of their somatic experiences, including detailed analysis of sensations (e.g., numbness), appraisals of such sensations, and possible somatosensory amplification (Barsky, 1992) resulting from negative interpretations. Patients often also need reassurance that the effects of hypnotically induced symptoms are temporary.

Symptom induction suggestions should typically closely follow the patient's symptom phenomenology. That is, a patient with left leg paralysis might be encouraged to develop right leg paralysis during hypnosis, whereas a patient with left hand numbness would receive suggestions for right hand numbness. Once a patient is able to voluntarily induce a similar symptom, hypnotic suggestions can begin to target the involuntary symptom. This is illustrated as follows, in an example of a person with right hand paralysis who has successfully established left hand paralysis during hypnosis:

Therapist: So now both of your hands are completely paralyzed, aren't they, Joe?

Patient: Yeah, I can't move either one.

Therapist: Good. Now, this is the third time that you have developed paralysis in your left hand using hypnosis, and you seem to be getting pretty good at making it impossible for that hand to move. And right now, you cannot move either of your hands. But as you've begun to learn, by drawing on your own resources and by listening to my suggestions, you've been able to, bit-by-bit, joint-by-joint, bring movement back into your left hand. This time, however, I would like to suggest that you will experience something a little different. Right now, I would like to suggest that movement will start to come back into both hands. Now, consciously, this may sound impossible, but you can trust your unconscious thoroughly in allowing movement to come back into your hands, even if you don't know exactly what you know that will allow you to do this. So without having to know, see if you can notice any muscles beginning to twitch ever so slightly—whether in your left hand or in your right hand. See if you can become curious which hand will move first: your right hand or your left hand. [*Left hand twitches slightly.*] Good, Joe, that's right, thank your left hand for its twitch, for the movement that is starting to come into both of your hands. And right now, I would like to suggest that you are becoming aware of what you are capable of, even if you don't know it consciously. You have the resources to move your hands and not to move your hands. Just be curious what your hands will do next: your left hand and your right hand.

Note that with this approach, the patient was able to move both hands following additional suggestions for sensations in the hands, small movements, and, eventually, gross movements.

Deconstructing Symptoms Using Hypnosis: Extending Erickson's Approach to Pain Control

For some patients, direct suggestions for increased comfort and decreased pain (as outlined previously) may be sufficient to satisfactorily control pain, and such suggestions may serve as a first line of treatment. However, other patients may not respond to straightforward intervention, particularly when their symptoms are related to underlying psychological problems or are of long-standing duration. Indeed, hypnotic interventions for chronic pain are often less effective than those that target more acute pain, possibly because chronic pain often co-occurs with psychological disorders, maladaptive beliefs about pain, and somatosensory amplification, aspects of chronic pain that many hypnotic treatments have failed to address (Patterson & Jensen, 2003).

Erickson (1983, Part IV) wrote an outstanding monograph on the use of hypnosis for pain control that contains many rich clinical insights and techniques relevant to the treatment of somatoform symptoms. Erickson suggested that therapists conduct a rather detailed analysis of each patient's somatic symptoms, including the location, duration, intensity, and character of uncomfortable sensations. From such an analysis, the therapist may begin to deconstruct the somatic experience and to target each element. This approach may also communicate that the clinician is quite interested in understanding the patient's physical difficulties. For example, for a patient with chronic knee pain, a detailed assessment might reveal that the patient experiences burning, throbbing pain in a five-inch radius circumferential to the left kneecap that intensifies when the knee is bent. The throbbing aspect of the pain is essentially present at all times, and its size does not change. At times, especially in the morning, the pain takes on a cold, piercing character, which lasts only a few minutes but causes the patient to sweat with discomfort. In addition, the knee pain has been present for 3 years and has gradually worsened over time despite analgesic medication.

Using information gathered from a detailed assessment of somatic sensations, the clinician may interact with specific aspects of symptoms, and hypnotic suggestions may be most effective when therapists adopt the patient's exact descriptive language. Extending the example provided, the clinician might ask the patient what aspect of the knee pain should be focused on first. Thereafter, the clinician may use creative suggestions to alter specific aspects of a patient's somatic symptoms, essentially embracing a "divide and conquer" strategy whereby successively small portions of the symptom phenomenology are addressed, thereby fostering the expectancy that pain is comprised of many smaller experiences and each of these can be improved in turn.

In terms of specific suggestions to address each component of a particular somatic symptom, Erickson (1983) encouraged clinicians to experiment creatively with a variety of suggestions and to monitor which suggestions were most successful in changing the patient's sensations. For example, if the patient reported a hot, burning pain in his foot, hypnotic suggestions could include (a) reducing the intensity of the heat to a pleasant warmth, (b) trying to shift the pain from one foot to the other, (c) attempting to increase or decrease the radius of pain (e.g., limiting pain to only the big toe), (d) converting the hot pain into a cold pain, or (e) offering a post-hypnotic suggestion for increasing comfort whenever the patient puts weight on his foot. In essence, the idea is that by altering patients' experience of a symptom, they can begin to understand that unpleasant somatic experiences are not immutable and can be brought under their control. In many of his writings (e.g., Haley, 1985), Erickson emphasized that many patients are not aware of what they can do, of what is possible; simply exploring the possibilities for change can bring about positive expectancies for symptom improvement.

Clinicians using such an approach should remember to praise the patients for any changes in sensation that they report during hypnosis. Even if patients report that the radius of sensation is enlarging (e.g., numbness is present in the right arm, not only the hand), therapists may wish to reframe the experience as indicative of the power of the patient's mind to control the size of the sensation. Many patients with long-standing medically unexplained symptoms may express urgency that the symptoms be eliminated entirely. Therapists should proceed cautiously with such requests and may benefit from a careful negotiation of the degree of reduction in symptom intensity required for patients to consider the symptom improved. For example, therapists might ask, "If we could reduce the numbness in your hands by 5%, would you feel that hypnosis had been worthwhile?" This is not to say that large improvements are not possible but rather to call into question the reasonableness of demands for outright symptom remission and to quantify treatment goals.

Using Hypnotic Age Regression to Explore the Origin of Somatic Symptoms

Some patients with medically unexplained symptoms are able to trace the onset of those symptoms to a particular day, time, or event. For example, Brown (2004) described a doctoral student whose writing arm became paralyzed shortly before his dissertation was due. Such symptomatology is consistent with the concept of conversion, whereby physical symptoms serve to reduce anxiety, presumably without conscious awareness of the psychological fear—in this case, the anxiety stemming from the dissertation project. However, many patients cannot identify a distinct occasion for the onset of their symptoms, and hypnosis may be useful in elucidating possible psychological antecedents of somatic symptoms. Hypnotic age regression suggestions may facilitate the treatment of medically unexplained symptoms in three ways: (a) by helping to identify salient experiences associated with the onset of physical symptomatology; (b) by facilitating the expression of painful emotions related to the onset of symptoms; and (c) by developing greater awareness of, and insight into, the psychological correlates of physical symptoms.

Age regression suggestions are unlikely to facilitate memory recovery more than direct questioning, and age regression should not be used to enhance recall (Lynn & Kirsch, 2006; see also chap. 29, this volume). Rather, we view hypnotic age regression suggestions as facilitative of deep introspection about past experiences and the identification of possible psychological factors that relate to symptoms. Although the conversion of psychological concerns into somatic manifestations may underlie some medically unexplained symptoms, it is unlikely that all such symptoms can be traced to a particular trauma or fear, and hypnosis should not be used in a quest to search for "the cause" of such symptoms.

Hypnotic age regression may also help to uncover unexpressed emotions associated with medically unexplained symptoms. For example, hypnotic exploration of a particular experience related to the emergence of somatoform symptomatology may reveal that the patient felt afraid but was unable to express her fear (e.g., during a rape). During hypnosis (or in psychotherapy, more broadly), patients can be encouraged to explore and reexperience difficult events on behalf of facilitating emotional processing, a common feature of many psychological interventions for anxiety and trauma (e.g., prolonged exposure; Foa et al., 1999). When a particular experience is likely associated with the onset or worsening of symptoms, patients may benefit from the therapist suggesting that expressing difficult or suppressed emotions may lead to symptom alleviation (Moene et al., 2003).

CLINICAL MATERIAL

Ann, a patient treated by Hallquist, was a 35-year-old Caucasian woman presenting with widespread severe chronic pain and numbness that began at age 14. At the time of treatment, Ann was diagnosed with fibromyalgia, IBS, paresthesias (i.e., sensations of numbness and tingling on the skin), dysesthesias (i.e., distortions of touch sensations that occur in the absence of tissue damage and include sensations such as burning, itching, and gnawing), and restless leg syndrome. As is common among patients with fibromyalgia, Ann experienced debilitating fatigue and sleep dysregulation. Ann also experienced migraine headaches several times per week, many of which lasted upward of 4 hours, despite medication. Ann reported acute abdominal cramping pain and constipation on a regular basis, which led to her IBS diagnosis. Ann scored a 27 on the Beck Depression Inventory—II (BDI–II; Beck, Steer, & Brown, 1996) at intake, indicating a moderate level of depression. She was particularly saddened about the reduction in routine physical activities (e.g., gardening, cooking, sexual intercourse) because of her level of chronic pain, as well as the distress she experienced related to her paresthesias.

Concomitant with psychotherapy, Ann was under the care of six physicians: a primary care physician, a neurologist, a gastroenterologist, a psychiatrist, an anesthesiologist, and an internist. She was prescribed 13 medications to treat symptoms of her various ailments but reported that these interventions had only been slightly helpful. The client had been on disability for 3 years preceding therapy. Prior to receiving disability compensation, Ann worked at a meat-packing plant, which she described as "backbreaking labor." At the time of treatment, Ann had been married to her second husband for approximately 5 years. She had two children, ages 9 and 11, from her first marriage, and she shared custody with her ex-husband, seeing her children roughly 4 days per week.

Ann identified three goals for treatment in the initial session: (a) to develop a regular sleep schedule and to go to bed mostly free from pain and restless legs; (b) to reduce or eliminate the widespread pain she felt in her body; and (c) to reengage in valued daily activities, including gardening, remodeling, and cooking. Psychotherapy was predominantly cognitive–behavioral in orientation and was informed by the treatment approach of Turk and others (e.g., Turk, 2002). Treatment included cognitive restructuring, identifying catastrophic automatic thoughts associated with pain, attention retraining, and hypnosis. Ann attended psychotherapy with Hallquist for 22 sessions over the course of 6 months. In the interest of relevance to our discussion, the present case example focuses only on how hypnosis was incorporated into her treatment.

At the outset of treatment, Ann was dubious about the value of psychotherapy. Specifically, she repeatedly said that her problems were medical and that only a medical doctor would be able to eliminate her pain and regulate her sleep. Further, Ann routinely expressed intense anger toward her doctors, whom she believed were not spending sufficient time to discover the source of her problems. At the outset of treatment, the client was deeply identified with her medical symptoms and expressed bouts of sadness as "a hormone imbalance" and periods of anxiety as "autonomic arousal."

Given Ann's deep-seated ambivalence about psychotherapy, treatment began with a discussion of how she could use hypnosis to reduce pain. Hypnosis was presented as a tool that Ann could learn and use whenever pain became overwhelming, as well as a skill that could help to calm her restless legs and improve her sleep. Although Ann expressed interest in symptom improvement, she voiced significant concerns about the use of hypnosis, stating that she feared that the therapist would try to take over her mind and that he would implant suggestions that she could not refuse. Consequently, I spent over 40 minutes discussing the procedure with Ann and told her that she would likely be even more aware than usual of her experience and would be free to accept or reject any hypnotic suggestions. I described hypnosis as a procedure in which I would offer suggestions on behalf of her goals and she would focus her attention on these suggestions. Further, I presented hypnosis as a medical intervention that had a neurological basis and cited empirical research that has supported the use of hypnosis in medical settings (e.g., Montgomery, David, Winkel, Silverstein, & Bovbjerg, 2002), as well as possible neurological mechanisms of hypnosis (Rainville, Duncan, Price, Carrier, & Bushnell, 1997). This "medicalized" presentation of hypnosis bolstered

Ann's confidence in the legitimacy of hypnosis and also provided a conceptualization that was congenial to her, given her extensive treatment experiences with medical professionals.

After Ann's concerns were resolved, she expressed optimism that hypnosis could help her to live with less pain and to sleep better. In terms of hypnotic work, in the second session, I began to address Ann's sleep dysregulation. Ann often experienced difficulty falling asleep at night and reported that she felt as though her hormones were keeping her active and awake, as if she had consumed a great deal of coffee. Ann said that she often failed to sleep at night for several consecutive days and experienced persistent fatigue throughout the day. Her insomnia led to frequent daytime naps, which may have perpetuated and exacerbated poor sleep at night. She also reported that her legs were especially restless at night and that her involuntary kicking sometimes woke her. In addition to developing a consistent sleep schedule and good sleep hygiene habits (e.g., only sleeping when tired; see Kryger, Roth, & Dement, 2005, for a full description of sleep hygiene), hypnosis was used to facilitate Ann's ability to relax and become sleepy at night.

Specifically, I asked Ann to identify a recent time when she had felt particularly sleepy and had fallen into a sound, restful sleep. I suggested that we explore what she knew about falling asleep and then use hypnosis to help her transfer this knowledge to evenings when sleep was difficult. Ann recalled a time a few weeks prior when she had been reading a book in the evening while taking a hot bath. After getting out of the bath, she had eaten a couple of cookies while reading in her rocking chair. Ann described feeling tired; that her limbs had felt warm, relaxed, and heavy; and that she had difficulty keeping her eyes open. I asked Ann to explore and describe her experience in great detail, and in so doing, I facilitated her experience of relaxation. As Ann described her experience of feeling sleepy, her eyes began to appear heavy and tired, which I commented on. I suggested that she could close her eyes and just allow herself to feel the warmth in her limbs, to feel the heaviness in her body and to notice her slow, deep breathing.

With her eyes closed, Ann described how she had stumbled from her chair to her bed and fallen into a deep sleep almost immediately. I asked her to slow down time a moment to notice and experience the sensations she felt just before she fell asleep. The hypnotic induction continued as follows:

> Good, Ann. Now I want you to take as much time as you need to notice each little detail: how you feel in your feet or in your toes, notice your breathing, notice the warmth in your body . . . feelings of heaviness . . . I wonder if you can notice whether your right arm feels heavier than your left, or is it the other way around? Just stay in contact with those feelings of sleepiness, of those few moments right before you fall asleep when you feel exactly what you feel, when your breathing is just so, when your body

is positioned just so in whatever position is most comfortable for you, when your hormones are just right and your nervous system is calm . . . in those few moments before you fall into a deep, restful sleep. . . . You sleep all night long so restfully and deeply . . . I wonder whether there are other sensations that you haven't yet considered . . . I wonder whether your unconscious, that part of yourself that has been with you your whole life, noticing, learning, knowing everything you know and perhaps a few things that you have forgotten . . . consciously . . . whether your unconscious can assist you now in connecting with the intention you brought with you to learn how much you know and have already learned and continue to learn about sleeping restfully, completely, and fully.

Without having to know, I wonder how your unconscious will assist you in sleeping restfully and learning all of the ways that are important for you to sleep . . . sleep . . . restfully, with the warmth in your arms and legs, and heaviness . . . your breathing deep and slow. And now, as you're beginning to feel relaxed and comfortable, your autonomic nervous system is winding down, your adrenaline is decreasing. I'd like to suggest that each time you lie down in your bed, you can feel the relaxation, warmth, and comfort you feel right now, that as soon as your head hits the pillow, your unconscious will assist you in developing just the right balance of hormones needed to sleep comfortably. Feel whatever best supports your falling into a deep, restful sleep, sleeping with a comfortable heaviness and calmness in your arms and legs.

Over the course of the following several weeks, Ann listened to a tape of this hypnotic intervention and reported that her sleep quality had improved to a considerable degree, such that she was sleeping through the night about 90% of the time. She said that her feelings of being "keyed up" had largely dissipated, although she continued to experience some involuntary kicking of her legs, which caused her to wake up at times. Nevertheless, the improvements in her sleep quality were associated with moderate improvements in her depressed mood: Her BDI–II score dropped from a 27 to a 20.

In view of her continuing difficulties with symptoms of restless leg syndrome, further hypnotic work focused specifically on the involuntary leg movements, as well as the dysesthesias she experienced in her feet and calves, which included sensations of burning, itching, and gnawing. Hypnotic suggestions focused on progressive muscle relaxation in her legs (involving first tensing the muscles and then relaxing) and increasing tolerance of the urge to move her legs. During hypnosis, I also asked Ann to flex and extend her legs and suggested that with each extension, her sense of comfort and calmness in the legs would increase. I encouraged Ann to reduce the restlessness to the degree that she chose, and many suggestions focused on reducing the severity of leg movements, from strong kicks to small twitches and jerks. Ann reported that suggestions for lessening of large movements and calming of her muscle fibers had reduced the intensity, but not the frequency, of her restless legs. Nevertheless, because the involuntary movements in her legs were smaller, she began to sleep better.

During Sessions 8 and 9, hypnotic treatment focused on reducing the dysesthesias in Ann's legs. Although several different hypnotic suggestions were incorporated in the hypnotic work (e.g., reducing the size of the affected regions and imagining cool water running over her legs), Ann particularly benefited from visualizing herself rubbing a soothing, cool balm on her legs that would relieve discomfort and create sensations of coolness and relaxation. During hypnosis, Ann visualized herself rubbing the cooling, soothing cream on her hands, and then she actively rubbed her legs while visualizing the cream penetrating deep into her muscles and bones. Using these suggestions, Ann was able to greatly reduce the burning and itching sensations in her legs, and these positive effects typically persisted for several hours after the hypnotic work. Indeed, Ann was able to implement these suggestions during self-hypnosis, which she found particularly helpful when her discomfort level was high.

As mentioned previously, Ann was diagnosed with IBS, and she experienced abdominal cramping and constipation. Beginning in Session 10, I used hypnosis to help Ann with her IBS symptoms. Suggestions were adapted from the Albany IBS Treatment Studies, which used a structured hypnotherapy treatment manual (Blanchard, 2000; Galovski & Blanchard, 1999). The focus of IBS-related suggestions was on enhancing feelings of comfort and warmth in the intestines, as well as developing more regular bowel patterns.

> Now that you are feeling more relaxed and calm in a comfortable state of hypnosis, I would like you to turn your attention toward your gut. Just pay attention to any sensations you notice in your stomach or your bowels. If you notice feelings of warmth or coolness, comfort or discomfort, whatever you feel, just notice it. Our minds have a fantastic ability to alter our experiences and our sensations. Perhaps you weren't aware of the sensations in the toes on your right foot, but when you direct your attention there, you become more aware of your experience. I don't know if you've had this experience before, but sometimes when you're really focused on a task, like when you're planting a flower bed, you may not notice when you accidentally scrape your hand on a tool, and it may be only much later that you realize that your hand was bleeding. Without even being aware of it, your mind can change the sensations you experience.
>
> Now, I would like you to place your right hand on your stomach and just let it rest comfortably there. Using the power of your mind but without having to know how it works, I would like to suggest that your hand is beginning to feel a bit warmer. Imagine that energy is flowing into your right hand, warming it, giving you a pleasurable sense of heat, like the feeling you get when you warm your hands by a campfire. If you're beginning to feel warmth in that hand, just nod your head a little bit right now. [*Patient nods.*]

Good, that's it, Ann. Now, I would like to suggest that your hand is heating up a bit more now, very comfortably warm, getting warmer, soothing warmth. And that warmth is starting to move from your hand into your stomach, into your bowels, very gradually. Slowly, just allow your hand to warm your tummy, giving you that warm, comfortable feeling you might get after eating a delicious bowl of chicken soup, warming every muscle, every fiber of your bowels. Your stomach and bowels are lined with smooth muscle that contracts ever so slightly to help move food and liquids through your gastrointestinal system. Unlike the muscles in your legs or fingers, smooth muscle moves without you even thinking about it. Your stomach and bowels can be trusted to digest food comfortably. Notice the soothing feeling in your bowels, the feelings of warmth and comfort. Just nod slowly if you're starting to feel that comfortable warmth in your gut. [*Patient nods.*]

That's great, Ann, you're starting to learn the power of your mind to direct its healing resources where you need them the most. The movement of food in your bowels is controlled by a rhythmic contraction of smooth muscle called peristalsis. . . . Food moves through your system so naturally, rhythmically, regularly. You're starting to learn the skill of hypnosis to bring comfort, warmth, and healing to your gut. . . . Imagine the rhythmic, regular, comfortable movements of your bowels supporting you digesting your food, assisting you without even being aware of it. Continue to feel that warmth in your hand radiating, moving into your stomach and bowels. Even if you don't know how consciously, I would like to suggest that your mind has the strength to bring relaxation and comfort to your bowel habits. You have the inner resources to bring control, strength, and comfort back to your bowels. I would like you to connect right now with a deep intention to soothe your gut and feel your determination to bring your gut under your control. And when you're ready to take your experience of hypnosis even deeper, I would like you to place your left hand on your tummy as well and really let yourself experience the healing warmth in your stomach.

We focused on hypnotic treatment of IBS symptoms for approximately five sessions, after which Ann reported that her constipation had decreased considerably. She stated that she continued to use the hand warming suggestions during self-hypnosis and found this intervention soothing. Ann nevertheless reported that abdominal cramping continued to be problematic, so hypnotic suggestions were developed for muscle relaxation and control of muscle spasms. Ann reported a mild decline in abdominal cramping, but these symptoms continued to trouble her.

In terms of her third goal for treatment, to reengage with daily activities, hypnotic treatment emphasized the utility of maintaining focus on tasks at hand, rather than becoming distracted or upset about pain or other uncomfortable sensations. I encouraged Ann to become absorbed and curious about each activity she engaged in. For example, when she gardened, I encouraged her to notice the feeling of the dirt, to become interested in the appearance of her flowerbed and to enjoy the warmth of the sun. By fostering interest in her environment, I hoped to reduce her preoccupation with somatic symptoms and to minimize negative appraisals of uncomfortable sensations. Ann was particularly distressed by frequent numbness in her hands and the sensation that they were asleep. Neurological evaluation ruled out the possibility of circulation problems, metabolic disorders, or other medical causes for these symptoms. Hypnotic suggestions for these paresthesias focused on increasing sensations in her hands, including warmth, relaxation, and reducing tingling and numbness.

Ann reported moderate reengagement with valued daily activities after three sessions of hypnotic work and psychotherapy that incorporated principles of contextual cognitive–behavioral therapy, which emphasizes acceptance of pain and a focus on goal-oriented activity in the presence of pain (McCracken, 2005). When her pain and fatigue were not severe, Ann experienced enjoyment during gardening, cooking, and remodeling. She replaced all of the baseboards in her living room, which had been a long-standing goal toward which Ann had made little progress. Nevertheless, Ann reported that pain and fatigue greatly curtailed her activities at least twice a week, and further psychological and hypnotic intervention did not succeed in improving her daily functioning.

As can be discerned from the interventions described, hypnosis was a cornerstone of psychological intervention with Ann. After experiencing early improvements in sleep quality using hypnosis, Ann reported considerable motivation for using hypnosis in the treatment of many of her symptoms. Using hypnotic strategies, Ann experienced reductions in paresthesias, dysesthesias, restless legs, pain, and IBS symptoms. One principle to be extracted from this case is that hypnosis should often address the most treatable symptoms first, reserving the most difficult symptoms for later work. Adopting this approach, Ann first improved her sleep quality, which seemed to be an easy target for early intervention. Indeed, hypnosis is commonly associated with relaxation, comfort, and a peaceful state of mind, all of which are typically conducive to sleepiness. By achieving early successes in therapy, the therapist builds the expectation that hypnosis will be a useful tool in treating other symptoms, thereby generating momentum and motivation for further hypnotic work.

Another theme that emerged from this case is the importance of custom tailoring hypnotic suggestions for each patient. With each focus of treatment, I listened carefully to Ann's descriptions of her symptoms and attempted to use her language when developing suggestions for symptom relief and personal growth. Indeed, because of her extensive contact with medical professionals and her degree of disease conviction, Ann's language frequently incorporated medical terminology, such as "esophageal reflux." Consequently, relevant medical terms such as "autonomic nervous system" and "peristalsis" were incorporated for two reasons: (a) to lend weight to the plausibility of hypnosis as a medical intervention and (b) to present suggestions that were consonant with Ann's perspective of her experience.

On termination, Ann's somatic symptoms had remitted considerably, and her quality of life was noticeably improved. Ann's sleep quality had improved, and she rarely had nights of insomnia. Although she continued to experience restlessness and twitching in her legs, the movements were much smaller and did not disturb her sleep. Symptoms of IBS were also improved: Ann said that she experienced constipation approximately once per week, whereas she reported near-daily constipation on intake. Abdominal cramping and pain were also lessened, although she experienced some pain after each meal. Chronic widespread pain related to fibromyalgia was reduced to some degree, although this was not detailed in this chapter. Strategies for pain reduction are covered in more detail in chapter 21 of this volume, and such strategies were used in the present case. Despite the many improvements observed in this case, Ann nevertheless continued to experience considerable fatigue, which limited her ability to complete daily tasks such as grocery shopping and cleaning. She also continued to report a moderate degree of hopelessness about her future, particularly her medical condition. Her BDI–II score on termination was a 10, indicating a mild level of depression.

RESEARCH AND APPRAISAL

As described earlier, hypnosis has been used to treat medically unexplained symptoms for decades. Moreover, Hilgard (1977, 1986) emphasized that medically unexplained symptoms and hypnotically induced somatic symptoms likely share similar dissociative processes, and thus, hypnosis may be particularly useful in treating somatoform disorders. Nevertheless, little empirical research has closely examined the efficacy of hypnosis for such disorders.

Of the syndromes characterized by medically unexplained symptoms, the efficacy of hypnosis has been best-demonstrated and studied for IBS. Hypnosis has emerged as an efficacious, cost-effective treatment for IBS in a number of independent clinical trials (Galovski & Blanchard, 1998; Gonsalkorale, 2006; Gonsalkorale, Houghton, & Whorwell, 2002; Palsson, Turner, & Johnson, 2002). In a recent review of trials using hypnosis for IBS, Whitehead (2006) found that 87% of patients, on average, showed significant improvement in IBS symptoms following hypnosis. Gonsalkorale, Miller, Afzal, and Whorwell

(2003) reported that 81% of patients who initially responded to hypnotherapy for IBS maintained treatment gains several years posttreatment, whereas 19% reported slight increases in IBS symptoms. Moreover, many patients who received hypnotic treatment for IBS previously failed to respond to other medical interventions, indicating that hypnosis may be a potent treatment option that should be routinely considered for patients with IBS.

Four studies (Llaneza-Ramos, 1989; Melis, Rooimans, Spierings, & Hoogduin, 1991; Spanos et al., 1993; ter Kuile et al., 1994) have found positive treatment effects for hypnosis for chronic tension headaches, which may be related to excessive stress. However, Spanos et al. (1993) demonstrated that a placebo group that received "subliminal reconditioning" (in which supposedly headache-reducing words were briefly flashed on the screen) benefited as much as those who learned hypnosis, suggesting that hypnosis may act as a nondeceptive placebo treatment (Kirsch, 1990). Moene et al. (2003) completed a randomized clinical trial in which 44 patients with conversion disorder were randomly assigned either to a hypnosis treatment protocol or a wait-list control condition. Behavioral observation and an interview measure of motor impairment both indicated that patients treated with hypnosis improved significantly over the course of 10 weekly sessions (Moene et al., 2003).

Although relatively little clinical research has been conducted on hypnotherapy as a treatment for fibromyalgia, which is characterized by chronic widespread pain of a medically unknown origin, recent experimental research provides promise that hypnosis may be useful in the treatment of this condition. Patients with fibromyalgia who completed a positron emission tomography scan (which produces a dynamic image of cerebral blood flow) following hypnotic analgesia suggestions reported less pain, and limbic regions involved with emotion and appraisal of experience showed significant alterations during hypnosis (Wik, Fischer, Bragée, Finer, & Fredrikson, 1999). In another study, a single session protocol including hypnotic suggestions for analgesia produced significant pain reductions among patients with fibromyalgia, although the duration of these decreases was not observed (Castel, Pérez, Sala, Padrol, & Rull, 2007).

In summary, several studies have provided preliminary evidence for the efficacy of hypnosis for somatoform disorders and medically unexplained symptoms. Nevertheless, the utility of hypnosis for disorders such as somatization disorder, pain disorder, and hypochondriasis is unknown, as is its efficacy for more isolated symptoms, such as paresthesias or dysesthesias. It is important to note that most of the extant studies of hypnosis for medically unexplained symptoms suffer from many of the problems that affect early treatment trials, such as small sample sizes and failure to compare hypnosis with another bona fide treatment option.

CONCLUSION

The available evidence suggests that hypnosis may be a promising and efficacious treatment for medically unexplained symptoms and somatoform disorders, although supporting empirical literature is limited at this time. Hypnotic interventions may be particularly well suited to the treatment of medically unexplained symptoms for a number of reasons. First, hypnosis and medically unexplained symptoms may be related to the unconscious process of generating sensory representations, which can at times be dissociated from volitional control (Brown, 2004). Hypnotic strategies may promote clients' perceptions of volitional control of their symptoms while also directly altering uncomfortable sensations. Hypnosis lends itself to being presented as a medical intervention, which provides an opportunity to validate clients' symptoms as medical rather than psychological in nature. More broadly, hypnosis is a cost-effective, flexible method that can enhance positive treatment expectances and facilitate the generalization of treatment gains to everyday life. We hope that this chapter inspires further clinical interventions for medically unexplained symptoms and promotes additional hypnosis treatment research on this topic.

REFERENCES

American Psychiatric Association. (1994). *Diagnostic and statistical manual of mental disorders* (4th ed.). Washington, DC: Authors.

Arnold, I. A., de Waal, M. W., Eekhof, J. A., & van Hemert, A. M. (2006). Somatoform disorder in primary care: Course and the need for cognitive–behavioral treatment. *Psychosomatics, 47*, 498–503.

Barsky, A. J. (1992). Amplification, somatization, and the somatoform disorders. *Psychosomatics, 33*, 28–34.

Barsky, A. J., & Borus, J. F. (1995). Somatization and medicalization in the era of managed care. *JAMA, 274*, 1931–1934.

Beck, A. T., Steer, R. A., & Brown, G. K. (1996). *Manual for the Beck Depression Inventory* (2nd ed.). San Antonio, TX: Psychological Corporation.

Benjamin S., & Eminson, D. M. (1992). Abnormal illness behaviour: Childhood experiences and long-term consequences. *International Review of Psychiatry, 4*, 55–70.

Blanchard, E. B. (2000). *Irritable bowel syndrome: Psychosocial assessment and treatment.* Washington, DC: American Psychological Association.

Breuer, J., & Freud, S. (1974). *Studies on hysteria* (J. Strachey & A. Strachey, Trans.). Harmondsworth, England: Penguin. (Original work published in 1895)

Briquet, P. (1859). *Traite clinique et therapeutique de l'hysterie* [Clinical traits and therapy of hysteria]. Paris: Bailliere & Fils.

Brown, R. J. (2004). Psychological mechanism of medically unexplained symptoms: An integrative conceptual model. *Psychological Bulletin, 130,* 793–812.

Castel, A., Pérez, M. Sala, J., Padrol, A., & Rull, M. (2007). Effect of hypnotic suggestion on fibromyalgic pain: Comparison between hypnosis and relaxation. *European Journal of Pain, 11,* 463–468.

Deary, V., Chalder, T., & Sharpe, M. (2007). The cognitive–behavioural model of medically explained symptoms: A theoretical and empirical review. *Clinical Psychology Review, 27,* 781–797.

Erickson, M. H. (1983). Healing in hypnosis: The seminars, workshops, and lectures of Milton H. Erickson: Vol. I (E. L. Rossi, M. O. Ryan, & F. A. Sharp, Eds.). New York: Irvington Publishers.

Faravelli, C., Salvatori, S., Galassi, F., Aiazzi, L., Drei, C., & Cabras, P. (1997). Epidemiology of somatoform disorders: A community survey in Florence. *Social Psychiatry and Psychiatric Epidemiology, 32,* 24–29.

Foa, E. B., Dancu, C. V., Hembree, E. A., Jaycox, L. H., Meadows, E. A., & Street, G. P. (1999). A comparison of exposure therapy, stress inoculation training, and their combination for reducing posttraumatic stress disorder in female assault victims. *Journal of Consulting and Clinical Psychology, 67,* 194–200.

Galovski, T. E., & Blanchard, E. B. (1998). The treatment of irritable bowel syndrome with hypnotherapy. *Applied Psychophysiology and Biofeedback, 23,* 219–232.

Gonsalkorale, W. M. (2006). Gut-directed hypnotherapy: The Manchester approach for treatment of irritable bowel syndrome. *International Journal of Clinical and Experimental Hypnosis, 54,* 27–50.

Gonsalkorale, W. M., Houghton, L. A., & Whorwell, P. J. (2002). Hypnotherapy in irritable bowel syndrome: A large-scale audit of a clinical service with examination of factors influencing responsiveness. *American Journal of Gastroenterology, 97,* 954–961.

Gonsalkorale, W. M., Miller, V., Afzal, A., & Whorwell, P. J. (2003). Long-term benefits of hypnotherapy for irritable bowel syndrome. *Gut, 52,* 1623–1629.

Haley, J. (1985). *Conversations with Milton H. Erickson, M.D.: Vol. I. Changing individuals.* New York: Triangle Press.

Hilgard, E. R. (1977). *Divided consciousness: Multiple controls in human thought and action.* New York: Wiley.

Hilgard, E. R. (1986). *Divided consciousness: Multiple controls in human thought and action* (Rev. ed.). New York: Wiley.

Horvath, A. O., & Bedi, R. P. (2002). The alliance. In J. C. Norcross (Ed.), *Psychotherapy relationships that work* (pp. 37–70). New York: Oxford University Press.

Janet, P. (1889). *L'automatisme psychologigue* [Psychological automatisms]. Paris: Alcan.

Kirmayer, L. J. (1988). Mind and body as metaphors: Hidden values in biomedicine. In M. Lock & D. Gordon (Eds.), *Biomedicine examined* (pp. 57–92). Dordrecht, the Netherlands: Kluwer Academic.

Kirsch, I. (1990). *Changing expectations: A key to effective psychotherapy*. Pacific Grove, CA: Brooks/Cole.

Kroenke, K., & Mangelsdorff, A. D. (1989). Common symptoms in ambulatory care: Incidence, evaluation, therapy, and outcome. *American Journal of Medicine, 86,* 262–266.

Kryger, M. H., Roth, T., & Dement, W. C. (Eds.). (2005). *Principles and practice of sleep medicine* (4th ed.). Philadelphia: Saunders.

Lipowski, Z. J. (1988). Somatization: The concept and its clinical application. *American Journal of Psychiatry, 145,* 1358–1368.

Llaneza-Ramos, M. L. (1989). Hypnotherapy in the treatment of chronic headaches. *Philippine Journal of Psychology, 22,* 17–25.

Looper, K. J., & Kirmayer, L. J. (2002). Behavioral medicine approaches to somatoform disorders. *Journal of Consulting and Clinical Psychology, 70,* 810–827.

Looper, K. J., & Kirmayer, L. J. (2004). Perceived stigma in functional somatic syndromes and comparable medical conditions. *Journal of Psychosomatic Research, 57,* 373–378.

Lynn, S. J., & Kirsch, I. (2006). *Essentials of clinical hypnosis: An evidence-based approach*. Washington, DC: American Psychological Association.

Lynn, S. J., & Rhue, J. W. (1994). *Dissociation: Clinical and theoretical perspectives*. New York: Guilford Press.

McCracken, L. M. (2005). *Contextual cognitive–behavioral therapy for chronic pain*. Seattle, WA: IASP Press.

Melis, P. M. L., Rooimans, W., Spierings, E. L. H., & Hoogduin, C. A. (1991). Treatment of chronic tension-type headache with hypnotherapy: A single-blind time controlled study. *Headache, 31,* 686–689.

Moene, F. C., Spinhoven, P., Hoogduin, K. A. L., & van Dyck, R. (2003). A randomized controlled trial of a hypnosis-based treatment for patients with conversion disorder, motor type. *International Journal of Clinical and Experimental Hypnosis, 51,* 29–50.

Montgomery, G. H., David, D., Winkel, G., Silverstein, J. H., & Bovbjerg, D. H. (2002). The effectiveness of adjunctive hypnosis with surgical patients: A meta-analysis. *Anesthesia and Analgesia, 94,* 1639–1645.

Palsson, O. S., Turner, M. J., Johnson, D. A., Burnett, C. K., & Whitehead, W. E. (2002). Hypnosis treatment for severe irritable bowel syndrome: Investigation of mechanism and effects on symptoms. *Digestive Diseases and Science, 47,* 2605–2614.

Patterson, D. R., & Jensen, M. P. (2003). Hypnosis and clinical pain. *Psychological Bulletin, 129,* 495–521.

Rack, S. K., & Makela, E. H. (2000). Hypothyroidism and depression: A therapeutic challenge. *Annals of Pharmacotherapy, 34,* 1142–1145.

Rainville, P., Duncan, G. H., Price, D. D., Carrier, B., & Bushnell, M. C. (1997, August 15). Pain affect encoded in human anterior cingulate but not somato-sensory cortex. *Science, 277,* 968–970.

Robbins, J. M., & Kirmayer, L. J. (1991). Cognitive and social factors in somatization. In L. J. Kirmayer & J. M. Robbins (Eds.), *Current concepts of somatization: Research and clinical perspectives* (pp. 107–141). Washington, DC: American Psychiatric Press.

Rohling, M. L., Binder, L. M., & Langhinrichsen-Rohling, J. (1995). Money matters: A meta-analytic review of the association between financial compensation and the experience and treatment of chronic pain. *Health Psychology, 14,* 537–547.

Smith, G. R., Monson, R. A., & Ray, D. C. (1986). Patients with multiple unexplained symptoms: Their characteristics, functional health, and health care utilization. *Archives of Internal Medicine, 146,* 69–72.

Spanos, N. P., Liddy, S. J., Scott, H., Garrard, C., Sine, J., Tirabasso, A., et al. (1993). Hypnotic suggestion and placebo for the treatment of chronic headache in a university volunteer sample. *Cognitive Therapy and Research, 17,* 191–205.

ter Kuile, M. M., Spinhoven, P., Linssen, A. C., Zitman, F. G., van Dyck, R., & Rooijmans, H. G. M. (1994). Autogenic training and cognitive self-hypnosis for the treatment of recurrent headaches in three different subject groups. *Pain, 58,* 331–340.

Toft, T., Fink, P., Oernboel, E., Christensen, K. S., Frostholm, L., & Olesen, F. (2005). Mental disorders in primary care: Prevalence and comorbidity among disorders: Results from the Functional Illness in Primary Care (FIP) study. *Psychological Medicine, 35,* 1175–84.

Turk, D. C. (2002). A cognitive–behavioral perspective on treatment of chronic pain patients. In D. C. Turk & R. J. Gatchel (Eds.), *Psychological approaches to pain management: A practitioner's handbook* (2nd ed., pp. 138–158). New York: Guilford Press.

Whitehead, W. E. (2006). Hypnosis for irritable bowel syndrome: The empirical evidence of therapeutic effects. *International Journal of Clinical and Experimental Hypnosis, 54,* 7–20.

Wik, G., Fischer, H., Bragée, B., Finer, B. & Fredrikson, M. (1999). Functional anatomy of hypnotic analgesia: A PET study of patients with fibromyalgia. *European Journal of Pain, 3,* 7–12.

Woolfolk, R. L., & Allen, L. A. (2007). *Treating somatization: A cognitive–behavioral approach.* New York: Guilford Press.

26

HYPNOSIS, EXERCISE, AND SPORT PSYCHOLOGY

AARON J. STEGNER AND WILLIAM P. MORGAN

Hypnosis has gained some notoriety in the realm of sport psychology as an instrument for performance enhancement. However, it is rarely used in this capacity (Liggett, 2000b). The application of hypnosis as a research tool within the more general field of exercise and sport science is also infrequent, despite a number of investigations establishing its usefulness in this area (Eysenck, 1941; Ikai & Steinhaus, 1961; Massey, Johnson, & Kramer, 1961; Morgan, Hirota, Weitz, & Balke, 1976; Morgan, Raven, Drinkwater, & Horvath, 1973). Hypnosis has often been advocated as a method of enhancing mental imagery (Liggett, 2000a; Newmark & Bogacki, 2005), increasing "flow" (Pates, Cummings, & Maynard, 2002; Pates, Oliver, & Maynard, 2001), and reducing precompetition anxiety (Newmark & Bogacki, 2005). However, there is little empirical evidence to support the influence of such strategies or efforts on athletic performance. At the same time, case studies and anecdotal reports of particular athletes who exhibit dramatic improvements in performance following hypnotic suggestion (Johnson, 1961a, 1961b; Morgan, 1980a, 1993) provide some evidence for the use of hypnosis as an ergogenic aid.

All clinical material has been disguised to protect patient confidentiality.

The lack of empirical support notwithstanding, it is remarkable that practitioners in the fields of sports medicine and sport psychology have not used hypnosis more frequently, because the difference between success and failure in competitive sport is often minuscule. It is not unusual in Olympic and international competition for the gold medal winner to be separated from those who failed to qualify for the final event by mere fractions of a second. Accordingly, any ergogenic procedure that might have the ability to enhance performance by even a small margin, providing it is legal, would be of potential value.

There are currently no regulations against the use of hypnosis by sport-governing bodies, such as the World Anti-Doping Agency (WADA), the National Collegiate Athletic Association (NCAA), or professional organizations, such as the American Psychological Association (APA) or the American College of Sports Medicine (ACSM). Nevertheless, it is not difficult to envision circumstances under which the use of hypnosis in the practice of sport psychology or sports medicine would be questionable from both an ethical and moral standpoint. In point of fact, WADA guidelines state that a substance or method is considered a candidate for the prohibited list if it meets any two of the following criteria: (a) It has the potential to enhance athletic performance, (b) it poses a health risk to those who use it, or (c) its use is considered contrary to the "spirit of sport" (WADA, 2003). Even though hypnosis is not explicitly named as a banned practice by any of the previously mentioned associations, its use with athletes in certain situations (e.g., pain management, fear and anxiety control, modulation of cardiovascular responses) could be regarded as an unfair advantage. It is thus imperative that psychologists who use hypnosis to treat athletes become familiar with the ethical and legal guidelines adopted by the APA ("Ethical Principles of Psychologists and Code of Conduct"; see APA, 2002), sport-governing bodies (e.g., NCAA, WADA), and sport science organizations (e.g., ACSM).

Hypnosis can also play an instrumental role in the laboratory. Typically, hypnosis has been used in exercise and sport science research in one of two ways. First, hypnosis can be used effectively to manipulate independent variables in exercise science experiments. Massey et al. (1961), for example, conducted an innovative experiment designed to account for the "psychological variable" of warming-up prior to exercise. Participants completed four bouts of a sprint task on a cycle ergometer under two conditions: (a) exercise testing following warm-up and (b) exercise testing without warm-up. Prior to testing, however, the participants were hypnotized and given a posthypnotic suggestion of amnesia regarding the pretest routine. In other words, the participants were presumably unaware of whether they had warmed up before the exercise test. Sprint times did not differ between the two conditions, and the absence of warm-up was not associated with injury. Related research by Smith and Bozymowski (1965) has shown that physical performance in such a setting is influenced by the participants' attitudes concerning the value and necessity of warm-up.

Second, exercise scientists can use hypnosis to better ascertain the true limits of human performance. Attempts to measure maximal physical performance are limited by inhibitory mechanisms. Furthermore, maximal or "supramaximal" efforts are governed by the extent to which disinhibition of these inhibitory mechanisms can be achieved. Ikai and Steinhaus (1961) demonstrated this phenomenon in a classic experiment that evaluated the influence of hypnotic suggestions, as well as other treatments designed to provoke disinhibition of inhibitory mechanisms (e.g., alcohol, amphetamines, loud noises), on maximal elbow flexion strength. Participants were trained to exert a maximal force against a dynamometer and demonstrated that "maximal" values could be enhanced significantly with each of these procedures. In other words, the researchers determined that the functional maximum obtained under usual testing procedures was actually a pseudomaximum and that participants were able to draw on considerable reserves. Although the effect of hypnosis was superior to the control condition, hypnotic suggestion did not differ significantly from gains observed with the other interventions.

Our examination of the use of hypnosis in exercise and sport settings begins with a selection of clinical cases drawn from the published literature. The application of hypnosis in these cases is based on the assumption that important information from an individual's past is sometimes not consciously available but can be accessed by means of hypnotic age regression. In the case of the competitive athlete, for example, information provided might be used to enhance performance or return to a previous level of performance that can no longer be achieved.

In this chapter, we also review three cases in detail related to the use of hypnosis as a performance enhancement technique. In each of the cases presented, the athlete in question experienced a decrement in performance and contacted, directly or through a referral, the second author (Morgan) to explore the possibility of using hypnosis to resolve the problem. These cases have been selected to highlight critical components of the effective use of hypnotic age regression in attempts to aid an athlete in returning to a previous level of performance. It is our position that efforts to retrieve repressed information should be nondirective, an approach based primarily on clinical reports described by Johnson (1961a, 1961b). In other words, rather than giving direct hypnotic suggestion designed to alter the athlete's biomechanics or competitive strategy, for example, the hypnotist should use a nondirective approach that relies on the athlete's recall and personal insights. In addition, we recommend a multidisciplinary approach that includes medical, physiological, and psychological components. It is our position that expertise in the use of hypnotherapy is necessary but not sufficient. Indeed, we propose that hypnotic applications should not be attempted in exercise and sport settings unless it can be shown that psycho-pathology does not exist and that the requisite physiological capacity is present.

The final section of this chapter provides a general overview of the use of hypnosis in sport and exercise science research. We will delve into some of the conflicting evidence and viewpoints in regard to the influence of hypnosis and hypnotic suggestion on exercise performance in a laboratory setting. This final section concludes with a summary of the findings of hypnosis research in exercise and sport science.

CLINICAL APPLICATIONS

Johnson (1961a) described one of the most widely cited hypnosis cases in sport psychology. A professional baseball player, whose batting average normally exceeded .300, had not had a hit for the last 20 times at bat, and neither he nor his coaches could detect any problems with his swing, stance, and so on. The frustrated player requested hypnosis to resolve the problem. During hypnosis, Johnson asked the player to explain his problem, and the player replied that he had no idea why he was in a slump. Johnson then told the player that he would gradually count from 1 to 10, and with each number, the player would become more and more aware of why he could no longer hit effectively. He also told the player that at the count of 10 he would have complete awareness of why he was in the slump. Johnson reported that at the count of 10, a look of incredulity came across the player's face, and he then provided a detailed analysis of his swing. This self-analysis included elaboration of specific problems that the player never disclosed prior to hypnosis. Johnson asked the player whether he wished to have immediate, conscious recall of his analysis or have the information "just come to him gradually" over time. The player replied that he would prefer to have this information come back to him over time. The player's slump ended at once, and he went on to complete the season with an impressive batting average of .400.

This particular case is instructive in several ways. First, it is widely recognized that athletes in various sports often have spontaneous remission of problems (e.g., "slumps"), and it would be difficult to argue that a hypnotic intervention was responsible for the resolution of a given problem. Second, the information gained in the hypnoanalysis done by Johnson was not available under nonhypnotic conditions. Third, according to Johnson, the player demonstrated unusual insight because he chose to have the wealth of biomechanical information return gradually. Once a complex motor skill has been learned, coaches often encourage athletes to "do it," rather than think about it. The situation is analogous to the problem of *paralysis through analysis,* which occurred when the frog of fable asked the centipede, "Pray tell, which foot do you move first?" As the story goes, the centipede was unable to resume normal locomotion once the question was considered. Fourth, at the completion of the season, the player thanked Johnson and was unable to accept the fact that he, not the hypnotist, had performed the analysis.

Little has been written about the use of psychodynamic approaches involving the use of hypnosis in sport and exercise psychology. However, Johnson (1961b) presented several case studies of performance decrements in sports as a consequence of aggression blockage. In each case, hypnotic age regression was used in an effort to retrieve important, previously unconscious or undisclosed material, which was followed by psychoanalytic interpretation and treatment. Also, posthypnotic suggestion was used to resolve the aggression conflicts. In one case, a cycle of aggression–guilt–aggression that impeded performance was identified. The athlete, a pitcher in baseball, performed well when aggressive affect dominated, but his performance fell when he experienced guilt and lacked aggression. After guilt feelings related to childhood incidents of aggression were identified and resolved, the aggression–guilt–aggression cycle was broken, and the pitcher's performance became more consistent.

Appel (1990) detailed the successful use of hypnosis in facilitating exercise performance in a physical rehabilitation setting. One case he described involved a 26-year-old graduate student who became wheelchair-bound as the result of a motor vehicle accident. For the 3 years since her accident she had been in physical therapy at an outpatient clinic learning to walk with the aid of braces and crutches, but progress in therapy had stalled. Her physical therapist was frustrated and felt that continued treatment would be of no value. According to the therapist, the patient exhibited an intense fear of falling, which was the primary obstacle to her progress. Her physiatrist, who believed that she was capable of learning to walk and that she could benefit from psychological intervention, referred her to Appel, a psychologist. Using age regression, Appel identified the source of the patient's anxiety as a fear of abandonment related to conflicts with, and unacknowledged anger toward, her mother. Following this revelation, the patient showed significant improvements in her physical therapy routines, and her physiatrist and therapist reported that her fear of falling no longer interfered with her rehabilitation.

Hanin (1978) showed that some athletes experience their best performances when precompetition anxiety is low, some when anxiety is high, and some when anxiety is intermediate. This finding is supported by empirical research involving athletes from various sports (Morgan, Brown, Raglin, O'Connor, & Ellickson, 1987; Morgan & Ellickson, 1989; Morgan, O'Connor, Ellickson, & Bradley, 1988; Raglin, 1992; Raglin, Morgan, & Wise, 1990; Raglin & Morris, 1994; Raglin & Turner, 1992, 1993; Turner & Raglin, 1996). Therefore, it would be inappropriate to assume that a single psychological intervention (i.e., to reduce or increase anxiety) would indiscriminately benefit all athletes. In addition, some people experience paradoxical anxiety and panic episodes during and following relaxation interventions (Borkovec et al., 1987; Heide & Borkovec, 1984). However, the mechanisms underlying relaxation-induced anxiety are not well understood.

The concept of a zone of optimal anxiety (ZOA) for athletes is well established (Hanin, 1978; Morgan & Ellickson, 1989; Raglin, 1992). Accordingly, it is imperative that efforts to manipulate precompetition anxiety (up or down) be individually tailored. The difficulty, of course, involves determining an athlete's ZOA. It is necessary to evaluate an athlete's anxiety level before many competitions to arrive at his or her ZOA. Alternatively, one might use hypnotic age regression to ascertain an athlete's anxiety levels before their best, usual, and worst performances. After the person's ZOA is determined, it would then be possible to establish, with autohypnosis or posthypnotic suggestion, a level of precompetition anxiety that falls within the athlete's optimal range. Although this approach is speculative, it is based on a sound theoretical rationale (Hanin, 1978) and on extensive empirical evidence of an indirect nature (Morgan, 1997; Raglin, 1992).

Despite the compelling support for the ZOA theory, sport psychologists are likely to be consulted about problems involving elevations, rather than decreases, in precompetition anxiety. Indeed, some athletes have been reported to be virtually incapacitated before competition, with anxiety attacks preventing customary levels of performance. Although an equal number of athletes may experience inadequately low levels of anxiety, this problem tends to be less apparent. Naruse (1965) presented one of the best discussions of how hypnosis can be used with athletes in the precompetitive setting. Naruse labeled intense anxiety in the precompetitive setting as *stage fright* and summarized the use of (a) direct hypnotic suggestions, (b) posthypnotically produced autohypnosis, and (c) self-hypnosis in conjunction with autogenic training and progressive relaxation in the treatment of anxiety states in athletes.

There are two important points to be made about Naruse's (1965) report. First, the athletes used in his study consisted of elite performers, and the results may not generalize to pre-elite or nonelite athletes. Second, the procedure used with a given athlete was determined on an individual basis. The unique nature of the athlete's stage fright and the individual's personality were considered together in deciding which procedure to use. Naruse's report could be particularly useful to hypnotherapists involved in the treatment of precompetition anxiety in athletes competing at the national or the Olympic level.

Vanek (1970) emphasized that attempts to manipulate anxiety levels before competition must be pursued with caution and that the psychologist should have a complete appreciation for the athlete's psychodynamics. As an example, Vanek described a heavyweight boxer who experienced an anxiety attack before an Olympic contest and then learned to control his anxiety with a nonhypnotic procedure known as the autogenic method (Garvin, Trine, & Morgan, 2001; Schultz & Luthe, 1969). The boxer then lost his match to an opponent he had previously beaten. Vanek reported that follow-up revealed that although the boxer typically experienced anxiety attacks before important competitions, he apparently performed well in this state. In retrospect, Vanek considered anxiety reduction to be inappropriate. This case serves to confirm the ZOA theory and underscores the point that it is inadvisable to use psychological procedures before competition without a careful evaluation.

Garver (1977) described a novel approach to the use of hypnotic control of arousal levels to enhance performance. This method requires that athletes establish a personal arousal scale ranging from 0 (the lowest possible level of arousal an athlete might experience) to 10 (the highest level) during hypnosis. The athlete is moved up and down this arousal scale to experience how different arousal intensities feel. The athlete's optimal level of arousal is defined as the sensations associated with a score of 5 on the scale. An effort is made to have the athlete perceive this optimal intensity level and use it as a posthypnotic cue during competition. Garver described cases of a gymnast and a golfer who experienced performance problems associated with elevated anxiety and anger, respectively. In these cases, posthypnotic cues and cognitive rehearsal were used to produce preferred arousal levels, which led to enhanced performance.

It is imperative that clinical application in any area be based on scientific evidence, but there is little clinical or systematic research on which to base interventions in the field of exercise and sport psychology. Although attempts have been made to apply the experimental literature to clinical settings, the ecological validity of such an approach remains to be demonstrated. In reviewing the case studies we summarize, it should be kept in mind that the applications are based on theoretical formulations rather than research evidence.

CLINICAL MATERIAL

The three cases we present involve individual athletes from the sports of distance running, baseball, and cycling. The first two cases, the distance runner and the baseball player, were first published in Morgan (1993), and the third case, the cyclist, was described in Morgan (2002). The hypnotic approach used relied on insight training through age regression and a nondirective procedure that builds on Johnson's (1961a, 1961b) case reports. Hanin's (1978) and Uneståhl's (1981) theories specify that optimal or ideal affective states characterize peak performance and that information about these ideal states can be recalled through hypnotic (Uneståhl, 1981) and nonhypnotic (Hanin, 1978) methods. In two of the three cases we present, age regression was instrumental in retrieving useful material. A multidisciplinary approach was used in each situation, and these case studies demonstrate that performance decrements in sports are sufficiently complex to rule out simplistic, unidimensional solutions. One of the current authors (Morgan) assumed responsibility in these cases for the hypnotic inductions.

Case 1: Distance Runner

This case represents a common problem in which an athlete is no longer able to perform at his or her customary level. This type of situation is considerably different from the case in which an athlete is performing at a given level and wishes to enhance his or her performance. In other words, the present case involved a situation in which an athlete previously performed at an elite level but was now unable to do so.

The case involved a 21-year-old distance runner who had previously established a school and conference record but was unable to replicate his performance. Indeed, the runner was not able to even complete many of his races, much less dominate a given competition. Problems of this nature are usually diagnosed as "staleness" in the field of sports medicine, and the only effective treatment appears to be rest (Morgan, Brown, et al., 1987). However, this was not the problem in the present case. The runner's ability to perform at his previous level was judged by the coach simply to reflect inadequate motivation and unwillingness to tolerate the distress and discomfort associated with high-level performance. However, the athlete reported that he was willing to do anything to perform at his previous level, and he felt that his principal problem stemmed from inadequate coaching. Although the athlete and the coach were both interested in the restoration of the runner's previous performance ability, they were clearly at odds with one another. Indeed, the conflict had reached the point where the two were unable to discuss the matter, and the runner had turned to his team physician for support. However, a thorough physical examination, including blood and urine chemistries routinely used in sports medicine, failed to reveal any medical problems.

The physician proposed hypnosis to resolve this problem, and the athlete was eager to try such an approach. However, it seemed appropriate to first evaluate the runner's physical capacity to ensure that he was actually capable of performing at the desired level. Because aerobic power is an important factor in successful distance running, the runner was administered a test of maximal aerobic power on a treadmill. This required that he run at a pace of 19.3 km/hour on the treadmill, and the grade was increased by 2% every minute until he could no longer continue. The runner achieved a peak, or maximal $\dot{V}O_2$, of 70 ml/kg·min by the 5th minute of exercise, and his ability to uptake oxygen fell during the 6th minute. In other words, a true physiological maximum, as opposed to a volitional or symptomatic maximum, was achieved. The recorded value of 70 ml/kg·min represents the average reported for elite distance runners (Morgan & Pollock, 1977), and the runner was therefore physiologically capable of achieving the desired performance level. However, our calculations revealed that it would be necessary for him to average 96% of his maximum throughout the event to replicate his record performance. This could potentially be problematic because exercise metabolites such as lactic acid begin to accumulate and to limit performance during prolonged exercise at 60% to 80% of maximum in most trained individuals. In other words, it would have been possible for this runner to perform at the desired level, but such an effort would be associated with considerable discomfort (i.e., pain).

The runner scored within the normal range on anxiety, depression, and neuroticism as measured by the State-Trait Anxiety Inventory (STAI; Spielberger, 1983), Depression Adjective Check List (Lubin, 1967), and Eysenck Personality Inventory (EPI; Eysenck & Eysenck, 1968), respectively. He scored significantly higher than the population norms on extroversion on the EPI, but this is a common finding among athletes (Morgan, 1980b). He was found to be hypnotizable following preliminary induction and deepening sessions, and he was eager to pursue "insight training" through hypnosis and deep relaxation. The runner was viewed as a good candidate for hypnosis for the following reasons: (a) No medical contraindications were detected, (b) he possessed the necessary physiological capacity to achieve success, (c) there were no psychological contraindications, and (d) he was highly hypnotizable.

The athlete was next age-regressed to the day of his championship performance, and he was instructed to describe the competition as well as any related events that he judged to be relevant. However, rather than telling him that "the race was about to begin" or instructing him in the customary "on your marks" command, he was asked to recall all events leading up to the race on that day. He was given the following instructions:

> For example, try to remember how you felt when you awakened that morning; your breakfast or any foods or liquids you consumed; the temperature before and during the race; the nature and condition of the course; interactions with your coach, teammates, and opponents; your general frame of mind, and then proceed to the starting line when you are ready.

The athlete's team physician and second author (Morgan) had previously asked the runner whether it would be acceptable for either or both of them to ask questions during the session, and the athlete had no objections. The athlete had a somewhat serious or pensive look, but within a few minutes he began to smile and chuckle, saying that he had false-started. When asked why this was so amusing, he replied that it was "ridiculous since there is no advantage to a fast start in a distance race." This event can be viewed as a critical incident because runners and swimmers in sprints and middle distance events will intentionally false start at times in an effort to reduce tension. Others will do this in an effort to upset or "unnerve" their opponents. However, as suggested in the runner's comment, this seldom happens in distance events. At any rate, his facial expression became serious once again, and his motor behavior (e.g., grimacing and limb movements) suggested the race had begun. The verbatim narrative follows:

> The pace is really fast. I'm at the front of the pack. I don't think I can hold this pace much longer, but I feel pretty good. The pace is picking up . . . I don't think I can hold it. . . . My side is beginning to ache. . . . I have had a pain in the side many times. It will go away if I continue to press. There . . . it feels good now. The pain is gone, but I'm having trouble breathing. I'm beginning to suck air. . . . The pain is unbearable. . . . I'm going to drop out of the race as soon as I find a soft spot. There's a soft, grassy spot up ahead. I'm going to stop and lay in the soft grassy spot. . . . Wait—I can't—three of my teammates are up on top of the next grade . . . .They are yelling at me to kick. I can't let them down. I will keep going. I'm over the hill now . . . on level grade. . . . It feels okay. . . . I'm all right. There's another hill up ahead. I don't like hills. . . . It is starting to hurt again. . . . I can't keep this up. . . . I'm going to find a soft spot again and stop. There's a spot ahead. . . . I'm going to quit. . . . I'm slowing down. . . . This is it. Wait, there—I see a television set about 10 feet off the ground at the top of the hill. . . . Hey, I'm on the TV, but this race isn't televised . . . but I can see myself clearly on the TV. . . . I'm not here anymore. . . . I'm on the TV. Now there's another TV but to the right of the first one. My parents are on that TV, and they are watching me run this race on the other TV. I can't stop now. I can't let them down. Got to keep going. I'm not here; I'm on TV. It's starting to feel better. I feel like I'm in a vacuum now. I can't feel anything. My feet aren't hitting the ground anymore. . . . I can't feel the wind hitting me. Hey, I'm a Yankee Clipper . . . I'm on the high seas. . . . I'm flying . . . the sails are full . . . the wind is pushing me . . . I'm going to blow out. . . . I'm going to kick. . . . I don't feel pain anymore. . . . This is going to be a PB, maybe a record. I'm flying now. There is no one in sight. This is my race. There's the tape— I'm almost there. The tape hit my chest. It feels weird . . . weird . . . weird . . . the tape feels weird. . . . That's the end . . . the end . . . the end . . . the end.

The runner appeared to be deeply relaxed at this point, and he had previously agreed to answer any questions we might have following his recall of the race. He was asked, "You almost dropped out of the race twice. Why didn't you simply slow your pace? Would that not have been better than quitting?" The runner replied without any hesitation as follows:

Oh, no, you really have to take pride in yourself to quit. You have to be a real man; it takes guts to quit. Anybody can continue and turn in a lousy performance. I have too much pride to do that. I would rather quit.

Although this view can be judged as somewhat unusual, it is noteworthy that he had dropped out of more races than he had completed during the present season.

The runner was asked to clarify the meaning of selected terms or phrases he had used, and then he was asked the following question: "Would you like to have complete recall for all of this information, or would you prefer to forget about it or, perhaps, have it come back to you gradually?" The decision to ask this question was based on the earlier demonstration by Johnson (1961a) that after hypnosis athletes sometimes do not wish to remember material they disclosed during hypnosis. The decision to ask whether he would prefer that this information gradually return was intended to prevent the athlete from becoming overwhelmed or further confused as a result of this previously undisclosed material. At any rate, the runner responded that he would like to have complete recall following the session. Hence, no effort was made to produce posthypnotic amnesia.

The runner was also asked during hypnosis whether he wished to continue with this program of insight training, and he replied that he would like to give this some thought. For this reason, posthypnotic suggestions designed to ensure adherence to future hypnotic sessions were not administered. In other words, posthypnotic suggestions designed to produce amnesia regarding the previously repressed material, as well as motivating instructions designed to ensure continuation, could have been, but were not, administered to the runner.

This case serves to illustrate several points that practitioners in sport psychology or sports medicine might wish to consider prior to using hypnosis with an athlete. First, it is important to initially obtain relevant information concerning the athlete's physiological, psychological, and medical state. Second, the decision to proceed with hypnosis should be made after obvious contraindications (i.e., pathophysiology, psychopathology) have been ruled out. Third, peak performance involving the transcendence of usual or customary levels can be associated with cognitive–perceptual processes of a remarkable nature. The record-setting performance of this athlete was found to be associated with considerable pain, but the runner was unaware of, or at least did not disclose, this pain experience under nonhypnotic conditions. However, the cognitive–perceptual experience was "replayed" during hypnotic age regression, and the runner achieved awareness of this experience following hypnosis. It is possible that conscious awareness of this previously repressed material may have provided the runner with insights he previously lacked. That is, the excruciating pain associated with his earlier record-setting performance had apparently been repressed, and the recall under hypnosis resulted in the runner's awareness of that pain.

The runner subsequently elected to terminate insight training, though this decision was not congruent with his initial statement that he would do anything to return to his previous level of performance. It should be kept in mind that although he did possess the physiological capacity necessary to perform at a high level, to do so would have been associated with considerable pain. Also, despite the fact that his subsequent performance did not improve, our subjective impression was that he had "come to terms" with the situation in the sense that he now had a better understanding of why he was unable to perform at his previous level. One interpretation of this outcome could be that the runner gained insight into the nature of his presenting symptom.

Fourth, it is noteworthy that the athlete's record performance was characterized by the cognitive strategy known as *dissociation* (Morgan 1984, 1997, 2001; Morgan, Horstman, Cymerman, & Stokes, 1983). Runners who use this strategy attempt to ignore sensory input (e.g., muscle pain, breathing distress) by thinking about other activities (i.e., distraction). Other runners have reported that they initiate "out-of-body" experiences by entering the body's shadow cast on the ground in front of them. Although dissociative cognitive strategies can clearly facilitate endurance performance (Morgan et al., 1983), it is not the preferred strategy of elite distance runners (Morgan & Pollock, 1977). Indeed, elite runners have been found to use a cognitive strategy known as *association*, which is based on systematic monitoring of physical sensations, rather than ignoring such input (Morgan et al., 1988; Morgan, O'Connor, Sparling, & Pate, 1987; Morgan & Pollock, 1977).

There is a possibility that this athlete could have been taught to use dissociation (Morgan, 1984) under hypnotic or nonhypnotic conditions in an effort to help him cope with the perception of pain during competition. It is also possible that such an approach would have led to enhanced performance, because (a) laboratory research has shown that such an approach is ergogenic (Morgan et al., 1983), and (b) the runner had actually experienced a form of dissociation during his record-setting performance. However, ignoring sensory input while performing at a high metabolic level in a sport contest is not without risk, and such an approach can lead to heatstroke, muscle sprains or strains, and stress fractures (Morgan, 1984). Cognitive strategies designed to minimize or eliminate the sensation of pain and discomfort during athletic competition and training should be used judiciously and with caution.

Case 2: Baseball Player

Hypnotic age regression was used to resolve a periodic problem experienced by a college baseball player who was an outfielder on a Division I team.

The player's team physician introduced him to the second author (Morgan) in the hope that hypnosis might be used to improve the player's batting performance. He was regarded as a strong hitter, with the exception that he would "bail out" of the batter's box at times when he was not in apparent danger of being hit by a pitched ball. He had been examined and treated by the team physician and found to be in good physical health, including unimpaired vision. The player was highly regarded by several professional baseball teams, and he stood a good chance of earning a professional contract following graduation in 2 months. He was highly motivated to solve his batting problem because several professional scouts had arranged visits to observe him play. The coach was somewhat frustrated about the situation, and his only approach had been to instruct the player to "hang in with the pitch." This instruction was of no help to the batter, and the exhortation seemed to exacerbate the problem. The player was deeply concerned about the possibility that he would bail out of the batter's box during the forthcoming visits by pro scouts. Because he had a .315 batting average despite bailing out of the batter's box periodically, it was decided that he would be a possible candidate for hypnoanalysis.

A battery of psychological questionnaires was administered, and he was found to score within the normal range on measures of state and trait anxiety (STAI; Spielberger, 1983); aggression (Thematic Apperception Test; Murray, 1971); tension, depression, anger, vigor, and confusion (Profile of Mood States; McNair, Lorr, & Dropplemann, 1992); and neuroticism–stability and extroversion–introversion (EPI; Eysenck & Eysenck, 1968). Also, his lie score on the personality inventory was not remarkable. This screening was followed by administration of the Harvard (Shor & Orne, 1962) and Stanford C (Weitzenhoffer & Hilgard, 1962) scales of hypnotizability on separate days. He was quite responsive, scoring 9 on the Harvard Scale and 10 on the Stanford C Scale.

On the basis of the earlier example described by Johnson (1961a), he was initially age-regressed to a recent game in which the problem occurred, and he was asked to describe the situation. He had previously agreed that he did not object to the team physician or hypnotist asking him questions as the analysis proceeded. The athlete was unable to provide any detail during this age regression that was not available prior to the hypnotic condition. The hypnotist indicated that he would count from 1 to 10 and that the player would have recall for relevant information that was not previously available when the number 10 was reached. This, too, was based on the earlier approach successfully used by Johnson (1961a). At the count of 10, the athlete began to shake his head from side to side, and he apologized for not remembering additional material. He was assured that such a response was not unusual, and he was given posthypnotic suggestions to the effect that he would feel relaxed and refreshed following the session. It also was emphasized that he would look forward to next week's session.

The player returned a week later, at which time a second age regression was used, but on this occasion, he was asked to go back in time and try to recall any events in his baseball career that were of particular importance to him. Within a brief period, he described an occasion during his 1st year at the university in which he was hit on the back as he turned in an attempt to avoid a pitched ball. He thought the ball was going to "break," but it did not, and as he turned away from the ball, his left scapula was hit and broken. It is remarkable that he had apparently forgotten or not discussed this event, because it was significant. He had never mentioned this incident to us during the nonhypnotic period. He then proceeded to describe a situation in high school when, as a pitcher, he had attempted to "dust off" a batter (i.e., throw at the batter rather than at the plate) to distract the batter and increase his apprehension about succeeding pitches. Unfortunately, he hit the batter in the head and effective protective equipment was not worn at that time. Although the injury was not serious, the batter did not return to the game, and the athlete reported that he felt badly about the event.

We felt that it would be inappropriate to administer suggestions designed to restrain him in the batter's box because of the potential for injury from a pitched ball. Rather, we asked the batter whether he wanted to have conscious recall of this previously undisclosed material following hypnosis. He indicated that he would like to recall all of the information, and he was then given the same concluding suggestions administered in the previous session.

In the next and final session, the athlete was asked following the induction to once again go back in time and recall events in his baseball career that had particular meaning for him. He responded to this request by saying the following:

> Okay, but I want to tell you something first. I think I have solved my "bailing out" problem. I have been using a closed stance, and I crowd the plate as much as possible in order to "control" the plate and reduce the pitcher's strike zone. All good batters do this, but you always run the chance of being "beaned." Therefore, I'm changing to an open stance with my left foot dropped back, so I will have a wide-open view of all pitches. I'm a good enough hitter that I can do that without hurting my average.

Because the athlete seemed to have gained insight and resolved the problem, we elected not to proceed with further age regression. We talked with him briefly about his decision, and he was encouraged to review this plan with his coach. He was then given posthypnotic suggestion so that he would feel relaxed, rested, and confident about his decision following the session. He also was encouraged to contact us if he had any further problems. This case can be judged as representing a successful resolution of a presenting symptom, because the batter's performance improved. He was no longer plagued with the problem of bailing out, he completed the remainder of the season with a .515 average, and his overall average ranked near the top for all Division I players that year.

Case 3: Cyclist

The following case report was originally published in a chapter titled "Hypnosis in Sport and Exercise Psychology" (Morgan, 2002). We include it here as an example of a situation in which hypnotherapy, as a treatment for a decrement in performance, would be inappropriate.

A 27-year-old competitive cyclist approached us with the request that hypnosis be used to resolve a problem he was experiencing with his training. He was unable to complete routine training rides of 50 km to 75 km, and he was concerned that he would not be able to compete effectively in a forthcoming national race. He completed a standard battery of psychological questionnaires, and the results were remarkable in that he was found to be depressed and anxious. Because of the elevated scores on these measures, it was felt that his performance problem should not be addressed with hypnoanalysis. He was referred to a clinical psychologist for evaluation and possible treatment. Not only did this assessment reveal that he was clinically depressed, but it also showed that crisis intervention was warranted. Therefore, he was referred to an outpatient psychiatry clinic where he was treated for several months. Treatment consisted of time-limited psychotherapy in concert with antidepressant drug therapy.

During the course of his psychotherapy, he continued to visit our physiology of exercise laboratory, where he had previously completed a test of maximal aerobic power on the bicycle ergometer. This test revealed that he had a peak $\dot{V}O_2$ of 66 ml/kg·min. He was retested using the same protocol, and the test was performed by the same laboratory technician who performed the earlier assessment. The cyclist's maximal capacity had fallen to 53 ml/kg·min. Because a reduction of 20% in actual physiological capacity is both atypical and remarkable, the cyclist was retested a week later to confirm these results. The second test yielded identical results, and these data served to confirm that the decision to use hypnosis in such a case was contraindicated. That is, he could no longer perform at his customary level because he no longer had the physiological capacity to do so. The unexplained reduction in $\dot{V}O_{2max}$ warranted further assessment, and he was referred for a complete physical examination, including routine blood and urine chemistries. All results were negative, with the exception that he seemed to have some suspicious chest sounds. For this reason, he was referred to the pulmonary function laboratory, where all test results were found to be negative.

The psychotherapy and drug therapy led to a reduction in this cyclist's anxiety and depression, and he was eventually able to resume customary levels of training. However, the 20% decrement in physical capacity was not restored, nor was he able to return to competitive cycling at the national level. The purpose of elaborating on this case study is threefold. First, the "motivational" problem was based on a profound and difficult-to-explain reduction in the cyclist's physiological capacity. Second, the use of hypnosis to treat this problem was contraindicated in our view owing to the demonstration of both psychopathology (i.e., anxiety and depression) and pathophysiology (i.e., reduced $\dot{V}O_{2max}$). Third, it is apparent in retrospect, and on theoretical grounds, that a multidisciplinary approach to these problems was, and is, the only defensible course of action.

RESEARCH AND APPRAISAL

Research involving the use of hypnosis in exercise and sport psychology has been largely restricted to laboratory experimentation in which attempts have been made to elucidate the effectiveness of hypnotic suggestion on the transcendence of baseline measures of physical capacity. There have been two principal methodological problems associated with the published literature that warrant mention from the outset. First, investigators have used laboratory tasks (e.g., grip strength, weight-holding endurance) under controlled conditions, and it is unlikely that any of this work possesses ecological validity and generalizability to complex sport skills performed by athletes in emotionally charged competitive settings. Second, there has been a tendency to contrast performances in the laboratory following hypnotic suggestion with control or baseline performances in which suggestion has not been used. This traditional research paradigm has been characterized by the confounding of state (i.e., hypnosis vs. control) and suggestion. With few exceptions, it has been difficult to delineate the effects due to hypnosis versus those due to suggestion, because hypnosis with suggestion has typically been contrasted with nonhypnotic interventions without suggestion. Furthermore, the influence of demand characteristics has been largely ignored in this research literature.

The first comprehensive review dealing with the influence of hypnotic suggestibility and transcendence of voluntary capacity was published by Hull (1933). Hull's principal conclusion was that existing evidence bearing on this question was contradictory. Furthermore, Hull explained the equivocal nature of this experimentation as being due to design flaws. Later reviews, by Gorton (1959), Johnson (1961b), Weitzenhoffer (1953), Barber (1966), Morgan (1972, 1980a), and Morgan and Brown (1983) were inconsistent regarding the ability of hypnotic suggestion to enhance physical performance.

Gorton (1959) indicated that reserves of muscular power exist but that these reserves are not usually available. Gorton proposed that hypnotic suggestion is capable of mobilizing these reserves through disinhibition of inhibitory mechanisms, with the result that muscular performance is enhanced. This proposal has appeal from a teleological standpoint because it is known that maximal contraction of muscle can result in serious injuries such as bone fractures, dislocations, and muscle tears and strains, as well as damage to ligaments and tendons. Evidence in support of this view is largely indirect, and it derives from complications associated with the use of electroconvulsive shock therapy (Gorton, 1959).

Other investigators have not been as enthusiastic as Gorton (1959) regarding the effectiveness of hypnosis in facilitating physical performance. Weitzenhoffer's (1953) review failed to support the belief that hypnotic suggestion can enhance muscular performance, which confirmed the position advanced by Hull (1933) 3 decades earlier. Weitzenhoffer reported that contradictory findings in this area might have been due to dissimilar designs across studies.

Johnson (1961b) reported that direct hypnotic suggestions designed to enhance muscular strength and endurance sometimes work but that suggestions of this type are not consistently effective, although hypnotic suggestions designed to decrease performance are far more likely to be effective. However, such an effect could be easily produced in the nonhypnotic state with cooperative individuals.

Barber (1966) presented the most critical review of research in this area and concluded that hypnosis without suggestions for enhanced performance did not influence muscular strength or endurance. Furthermore, Barber reported that motivational suggestions are generally capable of augmenting muscular strength and endurance in both nonhypnotic and hypnotic conditions and cautioned about the necessity of not confounding hypnosis and suggestion (e.g., including suggestions with hypnosis and no suggestions in waking control conditions).

It is important to keep in mind that the case studies described in this chapter are purely anecdotal in nature and that empirical evidence for the use of hypnosis as an ergogenic aid is sorely lacking. Despite the paucity of scientific research to support the use of hypnosis as a sport performance enhancement technique, it continues to be advocated as a method of augmenting mental imagery and precompetition relaxation (Dunlap, 2005; Liggett, 2000a; Newmark & Bogacki, 2005). The methodological issues cited earlier persist in this literature, as does the tendency to ignore the responsibility of practitioners to identify situations when the use of hypnosis may be contraindicated (e.g., when the patient/client has an existing psychopathology) or even reckless (e.g., when conducted without the collaboration of a trained medical professional).

Recent research has used hypnosis as a method of influencing independent variables in exercise science experimentation. It has been reported, for example, that hypnotic suggestion can influence cardiac output, heart rate, blood pressure, forearm blood flow, respiratory rate, ventilatory minute volume, oxygen uptake, and carbon dioxide production, at rest as well as during exercise (Morgan, 1985). It has further been shown that perception of effort can be systematically increased and decreased during exercise with hypnotic suggestion (Morgan, 1970, 1981; Morgan et al., 1973, 1976; Thornton et al., 2001; Williamson et al., 2001). Moreover, when exercise intensity is perceived as being more effortful, there is a corresponding elevation in physiological responses even though the actual workload remains unchanged.

A pair of studies by Williamson et al. (2001, 2002) has made use of this phenomenon and demonstrated the utility of hypnosis in the research setting to identify cortical brain regions associated with centrally modulated cardiovascular responses to exercise. The purpose of the first investigation by Williamson et al. (2001) was to alter perceived exertion during exercise through the use of hypnotic suggestion and examine the impact of doing so on brain regions previously associated with the central regulation of cardiovascular responses. Six high hypnotizable participants each completed three bouts of cycle ergometry exercise on separate days. The participants were hypnotized for the duration of each exercise bout, and intensity and duration were standardized across the trials. One session was designated as the control session and was conducted without suggestion, as exercisers perceived riding on an even grade. Effort sense was manipulated during the final 5 min of the remaining sessions by giving a suggestion of riding on either an uphill or downhill grade. Single-photon-emission computed tomography (SPECT) was used to evaluate changes in regional cerebral blood flow (rCBF) for particular areas of the brain thought to play a role in the central regulation of the cardiovascular system. Participants reported decreased ratings of perceived exertion (RPE) after receiving a suggestion of riding downhill in comparison with cycling on actual level grade. However, there were no differences in heart rate, blood pressure, or rCBF compared with the control session. Even so, the suggestion of riding uphill was associated with increases in RPE, heart rate, blood pressure, and rCBF in right insular and thalamus in comparison with the control session. These findings confirmed the influence of central command on cardiovascular responses to exercise and suggested that the insula and thalamus appear to be involved in the central regulation of the cardiovascular system.

The subsequent study (Williamson et al., 2002) also used SPECT technology and was designed to identify patterns of brain activation associated with the central regulation of the cardiovascular system. Both high and low hypnotizable participants were included in this study, which compared participants' responses with actual and imagined handgrip exercise. During hypnosis, each participant completed a 3-min session of static handgrip exertion at 30% of maximum voluntary contraction (MVC) and an equivalent session of imagined handgrip exercise at 30% MVC. A radioactive blood-flow tracer was administered during the final minute of the session, and SPECT imaging was initiated within 20 min of the real and imagined exercise bout. Although there were no differences between the two groups on the variables of interest during actual exercise, the high hypnotizable individuals demonstrated an increase in RPE, heart rate, and blood pressure during imagined handgrip exercise in comparison with the low hypnotizable participants. In addition, the high hypnotizable group exhibited a greater level of rCBF in the anterior cingulate and insular cortices, suggesting a role for these structures in the central modulation of the cardiovascular response to exercise.

Positron emission tomography has also been used to investigate the role of brain regions associated with the cardiorespiratory response to exercise (Thornton et al., 2001). This neuroimaging modality was used to identify brain structures that were activated during the imagery of cycling while under hypnosis. An activation map was created for the imagery condition and compared with activation elicited during volitional hyperventilation and imagery of "freewheeling downhill" conditions also conducted under hypnosis. The resulting contrasts identified a number of brain regions associated with the imagination of exercise (e.g., supplementary motor and premotor areas, thalamus, cerebellum) and the voluntary control of respiration (e.g., supplementary motor and lateral sensorimotor areas). Thornton et al. (2001) suggested that these areas might be responsible for a portion of the cardiorespiratory response to exercise that they attributed to a behavioral response rather than the actual bodily demand of the activity.

In an attempt to tackle one of the major criticisms of hypnosis research in exercise science—confounding hypnosis and suggestion—Williamson et al. (2004) conducted a supplementary study to examine the impact of hypnosis, without suggestion, on individuals' response to exercise. High and low hypnotizable participants completed 3 min of static handgrip exercise at 30% of MVC, once while under hypnosis without suggestion (i.e., "neutral hypnosis") and again without hypnosis. Regional cerebral blood flow was monitored via SPECT during both conditions. Heart rate, blood pressure, forearm muscle activity, force generation, and RPE were also collected during exercise. The only significant difference reported between conditions was an increase in rCBF in the occipital region for the hypnosis condition. There were no statistical differences between the two groups or conditions for the remaining variables. These results demonstrated a change in brain activation during exercise attributable to hypnosis. However, this difference in activation was not associated with any changes in forearm muscle activity, cardiovascular responses, or perceived effort during handgrip exercise. The authors concluded that hypnosis could be effectively used during exercise conducted for the purpose of research, without concern for altering the typical exercise response.

Although the conclusions drawn by Morgan (1980a, 1985) and Morgan and Brown (1983) in their reviews of the hypnosis research in exercise and sport science were originally penned more than 20 years ago, they still hold relevancy for investigators today. The following is a summary of those conclusions:

1. Although some investigators have reported that hypnosis per se has no influence on muscular strength and endurance, an equal number have found that hypnosis (without suggestion) can lead to both increments and decrements in muscular performance. The evidence in this area is equivocal.

2. Hypnotic suggestions designed to enhance muscular performance have generally not been effective, whereas suggestions designed to impair strength and endurance have been consistently successful.

3. Individuals who are not accustomed to performing at maximal levels usually experience gains in muscular strength and endurance when administered involving suggestions (Hilgard, 1965) during hypnosis. However, suggestions of a noninvolving nature are not effective when administered to the individuals who are accustomed to performing at maximal levels.

4. Efforts to modify performance on various psychomotor tasks (e.g., choice reaction time) have effects similar to those observed in research involving muscular strength and endurance. That is, efforts to slow reaction time are usually effective, whereas attempts to speed reaction time are not.

5. Case studies involving efforts to enhance performance in athletes by means of hypnosis appear to be universally successful. However, this observation should probably be viewed with caution because therapists and journals are not known for emphasizing case material depicting failures.

6. Hypnotic suggestion of exercise in the nonexercise state is associated with increased cardiac frequency, respiratory rate, ventilatory minute volume, oxygen uptake, carbon dioxide production, forearm blood flow, and cardiac output. These metabolic changes often approximate responses noted during actual exercise conditions.

7. Perception of effort during exercise can be systematically increased and decreased with hypnotic suggestion even though the actual physical workload is maintained at a constant level. Furthermore, alterations in effort sense (i.e., perceived exer-

tion) are associated with significant changes in physiological responses (e.g., ventilation).

CONCLUSION

Hypnosis has been used in the field of exercise and sport psychology for a number of years as a research tool in efforts designed to elucidate the mechanisms underlying physical performance. Also, there have been numerous clinical applications designed to enhance performance in sport settings, and these interventions have been based largely on theoretical formulations as opposed to empirical research evidence. These clinical applications have generally been successful, but there has been little attention paid to behavioral artifacts, such as expectancy effects, placebo effects, and demand characteristics in this work. Furthermore, there is evidence that effects obtained with these clinical applications exceed those that one might achieve with the same or comparable approaches in the absence of hypnosis.

Efforts to enhance athletic performance by increasing or decreasing precompetitive anxiety have usually not been effective. This can be explained by the observation that most athletes perform best within a narrow ZOA. Hence, efforts to decrease or increase anxiety in athletes should be discouraged unless the athlete's ZOA is known. It is noteworthy that hypnotic age regression offers considerable promise in defining an individual's ZOA. Furthermore, once this anxiety zone has been established, it can be reproduced with various hypnotic procedures.

An additional area in which hypnosis has proven to be effective in sport psychology involves the interpretation of decreased performance levels (i.e., slumps, failure) in previously successful athletes. Examples of nondirective hypnotic age regression are presented in this chapter, and these cases emphasize the importance of multidisciplinary approaches. In conclusion, direct hypnotic suggestions of enhanced performance are not likely to be successful, but there are a number of ways in which the hypnotic tool can be used effectively in exercise and sport psychology.

REFERENCES

American Psychological Association (2002). Ethical principles of psychologists and code of conduct. *American Psychologist, 57,* 1060–1073.

Appel, P. R. (1990). Clinical application of hypnosis in the physical medicine and rehabilitation setting: Three case reports. *American Journal of Clinical Hypnosis, 33,* 85–93.

Barber, T. X. (1966). The effects of hypnosis and suggestions on strength and endurance: A critical review of research studies. *British Journal of Social and Clinical Psychology, 5,* 42–50.

Borkovec, T. D., Mathews, A. M., Chambers, A., Ebrahimi, S., Lytle, R., & Nelson, R. (1987). The effects of relaxation training with cognitive or nondirective therapy and the role of relaxation-induced anxiety in the treatment of generalized anxiety. *Journal of Consulting and Clinical Psychology, 55,* 883–888.

Dunlap, E. M. (2005). Hypnosis and sport performance. In A. Barabasz & J. G. Watkins (Eds.), *Hypnotherapeutic techniques* (2nd ed., pp. 41–44). New York: Brunner-Routledge.

Eysenck, H. J. (1941). An experimental study of the improvement of mental and physical functions in the hypnotic state. *British Journal of Medical Psychology, 18,* 304–316.

Eysenck, H. J., & Eysenck, S. B. G. (1968). *Manual for the Eysenck Personality Inventory.* San Diego, CA: Educational and Industrial Testing Service.

Garver, R. B. (1977). The enhancement of human performance with hypnosis through neuromotor facilitation and control of arousal level. *American Journal of Clinical Hypnosis, 19,* 177–181.

Garvin, A. W., Trine, M. R., & Morgan, W. P. (2001). Affective and metabolic responses to hypnosis, autogenic relaxation, and quiet rest. *International Journal of Clinical and Experimental Hypnosis, 49,* 5–18.

Gorton, B. E. (1959). Physiologic aspects of hypnosis. In J. M. Schneck (Ed.), *Hypnosis in modern medicine* (pp. 246–280). Springfield, IL: Charles C Thomas.

Hanin, Y. L. (1978). A study of anxiety in sports. In W. F. Straub (Ed.), *Sport psychology: An analysis of athlete behavior* (pp. 236–249). Ithaca, NY: Movement.

Heide, F. J., & Borkovec, T. D. (1984). Relaxation-induced anxiety: Mechanisms and theoretical implications. *Behavioral Research and Therapy, 22,* 1–12.

Hilgard, E. R. (1965). *Hypnotic susceptibility.* New York: Harcourt, Brace & World.

Hull, C. L. (1933). *Hypnosis and suggestibility.* New York: Appleton-Century-Crofts.

Ikai, M., & Steinhaus, A. H. (1961). Some factors modifying the expression of human strength. *Journal of Applied Psychology, 16,* 157–163.

Johnson, W. R. (1961a). Body movement awareness in the nonhypnotic and hypnotic states. *Research Quarterly, 32,* 263–264.

Johnson, W. R. (1961b). Hypnosis and muscular performance. *Journal of Sports Medicine and Physical Fitness, 1,* 71–79.

Liggett, D. R. (2000a). Enhancing imagery through hypnosis: A performance aid for athletes. *American Journal of Clinical Hypnosis, 43,* 149–157.

Liggett, D. R. (2000b). *Sport hypnosis.* Champaign, IL: Human Kinetics.

Lubin, B. (1967). *Manual for the Depression Adjective Check Lists.* San Diego, CA: Educational and Industrial Testing Service.

Massey, B. H., Johnson, W. R., & Kramer, G. F. (1961). Effect of warm-up exercise upon muscular performance using hypnosis to control the psychological variable. *Research Quarterly of the American Association for Health, Physical Education & Recreation, 32,* 63–71.

McNair, D. M., Lorr, M., & Droppleman, L. F. (1992). *EITS manual for the Profile of Mood States.* San Diego, CA: Educational and Industrial Testing Service.

Morgan, W. P. (1970). Oxygen uptake following hypnotic suggestion. In G. S. Kenyon (Ed.), *Contemporary psychology of sport* (pp. 283–286). Chicago: Athletic Institute.

Morgan, W. P. (1972). Hypnosis and muscular performance. In W. P. Morgan (Ed.), *Ergogenic aids and muscular performance* (pp. 193–233). New York: Academic Press.

Morgan, W. P. (1980a). Hypnosis and sports medicine. In G. D. Burrows & L. Dennerstein (Eds.), *Handbook of hypnosis and psychosomatic medicine* (pp. 359–375). Amsterdam: Elsevier.

Morgan, W. P. (1980b). The trait psychology controversy. *Research Quarterly for Exercise and Sport, 51,* 50–76.

Morgan, W. P. (1981). Psychophysiology of self-awareness during vigorous physical activity. *Research Quarterly for Exercise and Sports, 52,* 385–427.

Morgan, W. P. (1984). Mind over matter. In W. F. Straub & J. M. Williams (Eds.), *Cognitive sport psychology* (pp. 311–316). Lansing, NY: Sport Science Associates.

Morgan, W. P. (1985). Psychogenic factors and exercise metabolism. *Medicine and Science in Sports and Exercise, 17,* 309–316.

Morgan, W. P. (1993). Hypnosis and sport psychology. In J. Rhue, S. J. Lynn, & I. Kirsch (Eds.), *Handbook of clinical hypnosis* (pp. 649–670). Washington, DC: American Psychological Association.

Morgan, W. P. (1997). Mind games: The psychology of sport. In D. R. Lamb & R. Murray (Eds.), *Perspectives in exercise science and sports medicine: Vol. 10. Optimizing sport performance* (pp. 1–62). Carmel, IN: Cooper.

Morgan, W. P. (2001). Psychological factors associated with distance running and the marathon. In D. Tunstall Pedoe (Ed.), *Marathon medicine 2000* (pp. 293–310). London: Royal Society of Medicine.

Morgan, W. P. (2002). Hypnosis in sport and exercise psychology. In J. L. Van Raalte & B. W. Brewer (Eds.), *Exploring sport and exercise psychology* (pp. 151–181). Washington, DC: American Psychological Association.

Morgan, W. P., & Brown, D. R. (1983). Hypnosis. In M. L. Williams (Ed.), *Ergogenic aids and sports* (pp. 223–252). Champaign, IL: Human Kinetics.

Morgan, W. P., Brown, D. R., Raglin, J. S., O'Connor, P. J., & Ellickson, K. A. (1987). Psychological monitoring of overtraining and staleness. *British Journal of Sports Medicine, 21,* 107–114.

Morgan, W. P., & Ellickson, K. A. (1989). Health, anxiety, and physical exercise. In C.D. Spielberger & D. Hackbart (Eds.), *Anxiety in sports: An international perspective* (pp. 165–182). Washington, DC: Hemisphere Publication Services.

Morgan, W. P., Hirota, K., Weitz, G. A., & Balke, B. (1976). Hypnotic perturbation of perceived exertion: Ventilatory consequences. *American Journal of Clinical Hypnosis, 18*, 182–190.

Morgan, W. P., Horstman, D. H., Cymerman, A., & Stokes, J. (1983). Facilitation of physical performance by means of a cognitive strategy. *Cognitive Therapy and Research, 7*, 251–264.

Morgan, W. P., O'Connor, P. J., Ellickson, K. A., & Bradley, P. W. (1988). Personality structure, mood states, and performance in elite male distance runners. *International Journal of Sport Psychology, 19*, 247–263.

Morgan, W. P., O'Connor, P. J., Sparling, B. P., & Pate, R. R. (1987). Psychological characterization of the elite female distance runner. *International Journal of Sports Medicine, 8*, 124–131.

Morgan, W. P., & Pollock, M. L. (1977). Psychologic characterization of the elite distance runner. *Annals of the New York Academy of Science, 301*, 382–403.

Morgan, W. P., Raven, P. B., Drinkwater, B. L., & Horvath, S. M. (1973). Perceptual and metabolic responsivity to standard bicycle ergometry following various hypnotic suggestions. *International Journal of Clinical and Experimental Hypnosis, 31*, 86–101.

Murray, H. A. (1971). *Thematic apperception test.* Cambridge, MA: Harvard University Press.

Naruse, G. (1965). The hypnotic treatment of stage fright in champion athletes. *International Journal of Clinical and Experimental Hypnosis, 13*, 63–70.

Newmark, T. S., & Bogacki, D. F. (2005). The use of relaxation, hypnosis and imagery in sport psychiatry. *Clinics in Sports Medicine, 24*, 973–977.

Pates, J., Cummings, A., & Maynard, I. (2002). The effects of hypnosis on flow states and three-point shooting performance in basketball players. *Sport Psychologist, 16*, 34–47.

Pates, J., Oliver, R., & Maynard, I. (2001). The effects of hypnosis on flow states and golf-putting performance. *Journal of Applied Sport Psychology, 13*, 341–354.

Raglin, J. S. (1992). Anxiety and sport performance. In J. O. Holloszy (Ed.), *Exercise and sport sciences reviews* (Vol. 20, pp. 243–274). Baltimore, MD: Williams & Wilkins.

Raglin, J. S., Morgan, W. P., & Wise, K. (1990). Pre-competition anxiety in high school girl swimmers: A test of optimal function theory. *International Journal of Sports Medicine, 11*, 171–175.

Raglin, J. S., & Morris, M. J. (1994) Precompetition anxiety in women volleyball players: A test of ZOF theory in a team sport. *British Journal of Sports Medicine, 28*, 47–51.

Raglin, J. S., & Turner, P. E. (1992). Predicted, actual, and optimal precompetition anxiety in adolescent track and field athletes. *Scandinavian Journal of Exercise and Science in Sports, 2*, 148–152.

Raglin, J. S., & Turner, P. E. (1993). Anxiety and performance in track and field athletes: A comparison of the inverted-U hypothesis with zone of optimal function theory. *Personality and Individual Differences, 14,* 163–171.

Schultz, J. H., & Luthe, W. (1969). *Autogenic Therapy. Vol. 1: Autogenic methods.* New York: Grune & Stratton.

Shor, R. E., & Orne, E. C. (1962). *Harvard Group Scale of Hypnotic Susceptibility.* Palo Alto, CA: Consulting Psychologists Press.

Smith, J. L., & Bozymowski, M. F. (1965). Effect of attitude toward warm-ups on motor performance. *Research Quarterly, 36,* 78–85.

Spielberger, C. D. (1983). *Manual for the State Trait Anxiety Inventory.* Palo Alto, CA: Consulting Psychologists Press.

Thornton, J. M., Guz, A., Murphy, K., Griffith, A. R., Pederson, D. L., Kardos, A., et al. (2001). Identification of higher brain centres that may encode the cardiorespiratory response to exercise in humans. *Journal of Physiology, 533,* 823–836.

Turner, P. E., & Raglin, J. S. (1996). Variability in precompetition anxiety and performance in collegiate track and field athletes. *Medicine and Science in Sports and Exercise, 28,* 378–385.

Uneståhl, L. E. (1981). *New paths of sport learning and excellence* [Monograph]. Orebro, Sweden: Orebro University, Department of Sport Psychology.

Vanek, M. (1970). Psychological problems of superior athletes: Some experiences from the Olympic Games in Mexico City, 1968. In G. S. Kenyon (Ed.), *Contemporary psychology of sport* (pp. 183–185). Chicago: Athletic Institute.

Weitzenhoffer, A. M. (1953). *Hypnotism: An objective study in suggestibility.* New York: Wiley.

Weitzenhoffer, A. M., & Hilgard, E. R. (1962). *Stanford Hypnotic Susceptibility Scale.* Palo Alto, CA: Consulting Psychologists Press.

Williamson, J. W., McColl, R., Mathews, D., Mitchell, J. H., Raven, P. B., & Morgan, W. P. (2001). Hypnotic manipulation of effort sense during dynamic exercise: Cardiovascular responses and brain activation. *Journal of Applied Physiology, 90,* 1392–1399.

Williamson, J. W., McColl, R., Mathews, D., Mitchell, J. H., Raven, P. B., & Morgan, W. P. (2002). Brain activation by central command during actual and imagined handgrip under hypnosis. *Journal of Applied Physiology, 92,* 1317–1324.

Williamson, J. W., McColl, R., Mathews, D., & Morgan, W. P. (2004). Does hypnosis alter cardiovascular responses or brain activation during handgrip exercise? *Hypnose und Kognition, 21,* 205–223.

World Anti-Doping Agency. (2003, March). *World anti-doping code.* Montreal, Canada: Author.

VI

ISSUES AND EXTENSIONS

27

ON A CLEAR DAY YOU CAN SEE FOREVER: HYPNOSIS IN THE POPULAR IMAGINATION

JUDITH PINTAR

From the 18th to the 21st century, mesmerism and hypnosis provided inspiration for creative expressions ranging from highly regarded works of literature to the most lowbrow of evening entertainment. Books, plays, and films have explored themes associated with mesmerism and hypnosis, both directly and obliquely. They have used humor and horror, revealing both fascination and wariness. The prevalence of hypnosis in a variety of media can be understood as cultural commentary on scientific and medical discovery; however, artistic expressions also fed back and influenced developments in fields of scientific inquiry, both mainstream and marginal. Assumptions about the nature of the hypnotic relation, the powers of the hypnotist, the personality characteristics of the subject, and the possibilities and limitations of the associated phenomena have all been amply addressed in a fluid discourse between people involved in what might appear to be separate spheres.

The complexity of the relationship between popular and scientific thought is fully embodied in the several remarkable careers enjoyed by the Nobel-prizewinning doctor, Charles Richet, whose work with techniques associated with both mesmerism and hypnosis were influential in late 19th-century France. Richet, who served as professor of physiology at the Faculty of Medicine in Paris, was also a poet who penned romantic novels under the name of Charles Epheyre. His novel, *Soeur Marthe* (1890), the story of a medical doctor who fell in love with the dissociated personality of a young neurotic woman he hypnotized, is a plot concept that provided Barbra Streisand with a star vehicle and an opportunity to sing *On a Clear Day You Can See Forever* (Lane & Lerner, 1969) 80 years later.

In this chapter, I survey the appearance of mesmerism and hypnosis in the popular imagination, from 18th-century poetry to 19th-century satire to 20th-century film. Hypnosis has proved to be a dependable element of plot and endlessly engaging as a theme, despite ubiquitous factual inaccuracies. This narrative legacy is thus double-edged: Although stereotypes and misconceptions about clinical hypnosis are perpetuated, its fascination is also preserved and renewed.

HYPNOSIS IN LITERATURE

Fiction writers, playwrights, poets, and, eventually, filmmakers have made use of mesmerism and hypnosis in stories that have been, by turns, romantic, fantastical, and nightmarish. Throughout the 19th and 20th centuries, fictional accounts of mesmerism and, later, hypnosis were frequently penned and enthusiastically received. Novelists credited magnetists and hypnotists of both the medical and stage variety with providing the inspiration for their stories. Some writers had witnessed performances, others read the available books on the subject, and some experimented with the techniques themselves, as both participants and practitioners.

Samuel Taylor Coleridge was considering mesmerism at the end of the 18th century in his poems "Rime of the Ancient Mariner" (1798/1857) and "Christabel" (1816/1869). Magnetic power provided a credible metaphor during this era for reflections on the inner workings of emotional and sexual relationships. In a poem by Percy Bysshe Shelley, "The Magnetic Lady to her Patient" (1822/1855), the "magnetizer" was a woman who tried to heal a man of his unrequited love for her:

> Sleep, sleep on! forget thy pain;
> My hand is on thy brow,
> My spirit on thy brain;
> My pity on thy heart, poor friend;
> And from my fingers flow
> The powers of life, and like a sign,
> Seal thee from thine hour of woe;
> And brood on thee, but may not blend
> With thine.

Shelley's poem is unusual for making the magnetizer female; for most of the 19th century, the relation of magnetizer to subject was accompanied by strongly gendered assumptions that emphasized male power and female passivity. A poem by Robert Browning, "Mesmerism" (1855), more typically suggested the potential for absolute control of a man's will and desire over a woman's body and her soul:

> Have and hold, then and there,
> Her, from head to foot
> Breathing and mute,
> Passive and yet aware,
> In the grasp of my steady stare—
> Hold and have, there and then,
> All her body and soul
> That completes my whole,
> All that women add to men,
> In the clutch of my steady ken—

In American literature, the dangers of mesmerism were addressed in the writings of Nathaniel Hawthorne, who was among the first Americans authors to make his interest in mesmerism central to plots and wider thematic concerns. His complicated musings revealed a man both intrigued and unsettled by the implications of the practice. When his fiancée, Sophia Peabody, revealed an interest in mesmerism as a treatment for her chronic headaches, his response was immediate and incontrovertible: "My spirit is moved to talk to thee today about these magnetic miracles, and to beseech thee to take no part in them" (as cited in Stoehr, 1978, p. 48). He explained the fear that lies behind his request:

> Supposing that this power arises from the transformation of one spirit into another, it seems to me that the sacredness of an individual is violated by it, there would be an intrusion into thy holy of holies—and the intruder would not by thy husband! Canst thou think, without a shrinking of thy soul, of any human being coming into closer communion with thee than I may?—than either nature or my own sense of right would permit me? (as cited in Stoehr, 1978, p. 48)

By the time the letter was written, Sophia, unbeknownst to Nathaniel, had already risked her "holy of holies." Prior to 1840, she was the frequent subject for Dr. Joseph Emerson Fiske, a successful dentist who heard a lecture on mesmerism in Salem, Massachusetts, in 1837. He began treating Sophia's headaches on what may even have been a daily basis, with apparent success, until her family relocated to Boston in 1840. It was then that she told Hawthorne that she had met with one Mrs. Cornelia Park, an old friend who had begun to dabble in mesmerism, and in response to that, Hawthorne sent back his dramatic reply.

Privately, Hawthorne admitted substantial curiosity about mesmerism and its potential for metaphysical discovery. He entitled a diary entry of 1842 "Questions as to unsettled points of History, and Mysteries of Nature, to be asked of a mesmerized person" (Stoehr, 1978, p. 52). However, horror won out over the potential for insight in his novels, a reflection of what appeared to be his assumption that the phenomena produced by mesmerism arises from the combination of a personally powerful mesmerist and a subject who has lost her will. In *The House of Seven Gables* (1851), Hawthorne created a mesmerist who controlled a young woman and brought about her death. In *The Blithedale Romance* (1852) he went further to suggest that the power of a mesmerist could actually destroy its subject's soul.

These novels also revealed Hawthorne's suspicion that the power of mesmerists was sexual in its essential nature. In both of these novels, the mesmerists were physically attractive, charismatic men, whereas their victims were equally attractive but powerless, and virginal, girls. Coupled with the idea that the power of mesmerism was a reflection of the mesmerist himself was the assumption that the personal characteristic of passivity is what makes hypnotic subjects susceptible to influence in the first place. Hawthorne perceived in the interpersonal relations of mesmerism a metaphor for wider human relations he saw operating in the world, not only between men and women but also between masters and slaves, a theme found in many of his novels (see Stoehr, 1978, p. 56).

In a similar vein, Herman Melville also used animal magnetism in *Moby Dick* (1851) as a metaphor to discuss power relations, particularly what a man must do to maintain control over the will of another:

> To accomplish his object Ahab must use tools; and of all tools used in the shadow of the moon, men are most apt to get out of order. He knew, for example, that however magnetic his ascendancy in some respects was over Starbuck, yet that ascendancy did not cover the complete spiritual man any more than mere corporeal superiority involves intellectual mastership; for to the purely spiritual, the intellectual but stand in sort of corporeal relation. Starbuck's body and Starbuck's coerced will were Ahab's, so long as Ahab kept his magnet at Starbuck's brain; still he knew that for all this the chief mate, in his soul, abhorred his captain's quest, and could he, would joyfully disintegrate himself from it, or even frustrate it (p. 208).

Unlike Melville, Hawthorne's interest in mesmerism was more metaphorical. The dangers he perceived in it, he viewed as literal possibilities. He was seemingly drawn to the darker aspect of magnetic power, associating mesmerism with witchcraft, and he often hinted at supernatural horrors at the edges of his human dramas.

Edgar Allan Poe explicitly expressed this potential for horror in a series of short stories written during the 1840s that addressed mesmerism, including "Mesmeric Revelation" (1844a), "Tale of Ragged Mountain" (1844b), and "Mesmerism in Articulo Mortis." The latter short story, which created substantial controversy, was originally published in *The American Review* as "The Facts of M. Valdemar's Case" (1845a). It presented the medical case of a dying man who allowed himself to be mesmerized to try to save his life but found his soul entrapped instead in a decomposing body. The tale was subsequently published in pamphlet forms as "Mesmerism in Articulo Mortis: An Astounding and Horrifying Narrative" (1845b) and as "Mesmerism, 'In Articulo Mortis,' An Astounding and Horrifying Narrative Shewing the Extraordinary Power of Mesmerism in Arresting the Progress of Death" (1846). The pamphlet style used in these publications and in translations in France, Germany, and Austria was meant to deliberately confound readers as to whether they were reading fiction or not. At first coyly sidestepping questions as to its factual basis, Poe eventually acknowledged it to be a hoax in his private correspondence.

Poe would no doubt be delighted to know that his intentional confusion regarding his actual views continues into the present day. In his story "Mesmeric Revelation" (1844a), Poe's prose was so authoritative and pedagogical in style that some commentators have interpreted his transmission of ideas found in the popular book, *Facts in Mesmerism* (Townshend, 1844), written by English minister Chauncy Hare Townshend, to mean that Poe may have personally believed that mesmerism allowed its participants to achieve transcendental insight. Others have been convinced of his cynicism (cf. Fuller, 1982, pp. 36–37; Tatar, 1978, pp.197–199). Certainly, Poe was unimpressed by the mesmeric trances of Andrew Jackson Davis who claimed to be channeling the Swedish mystic, Emanuel Swedenborg, wryly commenting, "There surely can *not* be more things in Heaven and Earth than are dreamt of (oh, Andrew Jackson Davis!) in *your* philosophy."(Poe, 1902, XIV, p. 173).

Charles Baudelaire (1821–1867), one of the early translators of Poe into French, seemed to take Poe as sympathetic to mesmerism and Swedenborgianism, but this may have been because within 19th-century French literature, the writings of Baudelaire and Balzac both explored its occult, supernatural possibilities (see Versluis, 2001). Balzac (1799–1850), for instance, addressed the mystical, rather than medical, forms of animal magnetism directly in 1842 in his novel *Ursule Mirout* (1841). The novels of another French author, Alexandre Dumas, in contrast to the work of Baudelaire and Balzac, were less mystical than psychological in their approach, and of course, his tales were more rollicking.

Dumas's view of mesmerism was colored by his acquaintance in Paris with Jose-Custodio de Faria, better known as Abbe Faria. Born in Goa of Indo-Portuguese ancestry, he was an ordained priest as well as a well-known demonstrator of mesmerism and somnambulistic sleep (see Carrer, 2005).

Dumas appropriated Faria's name and a dramatic episode in his life, incorporating them into his novel *The Count of Monte Cristo* (1846). Arrested in 1797 in Marseilles, the real Faria had been thrown into solitary confinement in the infamous Chateau d'If, the island prison with a breathtaking view of Marseilles. It was there that Faria claimed he had developed powerful techniques of self-suggestion.

Dumas explored the darker potentials of mesmerism in his novel *Memoirs of a Physician* (1847), in which he described the dangerous sexual control that a mesmerist may have over his subject and the phenomenon of hypnotically induced identity dissociation. In the story, a magnetizer married a woman while she was in her trance state, though she loathed him when she was awake. This exploration of identity prefigured the interest in the subject that reappeared later in the century in both medicine and literature.

Although novelists were commentators on the mesmerists with whom they shared their historical stage, they were sometimes also clearly participants in the magnetic movement as well. Alfred Lord Tennyson liked to mesmerize himself and wrote poetry while in a self-induced trance state. Another well-known literary practitioner of mesmerism was Charles Dickens, whose friendship with John Elliotson was intimate and long-standing; Elliotson was the godfather of Dickens's son Walter. Elliotson was a prominent doctor at London University, whose interest in mesmerism did much to popularize the technique but which also led to Elliotson's fall from the medical mainstream. The friendship between the doctor and the novelist began as early as 1838 when Dickens was a regular witness to the demonstrations of mesmerism occurring at London Hospital.

While traveling in the United States in 1842, Dickens began to practice magnetism with his own wife as his subject. His experiments became more deliberate and extensive a few years later when they were vacationing in Genoa. Between 1844 and 1845, he conducted a magnetic relationship with a Madame La Rue, the wife of a Swiss banker who was supposedly suffering from hysteria. Dickens's wife was disturbed by the unusual intimacy that developed between him and La Rue, and he eventually abandoned his practice (see Kaplan, 1975).

Although the novels of Dickens never addressed mesmerism as a central point of their plot, it appeared regularly in his stories as a device to explore the various uses of human will, both for good and evil. Magnetic themes can be identified in a host of his novels, from *Nicholas Nickleby* (1838–1839) to *Barnaby Rudge* (1840–1841), from *David Copperfield* (1849–1850) to his unfinished final novel, *The Mystery of Edwin Drood* (1870). Dickens used Elliotson as the model for the doctor in *Little Dorrit* (1855–1857), and Elliotson's daughter became the idealized character of Esther Sommerson in *Bleak House* (1852–1853). William Makepeace Thackeray (1811–1863), who dedicated

The History of Pendennis (1849–1850) to Elliotson to thank him for his medical care, also used the doctor as the basis for the character of Dr. Goodenough. Of course, not all literary treatments of mesmerists and hypnotists were as kind and flattering as these.

Satire and Science Fiction

By the end of the 19th century, generations of writers, both the celebrated and many less well known, had established mesmerism as a standard plot element and a literary trope. Writers could comfortably rely on the assumption that audiences would share basic knowledge of the vocabulary of mesmerism, its traditional techniques, the philosophical questions that adhered to it, and its mundane manifestations. The antics of traveling stage performers who mesmerized and hypnotized across the planet were captured in humorous accounts by authors on both sides of the Atlantic. Mark Twain in *Huckleberry Finn* (1884/1912) poked fun at their versatility:

> First they done a lecture on temperance; but they didn't make enough for them both to get drunk on. Then in another village they started a dancing-school; but they didn't know no more how to dance than a kangaroo does; so the first prance they made the general public jumped in and pranced them out of town. Another time they tried to go at yellocution; but they didn't yellocute long till the audience got up and give them a solid good cussing, and made them skip out. They tackled missionarying, and mesmerizing, and doctoring, and telling fortunes, and a little of everything; but they couldn't seem to have no luck. (p. 290)

During the 1870s, Gustave Flaubert penned in his novel *Bouvard and Pecuchet* (1881/1976) what must be the most concise, and certainly funniest, history of mesmerism ever published. Unfinished at his death, the novel is a broad and biting satire of 19th-century philosophical and popular thought. It dedicated several pages to mesmerism, memorably lampooning Franz Mesmer and his *baquet*, the tub of magnetized water Mesmer used in Paris to heal a room full of people at once. Participants would stand in a circle around it while he played to them on his glass harmonica. Flaubert's hapless mesmerizers did their best:

> To induce somnambulism they planned to construct a mesmeric tub. Pecuchet had already collected filings and cleaned a score of bottles when a scruple stopped him. Among the patients would come members of the fair sex.
> "And what shall we do if they are seized with attacks of erotic frenzy?"
> That would not have stopped Bouvard; but because of gossip and perhaps blackmail it was better to abstain. They contented themselves with a harmonica and carried it with them into people's houses, to the delight of the children.

One day when Migraine was worse they resorted to it. The crystalline notes exasperated him; but Deleuze tells you not to be frightened by complaints. The music continued.

"Enough, enough!" he cried.

"A little patience," replied Bouvard.

Pecuchet was tapping still faster on the strips of glass, the instrument was vibrating, and the poor man howling, when the doctor appeared, attracted by the noise.

"What, you again!" he cried, furious at finding them again with his patients.

They explained their magnetic method. Then he fulminated against magnetism, a lot of conjuring tricks, whose effects derive from the imagination. (Flaubert, 1881/1976, p. 190)

Flaubert went on to poke fun at the Swiss stage magician, Charles Lafontaine, with scatological glee. Lafontaine was famous for torturing his subjects to demonstrate their insensibility to pain and famously claimed to have mesmerized a lioness:

They did not have a lioness. Chance provided them with another animal.

Because next day at 6 o'clock, a ploughboy came to tell them that they were wanted at the farm, for a cow in a desperate state.

They ran.

The apple-trees were in blossom and the grass in the yard steamed under the rising sun. At the end of the pond, half covered with a cloth, a cow was lowing, shivering with the pails of water that had been thrown over it, and so immeasurably swollen that it looked like a hippopotamus . . . .

They rolled up their sleeves and placed themselves one at the horns, the other at the tail, and with great inward efforts and frantic gesticulation they spread out their fingers to pour out streams of fluid over the animal, while the farmer and his wife, their lad and some neighbours looked on almost in terror.

The rumblings that could be heard in the cow's belly made their own insides bubble. It broke wind. Then Pecuchet said:

"That opens the door to hope, there is a way out, perhaps."

The way out worked, hope gushed out in a tub full of yellow matter exploding like a bomb. Hearts were eased. The cow's swelling went down. An hour later, nothing showed.

It was not the effect of imagination, that was certain. (Flaubert, 1881/1976, p. 191)

Flaubert's fable deliberately conflated the work of medical mesmerists with the entrepreneurial entertainers who were mesmerizing across Europe at that time. Most 19th-century medical doctors and researchers rejected stage performers as charlatans, dismissing their performances outright as having nothing interesting to contribute to legitimate science. There were serious moves to standardize orthodox techniques during this period, but the medical men could not control the flooding of hypnotic ideas and techniques into popular culture as a source of entertainment (see Nadis, 2001). What went on onstage often found its way into the pages of a book.

Among the most influential of 19th-century stage hypnotists on the popular imagination was the Belgian-born Alfred d'Hont, who used the stage name Donato. He used his powerful gaze in an intimidating and frankly sexual way. One contemporary account (Spurling, 1998) described it as follows:

> Donato comes close, darts the piercing rays emanating from his eyes deep into the eyes of one of his subjects, who, almost immediately, against his own will, rises to his feet, walks, and, oblivious of himself, carries out . . . any order he is given. (p. 31)

Even when writers lampooned stage hypnotists as frauds, they betrayed their suspicion that there was an underlying sexual risk to impressionable young women that was dangerously real, a contradiction captured by Henry James, brother of pragmatist philosopher William James, in his short story, "Professor Fargo" (1874/1919):

> He fixed his eye for a moment on the young girl. She immediately looked up at him, rose, advanced, and stood before him. Her face betrayed no painful consciousness of what she was doing, and I have often wondered how far, in her strangely simple mood and nature, her consciousness on this occasion was a guilty one. I never ascertained. This was the most unerring stroke I had seen the Professor perform. The poor child fixed her charming eyes on his gross, flushed face, and awaited his commands. She was fascinated; she had no will of her own. "You'll be so good as to choose," the Professor went on, addressing her in spite of her deafness, "between your father and me. He says we're to part. I say you're to follow me. What do you say?"
>
> For all answer, after caressing him a moment with her gentle gaze, she dropped before him on her knees. The Colonel sprang towards her with a sort of howl of rage and grief, but she jumped up, retreated, and tripped down the steps of the platform into the room. She rapidly made her way to the door. There she paused and looked back at us. Her father stood staring after her in helpless bewilderment. (p. 122–123)

It was inevitable, perhaps, that an anonymous Victorian would eventually produce *The Power of Mesmerism: A Highly Erotic Narrative of Voluptuous Facts and Fancies, Printed for the Nihilists* (1880), which did not warn of, but rather celebrated, its pornographic possibilities. The volume was a precursor in its own right, as hypnosis quickly became established as a standard plot element in the adult film industry in the early 20th century and continues as such into the 21st century.

As new developments in hypnosis in both England and France in the 19th century pushed traditional associations with mesmerism into the background and began to strike up new paths in the popular imagination having to do with identity, these changes were reflected in literary changes in plot and themes. Novels of fantasy, horror, and science fiction during this period that explored darker themes associated with the dissociation of identity, though not directly with hypnosis, included most famously *The Strange Case of Dr. Jekyll and Mr. Hyde* (1886) by Robert Louis Stevenson and *The Picture of Dorian Grey* (1890) by Oscar Wilde. Many authors saw in disordered identity the fantastical and humorous possibilities as well. In a short story by Arthur Conan Doyle, "The Great Keinplatz Experiment" (1894/1989), a hypnotist inadvertently and unknowingly switched his own soul with his subject:

> "I see it all. Our souls are in the wrong bodies. I am you and you are I. My theory is proved—but at what expense! Is the most scholarly mind in Europe to go about with this frivolous exterior? Oh, the labours of a life-time are ruined!" and he smote his breast in his despair.
>
> "I say," remarked the real von Hartmann from the body of the Professor, "I quite see the force of your remarks, but don't go knocking my body about like that. You received it in excellent condition, but I perceive that you have wet it and bruised it and spilled snuff over my ruffled shirtfront."
>
> "It matters little," the other said moodily. "Such as we are so must we stay. My theory is triumphantly proved, but the cost is terrible." (p. 184)

H. G. Wells picked up the theme of the apparent power of hypnosis over memory in a wry short story, "A Tale of the Days to Come" (1897/1952), which reads like a contemporary film treatment. Wells described a hypnotist in the distant future who was hired to destroy the memories of the daughter of a man who did not approve of her boyfriend, a handsome flight attendant. The client wanted his daughter to marry instead a "very good friend of mine—Bindon of the Lighting Commission—plain little man, you know, and a bit unpleasant in some of his ways, but an excellent fellow really—an excellent fellow" (p. 737). The hypnotist assured him that it could be done. He ran a brisk business altering memories and emotions for his clients:

> In those days our business was scarcely thought of. I daresay if anyone had told them that in 200 years' time a class of men would be entirely occupied in impressing things upon the memory, effacing unpleasant ideas, controlling and overcoming instinctive but undesirable impulses, and so forth, by means of hypnotism, they would have refused to believe the thing possible. Few people knew than an order made during a mesmeric trance, even an order to forget or an order to desire, could be given so as to be obeyed after the trance was over. (p. 736)

Despite the manifest powers of hypnosis, love was victorious in the end. The broken-hearted flight attendant went by chance to the same hypnotist to have his memories of the girl excised and uncovered her father's scheme. He threatened violence until the man agreed to hypnotize the girl again to bring back her memories and her love.

The Trilby and Svengali Craze

The disappearance of hypnosis from the canonical center of the medical world at the turn of the 20th century was not accompanied by a corresponding decline in attention from popular culture. The widespread cultural awareness of literary themes associated with mesmerism and hypnosis laid the groundwork for the astonishing popular success of the novel *Trilby* (1894/1992), a tragic love story by George du Maurier, in which a charming girl of Irish descent, working in Paris as an artist's model, is exploited by a foreign Jew, the nefarious Svengali.

When du Maurier's novel became the world's first "best-seller," it appealed to a public that did not need the key features to be explained. Du Maurier (1894/1992) described the hypnotist using a plethora of anti-Semitic stereotypes:

> He was very shabby and dirty and wore a red beret and a large velveteen cloak, with a big metal clasp at the collar. His thick, heavy, languid, luster-less black hair fell down behind his ears on to his shoulders, in that musician-like way that is so offensive to the normal Englishman. He had bold, brilliant black eyes, with long heavy lids, a thin, sallow face, and a beard of burnt-up black, which grew almost from his under eyelids. . . . He went by the name of Svengali, and spoke fluent French with a German accent and humorous German twists and idioms, and his voice was very thin and mean and harsh, and often broke into a disagreeable falsetto. (p. 13)

His description of Trilby, in contrast, emphasized her innocence, despite the circumstances of her life:

> My poor heroine . . . had all the virtues but one; but the virtue she lacked (the very one of all that plays the title-role, and gives its generic name to all the rest of that goodly company) was of such a kind that I have found it impossible so to tell her history as to make it quite fit and proper reading for the ubiquitous young person so dear to us all. . . . Whether it be an aggravation of her misdeeds or an extenuating circumstance, no pressure of want, no temptations of greed or vanity, had ever been factors in urging Trilby on her downward career after her first false step in that direction—the result of ignorance, bad advice (from her mother, of all people in the world), and base betrayal. (p. 41)

The novel asserted that her susceptibility to mesmerism (conflated completely with hypnosis) was a reflection of her "impressionable nature":

> "He mesmerized you; that's what it is – mesmerism! I've often heard of it, but never seen it done before. They get you into their power, and just make you do any blessed thing they please—lie, murder, steal—anything! and kill yourself into the bargain when they've done with you! It's just too terrible to think of!" . . . Cold shivers went down Trilby's back as she listened. She had a singularly impressionable nature, as was shown by her quick and ready susceptibility to Svengali's hypnotic influence. (du Maurier, 1894/1992, p. 61)

When the girl was fully under his power, Svengali caused her personality to split, and in this dissociated state, she became a star, though her talent was wholly borrowed from him:

> I will tell you a secret. There were two Trilbys. There was the Trilby you knew, who could not sing one single note in tune. She was an angel of paradise. She is now! But she had no more idea of singing than I have of winning a steeplechase at the *Croix de Berny*. She could no more sing than a fiddle can play itself! She could never tell one tune from another—one note from the next. . . . But all at once—*pr-r-r-out! presto! Augenblick!* . . . with one wave of his hand over her—with one look of his eye—with a word—Svengali could turn her into the other Trilby, his Trilby—and make her do whatever he liked . . . you might have run a red-hot needle into her and she would not have felt it. He had but to say "*Dors!*" and she suddenly became an unconscious Trilby of marble, who could produce wonderful sounds—just the sounds he wanted, and nothing else—and think his thoughts and wish his wishes—and love him at his bidding with a strange, unreal factitious love . . . just his own love for himself turned inside out—*a l'envers*—and reflected back on him, as from a mirror . . . *un echo, un simulacre, quoi! pas autre chose!* . . . Ah monsieur, that Trilby of Svengali's! I have heard her sing to kings and queens in royal palaces! as no woman ever sung before or since. (du Maurier, 1894/1992, p. 352)

No one, least of all du Maurier, was ready for the story's phenomenal success. His granddaughter, novelist Daphne du Maurier described her grandfather as embarrassed by its success and his unwanted celebrity. "He felt it all rather vulgar" (Alexander, as cited in du Maurier, 1894/1982, p. 5). By February 1895, 200,000 copies of *Trilby* had been sold, and in that year it was swiftly issued in its seventh printing. Trilby's image, her face, her feet, her name were swiftly commodified, and an explosive industry began producing Trilby hats, Trilby shoes, Trilby candy, Trilby sausages, Trilby soap, Trilby toothpaste, a Trilby waltz, and ice cream in the shape of Trilby's feet (see Jenkins, 1998).

Most extravagant, perhaps, the Emerson Drug Company in Baltimore, Maryland, in 1895 released a several-page redaction of the story entitled

"The True Tale of Trilby Tersely Told" as an advertisement for Bromo-Seltzer, complete with du Maurier-like illustrations. The story's conclusion contains a moral:

> Yes, the world is full of Trilbys,
> Just as foolish, p'r'aps as she,
> Who when troubled with a headache
> Seek some silly remedy.
> Had she spurned Svengali's offer
> When her headache made her sick,
> And just taken Bromo-Seltzer,
> 'Twould have cured her just as quick.

In April 1895, the four-act play *Trilby* based on the novel, written by English-born former journalist, Paul M. Potter, premiered at the Garden Theater on Broadway, with Virginia Harned playing the role of Trilby and Wilton Lackaye as Svengali. Potter's play ran in the United States from 1895 to 1897. When his show opened in London at the Haymarket Theater later in the summer of 1895, it ran for 254 performances starring Sir Herbert Beerbohm Tree (1853–1917) as Svengali and Dorothea Beard as Trilby. By 1896, there were 24 different stage productions being shown across the United States. Productions in London and subsequently all across England enjoyed equally spectacular success.

Contemporary reviews of both the novel and the burgeoning stage productions suggested it was the audience that had been mesmerized, both figuratively and literally (Pick, 2000, p. 22). The stage productions were cast and sets designed to replicate du Maurier's illustrations as closely as possible. Because Trilby was both described and drawn with bare and unbound feet, Dorothea Beard was supposedly cast in part because of her long and straight toes (see Jenkins, 1998, p. 239). In fact, the play was much more truthful to its illustrations than to its plot.

Almost immediately, satirical and obscene parodies of the novel appeared on both sides of the Atlantic, including *Drilby Re-Versed* by Leopold Jordan (1895), *Frilby: An Operatic Burlesque, in Two Acts* by Frederic Almy, Walter Carey, John Bartow Olmstead, and Carleton Sprague (1895), *Thrilby in Two Acts* by Joseph Herbert (1895), and *Thrillby: A Shocker in One Scene and Several Spasms* by William Muskerry and F. Osmond Carr (1896). Many of these plays were making fun of the novel and also satirizing the practice of hypnosis. In the novel, as in the straight stage productions, hypnosis was always presented as real, but in the satires, it was a preposterous fraud that was exposed in the end. In *Thrillby* (Muskerry, 1896), the character of Svengali asked the mesmerized Trilby what she could see. She replied, "Well, candidly speaking, not much, beyond an inordinate quantity of 'No. 5' grease-paint, and a shocking bad wig" (as cited in Pick, 2000, p. 43).

Not all the comedy was benign. *Drilby Re-Versed* exploited racist stereotypes in its exaggerated characterization of "Zvengali" as a rapacious Jew (see Pick, 2000, p. 96). Du Maurier had always intended that Svengali be a foreign Jew, and literary critics, in discussing the anti-Semitic aspects of the story, have often suggested that the danger he represented was intended to be racial as well as sexual (Pick, 2000, p. 145). However, the novel also reflected issues of social class and social mobility. Trilby's vulnerability to Svengali's ambitions resulted in large part because of her low class status; the three young men who were in love with Trilby could not raise her far or fast enough to save her. In her hypnotized state she was only a pretender to a higher social class.

In sum, du Maurier's novel was not exceptional for its critical social commentary or even in its comprehension of hypnosis, as it was understood by the physicians of his time. The reason for the story's phenomenal success may be that in du Maurier's use of hypnosis, he was able to crystallize the central mythology that had developed over a century and stubbornly persisted in popular cultural understandings, despite medical and scientific arguments that had directly contradicted its central assertions. Everyone was familiar with the characters or at least with the qualities that made them believable: a personally powerful and ethically dubious (male) practitioner of the hypnotic arts who took emotional and sexual advantage of a gullible and passive (female) subject. His control over her memory and identity produced genius in her, but he exploited even this and eventually destroyed her.

Du Maurier died unexpectedly in 1896 with the Trilby craze still raging. He was overwhelmed by the attention he had received and became depressed and embarrassed by the hysterical reactions of the public. On his deathbed, he was said to have attributed his own demise to *Trilby*: "Yes [*Trilby*] has been successful; but the popularity has killed me at last" (as cited in Jenkins, 1998, p. 228).

HYPNOSIS IN FILM

As early as 1897, the pioneering French filmmaker George Melies made a silent film, *Le Magnetiseur*, which showed a hypnotist putting a girl in a trance to strip her of her clothes. It was released in the United States as *A Hypnotist at Work* and in the United Kingdom as *While Under a Hypnotist's Influence*. One of the earliest short films produced in the United States was made by Thomas Edison's Edison Manufacturing Company in 1899, entitled *The Mesmerist and the Country Couple*. The *Edison Films Catalog* from 1901 provided this description of the film:

> Mr. and Mrs. Hayseed have heard of this wonderful Professor and come
> to his office. They waken him from a trance, give him a fee, and he hyp-

notizes them. The stunts they do while under his influence would make the Sphinx laugh for joy. Hayseed stands on his head, balances himself on a chair, and takes off his clothes. Mrs. Hayseed also begins to disrobe, but she goes behind a screen. Her bare arm appears over the top, and she drops her clothes on the floor. It is a hair-raising moment to guess what she's going to do next. The mystical appearances and lightning changes are managed with wonderful cleverness. (pp. 84–85)

Other early short films made by Edison included *The Hypnotist's Revenge* (1903), *The Somnambulist* (1903), and *The Criminal Hypnotist* (1909).

In 1908, Somerset Maugham wrote his novel *The Magician* (1908), in which the character of the truly evil necromancer, Oliver Haddo, was supposedly modeled on the infamous occultist Aleister Crowley. It was brought to the silent screen in 1926. The tales of Sax Rohmer, the inventor of Fu Manchu whose evil power was hypnotic in nature, were transformed into a series of B-movie adaptations, with a variety of actors in the title role, including Harry Agar Lyons, Warner Oland, Boris Karloff, Henry Brandon, Manuel Requena, Christopher Lee, and Peter Sellers. Hypnosis was a staple of the horror-film genre throughout the 20th century, beginning with the classic *Cabinet of Doctor Caligari* (1919). "Split personality" stories involving hypnosis also were recurrently popular, including for example, *Woman of Mystery* (1914), *The Other Self* (1915), *The Two Souled-Woman* (1918), *The Poison Pen* (1919), and *The Untameable* (1923).

Many of the early short films involving hypnosis were based on stage plays. "The Case of Becky," written by Edward Locke (1912) and staged by David Belasco, for instance, was filmed twice: first in 1915, starring Blanche Sweet, and then again in 1924, starring Constance Binney in the title roles. The plot centered on a young woman who was the subject of an evil stage hypnotist. She developed a demonic dissociated personality that eventually endangered her soul. A "good" hypnotist engaged into a supernatural struggle with the evil Balsamo to save her. Balsamo was the name of Alexandre Dumas's antagonist in *Memoirs of a Physician* (1847), a character based on a real-life figure, Giuseppe Balsamo, a Sicilian occultist who used the pseudonym Count Allessandro di Cagliostro. Four period films telling the tale of an evil mesmerist named Cagliostro were released in 1910, 1920, 1928, and 1929. Orson Welles played Cagliostro in a more direct Dumas adaptation, *Black Magic* (1949).

The most famous split personality at the advent of filmmaking was, of course, Trilby. And though the commodification of Trilby products had waned as the century turned, the new filmmaking technologies were swiftly used to transform stage productions to screen. The first silent film productions based on du Maurier's *Trilby* appeared before the hypnosis films of either Melies or Edison. In the United States, the short piece *Trilby and Little Billee* was made in 1896. In the same year, a *Trilby Burlesque* dance number was filmed in the United Kingdom followed by another Trilby-inspired dance, featuring the Turkish belly dancer Ella Lola (born 1883), which was filmed in the United States in 1898.

A Danish *Trilby* was produced in 1908 and an Austro-Hungarian *Trilby* in 1912. England produced silent screen versions in 1912, 1913, and then again in 1914, in which Sir Herbert Beerbohm Tree reprised his stage role of Svengali with Viva Birkett as Trilby. The 1915 version in the United States, directed by Maurice Tourneur, likewise cast a stage star, Wilton Lackaye, as Svengali, as well as Clara Kimball Young as Trilby. Another English version was produced in 1922, and in the United States in 1923 there was a successful production starring Andrée Lafayette as Trilby and Edmond Carewe as Svengali. Directed by James Young (the husband of Clara Kimball Young, who had starred as Trilby in the 1915 version), the film received rave reviews. Its innovation was to film two different endings for the story: the traditional ending in which Trilby died and an alternative happy ending, in which she survived. Trilby silent screen parodies also made it to screen, including *The Adventures of Pimple-Trilby* (1914) and *Frilby Frilled* (1916).

Germany produced Trilby adaptations in 1914 and 1927, but both were entitled *Svengali*, an artistic change that was to become a distinct trend. There was a clear reason for the change. Although the novel had focused on the misadventures of the character of Trilby, in most stage versions she was upstaged by intense performances of the evil Svengali. Increasingly, the story was retold to shift attention from Trilby to the hypnotist. The best known Svengali was John Barrymore, who starred in the 1931 *Svengali*, directed by Archie Mayo. In this version, 17-year-old Marian Marsh (1913–2006), who had been a studio extra before being cast, played Trilby. A 1955 *Svengali* starred Donald Wolfit and Hildegarde Neff, whereas a made-for-television *Svengali* (1983) starred Peter O'Toole in the title role and Jodie Foster as his rock star protégée. Three years later, Jodie Foster reprised a Trilby-like character when she murdered a sexually deviant and Svengali-like husband in *Mesmerized* (1986).

Other films made use of a Svengali and Trilby motif in their plots, sometimes involving a young musician and a domineering mentor. The *Hypnotic Violinist* (1914) and *The Seventh Veil* (1945), starring James Mason, were of this variety. Sometimes only Svengali's name makes it into a film: the Three Stooges film, *Hocus Pokus* (1949), included a stage hypnotist named Svengarlic. Countless animated children's films and television programs have included the line, "You are getting sleeeeepy," ensuring that the cultural associations with hypnosis begin early.

Screenwriters and filmmakers have frequently found humor in hypnotic possibilities, including 21st-century films such as *The Curse of the Jade Scorpion* (2001) and *Shallow Hal* (2002). Surprisingly, several big screen musicals using hypnotic themes have also been produced: In *Carefree* (1938), Fred Astaire hypnotized Ginger Rogers, in *The Court Jester* (1956) Angela Lansbury hypnotized Danny Kaye so he can swordfight with Basil Rathbone, and *On a Clear Day You Can See Forever* (Lane & Lerner, 1969), Barbra Streisand was hypnotized and regressed to a past life, inspiring her doctor to fall in love with her dissociated self, even though he did not like her primary personality.

The use of hypnosis to explore the possibility of reincarnation regularly recurs, for instance, in *The Search for Bridey Murphy* (1956), *Audrey Rose* (1977), and *Dead Again* (1991). Its therapeutic possibilities have also been frequently and variously examined, as in *Spellbound* (1945), *The Three Faces of Eve* (1957), *Sybil* (1976), *Equus* (1977), and *Coach* (1978). Hypnosis has often been used as a dramatic plot device, with or without elements of the supernatural, as in *The Magician* (1959), *The Manchurian Candidate* (1962, 2004), and *Stir of Echoes* (1999). The uncertainty and ambiguities between the psychological and the supernatural aspects of hypnosis have been displayed in different ways in both *Agnes of God* (1986) and *K-Pax* (2001). Even animal magnetism periodically comes around again. A film starring Alan Rickman based on the life of Mesmer was released in 1994, and in 2006, a version of Poe's (1845a) short story, "The Facts of M. Valdemar's Case," was released as a horror film.

Arguably, the most intensely hypnotic film of all time is Werner Herzog's apocalyptic parable, *Heart of Glass* (1976). During the production, Herzog hypnotized most of his actors before filming them, eliciting performances often described by reviewers as "trancelike." His original intention was to attempt to hypnotize the viewing audience as well. He explained his plan in an interview with film critic Roger Ebert (2005):

> I actually had the idea that I would appear on screen myself and explain that I was the director and the scenes were shot under hypnosis: "And if you are willing to see the film under hypnosis, you should follow my advice now. I will ask you to look at something like a pencil, and don't remove your eyes, and listen to my voice and follow my words and follow my instructions." And of course I would tell the audience that at the end of the film they will return to the screen and softly wake up again.

Reviews are mixed as to the film's achievement, but no one disputes that the cinematography is mesmerizing.

HYPNOSIS AS METAPHOR

When mesmerism and hypnosis have been addressed in literature and film, the imperative to entertain the readership or viewing audience seems to supersede any attempt at accurate reflection of scientific research or actual clinical practice (see Barrett, 2006). Scanning the 2 centuries of fictional narratives, certain unambiguous patterns emerge. The imagined hypnotist, more often than not, is portrayed as personally powerful, or at least highly skilled, in a sometimes heroic, sometimes nefarious, and occasionally bumbling Svengarlic manner. The hypnotic subject is depicted as a comparatively weaker character who is naive, gullible, vulnerable, usually attractive, and who has been or will be victimized at some point in the story. The hypnotic experience involves a speedy induction of a trance state that appears to be closely related to sleep. In this state, participants display a variety of nonvolitional responses and may retrieve forgotten memories of their frequently traumatic past, including memories of past lives and alien abductions. They typically experience posthypnotic amnesia and respond to other posthypnotic triggers that suggest they can be made to commit acts against their will and inclination, even without their knowledge.

All of these strongly held popular associations have proved to be without empirical basis. Research on these issues has led to remarkable consensus: (a) Hypnotists need not be personally powerful or charismatic to be effective using hypnosis; (b) suggestibility is not correlated with gullibility or weakness; (c) the experience of "being hypnotized," even when it involves the subjective experience of being in a trance, is a state unrelated to sleep; and (d) hypnotic participants do not lose their personal will, even when they feel as though they are acting without volition (see Kirsch & Lynn, 1995).

Not surprisingly, the aspects of hypnosis that are still open to contentious debate are also presented unambiguously. Story lines dealing with the use of hypnosis to retrieve forgotten memories, for example, or to get in touch with dissociated personalities generally do not linger on the substantial controversy that has raged over these topics. Apart from made-for-television movies or sensationalist television shows, doubt about the accuracy of memories recovered through hypnosis or the diagnostic reality of multiple personalities emerging during therapy arises only as a plot device in thrillers or as a result of criminal deception, not scientific controversy.

Arguably, given the chronic inaccuracies in their presentation of fact, in literature and film, mesmerism and hypnosis are more compelling as ideas than as clinical techniques and psychological theories. The aspect of hypnosis that has been most persistent in the popular consciousness is the imagined relationship between hypnotists and their subjects. Regardless of the demonstrated efficacy of autosuggestion, few Hollywood films feature characters who use self-hypnosis to alleviate cravings for cigarettes. Even the mysteries of the hypnotically induced trance state, which have captivated generations of hypnosis researchers, have not provided the key attraction to storytellers.

Instead, novelists, poets, and filmmakers have portrayed in the intimate scene of the ritual induction of hypnosis a metaphor for human relations in which persuasion, seduction, control, and power are central to the interpersonal dynamic. Shelley, Hawthorne, Melville, Dickens, and Browning all used images of mesmerism to capture the struggles between good and evil that occur when people gain power over other human beings: slave owners over slaves, men over women, captains over crew, parents over children, ministers over their flocks, those who are loved over those who love them. In the 20th century, German writer Thomas Mann used hypnosis to illuminate the abuse of political power. In his short story, "Mario and the Magician" (1930), a family on holiday in Italy witnesses the performance of a stage hypnotist whose sadistic cruelty to the local people in his audience triggers violence. This parable of fascism remains as gripping now as it was when it was written; it was staged in 1992 by the Canadian Opera Company and again in 2005 by the Center for Contemporary Opera in New York City.

Reflecting on more than 300 years of hypnotic imagery in poetry, fiction, drama, and film, it is not at all clear whether the longevity of its appeal should be cause for celebration or lament. On the one hand, because of the power of expectancies on the hypnotic experience, the perpetuation of stereotypes and misconceptions about clinical hypnosis is significantly problematic. When research participants, medical patients, and psychotherapeutic clients show up in labs, waiting rooms, and offices, their first curiosities about hypnosis are less likely to have arisen from close readings of the luminaries of hypnotic theory than from what they have gleaned from *The Three Faces of Eve* and The Three Stooges, from *The Manchurian Candidate* and *The X-Files*, from Barbra Streisand and *The Bride of Fu Manchu*. Although popular attention to hypnosis has provoked seemingly undying fascination with the technique and its attendant phenomena, practitioners face the inescapable and not insubstantial task of allaying misplaced fears and clearing up factual inaccuracies before they can begin to work.

On the other hand, we live in a world in which parents sometimes abuse the power they have over their children, and religious leaders sometimes take advantage of the influence they have over their followers, and governments sometimes manipulate their citizens into violence and war. It can be argued that the burden of having to reshape clinical expectancies is outweighed by the fact that the subject of hypnosis has inspired discussion, persistently and across the centuries, of the philosophical and ethical questions surrounding suggestibility, persuasion, and the moral responsibilities that come with power.

REFERENCES

Almy, F., Carey, W., Olmstead, J. B., & Sprague, C. (1895). *Frilby: An operatic burlesque, in two acts*. Buffalo, NY: Peter Paul.

Anonymous. (1880). *The power of mesmerism: A highly erotic narrative of voluptuous facts and fancies, printed for the Nihilists*. London: n.p.

Balzac, H. d. (1900). *Ursule Mirouet* (C. Bell, Trans.). Philadelphia: Gebbie Publishing.

Barrett, D. (2006). Hypnosis in film and television. *American Journal of Clinical Hypnosis, 49*, 13–30.

Browning, R. (1855). Mesmerism. In R. Browning, *Men and women* (pp. 70–75). London: Chapman & Hall.

Carrer, L. (2005). *Jose Custodio de Faria: Hypnotist, priest, and revolutionary*. Victoria, British Columbia, Canada: Trafford.

Coleridge, S. T. (1857) *The rime of the ancient mariner*. London: Sampson Low. (Original work published 1798)

Coleridge, S. T. (1869). *Christabel and the lyrical and imaginative poems*. London: Sampson Low. (Original work published 1816)

Dickens, C. (1838–1839). *Nicholas Nickleby*. London: Chapman & Hall.

Dickens, C. (1840–1841). Barnaby Rudge: A tale of the riots of "eighty." Serialized in *Master Humphrey's Clock*. London: Chapman & Hall.

Dickens, C. (1849–1850). *David Copperfield*. London: Bradbury & Evans.

Dickens, C. (1852–1853). *Bleak house*. London: Bradbury & Evans.

Dickens, C. (1855–1857). *Little Dorrit*. London: Bradbury & Evans.

Dickens, C. (1870). *The mystery of Edwin Drood*. London: Chapman & Hall.

Doyle, A. C. (1989). The great Keinplatz experiment. In I. Asimov, M. H. Greenberg, & C. G. Waugh (Eds.), *Isaac Asimov presents tales of the occult*. Buffalo, NY: Prometheus Books. (Original work published 1894)

Du Maurier, G. (1982). *Svengali: George du Maurier's Trilby* (P. Alexander, Ed.). London: W. H. Allen. (Original work published 1894)

Du Maurier, G. (1992). *Trilby*. New York: J. M. Dent. (Original work published 1894)

Dumas, A. (1846). *The Count of Monte Cristo*. London: Chapman & Hall.

Dumas, A. (1847). *Memoirs of a physican*. London: G. Pierce.

Ebert, R. (2005, August 28). *A conversation with Warner Herzog*. Retrieved August 24, 2008 from http://rogerebert.suntimes.com/apps/pbcs.dll/article?AID=/20050828/PEOPLE/50828001

Edison Manufacturing Company. (1901, July). The mesmerist and the country couple. *Edison Films Catalog, 105*, 84–85.

Emerson Drug Company. (1895). *The true tale of Trilby tersely told* [Pamphlet]. Baltimore, MD: Author.

Epheyre, C. (1890). *Soeur Marthe*. Paris: Ollendorff.

Flaubert, G. (1976). *Bouvard and Pecuchet: A tragic–comic novel of a bourgeois life with the dictionary of accepted ideas* (A. J. Krailsheimer, Trans.). Baltimore, MD: Penguin Classics. (Original work published 1881)

Fuller, R. C. (1982). *Mesmerism and the American cure of souls*. Philadelphia: University of Pennsylvania Press.

Hawthorne, N. (1851). *The house of seven gables*. Boston: Ticknor, Reed & Fields.

Hawthorne, N. (1852). *The blithedale romance*. Boston: Ticknor, Reed & Fields.

Herbert, J. (1895). *Thrilby in Two Acts*. New York: Rosenfield Typewriting.

Herzog, W. (Producer & Director). (1976). *Heart of Glass* [Motion picture].

James, H. (1919). Professor Fargo. In H. James, *Travelling companions: Seven shorter tales*. New York: Liveright. (Original work published 1874)

Jenkins, E. (1998). Trilby: Fads, photographers, and "over-perfect feet." *Book History, 1*, 221–267.

Jordan, L. (1895). *Drilby re-versed*. New York: G. W. Dillingham.

Kaplan, F. (1975). *Dickens and mesmerism: The hidden springs of fiction*. Princeton, NJ: Princeton University Press.

Kirsch, I., & Lynn, S. J. (1995). The altered state of hypnosis: Changes in the theoretical landscape. *American Psychologist, 50*, 846–858.

Lane, B., & Lerner, A. J. (1969). On a clear day you can see forever. On *On a Clear Day You Can See Forever* [Original Soundtrack]. New York: Columbia Records.

Locke, E. (1912). The case of Becky. *Hearst's Magazine, 22*(2), 113.

Mann, T. (1999). Mario and the magician. In F. A. Lubich (Ed.) & H. T. Lowe-Porter (Trans.), *Death in Venice, Tonio Kroger, and other writings* (pp. 185–225).

Maugham, W. S. (1908). *The magician*. London: W. Heinemann.

Melville, H. (1851). *Moby-Dick; or, the whale*. New York: Harper & Brothers.

Muskerry, W. (1896). *Thrillby, a shocker in one scene and several spasm* [sic]. New York: T. H. French.

Nadis, F. (2001). Of horses, planks, and window sleepers: Stage hypnotism meets reform, 1836–1920. *Journal of Medical Humanities, 22*, 223–245.

Pick, D. (2000). *Svengali's web: The alien enchanter in modern culture*. New Haven, CT: Yale University Press.

Poe, E. A. (1844a). Mesmeric revelation. *Columbian Magazine, 2*, 67–70.

Poe, E. A. (1844b). A tale of the ragged mountains. *Godey's Lady's Book, 28*, 177–181.

Poe, E. A. (1845a). The facts of M. Valdemar's case. *The American Review*, 561–562.

Poe, E. A. (1845b). *Mesmerism in articulo mortis: An astounding and horrifying narrative* [Pamphlet]. London: Author.

Poe, E. A. (1846). *Mesmerism, "In articulo mortis," an astounding and horrifying narrative, shewing the extraordinary power of mesmerism in arresting the progress of death* [Pamphlet]. New York: Author.

Potter, P. M. (1895). *Trilby* [Play; 208 perf.]. Garden Theatre, New York.

Shelley, P. B. (1961). The magnetic lady to her patient. In T. Hutchinson (Ed.), *The complete poetical works of Percy Bysshe Shelley* (Vol. 3, pp. 223–225). New York: Oxford University Press. (Original work published 1822)

Smith, E. (n.d.) Trilby: A burlesque of the play of the same title. *English and American Drama of the Nineteenth Century*. Microform, 12.

Spurling, H. (1998). *The unknown Matisse: A life of Henri Matisse: The early years, 1869–1908*. New York: Knopf.

Stevenson, R. L. (1886). *The strange case of Dr. Jekyll and Mr. Hyde*. London: Longmans, Green.

Stoehr, T. (1978). *Hawthorne's mad scientists: Pseudoscience and science in nineteenth-century life and Letters*. Harnden, CT: Shoe String Press.

Tatar, M. M. (1978). *Spellbound: Studies on Mesmerism and literature*. Princeton, NJ: Princeton University Press.

Thackeray, W. M. (1849–1850). *The history of Pendennis*. London: Bradbury & Evans.

Townshend, C. H. (1844). *Facts in mesmerism, or animal magnetism: With reasons for a dispassionate inquiry into it*. London: Baillerie Press.

Twain, M. (1912). *The adventures of Huckleberry Finn*. London: Harper & Brothers. (Original work published 1884)

Versluis, A. (2001). *The esoteric origins of the American Renaissance*. New York: Oxford University Press.

Wells, H. G. (1952). A story of the days to come. In H. G. Wells, *Twenty-eight science fiction stories of H. G. Wells* (pp. 730–749). New York: Dover.

Wilde, O. (1890, June 20). The picture of Dorian Grey. *Lippincott's Monthly Magazine*, 3–100.

28

TRAINING ISSUES IN HYPNOSIS

DAVID M. WARK AND PETER B. BLOOM

Training health care professionals to use hypnosis in their clinical practices or in their research laboratories is a worthwhile, yet complex, undertaking. Licensed professionals such as dentists, nonpsychiatric physicians, nurse specialists, psychiatrists, psychologists, clinical social workers, and other qualified care providers may seek training in hypnosis to provide an efficient adjunct to their healing disciplines. During training these clinicians rightfully expect that hypnotic interventions they learn will "make sense" and be consistent with their basic training in their respective fields (Bloom, 2001). Training in hypnosis generates a new and wider view on how therapy works for most clinicians (Orne, Dinges, & Bloom, 1995). Respect for the symptom and its treatment; willingness to delay obtaining insight into the "deeper causes" of the illness (Bloom, 1994); creating measurable outcomes as the goals for therapy (Haley, 1963); and understanding patients as evolving, self-generating "open systems" (von Bertalanffy, 1968) are useful perspectives for the practitioner who studies hypnosis and its uses in therapy.

This chapter is an extension of earlier works on training professionals to use hypnosis (Bloom, 1993; 2001). The principles of adult education (Bloom, 1993; Carmichael, Small, & Regan, 1972; Coggeshall, 1965; Dryer, 1962; Hawkins & Kapelis, 1993; Knowles, 1980; Rodolfa, Kraft, Reilly, &

Blackmore, 1983) were offered as the foundation of training adult professionals. In this chapter, we review a current source for instructional content about hypnosis, then briefly review some principles of adult education and of adult learning styles. On the basis of these principles, we outline our approach to designing a practical training program that integrates the content and principles into a comprehensive workshop on clinical hypnosis. In the discussion of our experience, we frame our work in a series of "how to" questions and provide our best practice-based answers. We offer suggestions to the workshop director who has to think creatively with each new training assignment. As a context for our comments we have in mind the workshops sponsored by professional organizations worldwide, such as the American Society of Clinical Hypnosis, the Society for Clinical and Experimental Hypnosis, and the International Society of Hypnosis or any of the national components, and offered to licensed health service professionals.

HOW TO CHOOSE THE CONTENT OF A HYPNOSIS WORKSHOP

Until recently, there was no internationally recognized content for hypnosis training. In 1992, Cory Hammond and Gary Elkins began an international project to define the content of professional education in clinical hypnosis (Elkins & Hammond, 1998). They queried recognized hypnosis clinicians, teachers, and scientists of all theoretical orientations. Of the 109 respondents, 31% had earned diplomate status in their various disciplines, such as the American Boards of Clinical Hypnosis. These knowledgeable and advanced participants were asked, among other questions, to recommend the number of minutes to be devoted to each of 57 topics and whether the topic should be presented at a beginning, intermediate, or advanced level. The pooled and integrated responses showed that the respondents supported instruction organized into separate 20-hour basic and intermediate programs, each with specific recommended topics. Hammond and Elkins then developed learning objectives and offered recommended content for each topic at each level. This survey with its conclusions was published as the Standards of Training in Clinical Hypnosis (SOTCH; Hammond & Elkins, 1994).

The SOTCH is divided into chapters for the introductory and intermediate levels, each encompassing 20 hours. The 15 introductory-level sessions cover topics such as definition, history, and theories (Area 1); myths and misperceptions (Area 2); assessment (Area 3); hypnotic phenomena (Area 4); principles and processes of induction and realerting (Area 5); concepts of susceptibility (Area 9); ethics (Area 14), and so forth. At the intermediate level, there are 11 areas, such as advanced and specialized inductions (Area 1), hypnosis and memory: Age regression and trauma (Area 5), and insight-oriented and exploratory hypnotic techniques (Area 9). There are also recommended sessions on hypnotic strategies for concerns such as pain, anxiety, phobias, and habit disorders.[1]

Since 1998, 20-hour workshops that follow the SOTCH are requirements for membership in both the American Society of Clinical Hypnosis and the Society for Clinical and Experimental Hypnosis, the leading organizations for health service professionals in the United States. In 2006, the International Society of Hypnosis (ISH) adopted the SOTCH for an introductory workshop at its 17th International Congress of Hypnosis in Acapulco, Mexico. Other societies, both national and local, may, of course, use other content.

While it is widely used as a source of content for training, the SOTCH is in fact a work in progress. New research and practices have developed since 1998 when the SOTCH was published. For example, in the present version, there are no objectives or recommended content for the research on hypnosis using fMRI (Maquet et al., 1999; Rainville et al., 1999; Raz, Shapiro, Fan, & Posner, 2002), nor is there mention of the developing research on "consciousness" as a significant topic other than as "altered states of consciousness" (Rossi & Rossi, 2006). Likewise, there is scant mention of the growing body of data on empirically-based treatments using hypnosis (Barabasz, Olness, Boland, & Kahn, 2010; Wark 2008). All these advances and others are being considered for a revision of the SOTCH.

HOW ADULTS LEARN

The second major category to consider when planning training, after the content, is the participant. Learners come in many categories—experience/background, professional orientation, expectations, energy level, and intelligence. In this section we consider the special characteristics of education for adults, the way that teaching can be presented, and some of the styles by which adults learn.

The Principles of Adult Education

With the content of a training workshop defined, we now consider the nature of the participants in a workshop. As mentioned, we rely heavily on the concept of adult education, or *andragogy*, as described by Knowles (1980). We believe that if new knowledge is to be integrated by mature professional

---

[1]For further discussion of the ideas presented in paragraphs 1, 2, and 4, please see the introduction to chapter 2 (Bloom, 2001) of G. D. Burrows, R. O. Stanley, and P. B. Bloom (Eds.), *International Handbook of Clinical Hypnosis*.

participants, it must be congruent with their previous professional experience. There are four major assumptions underlying andragogy: (a) Adult learners become more self-directed as they mature, so they can be more responsible and active during the training workshop; (b) adult learners have a vast repertoire of experience that must be recognized and should be called on during training; (c) adults learners who enter further education do so voluntarily and are assumed to be ready for more education; and (d) adults learners are problem-oriented, so training should help solve problems. These assumptions do not imply any necessary set of practices but rather inform an approach to the teaching–learning process.

It follows then that in a typical adult learning seminar, the entire group can be conceptualized as equal participants. The only difference is that the leader is a little more equal because of advanced knowledge and experience; the participants are more equal than the leader in knowing their own life experiences and how they will incorporate what they learn into their practices. The playing field is level, and mutual respect provides the foundation of good learning for all (Bloom, 2001).

Adult education starts when the leader begins to conceptualize the people in the classroom as "participants" rather then "students." Each participant, now valued for his or her own experience, shares in the teaching and learning. We strongly believe that training workshops that regard the participants simply as students, in which information is imparted in a somewhat authoritative manner with the expectancy that "teacher knows best" (i.e., pedagogy), are less effective and risk failure to meet their objectives of adult education and the subsequent ability of the participants to use the material presented. The leader learns as well. Most seminars with adults vary, despite standard syllabi, because of the unique contributions of the participants (Hawkins & Kapelis, 1993). These variations, within a predetermined scheduling of topics, ensure a creative context for maximal learning time and again in our experience.

Certain practices are implicit in these principles. It is appropriate for the leader to make a professional introduction and then elicit the same information from the participants: who they are, the nature of their practice, and their approach to therapy. As the workshop develops, it is also important to check on the perceived relevance of the topics with participants to ensure a continuing good fit with their individual experience and goals. Thus, the life experience to date in each member of the workshop is a crucial variable in achieving a good adult educational outcome.

The Principles of Active Learning

Another important understanding of the adult learning process comes from the work of David Kolb (1984), who investigated active learning. His ideas are applicable to development of any new skill. According to Kolb, learners, such as those in hypnosis training, go through four active steps in developing their new knowledge and skills. The first step is a learner's *concrete experience* of something new. Being induced into hypnosis would be a concrete experience. The second stage is *reflective observation* of the experience. Watching a demonstration of an induction and discussing it later would be an appropriate example. The third step is *abstract conceptualization* about the experience, that is, creating a summary or theory. At this step, the participants would at least begin to forge new personal theories and ideas about hypnosis. The final step is *active experimentation*, testing out or extending the application of the theory to new situations. This step may be taken in a small group practice session, role-playing with other participants. The four steps are repeated as an adult learns. The active experimentation leads to a new concrete experience, and the process is repeated again and again in the image of a spiral, which will be the basis of our later discussion. Of course, there is no fixed starting place to the learning. The spiraling can begin at any point and continues through the workshop.

The Concept of Adult Learning Styles

Kolb's (1984) model represents adult learning using two dimensions. One dimension explains how a learner first grasps new information. The learning can be done by concrete experience or by abstract conceptualization. This vertical dimension comprises the feeling/touching ↔ thinking axis. The other dimension defines the way learners make use of newly grasped information. Some do it by observing carefully and some by hands on testing and manipulation. This second, horizontal dimension is the looking ↔ acting axis. The two dimensions intersect each other, creating four quadrants, each defining a distinct learning style. Participants can, of course, learn no matter how the material is presented. But they all have a favorite learning style with which they feel more comfortable.

Kolb (1984) has documented these four learning styles. Some people, for example, learn best by having a concrete experience and moving to reflective observation. Kolb calls this the *diverger* style, because such learners are most comfortable taking a concrete experience and looking at it from many perspectives, brainstorming, and generating many different ideas, often original, competitive, and, thus, divergent. Such people tend to study or work in the social sciences and mental health. Another group of learners is labeled *assimilators*, people who are particularly comfortable starting with abstract conceptualizations or theories, making an observation and then reflecting on what they see. They generate an overall theory that assimilates many observations. These people tend to work as researchers or academics in math, chemistry, or economics. Another identified learning styles is the *converger*, who takes abstract conceptualizations and moves by active experimentation to produce new results. These individuals tend to work as medical specialists and technologists. Finally, Kolb cites the *accomodator*, who likes to start with concrete experience and actively experiment, often with other people, to come up with cooperative new experiences. Not surprising, accomodators often work as nurses and medical therapists.

Although the conclusions about learning style and occupation are generalizations, there are some important implications of Kolb's work for teaching hypnosis. Any group of hypnosis workshop participants is likely to have a preponderance of divergers (e.g., psychologists, social workers, mental health specialists) and convergers (e.g., physicians, dentists, nurses, health science workers). Consider how these participants best learn a fundamental skill, such as doing a hypnotic induction: Each prefers to get his or her initial learning in different ways. Convergers may be more comfortable starting with an abstract summary of the principles of induction, such as a didactic lecture on pacing and leading, and then watching a demonstration. Divergers, however, will likely be more comfortable starting with a concrete experience of a hypnotic phenomenon. They may learn better in a group induction, with a suggestion for catalepsy. Then both divergers and convergers transform what they learn through reflective observation or small group practice. So both a skillful induction demonstration and discussion is important to meet the needs of participants with different styles in a workshop. The same considerations apply to the way diverse participants learn other topics: to assess susceptibility, elicit hypnotic phenomena, frame suggestions, teach a client to do self-hypnosis, and so forth.

One corollary of Kolb's notion is that the leader, as well as the participants, will have a personal learning style. Some leaders, for example, will be more comfortable giving an academic lecture on the concept of susceptibility as an individual difference. Others may prefer to use an experiential exercise, such as the Stanford Hypnotic Clinical Scale for Adults (Morgan & Hilgard, 1978–1979), to demonstrate the range of susceptibility. The same material can be introduced didactically or experientially; but there is no best way to do it. Of course, even though there may be a preponderance of participants with one learning style, all four will be represented in the workshop. One clear implication is that instructors should explicitly plan to present instruction using all the styles so that each learner will be comfortable.

This suggestion can also be applied within a session of instruction. For example, consider an abstract conceptual presentation on principles of induction. One instructional element is to explain the concept of *pacing* and propose as an example that operators track some physiological indicator, such as breathing. This would be an example of teaching by abstract conceptualization. Then, to extend the impact, an instructor can give an in-seat exercise for active experimentation. Participants can be asked to find a partner and select the role of either breather or watcher. The *breather* inhales and exhales normally, while mentally counting each cycle; the *watcher* silently counts each cycle. At the end of 1 minute, the members of each pair compare counts, which should be close. Then the participants swap roles and repeat the process. The participants can report their results, and the instructor responds and gives suggestions for better observation. The combination of abstract conceptualization, followed quickly by active experimentation, gives more participants a chance to learn the notion of pacing in a way that matches their favorite style.

HOW INFORMATION CAN BE ORGANIZED FOR ADULT LEARNING: THE SPIRAL CURRICULUM

After the content of instruction in a workshop has been chosen and the learners specified, the next question for a trainer to consider is how to organize and present that material in a way that supports various adult learning styles and facilitates transfer to professional practice. In other words, it is important to consider how to combine the principles of andragogy and learning style to produce an optimal training package for hypnosis.

We recommend what we call a *spiral curriculum* (Wark & Kohen, 2002). We assume that when new concepts are presented, participants' understandings are neither complete nor permanent; so material should be repeated. But for each repetition, the content is presented with more associations and more complexity. Each repetition can be thought of as a rising spiral: starting low and rising higher and higher, encompassing more and more. The spiral is repeated in as many levels as are appropriate, as the participants learn. The curriculum is designed to reach participants regardless of learning style, so there should be a combination of experience, demonstration, abstraction, and practice at each level; hence, the spiral curriculum.

Although the spiral has an educational focus, it is grounded in some well-known aspects of hypnosis. First, consider the basic principles of pace and lead. The group leader should *pace* participants by starting where they are, using their appropriate learning style. For some, starting with a concrete experience, such as a group trance, is appropriate. For others, an abstract conceptual approach, stressing history and theory, is a better place to start. In the SOTCH organization, the first topic encompasses the definition, history, and theories of hypnosis, but that does not mean it has to be presented as a workshop opener in every case. Indeed, there is good reason for presenting history and theory toward the end of the workshop, after the participants have learned something about hypnosis. The choice can be made after considering the preferences of all the participants in the class.

The hypnotic principle of *leading* is applied as the spiral workshop continues, offering the participants chances to practice and consider new applications. Finally, the instructor uses the principle of *utilization* to encourage the participants to strengthen their new skills and transfer them to outside practice. Each of the participants will develop in his or her own way. As an example of the spiral curriculum, consider Figure 28.1, outlining the schedule for an international congress in 2006. Notice how the spiral develops over time, systematically flowing through the stages of active learning.

Day 1 training models the basic notions of fixation of attention, induction, deepening, and alerting. In this case, the program is oriented toward divergers, those who prefer concrete experience before reflective observation. In this schedule, the participants start with a concrete experience of hypnotic phenomena. Specifically, they experience induction and suggestion for hands moving together as if magnetized, a regression to a safe place, and then realerting. The results are discussed and reflected on and the principles of induction are explained, and then there is another experiential exercise. After that, there is a demonstration of induction for more reflective observation. Next, summary presentations on the principles of induction are presented so the participants can develop their own abstract ideas of how hypnosis works. The day ends with a small group exercise in which the goals are to actively experiment with induction and realerting.

Day 2 is designed to go around the spiral one step higher into the hypnotic experience, the deepening of hypnosis. Participants start with some abstract conceptualizations of susceptibility. In that way, the curriculum paces the assimilators, who like to start with theory. The Day 1 concepts of induction and realerting are reviewed in the discussion. Some exercises are then done on techniques of deepening, and participants are given a chance to reflect on the process. With that background, the participants get didactic presentations on several applications, in this case, ego strength, stress management, and habit control. This is designed to integrate the material they have learned previously and to ensure it makes sense in a workshop small group practice. Day 2 ends with a review and then an active experimentation practice in induction and realerting, adding the new step of deepening.

Day 3 takes the spiral one level higher by adding techniques for hypnotic suggestion. In that context, participants get some didactic instruction on hypnotizability scales and then a demonstration of the Stanford Hypnotic Clinical Scale for Adults scale, which provides a variety of suggestions to produce hypnotic phenomena, such as ideomotor response, age regression, and hypnotic amnesia (Morgan & Hilgard, 1978–1979). Didactic material on manag-

SOTCH area	Topic	Content of instruction	Time (minutes)
		Day 1 Induction and realerting	
4	Welcome, introductions	Explain spiral model, obtain informed consent to induce hypnosis	30
5	Hypnotic phenomena	Group induction: eye closure, hands together, safe place regression, realert	30
4	Principles of Induction 1	Steps to facilitate hypnosis: expectation, fix attention, pace and lead, suggest, alert	30
6	Hypnotic phenomena	Group induction: eye fixation, catalepsy, alert, discuss	30
5	Demonstration of inductions	Demonstration and explanation	50
5	Principles of Induction 2	Reversed effort, positive suggestions, trance ratification, etc.	55
5	Principles of Induction 3	Review induction and alerting. Instructions for small group practice	15
8	Small group practice 1	Induction—realerting	75
		Day 2 Induction, deepening, and realerting	
9	Susceptibility 1	Hypnotic susceptibility and stages of hypnosis	30
9	Susceptibility 2	Techniques of deepening	45
10	Self-hypnosis:	How and what to teach	45
15	Application of hypnosis	Ego strengthening	45
15	Application of hypnosis	Hypnosis for stress management	45
15	Application of hypnosis	Hypnosis for habit control	45
5	Principles of induction	Review induction, deepening, realerting. Instructions for small group practice	15
8	Small Group Practice 2	Induction—deepening—testing depth—realerting	75
		Day 3 Induction, deepening, suggestions and realerting	
13	Introduction to scales	Advantages, limitations, and examples	40
7	Eliciting phenomena	The Stanford Adult Scale with 6 volunteers to demonstrate range of phenomena	40
2	Myths and misperceptions	Related to experiences in the practice exercises	40
12	Managing resistance	Resistance variables and appropriate therapeutic techniques	50
5	Principles of suggestion	Observation, utilization, direct versus indirect suggestions; examples	55
5	Orientation to small group	Review suggestions for small group practice	15
8	Small Group Practice 3	Induction—deepening—testing—suggesting phenomena—realerting	75
		Day 4 Integrated hypnosis	
11	Treatment planning	Integrating mental health and medical/dental perspective	120
15	How Dr. X does hypnosis	Personal reflections from a senior practitioner	35
1	History and theory	An overview related to the workshop experience	35
14	Ethics, certification	Concerns for your future and professional practice	
Total time			20 hours

Note. SOTCH = Standards of Training in Clinical Hypnosis.

Figure 28.1. Spiral curriculum for an introductory hypnosis workshop.

ing resistance comes next as background for instruction on how to frame hypnotic suggestions. The third small group practice is designed to use all of the material that had been presented at an earlier stage or lower spiral and includes induction, deepening, and suggestions to produce hypnotic phenomena.

Day 4 is focused on integrating the previous three spiral levels. Notice that the history of hypnosis and theory is presented at this point, after the participants have had a chance to learn background material that makes the history and theory more meaningful. Notice also that this is the part of the workshop when the participants connect with a senior practitioner who can model how to apply the new skills they have learned.

HOW PRACTICE GROUPS ARE PLANNED AND USED

The use of small group practice sessions is a fundamental part of all hypnosis training. Anecdotally, the group experience is often reported as having the greatest impact of any contact between a participant and a group leader in the whole workshop. In fact, most participants express their wish that there had been more practice time, so it is important that the practice facilitators be well prepared for the role. They should be seasoned clinicians, who know how to induce hypnosis, shape suggestions, and realert participants from hypnosis. In addition, they should be trained to help professionals who are strong in their own training to help them to add hypnosis to their skill set. Indeed, research has demonstrated that a facilitator with systematic training in leading small groups followed by 1 or 2 years experience leading groups produces a much better learning experience for the participants than a facilitator with many years of hypnotherapy experience but no leadership training.

HOW SMALL GROUP FACILITATORS CAN BE TRAINED

We offer some guidelines for training small group facilitators. First, the candidates for training should be seasoned practitioners, with several years of direct experience using hypnosis. During the facilitator training, they should have an opportunity to reflect on their own learning, including time to remember their own early training in the use of hypnosis. This reflection provides a basis for new learning and empathy that will be integrated into leading their small groups. The facilitator should also spend some time reviewing the concept of adult education and the stages of active learning as summarized in this chapter.

In addition, some time should be spent discussing the structure of the group practice activity to be used as part of the workshop. The actual structure varies from setting to setting. One model of small group training assumes that pairs of participants will alternate role-playing as operator and subject. That is, in a class of 10 participants, there will be 5 pairs; one member of the pair will be the subject, the other the operator. The role-playing takes place simultaneously with the facilitator observing, keeping the pairs on time, and intervening as needed. This system is efficient because one instructor can work with an unlimited number of participants.

However, we prefer an alternate structure if the number of participants is not overly large and if time permits. This alternate model assumes that all of the participants as a group will observe a pair of participants engaged in role-play induction and realerting. That is, in a class of 10 participants, 2 will be practicing and 8 will be observing the interaction. The facilitator leads a discussion of what transpires. The person who started as operator then becomes a subject, and a new operator takes over. Everyone observes the whole process. The observing participants are learning by reflective observation, whereas the role players are in active experimentation. We recommend this model for two reasons. First, the facilitator's wisdom becomes a relevant part of the learning for every participant. Second, there is much smaller chance of an untoward reaction or negative side effect. For example, the facilitator can be there to make sure that realerting takes place completely.

There should also be some instruction on the basics of small group dynamics. Participants enter with some anxiety about their performance. Indeed, some may feel that their professional competence is being judged, so the facilitator should learn to recognize the signs of anxiety that work against comfortable learning. One of the most common defenses by participants is to request that the facilitator "show us one more time" by modeling an induction. The result is to relieve the participants of their personal practice and leave less time for individual practice and experimentation. A solution to this example of participant hesitancy is to encourage the facilitators to take a few introductory minutes at the beginning of each practice session to tell the participants that there will be no demonstrations and that all discussions will occur in response to the participants' practice experience. Such remarks also reduce anxiety by giving some clear structure to the practice sessions.

Small group facilitators should be instructed in how to move participants through the stages of adult learning during the processing role-play. For example, when participants are processing an induction, the facilitator can ask, "What did you see?" (i.e., reflective observation). The next question could then be, "What do you think is happening?" (i.e., abstract conceptualization). And, of course, the next question might be, "How would you respond?" or "What would you do differently?" (i.e., active experimentation). In other words, the facilitator can learn how to use the small group exercises to move all the participants through the learning stages.

Finally, in accordance with the general principles of active adult learning, there should be role-play practice sessions in which the participants actively experiment with being participants and facilitators. For an extensive and comprehensive overview and training model curriculum, see Wark and Kohen (1998).

HOW PRACTICE GROUPS ARE INTEGRATED INTO THE SPIRAL CURRICULUM

Notice in Figure 28.1 how the small group exercises function in the spiral curriculum. At Spiral Level 1, the concepts of induction, pacing, leading, and informing clients are introduced. There are lectures, exercises, and demonstration of induction. Some trainers suggest only one induction at this point, whereas some offer two or three to demonstrate a range of options. Eventually, the participants get a chance for active experimentation in a supervised practice group, in which participants get time to role-play as operator and client. There are specific goals for each small group practice session. Specifically, the goals for Spiral Level 1 are as follows:(a) Establish rapport with a role-play client, (b) do an induction using one of the techniques demonstrated in the large group sessions, (c) realert from hypnosis, and (d) receive and give feedback on the experience.

At Spiral Level 2, earlier concepts are reviewed and practiced, and the concept of deepening is presented and used in the second small group practice session, again with explicit goals, which include induction, deepening, and then realerting, in the following sequence: (a) Establish rapport with a role-play client, (b) do an induction using one of the techniques demonstrated in the large group sessions, (c) deepen the hypnosis using a technique demonstrated in the large group session, (d) test for depth of hypnosis, (e) realert from hypnosis, and (f) receive and give feedback on the experience.

Finally, in Spiral Level 3, certain hypnotic phenomena are discussed and demonstrated. In the third small group, the participants again practice induction and deepening but add an exercise in eliciting at least one advanced hypnotic phenomenon. And again they get feedback, in the sequence that follows: (a) Establish rapport with a role-play client; (b) do an induction using one of the techniques demonstrated in the large group sessions; (c) deepen the hypnosis using a technique demonstrated in the large group session; (d) test for depth of hypnosis; (e) foster the transition and suggest one or more phenomena, using hypnotic language; (f) realert from hypnosis; (g) receive and give feedback on the experience.

Then, at Spiral Level 4, techniques such as introducing hypnosis to clients, susceptibility testing, treatment planning, formulating suggestions, and managing resistance are presented. With the background from the first four spirals, students are well prepared to consider ideas such as self-hypnosis and specific techniques for presenting problems.

HOW HYPNOSIS TRAINING CAN BE EVALUATED

Evaluation of introductory hypnosis workshops is a complex topic. One issue is testing the participant's grasp of fact and concepts. Often, this didactic material has to be accessed to meet the requirements for continuing education credits. The usual way of constructing this evaluation (i.e., multiple-choice, true/false items) is not covered in this chapter. An excellent source is Haladyna, Downing, and Rodriguez (2002).

A second issue for evaluation is the participant's behavioral performance of skills such as observation, pacing, leading, deepening, and realerting. These skills can best be evaluated in the context of an active experimentation group session. Indeed, by using a checklist such as that in Figure 28.2, an observer or the facilitator can give the role-playing operator immediate feedback and use that as a springboard for discussion.

A third issue is the subjective evaluation of the small group process by the participants. Do they believe they have acquired the rudiments of hypnosis from the small group session? Have the participants absorbed their training, and can they apply it properly? That is, do they think they can transfer the skills they have gained from the training back to their professional life? That assessment can be made from items such as those in Figure 28.3.

A fourth issue is the evaluation of the practice group facilitators. Have they absorbed the material they were exposed to in the training session? Do they understand the structure of the small group and how it relates to the overall spiral well enough to explain the session objectives to the participants? Do they structure time so that everyone has a chance to practice? Can the participants use the feedback that they received in the small group? Perhaps most important, did they help the participants learn about hypnosis? That general line of assessment can be made using items such as those in Figure 28.4.

Another target for evaluation is the teaching faculty. They deserve valid and reliable feedback on their efforts. Generic or global items are of little value. They may give some ego satisfaction to the instructor who gets the highest rating for workshop, but they do not help an instructor improve skills nor do they guide the workshop director to find ways to raise the level of the teaching faculty. We think the best way to evaluate instructors is to tie the evaluation to the measurable objectives for each lesson. If the objective is to perform a catalepsy induction, can the participants do so after the instructor has lectured and demonstrated it? If the objective is to list three types of hypnosis theory,

Techniques for developing good rapport

Yes___ No___ Operator exchanges names with subject.
Yes___ No___ Operator asks about favorite relaxing places (comfort).
Yes___ No___ Operator asks about contact lenses, images to avoid (safety).
Yes___ No___ Operator uses the client's primary representation system (i.e., visual, auditory, kinesthetic).

Visual contact

___ Approximate % of time eyes oriented to client during induction.

Voice

Yes___ No___ Pauses paced to subject's breathing.

Pacing physiological response

___ Approximate % of comments that refer to observable behavior.
Yes___ No___ Comments on relaxation are paced with exhalation.

Leading suggestions

Yes___ No___ Suggests learner images a safe place.
Yes___ No___ Suggests appropriate visual imagery (e.g., "You may see . . . ").
Yes___ No___ Suggests appropriate auditory imagery (e.g., "You may hear . . . ").
Yes___ No___ Suggests appropriate kinesthetic imagery (e.g., "You may feel . . . ").

Realert choice

Yes___ No___ Operator directs realerting by suggestions paced to inhalation.
Yes___ No___ Operator suggests subject direct the realerting process.
Yes___ No___ Subject fully alerted and oriented.

Figure 28.2. Checklist for small group practice induction and realerting.

Circle the number that describes your reaction to this practice session.

1. By the end of this practice session, I had learned

1   2   3   4   5   6   7

A little new information   Some new information   A lot of new information
about hypnosis   about hypnosis   about hypnosis

2. By the end of this practice session, I was able to use the new skills

1   2   3   4   5   6   7

Not satisfactorily for me   Satisfactorily for me   Very satisfactorily for me

3. By the end of this practice session, I felt

1   2   3   4   5   6   7

Low confidence about   Usual confidence about   High confidence about
my ability to use   my ability to use   my ability to use
hypnosis in my practice   hypnosis in my practice   hypnosis in my practice

Figure 28.3. Evaluation of the small group practice sessions.

Circle a number that describes how your small group practice facilitator did the following:

1. Explained the session objectives

| 1 | 2 | 3 | 4 | 5 | 6 | 7 |

Did not explain   Partially explained   Completely explained

2. Gave feedback to us

| 1 | 2 | 3 | 4 | 5 | 6 | 7 |

Few learners got feedback   Most learners got feedback   Every learner got feedback

3. Helped us give feedback to each other

| 1 | 2 | 3 | 4 | 5 | 6 | 7 |

Few learners got feedback   Most learners got feedback   Every learner got feedback

4. Made sure we had time to practice

| 1 | 2 | 3 | 4 | 5 | 6 | 7 |

Few learners practiced   Most learners practiced   Every learner practiced

Figure 28.4. Evaluation of the small group facilitators.

can the participants do that? It is also desirable to arrange feedback on specific teaching skills. Is the instructor talking too fast or too slow for most of the students? Does the instructor give too many or too few examples? Are there too many main ideas without appropriate illustration and example? The results of these questions can provide useful feedback. At the end of each session, students can be asked to evaluate how well the instructor met the objectives and how the instructor did on specific presentation items. Figure 28.5 gives examples of evaluation from a workshop on alert hypnosis.

CONCLUSION

Training in hypnosis rests on several theoretical and practical foundations. Adult education (i.e., andragogy) is strikingly different from preadult education (i.e., pedagogy). Preadult students have become the adult participants in a group learning experience with all their life experiences to date determining what will be learned and what will be discarded from the workshop presentations. In addition to these differences, the learning styles of adults differ substantially from one adult to another and must be acknowledged

I'm not sure I know how to do it at all	I can do it but not well	I can do it somewhat	I can do it adequately	I can do it well	I can do it very well
0	1	2	3	4	5

Using the above definitions, circle a number from 0 to 5 for each objective to indicate how well the speaker prepared you to meet it.

Objective		How well you can meet it				
1. Enter alert hypnosis.	0	1	2	3	4	5
2. Deepen alert hypnosis.	0	1	2	3	4	5
3. Listen while in alert hypnosis.	0	1	2	3	4	5
4. Teach a client to enter and use alert hypnosis.	0	1	2	3	4	5

Circle a number to indicate how you rate each of the instructor characteristics listed below:

	For me too slow		For me just right		For me too fast
Speaker's rate of delivery	1	2	3	4	5

	Too few		Just right		Too many
Important ideas in the session	1	2	3	4	5

	Too few		Just right		Too many
Teaching examples in the session	1	2	3	4	5

	Too few		Just right		Too many
Practice exercises in the session	1	2	3	4	5

Figure 28.5. Instructor feedback for alert hypnosis: Theory and applications.

and worked with simultaneously in a continuing education program, such as a workshop on learning how to use hypnosis in one's practice or laboratory. Finally, the repetitive spiral curriculum offers a practical approach to conveying new knowledge and skills to adult professionals who come to learn better ways to solve problems in their clinical practices and research laboratories.

We believe that by embracing these concepts, clinicians and researchers leading introductory, intermediate, and advanced workshops in hypnosis will more effectively impart useful knowledge that will actually be used by participants from different disciplines in their professional work. We also believe that, if done well, training licensed professionals in hypnosis creates a solid core of colleagues who are then prepared to take advantage of and use the advanced material presented throughout this volume. In fact, by describing these practical aspects of our training workshops with thoughtful course outlines and obligatory ongoing feedback, we hope we have contributed to the betterment of our field. Finally, although we believe that the use of hypnosis remains in its infancy in mainstream health care, our hope is that we have contributed to its eventual maturity.

REFERENCES

Barabasz, A. F., Olness, K., Boland, R., & Kahn, S. (2010). *Medical hypnosis primer: Clinical and research evidence*. New York: Routledge/Taylor & Francis

Bloom, P. B. (1993). Training issues in hypnosis. In J. Rhue, S. J. Lynn, & I. Kirsch (Eds.), *Handbook of clinical hypnosis* (pp. 673–690). Washington, DC: American Psychological Association.

Bloom, P. B. (1994). Is insight necessary for successful treatment? *American Journal of Clinical Hypnosis, 36,* 172–174.

Bloom, P. B. (2001). Training in hypnosis. In G. D. Burrows, R. O. Stanley, & P. B. Bloom (Eds.), *International handbook of clinical hypnosis* (pp. 19–32). New York: Wiley.

Carmichael, H. T., Small, S. M., & Regan, P. E. (1972). *Prospects and proposals: Lifetime learning for psychiatrists*. Washington, DC: American Psychiatric Association.

Coggeshall, L. T. (1965). *Planning for medical progress through education*. Evanston, IL: Association of American Medical Colleges.

Dryer, B. V. (1962). Lifetime learning for physicians. *Journal of Medical Education, 37,* 1–334.

Elkins, G. R., & Hammond, D. C. (1998). Standards of training in clinical hypnosis: Preparing professionals for the 21st century. *American Journal of Clinical Hypnosis, 41,* 55–64.

Ginandes, C., Brooks, P., Sando, W., Jones, C., & Aker, J. (2003). Can medical hypnosis accelerate postsurgical wound healing? Results of a clinical trial. *American Journal of Clinical Hypnosis, 45,* 333–351.

Haladyna, T. M., Downing, S. M., & Rodriguez, M. C. (2002). A review of multiple-choice item-writing guidelines for classroom assessment. *Applied Measurement in Education, 15,* 309–334.

Haley, J. (1963). *Strategies of psychotherapy*. New York: Grune & Stratton.

Hammond, D. C., & Elkins, G. R. (1994). *Standards of training in clinical hypnosis*. Bloomingdale, IL: American Society of Clinical Hypnosis Press.

Hawkins, R. M. F., & Kapelis, L. (1993). Teaching hypnosis: The andragogy and direct-teaching models. *Australian Journal of Clinical and Experimental Hypnosis, 21,* 37–43.

Knowles, M. S. (1980). The modern practice of adult education: From pedagogy to andragogy (Rev. ed.). Chicago: Follett.

Kolb, D. A. (1984). *Experiential learning: Experience as the source of learning and development*. Englewood Cliffs, NJ: Prentice-Hall.

Lang, E. V., Benotsch, E. G., Fick, L. J., Lutgendorf, S., Berbaum, M. L., Berbaum, K. S., et al. (2000, April 29). Adjunctive nonpharmacological analgesia for invasive medical procedures: A randomised trial. *The Lancet, 355*, 1486–1490.

Maquet, P., Faymonville, M. E., Degueldre, C., Delfiore, G., Franck, G., Luxen, A., & Lamy, M. (1999). Functional neuroanatomy of hypnotic state. *Biological Psychiatry, 45*, 327–33.

Morgan, A., & Hilgard, J. (1978–1979). The Stanford Hypnotic Clinical Scale for Adults. *The American Journal of Clinical Hypnosis, 21*, 134–147.

Orne, M. T., Dinges, D., & Bloom, P. B. (1995). Hypnosis. In H. I. Kaplan & B. J. Sadock (Eds.), *Comprehensive textbook of psychiatry* (pp. 1807–1821). Baltimore, MD: Williams & Wilkins.

Rainville, P., Hofbauer, R. K., Paus, T., Duncan, G. H., Bushnell, M. C., & Price, D. D. (1999). Cerebral mechanisms of hypnotic induction and suggestion. *Journal of Cognitive Neuroscience, 11*, 110–125.

Raz, A., & Shapiro, T. (2002). Hypnosis and neuroscience: A cross talk between clinical and cognitive research. *Archives of General Psychiatry, 59*, 85–90.

Raz, A., Shapiro, T., Fan, J., & Posner, M. (2002). Hypnotic suggestion and the modulation of Stroop interference. *Archives of General Psychiatry, 59*, 1155–1161.

Rodolfa, E. R., Kraft, W. A., Reilly, R. R., & Blackmore, S. H. (1983). The status of research and training in hypnosis at APA accredited clinical/counseling psychology internship sites: A national survey. *International Journal of Clinical and Experimental Hypnosis, 31*, 284–292.

Rossi, E. L., & Rossi, K. L. (2006). The neuroscience of observing consciousness and mirror neurons in therapeutic hypnosis. *American Journal of Clinical Hypnosis, 48*, 263–78.

von Bertalanffy, L. (1968). *General system theory*. New York: Braziller.

Wark, D. M. (2008). What can we do with hypnosis? A brief note. *American Journal of Clinical Hypnosis, 51*(1), 30–36.

Wark, D. M., & Kohen, D. P. (1998). Facilitating facilitators' facilitation: Experience with a model for teaching leaders of hypnosis practice groups. *American Journal of Clinical Hypnosis, 41*, 75–81.

Wark, D. M., & Kohen, D. P. (2002). A spiral curriculum for hypnosis training. *American Journal of Clinical Hypnosis, 45*, 119–128.

29

HYPNOSIS AND MEMORY: THEORY, LABORATORY RESEARCH, AND APPLICATIONS

GIULIANA MAZZONI, MICHAEL HEAP, AND ALAN SCOBORIA

The complex and intriguing relationship between hypnosis and memory started to develop more than a century ago, when psychiatrists and therapists began to use hypnosis as a tool to help patients recover memories of traumatic childhood events, which were considered the cause of adult psychological or psychiatric symptoms. Janet (1889/1973) was one of the first therapists to conjecture that hypnosis and its ancillary technique, age regression, could help uncover traumatic childhood images and memories. Freud (1896/1962) used hypnosis and age regression when he still believed that current symptoms were created by real childhood traumatic experiences.

Following this lead, hypnosis has received considerable attention over the years as a method of enhancing memory reports. Freud's initial view, that memories recovered in therapy represent real early experiences, was resurrected in the second part of the 20th century by therapists claiming that memory work conducted in hypnosis helps to bring memories of actual traumatic episodes into awareness. Many modern psychodynamic therapists still consider hypnosis a viable tool for uncovering memories, unconscious phenomena, and personality dynamics. Haward and Ashworth (1980) reported hypnosis can "induce a mental state which facilitates recall and enables the subject to produce more information than he would be able to provide in the so-called waking state" (p. 471). This process has been popularized in books such as *Rebel Without a Cause* (Lindner, 1944), the story of a psychopath who through age regression was able to identify the initial trauma responsible for his pathology.

For the lay person, the belief that hypnosis provides substantial help to memory remains rather popular. For instance, Whitehouse, Orne, Orne, and Dinges (1991) found that 93% of college-age participants reported that hypnosis enhances memory retrieval. More than a decade later, Green (2003) reported that, on average, college students are in reasonably close agreement with the statement that "Hypnosis can make subjects remember things that they could not normally remember."

As hypnosis has become viewed as a useful and effective tool to enhance memory, it has been used not only in therapeutic practice but also in the forensic arena to help enhance witnesses' memories. At the same time, research has uncovered a variety of potential negative effects of hypnosis, which can impair the accuracy of what is remembered, to the point of inducing false memories of events that had not happened.

Hypnosis is also well known for being an effective way of reducing recall by inducing amnesia of experienced events. The phenomenon of posthypnotic amnesia is one component of hypnotic suggestibility and represents one of the criteria by which individuals with a high level of hypnotic suggestibility are screened from the rest of the population. The ability to forget on request, although present in only a small minority of the population, represents a rather intriguing aspect of the human mind. Some recent experimental work on inhibitory processes in memory (Anderson & Green, 2001) has garnered attention for showing that intentional forgetting occurs. A better understanding of posthypnotic amnesia can help toward a better understanding not just of hypnosis but also of memory mechanisms responsible for inhibition and suppression. This complex three-legged relationship between hypnosis and memory is the object of this chapter, which illustrates the state of the research in these three areas.

We review some of the extensive amount of research that over the years has demonstrated that hypnosis represents a dangerous technique when used to try to resurrect memories of the past. Some claim that the dangers are limited to neutral autobiographical and more generally episodic memories. Given the mixed evidence on whether traumatic autobiographical memories are encoded and/or retrieved differently from nontraumatic memories, the review does not take a specific stance on this topic. Even if these memories are encoded differently, the evidence for the danger of using hypnosis as a memory aid for nontraumatic neutral or mildly unpleasant autobiographical events is unequivocal. Conversely, the usefulness of hypnosis as an aid to remembering traumatic experiences has not been demonstrated. In this chapter, we also review the research on hypnosis and forgetting. In much of the recent work in this area, forgetting is hypothesized to be due to inhibition. This contention remains controversial, however, with some researchers claiming that inhibitory processes in memory have not yet been convincingly demonstrated. In this chapter, we do not take a stance on this issue either.

MEMORY ENHANCEMENT

It is often claimed that hypnosis can be used to enhance performance in a range of behavioral and cognitive skills and tasks. The simplest procedures entail hypnotizing the person and giving him or her injunctions and suggestions aimed at promoting greater competence, strength, motivation, efficiency, concentration, and so on. Memory is one area of human performance that has received particular attention. Indeed, there is a long-held popular belief that simply recalling events while hypnotized, without motivating instructions or suggestions, yields more detailed and accurate memories than when recalling the same events without hypnosis.

In laboratory investigations of this claim, the material to be recalled may be autobiographical events, sometimes from the person's remote past, or new material selected by the investigator, such as filmed scenes, spoken stories, and word lists, presented prior to hypnosis. In addition to hypnosis and nonhypnosis conditions and the meaningfulness of the material, other variables and conditions investigated have been hypnotizability, the presence of arousal or stress, the inclusion or exclusion of motivating instructions, and the length of time between exposure to the material and recall.

In addition to the research we have discussed, which is summarized shortly, there is the procedure known as *age regression*, whereby participants, including patients, are asked to "go back in time" (e.g., as the hypnotist counts down from their present age) and "relive" some childhood event. Sometimes, notably in the clinical setting, this would involve memories in the womb and beyond. The experience can be profound and vivid for many people. Some early research suggested that, unlike their attempts to recall the events in question in "the waking state," participants undergoing age regression are able to recall a wealth of accurate information, much of which they had "forgotten." For example in a well-known study, True (1949) claimed that when they were age regressed, the participants were able to name the day of the week on which a childhood birthday took place.

Subsequent, better-controlled studies have failed to replicate these findings; the reader is referred to the influential review of Nash (1987) for a summary of this research. It suffices to say that there is no convincing evidence that participants in any real psychological or physical sense regress to an earlier stage of development or that accurate childhood memories are uniquely retrieved by this procedure.

Hypnotic hypermnesia for more recent events has been the subject of investigation for many years now. In a review of laboratory studies and accounts of forensic cases in which hypnosis has been used to attempt to enhance eyewitness recall, Relinger (1984) concluded that hypnosis is more likely to facilitate the *free recall* of meaningful material (e.g., live or filmed scenes such as simulated crimes) than material such as word lists or nonsense syllables. For example, in one of the more contemporary studies in Relinger's review, De Piano and Salzburg (1981) examined recall of three films: one "neutral" (i.e., horses running), one designed to induce sexual arousal, and a third designed to induce "traumatic arousal" (i.e., a lobotomy). Recall was better with a hypnotic induction than with task-motivating instructions alone. However, these findings were not modified by the participants' level of arousal. A later study by Stager and Lundy (1985) demonstrated enhanced recall by hypnotized, highly susceptible individuals for a film presented a week previously. Some studies have reported corresponding improvements in the recall of less meaningful material; for example, Shields and Knox (1986) used word lists and obtained the effect for words processed at the "deep" level as opposed to the "shallow" level. *Deeply processed words* are those for which the subject is instructed to make a semantic decision when the word is presented (e.g., rating how pleasant or unpleasant it is). In the case of *shallow processing*, the decision is based on some structural attribute, such as whether the word contains a certain letter.

Wagstaff and Mercer (1993) were unable to replicate Shields and Knox's findings. Their experiment differed in a number of respects from Shields and Knox's, notably in that participants were not informed that the experiment was an investigation of hypnosis. Wagstaff and Mercer expressed a concern that has often been raised about studies of performance enhancement in hypnotized participants, namely that if they are aware that hypnosis is under investigation they may hold back on their performance until the hypnosis condition.

In a meta-analysis of 24 studies, Steblay and Bothwell (1994) found evidence for superior recall in hypnosis in response to neutral questions when a delay of at least 24 hours between event and recall attempt was imposed. However, the authors concluded that this finding must be tempered by two major considerations: (a) Confidence intervals for these effects were large and encompassed zero, suggesting considerable unaccounted variability, and (b) any benefit for hypnosis was limited to delays of 1 to 2 days. Even a 1-week delay reversed the effect to favour control participants. When considering inaccurate recollections, Steblay and Bothwell reported that relative to waking conditions, hypnosis produces more recall errors, more intrusions of uncued errors, and higher levels of memories for false information relative to non-hypnotic methods. Later reviews (Kebbell & Wagstaff, 1998; E. C. Orne, Whitehouse, Dinges, & Orne, 1996) confirmed the conclusion that hypnosis does not offer recall advantages beyond waking conditions, and although hypnosis can result in an increase of accurate memories, this is more than compensated for by an increase in inaccurate memories.

In fact, the outcome of research on this topic has been far from conclusive (see reviews by Erdelyi, 1994; Wagstaff, 1999). Absence of a clear specific effect of hypnosis on recall has been reported in a number of laboratory studies, including Register and Kihlstrom (1987), using words and pictures as the materials to be recalled; Dywan (1988), using drawings of common objects; and Lytle and Lundy (1988), using filmed material.

Consistent with Relinger's (1984) review, Erdelyi (1994) concluded that hypnotic hypermnesia is evident for the free recall of "high sense" material (e.g., poetry, pictures, films) as opposed to, say, recognition memory for lists of words or syllables. However, the evidence suggests that, in addition to a nonspecific, repeated retrieval effort, the procedure encourages participants to increase their reporting of information; thus, an increase in correct responses is offset by an increase in false responding, leaving accuracy unchanged. Another effect is that hypnotized participants appear to have more confidence in the validity of their memories, whether or not they are accurate (Erdelyi, 1994; Sheehan, 1988).

In conclusion, we should first acknowledge that any plausible attempt to assist an individual's memory of some specific event might prove productive. Hypnosis may seem a reasonable way of doing this, and it may be that particular individuals find this approach conducive. Indeed, Wagstaff, a critic of the use of hypnosis for memory enhancement, nevertheless acknowledges that some components of hypnosis, such as relaxation, focused attention, and context reinstatement through imagery, may facilitate recall (Wagstaff, 1999). He and his colleagues (e.g., Wagstaff, Cole, Wheatcroft, Marshall, & Barsby, 2007) have demonstrated significant memory enhancement with no increase in false positive errors when nonhypnotic procedures that combine these key elements are used to aid recall.

However, the prevailing opinion now seems to be that beyond this, hypnosis does not have any specific facilitative effect on memory, and there is little theoretical justification for insisting on this technique to aid recall. Moreover, there are problems of an increase in false or inaccurate memories and the individual's enhanced, but unwarranted, confidence in the veracity of his or her recollections. This has obvious implications when hypnosis is used in the interrogation of eyewitnesses in forensic cases, an application that goes back over 150 years (Gravitz, 1983) but which has declined in recent years (see Wagstaff, 1999) in favor of nonhypnotic approaches, such as the "cognitive interview" (R. P. Fisher & Geiselman, 1992; for recent reviews of use of hypnosis in eyewitness testimony, see Lynn, Boycheva, Deming, Lilienfeld, & Hallquist, 2009; Mazzoni & Lynn, 2007).

HYPNOSIS AND THE CREATION OF FALSE MEMORIES

Contrary to the lay view that memory produces accurate mental representations of experienced events, cognitive scientists agree that memory is a fallible and pliable construction strongly influenced by current beliefs, feelings, expectations, images, and guesses about past events (Conway & Pleydell-Pearce, 2000; Loftus, 2003; Mazzoni & Kirsch, 2002; Schacter, 1999). Most agree that even the most ordinary memories are comprised of accurate and inaccurate recollections.

In this light, it comes as no surprise that suggestive procedures, hypnosis being just one of them, have powerful distorting effects on the content of recollections. In interpreting the experimental data, it is important to consider the difference between the amount of material that is recalled and the accuracy of what is recalled. Work conducted in clinical settings aimed at uncovering forgotten past events under hypnosis has long been recognized as eliciting new and, in many instances, inaccurate or completely false memories. Research has clearly demonstrated that hypnosis can lead people into believing and remembering facts that did not occur, an outcome that poses serious challenges both for clinical practice and the legal system.

The Clinical Dimension

Hypnosis has been used extensively for memory recovery not only in the specialized field of hypnotherapy but also in mainstream psychotherapy. Yapko (1994) conducted a survey of over 850 psychotherapists in private practice, which revealed unexpectedly high rates of endorsement of beliefs concerning hypnosis as a way to enhance memory. More than 30% of the therapists believed that "When someone has a memory of a trauma while in hypnosis, it objectively must actually have occurred," and more than 50% claimed that "Hypnosis can be used to recover memories of actual events as far back as birth."

In 1995, Poole, Lindsay, Memon, and Bull reported the results of an extensive survey revealing that memory work in therapy aimed at recovering forgotten memories was rather widespread. At least 25% of licensed clinical psychologists in the United States and Great Britain indicated that memory recovery is an important component of therapy, and hypnosis, as well as guided imagery, should be used to facilitate retrieval of repressed memories.

Partially in line with these views, the American Society of Clinical Hypnosis (ASCH; 1995) issued guidelines for clinical hypnosis aimed at memory improvement or recovery (Hammond et al., 1995). The guidelines suggested that when therapists used procedures that were not leading, hypnosis posed no special risk of false memories, the assumption being that leading questions (see Loftus, 2005), but not hypnosis, have major distorting effects on memory.

The belief that events can reside in the unconscious and be accessed only by way of special memory recovery techniques is still prevalent among certain therapists. These clinicians claim that many forms of psychological problems are manifestations of repressed or dissociated memories of traumatic abuse and neglect during childhood (for a review, see Lynn, Knox, Fassler, Lilienfeld, & Loftus, 2004). According to these therapists, hypnosis and age regression represent roads to the retrieval of buried memories, which in turn help patients heal by bringing the memories into conscious awareness (e.g., Bass & Davis, 1988; Blume, 1990; Herman, 1992; Terr, 1994).

As recently as 2006, for example, following 3 years of therapy that included memory work conducted with relaxation, guided imagery and hypnosis, a young woman in her late 20s finally recovered memories of 5 consecutive years of sexual abuse perpetrated by a priest when she was a child (*State v. Govoni*, 2008). It is interesting that she became able to report extremely vivid and detailed day-to-day memories of unusual and striking precision. She was able to remember exact details of what she wore on different days, what she read, the weather, and the exact words of hundreds of conversations, in addition to odd visual details such as where the sunlight hit the wall, how the shadows played on the stairs, and so forth.

This is just one of many examples of the fact that clinical practice hypnosis is still used for memory recovery, with little consideration for the relatively large amount of data showing the dangers of this use. Oddly, the idea of hypnosis as a powerful tool to uncover buried memories has always coexisted with the awareness that in psychotherapy, hypnosis can (and sometimes should) be used to intentionally create what are called *pseudomemories* (Laurence & Perry, 1983), that is, false memories intentionally proposed by the therapist with the purpose of removing psychological symptoms caused by past traumatic events (see McConkey, Barnier, & Sheehan, 1998). The traumatic component of the event is replaced with neutral or positive elements. For example, Bernheim (1888/1973a) used hypnosis to create perceptions and memories that he dubbed "retroactive hallucinations." Janet (1894) substituted neutral or positive images instead of traumatic ones, as in the famous case of Marie, in which he transformed the traumatic memory of a facial deformity with the pseudomemory of a pleasant face, ridding the patient of the symptoms apparently caused by the actual experience.

The ASCH guidelines released in 1995 acknowledged that hypnosis could create intentional pseudomemories. Nonetheless, hypnosis was still recommended as a tool for memory recovery, overlooking the fact that it can also cause unintentional false memories. We see shortly how this advice was rather ill founded.

Over the years, many academic psychologists (e.g., Karlin, Kihlstrom, Laurence, Lynn, Nash, E. C. Orne, M. T. Orne, Perry) have argued against the use of hypnosis for memory recovery and highlighted instead its potential in increasing suggestibility and influencing false memory creation in psychotherapeutic and forensic contexts. One recent issue in the controversy over the use of hypnosis and memory recovery procedures involves what can be described as an explosion of cases of dissociative identity disorder (DID, formerly known as multiple personality disorder; American Psychiatric Association, 1994). Critics of DID have contended that the rise of reported cases during the 1970s and 1980s (by 1986 the number had increased to nearly 6,000) were produced by iatrogenic psychotherapy techniques (see Lilienfeld et al., 1999). At the turn of the 21st century, the number of reported cases of DID, although difficult to accurately determine, has been estimated at 40,000. Lawsuits against therapists for malpractice in "creating" rather than "discovering" multiple personalities paralleled the increase in the diagnosis of DID, and the use of hypnosis to facilitate access to "alter" personalities was frequently at the center of contention.

Currently, it is accepted in the research community that the clinical use of hypnosis as a tool to uncover memories in therapy is potentially dangerous, specifically when therapists interpret pseudomemories, often vivid and convincing mental experiences, as portraying real events.

The Research Dimension

The possibility of creating false memories in hypnosis was identified as early as the late 19th century. In a now-classic demonstration, Bernheim (1891/1973b) suggested a false event to a patient (i.e., that she had gone to the bathroom four times, and on her last visit she had fallen and hit her nose). The patient remembered the suggested event and reported using the bathroom, explaining that it was because of diarrhea, and mentioned falling on the fourth visit and hitting her nose. After hypnosis, Bernheim apparently could not shake her belief in the memory (Lynn, Boycheva, Deming, Lilienfeld, & Hallquist, 2009). In line with Bernheim's findings, the belief in the beneficial influence of hypnosis on memory has been drastically challenged by a sizeable body of research that consistently, convincingly, and rather unequivocally showed the lack of benefit and possible detrimental effect of hypnosis on memory.

By the late 1970s and early 1980s, a growing number of reports began to appear (M. T. Orne, 1979). Among these, Laurence and Perry's (1983) is one of the most dramatic empirical demonstrations of the production of a false memory in hypnosis. In their study, while hypnotized, highly suggestible participants were regressed to a night of the previous week and received the suggestion that a loud noise awakened them. If they reported having heard the suggested noise, they were asked to describe it in detail. Indeed, 63% of the participants accepted the suggestion and reported hearing the noise. Of these, 76% subsequently developed false memories of the noise. Half of these remembered the noise clearly and were convinced that it had actually happened, whereas the others reported being somewhat confused about the source of the noise.

In the same year, Dywan and Bowers (1983) determined that a twofold increase in the number of accurate items reported when memories were elicited in hypnosis was more than offset by a threefold increase in the number of errors compared with the error rate in nonhypnotic controls. In two related studies (Dinges et al., 1992; Whitehouse, Dinges, Orne, & Orne, 1988) that evaluated hypermnesia with response productivity controlled by means of a forced-choice recall procedure, hypnosis did not produce enhanced recall beyond nonhypnotic hypermnesia. In fact, in one of the studies (Dinges et al.), hypnosis not only failed to enhance retrieval of correct items, but it also increased the production of incorrect information.

Very early memory reports are also vulnerable to suggestive influences through hypnosis and a variety of other suggestive procedures (e.g., dream interpretation: Mazzoni, Loftus, Seitz, & Lynn, 1999; imagery: Mazzoni & Memon, 2003). For example, Malinoski, Lynn, and Sivec (1997) interviewed 40 hypnotized and 40 nonhypnotized participants about their earliest memories. The first time that participants were asked to report their earliest memory, only 3% of the nonhypnotized participants recalled a memory earlier than 2 years. This is in clear contrast with the 23% of hypnotized participants who reported a memory earlier than age 2 (and 20% earlier than 18 months). After the second interview, only 8% of nonhypnotized participants reported a memory earlier than 2 years), whereas 35% of hypnotized participants reported memories earlier than 18 months (30% earlier than a year).

In another study of hypnosis and early memory (Marmelstein & Lynn, 1999), participants reported earlier memories during hypnosis than they did prior to both hypnosis and (nonhypnotic) instructions to recover memories over a 2-week period. Whereas one third of participants reported memories prior to the cutoff of infantile amnesia (i.e., age 2) after nonhypnotic suggestions that they could recall earlier memories, two thirds of hypnotized participants reported such memories.

Some major reviews of the research conducted through the mid 1990s confirmed the potentially deleterious effect of hypnosis on memory (Erdelyi,

1994; Nash, 1987). Narratives obtained after age regression can be dramatic and compelling and contain visual and emotional details that make the "memories" feel true to not only the individual but also external evaluators. Nonetheless, Nash's review of over 100 studies on age regression as a tool to recover memories found no evidence that the memories of hypnotized adults correspond to actual child experiences. In other words, a sizeable percentage of the new material recalled while in hypnosis is false.

More recent work is aimed at understanding whether expectancy and warnings moderate the negative effect of hypnosis on memory. In the common memory-enhancing suggestion, participants are told that memories will come to mind effortlessly, without intentional control. Burgess and Kirsch (1999) found that under this condition, highly suggestible participants reported more memories, but these tended to be confident errors that were retained after hypnosis. When the suggestion contained warnings about the creation of false memories in hypnosis, fewer inaccurate memories were reported after hypnosis. However, the effect of the warning during hypnosis was minimal. Of further note, in no instance did hypnotic induction produce an increase in memory accuracy when compared with performance in controls.

Although in another study warnings minimized memory distortions during but not after hypnosis (Green, Lynn, & Malinoski, 1998), the Burgess and Kirsch results were in part confirmed by a study showing that challenging the new memories reported in hypnosis does not seem to work (Bryant & Barnier, 1999). The authors found that highly suggestible participants retracted memories retrieved after a suggestion only when they were not hypnotized. The challenge produced no retraction of newly created memories when high suggestible participants were still in hypnosis. It thus seems that the expectancy for memory enhancement in hypnosis is not easy to challenge, and highly suggestible individuals maintain and believe in their newly created memories.

The Issue of Confidence

The most frequently reported problem is that while in hypnosis, witnesses may erroneously report items that they would normally reject on the basis of uncertainty (see, for example, Diamond, 1980; Krass, Kinoshita, & McConkey, 1989; Laurence & Perry, 1988; M. T. Orne, 1979; M. T. Orne, Soskis, Dinges, & Orne, 1984; Perry, Orne, London, & Orne, 1996; Scoboria, Mazzoni, Kirsch, & Milling, 2002; Wagstaff, 1982 1989, 1999). Indeed, a number of these studies have shown that hypnosis is associated with enhanced confidence in responses, whether they are correct or erroneous. This is one of the issues that led to the ruling that hypnosis should be inadmissible in court, as it was presumed that jurors would be compelled by the confidently held testimony emerging from hypnosis (Scheflin, Spiegel, & Spiegel, 1999).

Another approach is to consider whether hypnosis leads to a more liberal response set. The argument is that hypnosis produces a criterion shift, resulting in poorer candidate responses being accepted because they are considered of higher quality (i.e., presumably due to the facilitative power of hypnosis). Some research has shown that hypnosis does affect response bias for perception (Jones & Spanos, 1982; Naish, 1985; Reed, Kirsch, Wickless, Moffitt, & Taren, 1996; Spanos, Burgess, Cross, & MacLeod, 1992) and memory (Dinges et al., 1992; Murrey, Cross, & Whipple, 1992); however, other recent work has failed to document such an effect for eyewitness memory (Scoboria, Mazzoni, & Kirsch, 2006, 2008). It is presently unclear to what degree differences in methods between studies may account for this discrepancy.

The Forensic Side

In the courtroom, the status of hypnosis as a memory-enhancing technique has fluctuated greatly. At the end of the 1800s, a famous verdict (*People v. Eubanks,* 1897) established that hypnotism was not recognized by the U.S. law, a precedent for per se inadmissibility, by which no testimony elicited with hypnosis could be heard in court. That was also the time in which Bernheim, foreseeing future concerns in forensic contexts, succeeded in suggesting a false memory of a rape, which the subject was willing to discuss with a representative of the law (see Rosen, Sageman, & Loftus, 2004).

Only in the second half of the 20th century was the status of hypnosis in the courtroom reversed, and testimony elicited in hypnosis was deemed acceptable as long as no suggestion or leading or misleading questions were added (*Harding v. State,* 1968). Experimental research in hypnosis enhanced the scientific respectability of the discipline, and data demonstrating the positive effect of hypnosis on memory helped extend its use as a memory-enhancing technique also in the forensic context.

The practice of hypnotizing witnesses for memory recovery and enhancement became popular during these years. Forensic hypnosis was especially popular in the late 1970s and early 1980s, when many books and papers supporting its use in police investigations were published (Haward & Ashworth, 1980; Hibbard & Worring, 1981; Kleinhauz, Horowitz, & Tobin, 1977; Reiser et al., 1980). According to Wagstaff (1999), published accounts likely underestimated the use and extent of hypnosis in police interrogations during this time period. He reported that one British investigator (Haward, 1988), who used hypnosis in forensic contexts for 30 years, conducted 17 interrogations in 1 week at the request of police. In certain cases, hypnotically elicited recall was even seen as more reliable of fact than actual physical evidence (Perry et al., 1996).

However, when practitioners and researchers started casting doubts on the accuracy of material remembered in hypnosis, the status of hypnosis in the courtroom was destined to change again (Heap, 2008). A steady stream of studies started challenging the reliability of hypnotically augmented recall, and the pendulum swung back to a final status of per se inadmissibility, which is still present in many states in the United States. Although sparked by one of many instances of misuse of hypnosis (in *People v. Shirley*, 1982, a lay person with vested interests in the case performed the hypnotic induction and helped the witness recover memories), the California Supreme Court ruled on the basis of a review of the literature on hypnosis and memory that the testimony elicited with the help of hypnosis was not reliable. The excessive cost of any case-by-case analysis of hypnotic procedures justified a per se rule of inadmissibility. More recently, the Supreme Court of Canada barred the admissibility of posthypnotic testimony (*R. v. Trochym*, 2007). It is noted that this has not been the sole approach to the admissibility of hypnosis. For example, about one third of U.S. State jurisdictions and U.S. federal courts use a *totality of the circumstances* rule by which the circumstances and characteristics of the hypnotic procedure are evaluated prior to admission to testimony (Scheflin et al., 1999).

This is the current state of affairs, in spite of more recent findings showing that hypnosis is not necessarily more detrimental than other more common procedures used during interrogation. Recent work that has more directly contrasted the effects of hypnosis with other memory distorting procedures indicates that the risks of hypnosis are, at least under some circumstances, of somewhat lower magnitude. Scoboria et al. (2002) showed in a study of responses to questions about an audiotaped narrative, that whereas hypnosis resulted in lowered response accuracy and lower "don't know" response rates than nonhypnotized individuals, the effects of asking misleading questions were even greater. These results were not mediated by the hypnotic responsiveness of participants. This is notable, because no jurisdiction bars admission of testimony following biased questioning; rather, it is assumed that cross-examination will challenge the quality of the evidence. A follow-up study confirmed the negative effects of misleading questioning on responses to questions and further showed that misleading questioning negatively affected recognition memory, whereas the negative impact of hypnosis was not replicated (Scoboria et al., 2006).

A recent study (Scoboria et al., 2008) reaffirmed the negative effects of misleading questioning and no overt effect of hypnotic induction for questions about a videotaped scene (again, hypnotic responsiveness was not related to memory performance). When "don't know" responses made to delayed questions were queried, a covert effect of hypnosis emerged by which hypnotized individuals rejected information as having been absent, when in fact it was present in the video stimulus. When accuracy was adjusted to account for this, the negative effects of misinformation and hypnosis were about equal. This is interesting, as it appears that hypnotized individuals lost access to material which had been presented, which led them to incorrectly state that they had never seen the information. This suggests that the negative effects of hypnosis on memory might be subtler and can, at times, only be observed through careful investigation of the meaning of responses that individuals provide. The authors speculated that hypnosis might affect metacognitive processes, the manners by which the quality of candidate responses are evaluated (i.e., confidence in responses, feeling of knowing). This is an approach which has not been taken in research on hypnosis and memory to date and may shed light on the inconsistent results regarding the impact of hypnosis on recall accuracy as well as on the confidence findings discussed previously.

In another study, the impact of hypnosis on memory was found to be less than that of witness preparation, another common practice in the legal system (Spanos, Quigley, & Gwinn, 1991). Work by Neuschatz, Lynn, Benoit, and Fite (2003) used the Deese–Roediger–McDermott paradigm, in which lists of related words are presented (e.g., night, dream, tired, pillow), leading to falsely recalling and recognizing a nonpresented critical word (e.g., sleep). In the study the authors failed to find any difference between hypnotized and nonhypnotized participants (i.e., those who were medium and highly hypnotizable) on false recognition of critical lures or in confidence in recognized material. The authors interpreted this as demonstrating no disadvantage, but also no advantage, of hypnosis on more basic memory processes.

Thus, across all of these studies, no advantage of hypnosis in enhancing memory was observed. These findings indicate that there is no excessive risk associated with hypnosis when contrasted with other memory distorting techniques (i.e., misinformation, witness preparation) but also no advantage for using hypnosis for memory refreshment. Thus, there seems little reason to use hypnosis for memory refreshment.

MEMORY INHIBITION

In this section, we are mainly concerned with the inhibition of memory processes by means of explicit hypnotic suggestion. It is necessary, however, to say a little about the occurrence of posthypnotic amnesia (PHA) when there has been no direct or indirect suggestion by the hypnotist.

Spontaneous Posthypnotic Amnesia

Throughout the history of hypnosis, reference has been made to the spontaneous occurrence of PHA (i.e., with no explicit suggestion to forget) for events that occurred during hypnosis. The amnesia may be dense or selective and the material may subsequently be recalled (i.e., the amnesia is *breached* or remain "forgotten"). The amnesia must not be explained by simple forgetting or a failure of registration. In the latter case, for example, a participant may not recall the hypnotist's words or directions simply because he or she was not attending to them at the time.

There appears to be a consensus that spontaneous PHA occurs only in a small minority of participants. For example, Hilgard and Cooper (1965) found that although 35% of the participants exhibited suggested amnesia, only 7% had spontaneous amnesia. Explanations have included reference to compliance (Wagstaff, 1977), expectation (Young & Cooper, 1972), and proneness to repression (Kunzendorf & Benoit, 1985–1986). However, more recent work (e.g., Simon & Saltzburg, 1985) does not suggest that either compliance or expectation is a major influence on the spontaneous occurrence of PHA.

Barber (1999) referred to work by Barrett (1990, 1996), who identified a small proportion of excellent hypnotic participants (i.e., just 15 out of 1,200) whom Barber labeled *amnesia prone* (i.e., in preference to Barrett's term "dissociaters"), 60% of whom exhibited spontaneous PHA and all of whom exhibited total suggested PHA. Typically, when alerted from hypnosis, these participants appeared confused and disoriented. They also reported amnesic experiences in their everyday lives, tended to forget their dreams, and had poor recall of their childhood. These participants differed from a small number of excellent hypnotic subjects who were "fantasy prone" and who did not exhibit spontaneous PHA and had good recall of childhood events. Barber also identified a third group of highly susceptible participants who are neither amnesia prone nor fantasy prone and are characterised by positive expectations and beliefs about hypnosis. Barber's three categories have not been universally accepted (e.g., Lynn, Meyer, & Shindler, 2004).

Spontaneous PHA is much less researched than suggested PHA, and there as yet appears to be no consensus concerning its properties and possible underlying mechanisms. There also appears to be little guidance available from laboratory research on memory and forgetting generally.

Suggested Posthypnotic Amnesia

The more common type of PHA studied in the literature is the amnesia that is specifically suggested by the hypnotist. The suggestion is that the participant will not recall the information targeted until he or she is alerted from hypnosis and not until the hypnotist has provided a signal, the *reversal cue* (which he or she specifies) for the memories to return.

The material to be forgotten may be items learned or experienced during hypnosis or information learned prior to hypnosis, such as word lists and even autobiographical events (e.g., Barnier, Bryant, & Briscoe, 2001). The suggested amnesia may be highly selective (e.g., for particular semantic categories in a word list) or be a "blanket" amnesia, as exemplified by the twelfth and last item of Form C of the Stanford Hypnotic Susceptibility Scale (SHSS:C; Weitzenhoffer & Hilgard, 1962), in which the request is to forget everything that has happened during hypnosis.

Many, though not all, responsive participants experience the amnesia as involuntary. The amnesia may be complete, partial, or absent; this is related to the subject's measured hypnotic susceptibility. For example, in the normative data for the SHSS:C provided by Weitzenhoffer and Hilgard (1962), 27% of the undergraduate students passed the amnesia suggestion to criterion (i.e., a maximum of 3 items recalled), the point biserial correlation with the total score for the other 11 items being .85.

General Theories of Posthypnotic Amnesia

Theoretical explanations of PHA have traditionally been couched in terms of some general theory of hypnosis, in which one pivotal idea or set of ideas accounts for all hypnotic phenomena. In the words of Ernest Hilgard (1991), PHA is part of the "domain of hypnosis." That this is the case is not inevitable, but one fact should persuade us, namely the high correlation, mentioned earlier, between the criterion for PHA and hypnotic susceptibility measured independently of PHA.

The simplest explanation for PHA is that the participant is being compliant: He or she is able to recall the target material but, to meet the hypnotist's demands, voluntarily delays reporting it until the reversal cue is given. Wagstaff (2004) considered that compliance is an important component in explaining PHA but also allows for the subject's deliberate use of cognitive strategies, notably self-distraction, that inhibit the process of retrieval. These processes, *strategic enactment*, are fundamental to the model elaborated by Spanos (1991), whereas for Kirsch (1991) the pivotal process is response expectancy, whereby the expectations implicitly and explicitly generated by the context (and the participants' existing beliefs) are the determinants of successful hypnotic responding.

According to these theories, the fact that some participants describe their amnesia as "involuntary" is explained by a process of attribution: The hypnotic context and the expectations created by the hypnotist may encourage those participants who are particularly adept in producing PHA to experience it as involuntary or as something that happens to them rather than something that they do. This insistence that PHA is something the subject does characterizes the approach of Sarbin and Coe (see Coe, 1989), which conceives of the good hypnotic subject as one who is best able to involve himself or herself in imaginative processes to enact the role demanded in the hypnotic context (e.g., laboratory, clinic, stage show). It is interesting, however, that they find it useful to invoke the concepts of deception and self-deception. With reference to PHA, for example, they do not seek an explanation in terms of memory mechanisms; rather, the responsive subject is one whose degree of involvement in imaginings (Sarbin & Coe, 1972) is such as to persuade them of the reality of their experience (i.e., of amnesia).

One of the central concepts of the neodissociation approach of hypnosis is the *amnesic barrier* (Hilgard, 1986). In brief, that part of the *executive ego* that controls the subject's responses to hypnotic (including posthypnotic) suggestion at any time—or the inhibition of the retrieval process in the case of PHA—is denied conscious representation by the formation of an amnesic barrier. The hypnotized subject is aware only of the responses and not the cognitive activity by which they are brought about; hence, he or she experiences them as involuntary. These theories, informed by processes such as compliance, strategic enactment, response expectancy, and role enactment, do not stipulate that, at the time the PHA suggestion is administered, the participant must be in a special state of hypnosis for the suggestion to take effect (or to be more likely to lead to the required response).

There is some variability of opinion in the theoretical literature as to whether Hilgard's (1986) theory is to be interpreted as a "special state" theory. Hilgard adopted a broader definition of dissociation than earlier theorists such as Janet, namely one that underlies a range of everyday phenomena and not simply pathological conditions. However, he was clear that some important change is happening when a person is subjected to a traditional hypnotic induction. He said the following:

> Looked at in other ways, we find that hypnotic procedures are designed to produce a readiness for dissociative experiences by disrupting the ordinary continuities of memories and by distorting or concealing reality orientation through the power that words exert by direct suggestion, through selective attention or inattention and through stimulating the imagination appropriately. (p. 226)

Whatever the case, evidence has accumulated to suggest that inducing the hypnotic state does not actually lead to an increased probability of responding over and above that of nonspecific effects such as enhanced expectation and commitment on the subject's part (Kirsch, 1997).

The *dissociated control* model (Woody & Bowers, 1994) is now probably the most influential state theory of hypnosis (see chap. 6, this volume). Briefly, in this model, the process of hypnotizing the subject disengages the frontal lobe executive control system from its influence on lower-level cognitive structures, and the behavior and experiences of the hypnotized subject are automatically triggered by the hypnotist's suggestions and are thus experienced by the subject as involuntary. In this respect, during hypnosis, the susceptible subject behaves like a patient with frontal lobe impairment, responding in a genuine involuntary manner to the suggestions and instructions of the hypnotist. Normal functioning is restored when the subject is alerted from hypnosis.

Unlike *nonstate* or sociocognitive approaches, theories that do depend on the concept of a hypnotic state to explain the experiences and behavior of participants during hypnosis need further elaboration to account for posthypnotic responding such as PHA, because, at that point, the subject has, by definition, been brought out of the hypnotic state. It is not clear from the dissociated control model what is happening when the "dehypnotized" subject is struggling to retrieve material targeted by a PHA suggestion yet in all other respects is behaving "normally" again. These apparently wide differences in the major theories about hypnosis have not proved too great an impediment to the investigation of PHA; the current consensus is that PHA seems to be a genuine phenomenon with properties that are replicable and not simply a product of the social demands on the participant. We now briefly examine some of the major properties of PHA and their implications.

Explicit and Implicit Memory

Although it appears that amnesic participants are consciously unable to recall the target material, its presence in memory is manifested implicitly. For example, in contrast to their reaction to new material, participants show an electroencephalographic response when presented with items from a word list for which they deny any conscious recall (Allen, Iacono, Laravuso, & Dunn, 1995; Schnyer & Allen, 1995) and such material still has the potential to interfere with the participant's recall of a word list presented earlier that is not included in the amnesia suggestion (Coe, Basden, Basden, & Graham, 1976). Indeed, the target material, although seemingly not available for explicit free recall or recognition, nevertheless is manifest in a range of indices of implicit memory, such as word associations and the completion of word fragments.

This is now a well established finding (e.g., Barnier et al., 2001; David, Brown, Pojoga, & David, 2000; Kihlstrom, 1980) and has constituted a major consideration for attempts to understand the mechanisms of PHA. For example, Kihlstrom (2003) considered that the differential effects of PHA on explicit and implicit memory can be understood in terms of the theory proposed by Mandler (1980) as follows:

> Recognition can be mediated by two quite different processes: retrieval, which is closely related to explicit memory and familiarity, which is closely related to implicit memory. . . . Where amnesia impairs explicit memory but spares implicit memory, subjects can use a priming-based

feeling of familiarity to make relatively accurate recognition judgments. (p. 176)

Kihlstrom draws comparisons with posthypnotic amnesia and organic amnesic syndromes in which explicit memory is impaired but implicit memory remains intact. From a rather different perspective, Huesmann, Gruder, and Dorst (1987) have constructed an *output inhibition* model in which, under the influence of the suggestion of PHA, "forbidden" information is allowed into working memory but is tagged so that, while it is able to influence new learning and other behavior, it cannot be outputted explicitly.

Disrupted Memory Retrieval Strategies

There is laboratory evidence, originating in experiments by Evans and Kihlstrom (1973) and Kihlstrom (1977), that PHA is associated with a breakdown of normal retrieval strategies. This evidence is derived from the apparent lack of structure in the material that is recalled. For example, under normal conditions, the chronological sequence of a series of items will tend to be reflected in how the material is recalled (*seriation*), and semantically related items will often be recalled in clusters. Individuals may also adopt their own strategies for organizing recall (*subjective organization*). According to Wilson and Kihlstrom (1986), PHA is associated with a disruption of the temporal organization of events in memory (leaving clustering and subjective organization intact).

Spanos, MacLean, and Bertrand (1986), Coe (1989), and others have challenged these conclusions and the experiments on which they are based. First, early studies confounded the presence of PHA with hypnotic susceptibility, and it may be that any effect on organization of recall may be due to susceptibility rather than a specific property of amnesia. Second, the effect for temporal organization appears to be at best weak and inconsistent; it may only apply for those participants who display a marked tendency for temporal organization in their recall of ordered items and may not be a major characteristic of PHA generally (Spanos et al., 1986). Third, there is evidence of an amnesia-specific disruption of clustering and subjective organization for PHA (e.g., Spanos & D'Eon, 1980). Both Spanos et al. (1986) and Wagstaff (1981) concluded that disruption of retrieval strategy is a consequence of the response strategies that participants adopt when they are instructed to forget information that they would normally retain in memory.

It is not our purpose here to attempt to resolve this controversy; indeed, it is likely that a resolution will be a long time coming. One obvious difficulty for this research is that the various hypotheses can only be tested with partially amnesic participants because those with high levels of amnesia would show little or no recall of the target material. Perhaps further research, comparing PHA with nonhypnotic methods of memory suppression, such as directed forgetting (discussed later), will assist in clarifying the issue.

The Role of the Reversal Cue

Another important topic of investigation is the significance and mode of operation of the reversal cue itself. What actually happens when the cue is administered? A neodissociation model would refer to the lifting of amnesic barriers that separate the memories from conscious expression. The dissociated control theory of Woody and Bowers (1994) would refer to the reengagement of the subject's supervisory control system in the process of memory retrieval. In the case of a model based on sociocognitive processes such as compliance (Wagstaff, 1981), strategic enactment (Spanos et al., 1991), or role enactment (Sarbin & Coe, 1972), the reversal cue signals the message that participants can stop whatever they are doing to inhibit recall or reporting of the target material and declare everything they can remember (see chap. 7, this volume).

Traditionally, proponents of dissociation theories have assigned a more potent role to the reversal cue than have those in favor of sociocognitive models; they have insisted that PHA remains robust prior to the cue to recall and cannot be breached. For example, Kihlstrom, Evans, Orne, and Orne (1980) examined, among other things, appeals to the amnesic participant to exercise more effort to recall or to be more honest during the PHA period. Although some individuals did breach their amnesia, it was concluded from this study that this was due to the natural remission of PHA over time (Kihlstrom, 1978). Later studies have made stronger demands on the amnesic participants to breach their PHA prior to the reversal cue. Methods used have included strong exhortations to the participants to be completely honest (Coe & Yashinski, 1985); a "lie detector" condition in which participants are attached to a device, which, they are told, reveals whether they are lying (Coe & Sluis, 1989; Coe & Tucibat, 1988, as cited in Coe, 1989); and participants being shown a videotape replay of the hypnosis session and being asked whether they are able to recall anything else (Coe & Sluis, 1989). Another method used by Silva and Kirsch (1987) is rehypnotizing amnesic participants and informing them that they will be placed in a "deep hypnotic state" in which they will remember either more or fewer of the items.

Once in these conditions, the reversal cue is given to participants and recall is tested again. These experiments revealed that hypnotized participants who show amnesia will breach their amnesia under strong demands to do so before the identified reversal cue is given. However, it appears that those participants who rate their amnesia as involuntary (i.e., they do not feel in control of their remembering) are more resistant to breaching (cf. Coe &

Tucibat, 1988, as cited in Coe, 1989). Also, often enough, there are one or two individuals in these experiments who do not breach at all.

These results have been interpreted as evidence that hypnotic participants displaying suggested PHA have control over the retrieval process (e.g., Coe, 1989); this in turn has been interpreted in favor of sociocognitive theories. In fact, all theoretical approaches in recent years should be able to acknowledge the fact that the hypnotic participant is sensitive to the demands and expectations created by the hypnotic context and, specifically, by the hypnotist. There are no pressing theoretical reasons why exhortations and inducements to recall should not be perceived by the hypnotic participants in a way similar to the reversal cue (i.e., as signifying that the amnesic period is at an end and recall is now expected). Such an interpretation is consistent with the results and conclusions of laboratory experiments on posthypnotic suggestion generally (Barnier & McConkey, 1998; S. Fisher, 1954; Spanos, Menary, Brett, Cross, & Ahmed, 1987), namely that whatever the preferred theoretical explanation, important determinants of responding are the demands and expectations explicitly and implicitly cued by the context, both general and specific.

What happens if the reversal cue is not given? Some authors (e.g., Kihlstrom, Easton, & Shor, 1983) consider that there is a natural tendency for the amnesia to dissipate with time. In terms of the neodissociation model, this would involve the spontaneous relaxing of amnesic barriers. The mechanism according to the dissociated control model would be the gradual reinstitution of supervisory system control over the recall process.

There is indeed laboratory evidence that without any pressure to recall, and prior to the administration of the reversal cue, the strength of the amnesia declines somewhat and participants report more material on retest prior to the cancellation of the amnesia. One explanation of this is that the effect of retesting the participant itself prompts further recall; Dubreuil, Spanos, and Bertrand (1983) showed that the expectation to recall either more or less on retest has the corresponding effect on performance. Results of experiments by Coe and colleagues (see Coe, 1989, for a summary of these) have demonstrated that the amnesia dissipates with attempts to recall by those participants who rate their amnesia as voluntary, whereas involuntary controls do not do so, except under strong pressures to breach.

It may be that one effect of the passage of time is that it acts in a similar way to the reversal cue and pressures to breach, as we suggested. There may be a tendency for participants to feel less committed to maintaining the amnesia as time progresses; that is, there is a weakening in the demands participants experience on them to remain amnesic, particularly if the automatic quality of the amnesia is illusory and cognitive effort is required. Admittedly, it would be difficult to distinguish experimentally such an explanation from one based on, say, weakening of the dissociation mechanism, but like breaching, the explanation itself need not have any serious theoretical implications.

The Relationship of Posthypnotic Amnesia to Other Types of Memory Inhibition

It is important that an understanding of PHA is consistent with and informed by theories and evidence from mainstream cognitive psychology concerning other forms of memory inhibition. For example, in the case of *directed forgetting* (DF), participants are exposed to some material, say a list of words, which they may or may not be required to learn and are then instructed to forget it (Bjork, 1970; Epstein, 1972). *Motivated forgetting*, however (e.g., Brewin & Andrews, 1998), is a term that represents a more refined version of Freud's idea of repression and generally refers to processes that enable an individual to inhibit memories of unpleasant and traumatic events. Associated with this are the concepts *repressive coping style* and *repressor*. The characteristics of repressors are that, despite physical evidence of anxiety, they tend to deny or minimise negative emotional states; they are motivated to present well socially and are less likely than others to remember negative autobiographical memories (see Eysenck, 1997).

So far, there is only limited laboratory research comparing PHA with other forms of memory inhibition, and this is restricted to DF. Collectively, the results of these studies suggest that DF and PHA leave implicit memory intact but involve different mechanisms (Basden, Basden, Coe, Decker, & Crutcher, 1994; Coe et al., 1988; David et al., 2000).

The Relationship of Posthypnotic Amnesia to Functional Memory Loss

Some writers (e.g., Barnier, 2002; Kihlstrom & Schacter, 1995) have remarked on the similarities between functional amnesia and PHA, notably the sparing of implicit memory and the contextual influences on the amnesia and its temporary nature. Hilgard (1986) considered that PHA and the Freudian concept of repression have much in common but noted one obvious disparity; namely that, unlike repression, in the case of PHA the target material is unrelated to any emotional concerns or conflicts experienced by the participant. At present, perhaps under the catalyzing influence of the "false memory" controversy, the idea of extensive repression of traumatic memories is viewed with considerable skepticism (e.g., Kihlstrom, 2002). Currently, many writers, especially those from the clinical disciplines, feel more comfortable with the concept of dissociation, although motivated forgetting (Brewin & Andrews, 1998) may command more support from within mainstream cognitive psychology.

To what extent can laboratory studies of PHA elucidate the mechanisms of functional amnesia? Probably, we should include in our question other memory inhibition procedures such as directed and motivated forgetting and repressive coping style. Collectively, they may provide valuable insights into cognitive mechanisms that may underpin functional amnesic disorders, but as always, laboratory investigations are severely limited by the kinds of material and experiences to which their participants may be subjected.

Possible Neural Mechanisms

Recently, Mendelsohn, Chalamish, Solomonovich, and Dudai (2008) presented the results of functional magnetic resonance imaging (fMRI) brain scans in participants given a PHA suggestion. The target material was a documentary film that participants had viewed a week previously. Analysis of scans taken during the PHA period and following memory recovery revealed a difference between those participants who were responsive to the suggestion of PHA and those who were not. These differences extended over occipital, temporal, and prefrontal areas. The authors considered that the simultaneous lifting of the amnesia and the restoration of brain activity in those regions that are crucial for retrieval strongly suggests that memory suppression occurred at early stages of the retrieval process. They indicated that the amnesia induced by the posthypnotic suggestion "affects an executive pre-retrieval monitoring process, which produces an early decision on whether to proceed or not on retrieval, and in case of a [question about the movie], aborts the process" (p. 165).

These results should, for the time being at least, be interpreted with caution for a number of reasons. First, reliable inferences concerning the cognitive processes underlying different patterns of brain activity are not easy to draw (see Uttal, 2001). Second, there are considerable variations in patterns of activity across individuals responding to the same experimental demands, and this is likely to be the case with hypnosis and suggestions for PHA, to which participants respond in varying ways. Also to be taken into consideration is the confounding of the presence of PHA and high hypnotic susceptibility.

Notwithstanding these caveats, it is likely that similar studies will, in the fullness of time, assist in understanding the cognitive processes involved in PHA and how these are distinguished from other forms of memory inhibition. In this context, it is worth noting that Anderson et al. (2004) and Depue, Curran, and Banich (2007) obtained fMRI scans of participants following instructions not to think about certain targeted words and pictures and claimed to have identified the neural systems underlying memory suppression. Like the Mendelsohn et al. (2008) study cited earlier, these experiments were heralded in the media as providing the neural basis for Freud's theory of repression. The earlier of these two studies has been subjected to skeptical criticism by Hayne, Garry, and Loftus (2006). One major problem is that the DF paradigm (i.e., "think/no-think") adopted by Anderson et al. (2004) produces only small and unstable decrements in recall that have been difficult to replicate (Bulevich, Roediger, Balota, & Butler, 2006). It is also unlikely that these kinds of laboratory investigations of voluntary memory suppression have much to say about the Freudian theory of repression (Kihlstrom, 2002).

Posthypnotic Amnesia: Summary

Over the last 40 years, an impressive body of knowledge has accumulated on suggested PHA and there are signs of an emerging consensus. Broadly speaking, it does appear that some form of retrieval or output inhibition is occurring with many responsive participants, to the extent that they are not aware of the material they are consciously endeavouring to recall; yet the material is clearly present in implicit memory.

A satisfactory account of PHA must be grounded in mainstream cognitive science and, most important, be consistent with current knowledge concerning human memory and robust models based on this knowledge. Its relationship with other types of memory inhibition needs to be fully explored and formalized. The existing evidence suggests that it is related to directed forgetting, though it has its own unique features. It is critical to consider that those individuals who are particularly responsive to the suggestion of PHA are in the minority and are highly hypnotizable (i.e., as defined by their scores on standard scales). Any model of PHA must take this into account, and there should be much common ground with explanations of other hypnotic phenomena. For example, the dissociation between performance on tests of explicit and implicit memory that is evident with PHA is mirrored by the performance of high hypnotizables for suggested deafness (e.g., Barber & Calverley, 1964) and negative hallucinations (M. T. Orne, 1962). The relationship of PHA to clinical memory disorders is also an important topic for further investigation.

Finally, Coe's insistence (e.g., Coe, 1989) that PHA is something participants do rather than something that happens to them seems apposite in the light of the accumulated evidence. We might specify this further and say it is something many highly hypnotizable individuals do. This is perhaps not so controversial and not so inconsistent with state or special process models of hypnosis.

CONCLUSION

Hypnosis, which represents a powerful tool to induce a variety of experiences and behaviors (e.g., profound analgesia, automatic movements, partial paralyses), also has remarkable effects on memory that include increasing the amount of material recalled and producing selective amnesia. Substantial research has been conducted on the enhancing effect of hypnosis on memory. The belief that in hypnosis one can recover memories that would otherwise be inaccessible has a long history and is still rather common, not only among laypeople but also among therapists. Indeed, survey research indicates that hypnosis and guided imagery are used relatively often to access buried memories of personal events (Poole et al., 1995).

Evidence regarding whether hypnosis enhances memory is at best inconclusive. Although the amount of material recalled may be increased, this comes at the expense of accuracy, and no data support the idea of hypnosis facilitating the retrieval of otherwise inaccessible personal memories. On the contrary, false but believed personal memories can be easily created if hypnosis is used as a tool to recover past autobiographical events. These findings have promoted the decision to bar hypnotically elicited memories from the courtroom, although recent research has shown that hypnosis is not more detrimental than other techniques used when interrogating witnesses (e.g., asking misleading questions; Scoboria et al., 2002).

Hypnosis can also be used to create the experience of amnesia in highly suggestible individuals. Researchers investigating the locus of forgetting show that although the material is not accessible intentionally, it is still retained in implicit memory. Examining the extent to which hypnotic amnesia parallels other forms of experimentally induced forgetting has also proven fruitful. Probably the best way to investigate hypnotic amnesia is through neuroimaging studies, which only recently have started to shed light on this fascinating but still poorly understood phenomenon.

REFERENCES

Allen, J. J., Iacono, W. G., Laravuso, J. J., & Dunn, L. A. (1995). An event-related potential investigation of posthypnotic recognition amnesia. *Journal of Abnormal Psychology, 104*, 421–430.

American Psychiatric Association. (1994). *Diagnostic and statistical manual of mental disorders* (4th ed.). Washington, DC: Author.

Anderson, M. C., & Green, C. (2001, March 15). Suppressing unwanted memories by executive control. *Nature, 410*, 366–369.

Anderson, M. C., Ochsner, K. N., Kuhul, B., Cooper, J., Robertson, E., Gabrieli, S. W., et al. (2004, January 9). Neural systems underlying the suppression of unwanted memories. *Science, 303*, 232–235.

Barber, T. X. (1999). A comprehensive three-dimensional theory of hypnosis. In I. Kirsch, A. Capafons, E. Cardeña-Buelna, & S. Amigó (Eds.), *Clinical hypnosis and self-regulation: Cognitive–behavioral perspectives* (pp. 21–48). Washington, DC: American Psychological Association.

Barber T. X., & Calverley, D. S. (1964). Experimental studies in "hypnotic" behavior: Suggested deafness evaluated by delayed auditory feedback. *British Journal of Psychology, 55,* 439–446.

Barnier, A. J. (2002). Posthypnotic amnesia for autobiographical episodes: A laboratory model of functional amnesia? *Psychological Science, 13,* 232–237.

Barnier, A. J., Bryant, R. A., & Briscoe, S. (2001). Posthypnotic amnesia for material learned before or during hypnosis: Explicit and implicit memory effects. *International Journal of Clinical and Experimental Hypnosis, 49,* 28–304.

Barnier, A. J., & McConkey, K. M. (1998). Posthypnotic responding: Knowing when to stop helps keep it going. *International Journal of Clinical and Experimental Hypnosis, 46,* 204–219.

Barrett, D. (1990). Deep trance subjects: A schema for two distinct subgroups. In R. G. Kunzendorf (Ed.), *Mental imagery* (pp. 101–112). New York: Plenum Press.

Barrett, D. (1996). Fantasizers and dissociaters: Two types of high hypnotizables, two different imagery styles. In R. G. Kunzendorf, N. P. Spanos, & B. Wallace (Eds.), *Hypnosis and imagination* (pp. 123–135). Amityville, NY: Baywood Publishing.

Basden, B. H., Basden, D. R., Coe, W. C., Decker, S., & Crutcher, K. (1994). Retrieval inhibition in direct forgetting and posthypnotic amnesia. *International Journal of Clinical and Experimental Hypnosis, 42,* 184–203.

Bass, E., & Davis, L. (1988). *The courage to heal: A guide for women survivors of child sexual abuse.* New York: Harper & Row.

Bernheim, H. (1973). *Hypnosis and suggestion in psychotherapy* (C. Herter, trans.). New York: Jason Aronson. (Original work published 1888)

Bernheim, H. (1980). *New studies in hypnotism* (R. S. Sandor, trans.). New York: International University Press. (Original work published as *Hypnotisme, Suggestion, Psychothérapie: Études Nouvelles,* 1891)

Bjork, R. A. (1970). Positive forgetting: The noninterference of items intentionally forgotten. *Journal of Verbal Learning and Verbal Behavior, 9,* 255–268.

Blume, E. S. (1990). *Secret survivors: Uncovering incest and its aftereffects in women.* Oxford, England: Wiley.

Brewin, C. R., & Andrews, B. (1998). Recovered memories of trauma: Phenomenology and cognitive mechanisms. *Clinical Psychology Review, 18,* 949–970.

Bryant, R. A., & Barnier, A. J. (1999). Eliciting autobiographical pseudomemories: The relevance of hypnosis, hypnotizability, and attributions. *International Journal of Clinical and Experimental Hypnosis, 47,* 267–283.

Bulevich, J. B., Roediger, H. L., Balota, D. A., & Butler, A. C. (2006). Failures to find suppression of episodic memories in the think/no-think paradigm. *Memory & Cognition, 34,* 1569–1577.

Burgess, C., & Kirsch, I. (1999). Expectancy information as a moderator of the effects of hypnosis on memory. *Contemporary Hypnosis, 16,* 22–31.

Coe, W. C. (1989). Posthypnotic amnesia: Theory and research. In N. P. Spanos & J. F. Chaves (Eds.), *Hypnosis: The cognitive–behavioral perspective* (pp. 110–148). Buffalo, NY: Prometheus Books.

Coe, W. C., Basden, B. H., Basden, D. R., & Graham, C. (1976). Posthypnotic amnesia: Suggestions of an active process in dissociative phenomena. *Journal of Abnormal Psychology, 85,* 455–458.

Coe, W. C., & Sluis, A. (1989). Increasing contextual pressures to breach posthypnotic amnesia. *Journal of Personality and Social Psychology, 57,* 885–894.

Coe, W. C., & Yashinski, E. (1985). Breaching posthypnotic amnesia: Volitional experiences and their correlates. *Journal of Personality and Social Psychology, 48,* 716–722.

Conway, M. A., & Pleydell-Pearce, C. W. (2000). The construction of autobiographical memories in the self-memory system. *Psychological Review, 107,* 261–88.

David, D., Brown, R., Pojoga, C., & David, A. (2000). The impact of posthypnotic amnesia and directed forgetting on implicit and explicit memory: New insights from a modified process dissociation procedure. *International Journal of Clinical and Experimental Hypnosis, 48,* 267–289.

De Piano, F. A., & Salzburg, H. C. (1981). Hypnosis as an aid to recall of meaningful information presented under three types of arousal. *International Journal of Clinical and Experimental Hypnosis, 29,* 383–400.

Depue, B. E., Curran, T., & Banich, M. T. (2007, July 13). Prefrontal regions orchestrate suppression of emotional memories via a two-phase process. *Science, 317,* 215–219.

Diamond, B. L. (1980). Inherent problems in the use of pretrial hypnosis on a prospective witness. *California Law Review, 68,* 313–349.

Dinges, D. F., Whitehouse, W. G., Orne, E. C., Powell, J. W., Orne, M. T., & Erdelyi, M. H. (1992). Evaluating hypnotic memory enhancement (hypermnesia and reminiscence) using multitrial forced recall. *Journal of Experimental Psychology: Learning, Memory, and Cognition, 18,* 1139–1147.

Dubreuil, D. L., Spanos, N. P., & Bertrand, L. D. (1983). Does hypnotic amnesia dissipate with time? *Imagination, Cognition, and Personality, 2,* 103–113.

Dywan, J. (1988). The imagery factor in hypnotic hypermnesia. *International Journal of Clinical and Experimental Hypnosis, 36,* 312–326.

Dywan, J., & Bowers, K. S. (1983, December 2). The use of hypnosis to enhance recall. *Science, 222,* 184–185.

Epstein, W. (1972). Mechanisms of directed forgetting. In G. H. Bower (Ed.), *The psychology of learning and motivation: Advances in research and theory* (Vol. 6, pp. 147–191). New York: Academic Press.

Erdelyi, M. W. (1994). The empty set of hypermnesia. *International Journal of Clinical and Experimental Hypnosis, 42,* 379–390.

Evans, F. J., & Kihlstrom, J. F. (1973). Posthypnotic amnesia as disrupted retrieval. *Journal of Abnormal Psychology, 82,* 317–323.

Eysenck, M. J. (1997). *Anxiety and cognition: A unified theory*. Hove, England: Psychology Press.

Fisher, R. P., & Geiselman, R. E. (1992). *Memory enhancing techniques for investigative interviewing: The Cognitive Interview*. Springfield, IL: Charles C Thomas.

Fisher, S. (1954). The role of expectancy in the performance of posthypnotic behavior. *Journal of Abnormal Psychology, 49*, 503–507.

Freud, S. (1962). The psychical mechanism of forgetfulness. In J. Strachey (Ed. & Trans.), *The standard edition of the complete works of Sigmund Freud* (Vol. III, pp. 287–301). London: Hogarth Press. (Original work published 1896)

Gravitz, M. A. (1983). An early case of investigative hypnosis: A brief communication. *International Journal of Clinical and Experimental Hypnosis, 31*, 224–226.

Green, J. P. (2003). Beliefs about hypnosis: Popular beliefs, misconceptions, and the importance of experience. *International Journal of Clinical and Experimental Hypnosis, 51*, 369–381.

Green, J. P., Lynn, S. J., & Malinoski, P. (1998). Hypnotic pseudomemories, prehypnotic warnings, and the malleability of suggested memories. *Applied Cognitive Psychology, 12*, 431–444.

Hammond, D. C., Garver, R. B., Mutter, C. B., Crasilneck, H. B., Frischholz, E., Gravitz, M. A., et al. (1995). *Clinical hypnosis and memory: Guidelines for clinicians and for forensic hypnosis*. Des Plaines, IL: American Society of Clinical Hypnosis Press.

Harding v. State, 5 Md.App. 230, 246 A.2d 302 (1968).

Haward, L. R. C. (1988). Hypnosis by the police. *British Journal of Experimental and Clinical Hypnosis, 5*, 33–35.

Haward, L. R. C., & Ashworth, A. (1980, August). Some problems of evidence obtained by hypnosis. *Criminal Law Review*, 469–485.

Hayne, H., Garry, M., & Loftus, E. F. (2006). On the continuing lack of evidence for repressed memories. *Behavioral and Brain Sciences, 29*, 521–522.

Heap, M. (2008). Hypnosis in the courts. In M. Nash & A. J. Barnier (Eds.), *The Oxford Handbook of Hypnosis* (pp. 745–766). Oxford, England: Oxford University Press.

Herman, J. L. (1992). *Trauma and recovery*. New York: Basic Books.

Hibbard, W. S., & Worring, R. W. (1981). *Forensic hypnosis: The practical application of hypnosis in criminal investigation*. Springfield, IL: Thomas.

Hilgard, E. R. (1986). *Divided consciousness: Multiple controls in human thought and action*. New York: Wiley.

Hilgard, E. R. (1991). A neodissociation interpretation of hypnosis. In S. J. Lynn & J. W. Rhue (Eds.), *Theories of hypnosis: Current models and perspectives* (pp. 83–104). New York: Guilford Press.

Hilgard, E. R., & Cooper, L. M. (1965). Spontaneous and suggested posthypnotic amnesia. *International Journal of Clinical and Experimental Hypnosis, 13*, 261–274.

Huesmann, L. R., Gruder, C. L., & Dorst, G. (1987). A process model of posthypnotic amnesia. *Cognitive Psychology, 19*, 33–62.

Janet, P. (1889). *L'automatisme psychologique* [*Psychological automation*]. Paris: Felix Alcan.

Janet, P. (1894). Histoire d'une idée fixe [History of fixed ideas]. *Revue Philosophique, 37*(1), 121–163.

Jones, B., & Spanos, N. P. (1982). Suggestions for altered auditory sensitivity, the negative subject effect, and hypnotic susceptibility: A signal detection analysis. *Journal of Personality and Social Psychology, 43*, 637–47.

Kebbell, M. R., & Wagstaff, G. F. (1998). Hypnotic interviewing: The best way to interview eyewitnesses? *Behavioral Sciences and the Law, 16*, 115–129.

Kihlstrom, J. F. (1977). Models of posthypnotic amnesia. *Annals of the New York Academy of Sciences, 296*, 284–301.

Kihlstrom, J. F. (1978). Context and cognition in posthypnotic amnesia. *International Journal of Clinical and Experimental Hypnosis, 26*, 246–257.

Kihlstrom, J. F. (1980). Posthypnotic amnesia for recently learned material: Interactions with "episodic" and "semantic" memory. *Cognitive Psychology, 12*, 227–251.

Kihlstrom, J. F. (2002). No need for repression [Comment on "Inhibitory processes and the control of memory retrieval" by B. J. Levy & M. C. Anderson]. *Trends in Cognitive Science, 6*, 502.

Kihlstrom, J. F. (2003). The fox, the hedgehog, and hypnosis. *International Journal of Clinical & Experimental Hypnosis, 51*, 166–189.

Kihlstrom, J. F., Easton, R. D., & Shor, R. E. (1983). Spontaneous recovery of memory during posthypnotic amnesia. *International Journal of Clinical and Experimental Hypnosis, 31*, 309–323.

Kihlstrom, J. F., Evans, F. J., Orne, E. C., & Orne, M. T. (1980). Attempting to breach posthypnotic amnesia. *Journal of Abnormal Psychology, 89*, 603–616.

Kihlstrom, J. F., & Schacter, D. L. (1995). Functional disorders of autobiographical memory. In A. Baddeley, B. A. Wilson, & F. Watts (Eds.), *Handbook of memory disorders* (pp. 337–364). London: Wiley.

Kirsch, I. (1991). The social learning theory of hypnosis. In S. J. Lynn & J. W. Rhue (Eds.), *Theories of hypnosis: Current models and perspectives*, (pp. 439–466). New York: Guilford Press.

Kirsch, I. (1997). Suggestibility or hypnosis: What do our scales really measure? *International Journal of Clinical and Experimental Hypnosis, 45*, 212–225.

Kleinhauz, M., Horowitz, I., & Tobin, T. (1977). The use of hypnosis in police investigation: A preliminary communication. *Journal of the Forensic Science Society, 17*, 77–80.

Krass, J., Kinoshita, S., & McConkey, K. M. (1989). Hypnotic memory and confident reporting. *Applied Cognitive Psychology, 3*, 35–51.

Kunzendorf, R. G., & Benoit, M. (1985–86). Spontaneous posthypnotic amnesia and spontaneous rehypnotic recovery in repressors. *Imagination, Cognition, and Personality, 5*, 303–310.

Laurence, J., & Perry, C. (1983, November 4). Hypnotically created memory among highly hypnotizable subjects. *Science, 222*, 523–524.

Lilienfeld, S., Lynn, S. J., Kirsch, I., Chaves, J., Sarbin, T., Ganaway, G., & Powell, R. (1999). Dissociative identity disorder and the sociocognitive model: Recalling the lessons of the past. *Psychological Bulletin, 125*, 507–523.

Lindner, R. (1944). *Rebel without a cause*. New York: Grune & Stratton.

Loftus, E. F. (2003). Make-believe memories. *American Psychologist, 58*, 867–873.

Loftus, E. F. (2005). Planting misinformation in the human mind: A 30-year investigation of the malleability of memory. *Learning & Memory, 12*, 361–366.

Lynn, S. J., Boycheva, E., Deming, A., Lilienfeld, S. O., & Hallquist, M. N. (2009). Forensic hypnosis: The state of the science. In J. Skeem, K. Douglas, & S. O. Lilienfeld (Eds.), *Psychological science in the courtroom: Controversies and consensus*. New York: Guilford.

Lynn, S. J., Knox, J. A., Fassler, O., Lilienfeld, S. O., & Loftus, E. F. (2004). Memory, trauma, and dissociation. In G. M. Rosen (Ed.), *Posttraumatic stress disorder: Issues and controversies* (pp. 163–186). New York: Wiley.

Lynn, S. J., Meyer, E., & Shindler, K. (2004). Clinical correlates of high hypnotizability. In M. Heap, D. Oakley, & R. Brown (Eds.), *The highly hypnotizable person* (pp. 187–212). London: Brunner-Routledge.

Lytle, R. A., & Lundy, R. M. (1988). Hypnosis and the recall of visually presented material: A failure to replicate Stager and Lundy. *International Journal of Clinical and Experimental Hypnosis, 36*, 327–335.

Malinoski, P., Lynn, S. J., & Sivec, H. (1998). The assessment, validity, and determinants of early memory reports: A critical review. In S. J. Lynn & K. M. McConkey (Eds), *Truth in memory* (pp. 109–136). New York: Guilford Press

Mandler, G. (1980). Recognizing: The judgment of previous occurrence. *Psychological Review, 87*, 252–271.

Marmelstein, L., & Lynn, S. J. (1999). Expectancies, group, and hypnotic influences on early autobiographical memory reports. *International Journal of Clinical and Experimental Hypnosis, 47*, 301–319.

Mazzoni, G., & Kirsch, I. (2002). Autobiographical memories and beliefs: A preliminary metacognitive model. In T. J. Perfect & B. L. Schwartz (Eds.), *Applied metacognition* (pp. 121–145). New York: Cambridge University Press.

Mazzoni, G., Loftus, E. F., Seitz, A., & Lynn, S. J. (1999). Changing beliefs and memories through dream interpretation. *Applied Cognitive Psychology, 13*, 125–144.

Mazzoni, G., & Lynn, S. J. (2007). Using hypnosis in eyewitness memory: Past and current issues. In M. P. Toglia, J. D. Read, D. F. Ross, & R. C. L. Lindsay (Eds.), *The handbook of eyewitness psychology. Vol. I: Memory for events* (pp. 321–338). Mahwah, NJ: Erlbaum.

Mazzoni, G., & Memon, A. (2003). Imagination can create false memories. *Psychological Science, 14*, 186–188.

McConkey, K. M., Barnier, A. J., & Sheehan, P. W. (1998). Hypnosis and pseudomemory: Understanding the findings and their implications. In S. J. Lynn & K. McConkey (Eds.), *Truth in memory* (pp. 227–259). New York: Guilford Press.

Mendelsohn, A., Chalamish, Y., Solomonovich, A., & Dudai, Y. (2008). Mesmerizing memories: Brain substrates of episodic memory. *Neuron, 57,* 159–170.

Murrey, G. J., Cross, H. J., & Whipple, J. (1992). Hypnotically created pseudomemories: Further investigation into the "memory distortion or response bias" question. *Journal of Abnormal Psychology, 101,* 75–77.

Naish, P. L. (1985). Is a signal detection account of hypnosis supportable? *British Journal of Experimental and Clinical Hypnosis, 2,* 147–150.

Nash, M. (1987). What, if anything, is regressed about hypnotic age regression? A review of the empirical literature. *Psychological Bulletin, 102,* 42–52.

Neuschatz, J. S., Lynn, S. J., Benoit, G. E., & Fite, R. (2003). Hypnosis and memory illusions: An investigation using the Deese/Roediger and McDermott paradigm. *Imagination, Cognition and Personality, 22,* 3–12.

Orne, E. C., Whitehouse, W. G., Dinges, D. F., & Orne, M. T. (1996). Memory liabilities associated with hypnosis: Does low hypnotizability confer immunity? *International Journal of Clinical and Experimental Hypnosis, 44,* 354–369.

Orne, M. T. (1962). Hypnotically induced hallucinations. In L. J. West (Ed.), *Hallucinations* (pp. 211–219). New York: Grune & Stratton.

Orne, M. T. (1979). The use and misuse of hypnosis in court. *International Journal of Clinical and Experimental Hypnosis, 27,* 311–341.

Orne, M. T., Soskis, D. A., Dinges, D. F., & Orne, E. C. (1984). Hypnotically induced testimony. In G. L. Wells & E. F. Loftus (Eds.), *Eyewitness testimony: Psychological perspectives* (pp. 171–213). New York: Cambridge University Press.

People v. Eubanks, 49 P 1049 (Cal. 1897).

People v. Shirley, 641 P.2d 775 (Cal.) cert. denied, 439 U.S. 860 (1982).

Perry, C. W., Orne, M. T., London, R. W., & Orne, E. C. (1996). Rethinking per se exclusions of hypnotically elicited recall as legal testimony. *International Journal of Clinical and Experimental Hypnosis, 44,* 66–81.

Poole, D. A., Lindsay, D. S., Memon, A., & Bull, R. (1995). Psychotherapy and the recovery of memories of childhood sexual abuse: U.S. and British practitioners' opinions, practices, and experiences. *Journal of Consulting and Clinical Psychology, 68,* 426–437.

R. v. Trochym, 2007 SCC 6, [2007] 1 S.C.R. 239.

Reed, S. B., Kirsch, I., Wickless, C., Moffitt, K. H., & Taren, P. (1996). Reporting biases in hypnosis: Suggestion or compliance? *Journal of Abnormal Psychology, 105,* 142–145.

Register, P. A., & Kihlstrom, J. F. (1987). Hypnotic effects of hypermnesia. *International Journal of Clinical and Experimental Hypnosis, 35,* 155–170.

Reiser, M. et al. (1980). Symposium—Forensic Hypnosis: 22nd Annual Scientific Meeting of the American Society of Clinical Hypnosis, November 16, 1979, San Francisco, California. *American Journal of Clinical Hypnosis, 23*, 73–118.

Relinger, H. (1984). Hypnotic hypermnesia: A critical review. *American Journal of Clinical Hypnosis, 26*, 212–225.

Rosen, G. M., Sageman, M., & Loftus, E. (2004). A historical note on false traumatic memories. *Journal of Clinical Psychology, 60*, 137–139.

Sarbin, T. R., & Coe W. C. (1972). *Hypnosis: A social psychological analysis of influence communication.* New York: Holt, Rhinehart & Winston.

Schacter, D. L. (1999). The seven sins of memory: Insights from psychology and cognitive neuroscience. *American Psychologist, 54*, 182–203.

Scheflin, A. W., Spiegel, H., & Spiegel, D. (1999). Forensic uses of hypnosis. In A. S. Hess & I. B. Weiner (Eds.), *Handbook of forensic psychology* (2nd ed., pp. 474–498). New York: Wiley.

Schnyer, D. M., & Allen, J. J. (1995). Attention related electroencephalographic and event-related potential predictors of responsiveness to suggested posthypnotic amnesia. *International Journal of Clinical & Experimental Hypnosis, 43*, 295–315.

Scoboria, A., Mazzoni, G., & Kirsch, I. (2008). "Don't know" responding to answerable and unanswerable questions during misleading and hypnotic interviews. *Journal of Experimental Psychology: Applied, 14*, 225–265.

Scoboria, A., Mazzoni, G., & Kirsch, I. (2006). Effects of misleading questions and hypnotic memory refreshment on memory reports: A signal detection analysis. *International Journal of Clinical and Experimental Hypnosis, 54*, 340–359.

Scoboria, A., Mazzoni, G., Kirsch, I., & Milling, L. S. (2002). Immediate and persisting effects of misleading questions and hypnosis on memory reports. *Journal of Experimental Psychology: Applied, 8*, 26–32.

Sheehan, P. W. (1988). Memory distortion in hypnosis. *International Journal of Clinical and Experimental Hypnosis, 36*, 296–311.

Shields, I. W., & Knox, V. J. (1986). Level of processing as a determinant of hypnotic hypermnesia. *Journal of Abnormal Psychology, 95*, 358–364.

Silva, C. E., & Kirsch, I. (1987). Breaching hypnotic amnesia by manipulating expectancy. *Journal of Abnormal Psychology, 96*, 325–329.

Simon, M. J., & Salzberg, H. C. (1985). The effect of manipulated expectancies on posthypnotic amnesia. *International Journal of Clinical and Experimental Hypnosis, 33*, 40–51.

Spanos, N. P. (1991). A sociocognitive approach to hypnosis. In S. J Lynn & J. W. Rhue (Eds.), *Theories of hypnosis: Current models and perspectives* (pp. 324–361). New York: Guilford Press.

Spanos, N. P., Burgess, C. A., Cross, P. A., & MacLeod, G. (1992). Hypnosis, reporting bias, and suggested negative hallucinations. *Journal of Abnormal Psychology, 101*, 192–199

Spanos, N. P., & D'Eon, J. L. (1980). Hypnotic amnesia, disorganized recall and inattention. *Journal of Abnormal Psychology, 89,* 744–750.

Spanos, N. P., MacLean, J. M., & Bertrand, L. D. (1986). Serial organization during hypnotic amnesia under two conditions of item presentation. *Journal of Research in Personality, 21,* 361–374.

Spanos, N. P., Menary, E., Brett, P. J., Cross, W., & Ahmed, Q. (1987). Failure of hypnotic responding to occur outside the experimental setting. *Journal of Abnormal Psychology, 96,* 52–57.

Spanos, N. P., Quigley, C. A., & Gwynn, M. I. (1991). Hypnotic interrogation, pre-trial preparation, and witness testimony during direct and cross-examination. *Law & Human Behavior, 15*), 639–653.

Stager, G. L., & Lundy, R. M. (1985). Hypnosis and the learning and recall of visually presented material. *International Journal of Clinical and Experimental Hypnosis, 33,* 27–39.

Steblay, N. M., & Bothwell, R. K. (1994). Evidence for hypnotically refreshed testimony: The view from the laboratory. *Law & Human Behavior, 18,* 635–651.

Terr, L. (1994). *Unchained memories: True stories of traumatic memories, lost and found.* New York: Basic Books.

True, R. M. (1949, December 2). Experimental control in hypnotic age regression states. *Science, 110,* 583–584.

Uttal, W. R. (2001). *The new phrenology: The limits of localizing cognitive processes in the brain.* Cambridge, MA: MIT Press.

Wagstaff, G. F. (1977). Experimental study of compliance and posthypnotic amnesia. *British Journal of Social and Clinical Psychology, 16,* 225–228.

Wagstaff, G. F. (1981). *Hypnosis, compliance, and belief.* New York: St. Martin's Press.

Wagstaff, G. F. (1982). Hypnosis and recognition of a face. *Perceptual and Motor Skills, 55,* 816–818.

Wagstaff, G. F. (1989). Forensic aspects of hypnosis. In N. P. Spanos & J. F. Chaves (Eds.), *Hypnosis: The cognitive–behavioral perspective* (pp. 340–357). Amherst, NY: Prometheus Books.

Wagstaff, G. F. (1999). Hypnosis and forensic psychology. In I. Kirsch, A. Capafons, E. Cardeña-Buelna, & S. Amigó (Eds.), *Clinical hypnosis and self-regulation: Cognitive–behavioral perspectives* (pp. 277–310). Washington DC: American Psychological Association.

Wagstaff, G. F. (2004). High hypnotizability in a sociocognitive framework. In M. Heap, D. Oakley, & R. Brown (Eds.), *The highly hypnotizable person* (pp. 85–114). London: Brunner-Routledge.

Wagstaff, G. F., Cole, J., Wheatcroft, J., Marshall, M., & Barsby, I. (2007). A componential approach to hypnotic memory facilitation: Focused meditation, context reinstatement and eye movements. *Contemporary Hypnosis, 24,* 97–108.

Wagstaff, G. F., & Mercer, K. (1993). Does hypnosis facilitate memory for deep processed stimuli? *Contemporary Hypnosis, 10,* 59–66.

Weitzenhoffer, A. M., & Hilgard, E. R. (1962). *Stanford Hypnotic Susceptibility Scale, Form C*. Palo Alto, CA: Consulting Psychologists Press.

Whitehouse, W. G., Dinges, D. F., Orne, E. C., & Orne, M. T. (1988). Hypnotic hypermnesia: Enhanced memory accessibility or report bias? *Journal of Abnormal Psychology, 97*, 289–295.

Whitehouse, W. G., Orne, E. C., Orne, M. T., & Dinges, D. F. (1991). Distinguishing the source of memories reported prior waking and hypnotic recall attempts. *Applied Cognitive Psychology, 5*, 51–59.

Wilson, L., & Kihlstrom, J. F. (1986). Subjective and categorical organization of recall in posthypnotic amnesia. *Journal of Abnormal Psychology, 95*, 264–273.

Woody, E. Z., & Bowers, K. S. (1994). A frontal assault on dissociative control. In S. J. Lynn & J. W. Rhue (Eds.), *Dissociation: Clinical and theoretical perspectives* (pp 52–79). New York: Guilford Press.

Yapko, M. D. (1994). Suggestibility and repressed memories of abuse: A survey of psychotherapists' beliefs. *American Journal of Clinical Hypnosis, 36*, 194–208.

Young, J., & Cooper, L. M. (1972). Hypnotic recall amnesia as a function of manipulated expectancy. *Proceedings of the 80th Annual convention of the American Psychological Association, 7*, 857–858.

30

THE CULTURAL CONTEXT OF HYPNOSIS

ETZEL CARDEÑA AND STANLEY KRIPPNER

In the diverse world in which we live, hypnosis practitioners, researchers, and theoreticians need to become culturally competent; thus, this chapter focuses on major cross-cultural issues in this area. We begin with a discussion of hypnosis as a construct specific to our postmodern Western culture, which cannot just be transplanted into other cultures. Nonetheless, we also consider healing practices in other settings that can be partly analyzed according to some of the variables inherent to our notion of hypnosis. Thus, we provide a summary and more detailed discussion of practices in other cultures that share some resemblances with the dynamics of hypnosis.

Culture has been defined as "the organized system of knowledge and beliefs that allows a group to structure its experiences and choose among alternatives" (Tseng, 1997, p. 4). Over the course of our lives, we are immersed in a specific culture. Its concepts are multilayered and complex, and any notion of an easily definable culture is misleading. There are groups that can be more (e.g., some

The authors dedicate this chapter to the memory of David Bakan, the quintessential wise man, and thank Wendy Cousins, Rosemary Coffey, Jeffrey Kirkwood, and Devin Terhune for their editorial assistance. Stanley Krippner expresses his gratitude to the Saybrook Graduate School's Chair for the Study of Consciousness for supporting his participation in the preparation of this chapter.
All clinical material has been disguised to protect patient confidentiality.

tribes) or less (e.g., New York City inhabitants) homogeneous, more (e.g., the Hassidim) or less (e.g., "metrosexual" males) traditional, more (e.g., traditional Japanese) or less (e.g., urban U.S. citizens) communal, and, in the case of immigrants, more or less acculturated to their new homeland. Even within a culture there are important socioeconomic differences that may, for instance, make the experience of an inner city African American more similar to that of a denizen of a Brazilian *favela* than that of his or her wealthy suburb counterpart.

This chapter is part of a larger debate about the very definition of hypnosis. The different perspectives presented herein help shed light on our understanding of the way hypnosis functions in clinical settings in Western and other cultures. For example, it is important to note that cultural analyses are often framed within *etic* (i.e., reputedly universal) or *emic* (i.e., culturally relative) explanations and constructs. The former are typically based on Western rationality and are context-poor, whereas the latter tend to include a richer discussion of specific personal, historical, and cultural circumstances; that is, they are more "thick" in anthropological terms. Research shows that etic explanations are neither obvious nor easy to establish (e.g., van Duijl, Cardeña, & de Jong, 2005). We aim to keep these considerations in mind as we discuss the cultural construct known as hypnosis. Disregarding cultural variables may produce implausible conclusions such as accepting that individuals who show impressive hypnotic-like phenomena (e.g., analgesia) in the midst of a *Thaipusam* ritual, which involves body mutilations, piercings, and alterations of consciousness, are "low hypnotizables" because they scored below average on a Western measure of hypnosis that had not been validated in their culture (Kok, 1989).

We focus here on hypnotic and hypnotic-like phenomena in non-Western cultures rather than comparing hypnotizability evaluations in Western countries (e.g., Cardeña, Kallio, Terhune, & Buratti, 2007; Perry, Nadon, & Button, 1997). The value of a truly cross-cultural approach is to understand the range of individual and social variation in the scientific search for an understanding of human capacities (Price-Williams, 1975). In this chapter, we discuss the similarities and differences between hypnotic virtuosos (i.e., the approximately 2%–3% of people most responsive to hypnotic suggestions) and shamans and describe the hypnotic-like aspects of native healing procedures, while only incidentally making interpretive analyses of the procedures from the standpoint of Western science and therapy. After general discussions, we present specific examples of convergences and divergences between hypnosis and some indigenous healing practices.

Most illnesses in a society, as well as alleged changes in consciousness, are socially constructed, at least in part. Because some native models of healing assume that practitioners, to be effective, must shift their attention and awareness (e.g., "journeying to the upper world," "traveling to the lower world," "incorporating spirit guides," "conversing with power animals," "retrieving a lost soul"), the hypnosis literature can illuminate these processes and be illuminated by them. We include within the rubric of shamans both those who manifest the classical "soul journey" and those who can be "possessed by the spirits" in a controlled way (Cardeña, 1996). We also note that some critics continue to question the effectiveness of native healers, perhaps because of their dislike of the spiritual aspects of the treatment, including the notion of incorporeal spirits.

More than 2 decades ago, Locke and Kelly (1985) provided a valuable framework for understanding how cultural variables undergird states of consciousness. In their model, culture shapes an experience through a number of interrelated processes, including *ethnoepistemology* (i.e., the basic metaphysical and epistemological axioms held by a culture, such as whether shamanic experiences refer to "another reality" or are just fantasy); its signs, symbols, and metaphors (e.g., indicators of special powers or attributes, such as a shaman holding a magical pouch or a physician having an MD from Harvard); predisposing factors (e.g., having been socialized by the media or rituals to have specific expectations about what may happen in hypnotic or *vodou* contexts); situational factors (e.g., the general context of a hypnosis experiment or a ritual); and the specific patterning of experiential, behavioral, and phenomenological changes (e.g., the hypnotic suggestions themselves or specific drumming beats in a *vodou* ceremony). This framework will help us understand better in what ways mesmerism, hypnosis, and possibly related phenomena such as shamanism are similar or differ from one another.

The term *hypnosis* is often used to refer to a variety of structured, goal-oriented procedures in which suggestions for somatic or psychological changes are provided by another person, a mechanical device, a conducive environment, or by oneself. These procedures often attempt to blur, focus, or amplify attention or mentation (e.g., imagination, intention) to produce suggested or spontaneous behaviors or experiences. Barber (1984) defined *hypnosis* as a procedure that includes disregarding extraneous concerns and focusing on specific suggestions to alter one's experience, behavior, and/or physiology. This mostly atheoretical formulation allows us to more easily look at the hidden cultural variables in hypnosis (Cardeña, 1999).

It is common, although arguable, to state that what we now term *hypnosis* had its modern birth in the theory and practice of mesmerism as first enunciated by Franz Anton Mesmer in the 18th century, yet at the same time trace its historical roots back to tribal rites and shamanic practices (Brown & Fromm, 1986, p. 3). For example, Agogino (1965) stated that, "the history of hypnotism may be as old as the practice of shamanism" (p. 31). He added that priests in the healing temples of Asclepius (beginning in the 4th century BC) induced their clients into "temple sleep" by "hypnosis and autosuggestion" and that the ancient druids chanted over their clients until the desired effect was obtained. Vogel (1970/1990) pointed out that native healers used herbs in pre-Columbian Central and South America to enhance verbal suggestion. How can we make sense of such disparate statements?

One way is by following Locke and Kelly's (1985) model and proposing that although the specific patterning of experience in hypnosis (e.g., suggestion) has precedents, the ethnoepistemology of hypnosis as a secular process involving a "natural" mechanism (i.e., in the case of Mesmer, a proposed "animal magnetism"; in the case of the Abbé Faria and others, the use of psychosocial variables such as suggestions) may be traced back to Mesmer. Even earlier discussants of what was then considered demonic possession pointed to suggestions and other psychosocial variables rather than metaphysical explanations (Duncan, 1634, as cited in de Certeau, 2000). Laurence and Perry (1988) mentioned that mesmerism was in fact heir to the exorcist practices of the time although couched in the scientific terms of the time. The emotional and social displays during Mesmer's healings, so different from the physically passive and isolated contemporary practice of hypnosis, were also likely influenced by other religious ecstatic movements in Europe (Rosen, 1969). How the original theory and practices of mesmerism were transformed into contemporary hypnosis would require a whole volume, but the interested reader can consult excellent histories of hypnosis (e.g., Gauld, 1992; Laurence & Perry, 1988).

What we now call hypnosis is embedded in a network of implicit meanings and ontological assumptions about the nature of reality and of hypnosis itself (e.g., E. R. Hilgard, 1973). Too often authors commit the categorical fallacy (Kleinman, 1988) of using Western constructs such as hypnosis or trance and superimposing them on other cultures without first evaluating whether such constructs are valid or reliable in their new environment. Even though within our own specific culture there are disagreements as to the basic nature of hypnosis (Lynn & Rhue, 1991), some authors will use the term as a facile explanation for manifestations in other cultures or conclude that "clinical hypnosis . . . is simply a cultural and historical adaptation of shamanism" (Overton, 1998, p. 151), although it would be questionable even to use it as a descriptive term in other cultural contexts than in the current Western one.

Trance is good example of a term that is often used as a cross-cultural explanatory term despite its many meanings, even within our own cultural framework. Although the term is often assumed to connote some kind of etic category, perhaps of a biological predisposition to "enter" into a hypnotic state, Exhibit 30.1 shows that there are multiple meanings of trance just within the English language. Directly transferring such an ambiguous concept to other cultures disregards its semantic networks and intertextuality and fails to provide any real explanation of it. Gergen (1985) observed that the terms

EXHIBIT 30.1
The Senses of *Trance*

Oxford English Dictionary (1st ed.) sense	Quotations from the psychological/ anthropological literature
1. "great apprehension or dread of coming evil . . . ; to pass, depart (esp. from life), to die . . . to benum or be numbed by fear or cold . . . to pass over, cross."	none
2. "A state of extreme apprehension or dread; a state of doubt or suspense."	Agitated states, possession crises (Rouget, 1985); wondering (Shor, 1962)
3. "An unconscious or insensible condition, a swoon, a faint; in mod. Use, a state characterized by a more or less prolonged suspension of consciousness and inertness to stimulus; a cataleptic or hypnotic condition."	various anesthetic and amnestic phenomena; unresponsiveness to stimulation (Henney, 1974; Besmer, 1983); regional or non-connective consciousness (O'Shaughnessy, 1972); Generalized Reality Orientation (Shor, 1959)
4. "An intermediate state between sleeping and waking; half conscious or half-awake condition; a stunned or dazed state."	"a sleeplike state such as that of deep hypnosis" (Gowan, 1975, p. 35)
5. "A state of mental abstraction from external things; absorption, exaltation, rapture, ecstasy."	the trait of absorption (Tellegen & Atkinson, 1974) religious ecstasy (Rouget, 1985)
6. (an attribute in such compounds as) "trance-coma, -medium, -sleep, -state; trance-bound, like"	

Note. Representative quotations from the psychological or anthropological literature (based on Cardeña, 1990; see also Rouget, 1985).

in which the world is understood are social artifacts, "products of historically situated interchanges among people" (p. 267).

Much theory and research data suggest that the response to hypnosis involves various interpersonal, sociocultural, and cognitive factors (e.g., Shor, 1962; Woody, Bowers, & Oakman, 1992). Among them are behaviors and experiences that reflect expectations and role enactments on the part of the "hypnotized" individuals or groups, who attend to their own personal needs and to implicit or explicit interpersonal or situational cues that shape their responses (Barber, 1969; Brown & Fromm, 1986; Spanos & Chaves, 1989). Other research data have emphasized the part that attention (whether it is diffuse, concentrated, or expansive) plays in hypnosis, by enhancing the salience of the suggested task or experience (Balthazard & Woody, 1992; Krippner & Bindler, 1974).

The hypnosis literature has underscored the interaction of several variables in hypnosis and can help our understanding of healing indigenous practices that involve either overt or covert suggestive and motivational dynamics.

However, to use the term *hypnosis* to describe exorcisms, the laying-on of hands, dream incubation, and the like does an injustice to the varieties of cultural experience and their historic roots. Hypnosis and a putative hypnotic state have been too often reified (Spanos & Chaves, 1991, p. 71), distracting serious investigators from investigating ingenious uses of human imagination and motivation that are worthy of study in their own right. Nonetheless, a survey of the social science literature, as well as our observations in several traditional societies, suggests that there are frequently elements of native healing procedures that can be termed hypnotic-like. Alterations in consciousness (i.e., observed or experienced changes in people's patterns of perception, affect, or cognition, especially awareness, attention, and memory) are sanctioned and deliberately fostered by virtually all indigenous groups. For example, Bourguignon and Evascu (1977) found that 89% of 488 sampled societies displayed socially approved altered states of consciousness. The ubiquitous nature of hypnotic-like procedures in native healing is also the result of the ways in which human capacities, such as the abilities to strive toward a goal and imagine a suggested experience, can be channeled and shaped differentially by social interactions (Murphy, 1947, chap. 8).

Concepts of sickness and of healing are also socially constructed and represented in various ways. The models found in traditional cultures frequently identify such etiological factors of sickness as "soul loss," "breach of taboo," spirit "possession," "intrusion," or "invasion," all of which are diagnosed, at least in part, by observable changes in the victims' behavior as related to their mentation or mood (Frank & Frank, 1991, chap. 5), a concept also present in Western history (see Sluhovsky, 2007). Similarly, the alterations in consciousness identified by Bourguignon and Evascu (1977) are shaped by historical and social forces within a culture. For example, there is no Western equivalent of *wagumuma*, a Japanese emotional disorder characterized by childish behavior, emotional outbursts, apathy, and negativity. *Susto* is a malaise, commonly referred to in several parts of Latin America, thought to be caused by a shock or fright and often connected with breaking a spiritual taboo. Conversely, some Western eating disorders can be considered "culture-bound" (Keel & Klump, 2003).

Cross-cultural studies of native healing have only started to take seriously the importance of understanding indigenous models of sickness and treatment, perhaps because of the prevalence of behavioral, psychoanalytic, and medical models, which have not been sympathetic to the explanations offered by traditional practitioners (Ward, 1989). Kleinman (1980) commented that the habitual, and frequently unproductive, way researchers try to make sense of healing, especially indigenous healing, is by speculating about psychological and physiological mechanisms of therapeutic action. These are then applied to case material in an ethnocentric fashion that explains particular instances exclusively according to etic principles. The latter are primarily derived from the concepts of biomedicine and individual psychology. By reducing healing to the language of biology, other human aspects such as its psychosocial and cultural significance are eliminated, leaving behind something that can be expressed in biomedical terms but that disregards the language of experience, which is a major aspect of healing.

An example of Kleinman's (1980) observation is the overly facile equation of the Eskimo *pibloktoq* (in which individuals tear off their clothes and wander aimlessly in inclement environments) with a "hysterical disorder" (Gussow, 1985). In much the same way, *hsieh-ping*, a Taiwanese condition marked by disorientation and auditory hallucinations, has been considered a "depressive condition" (Hughes, 1985). Ward (1989) remarked that in both instances, it is prematurely assumed that Western classifications of mental disorders are universal, even though their manifestations may be shaped by culture. Gergen (1990) warned against using these terms as if they depicted actual occurrences; the vocabulary of the mental health professions serves "to render the alien familiar, and thus less fearsome" (p. 358).

CLINICAL AND FORENSIC APPLICATIONS

Although not without its limitations (Cardeña, 1995), Winkelman's (1992) important typology, based on archival data from dozens of traditional societies, identifies four general groups of spiritual practitioners: shamans and shamanic healers, priests and priestesses, mediums and diviners, and malevolent practitioners (some culture may have more nuanced typologies, such as the 40 different types of Náhuatl healers in ancient México or the current variations of healers and shamans in the Sierra Mazateca; Miranda, 1997). With the exception of priests and priestesses, at least some of these practitioners purportedly cultivate the ability to regulate or shift their patterns of perception, affect, and cognition for benevolent (e.g., healing or divining) or malevolent (e.g., casting spells or hexing) purposes. Of the four groups, shamanism bears the greatest similarity with Western hypnosis, although there are also important differences. For instance, although shamans primarily seek to affect their own state of consciousness, hypnotists primarily seek to affect their clients or research participants.

Shamanism and Hypnosis

Hypnotic-like procedures are often apparent in the healing practices of native shamans. Shamans can be defined as socially sanctioned practitioners who claim to voluntarily regulate their states of consciousness so as to access information not ordinarily available, using it to facilitate appropriate behavior and healthy development, as well as to alleviate stress and sickness among members of their community or the community as a whole. In this chapter, we include within the rubric of shamans both those who manifest the classical soul journey as well as those who can be possessed by the spirits in a controlled way (Cardeña, 1996).

Among the shaman's many roles, that of healer is the most common. Shamanic healing procedures may be highly scripted in a manner similar to the way that hypnotic procedures are carefully sequenced and structured. The expectations of the shaman's or hypnotist's clients can enable them to decipher task demands, interpret relevant communications appropriately, and translate the practitioner's suggestions into personalized perceptions and images.

Shamans themselves display what Kirsch (1990), in discussing the hypnosis literature, called *learned skills*: Their introduction to hypnotic-like experiences during their initiation and training generalizes to later sessions, and they can ultimately engage in *soul journeying*, or invite spirits to possess them. For instance, Japanese shamans of the Tohoku region believe that they can contact the Buddhist goddess Kan'non, who assists with their diagnosis, producing visual or auditory imagery that the shaman experiences and reports. This is an example of the "translation" that characterizes both hypnotic sessions and shamanic imagination. Achterberg (1985) studied these shamanic translations and considers dreams, visions, and similar processes a venerable source of vital information about human health and sickness, as Jung proposed earlier on (Jung, 1966). So ubiquitous is their process of gleaning pertinent information from fantasy-based symbols and metaphors that Krippner (1987) suggested that shamans, as a group, might be considered "fantasy prone."

A systematic comparison between shamans and hypnotic virtuosos reveals both similarities and differences (Cardeña, 1996):

- The proposed typology of high hypnotizables as either fantasy prone or dissociator virtuosos (Barrett, 1990) is similar to that of "classical" shamans and "mediums" (Eliade, 1964; Winkelman, 1992).
- Hypnotizability shows a genetic contribution (Lichtenberg, Bachner-Melman, Ebstein, & Crawford, 2004; Morgan, 1973), and family incidence has been found among various types of healers (Campos Navarro, 1997; Eliade, 1964).
- The developmental paths for high hypnotizability of either punishment (or trauma) or encouragement of fantasy (J. Hilgard, 1979) have a parallel in the described common history of illness and training of imagination among shamans (Halifax, 1980; Noll, 1985).

- Hypnotic virtuosos often have a propensity for the arts and for cognitive flexibility (J. Hilgard, 1979), as do shamans (Cardeña & Beard, 1996; Shweder, 1972).
- Many, but not all (e.g., mention of plants and animals), of the phenomena reported in shamanism, such as kaleidoscopes and out-of-body experiences (Lewis-Williams & Pearce, 2005), are also mentioned spontaneously by hypnotic virtuosos (Cardeña, 2005).
- Hypnosis and shamanism have been associated with reputed parapsychological events (Angoff & Barth, 1973; Stanford, 1992).

There are, however, important sociocultural differences. Whereas hypnosis typically occurs within a one-on-one clinical or research individual setting and has a secular ethnoepistemology, shamanism usually occurs in a social, ritual context of service, embedded within a metaphysical framework (Cardeña, 1996).

Induction Procedures

Furst (1977) described procedures by which North American Native Americans sought alternative states of consciousness: "psychoactive plants, animal secretions, fasting, thirsting, self-mutilation, exposure to the elements, sweat lodges, sleeplessness, incessant dancing, bleeding, plunging into ice-cold pools, and different kinds of rhythmic activity, self-hypnosis, meditation, chanting, and drumming" (p. 70; see also Ludwig, 1966). Furst used nonindigenous concepts (e.g., "self-hypnosis," "trance," "meditation") that may not be directly comparable with the original experiences and went on to describe the use of "ecstatic trance" to determine the experients' relationship with the unseen forces of the universe. Nonetheless, analogous hypnotic practices are the various nondirective, permissive procedures in which hypnotized clients use their own fantasy and imagery to work toward the desired goals (e.g., Kroger, 1977, chap. 14).

Alaskan Inuit shamans claim to journey to the spirit world during a ceremony conducted in a darkened igloo while they, stripped naked, sing and beat drums (Rogers, 1982, p. 124). Rogers (1982) claimed that the shaman's use of rhythmic drumming and monophonic chanting induces "self-hypnosis" (apparently because of their goal-directed nature) while also placing the client "in a hypnotic trance in which the suggestions of recovery and cure are given" (p. 143). Although drumming is a common feature in shamanism, Rouget (1985) criticized the theory that a simple "acoustic driving" of the brain by drumbeats can explain the alterations of consciousness observed. He asserted that attempts to explain a universal "trance mechanism" in terms of music alone are faulty because ritual leaders and musicians do not enter these states unintentionally. A person must be willing to "fall into a trance," know the pertinent cultural techniques of music and singing, and be cognitively prepared for the alteration in consciousness (pp. 167–183, 315–326). In the case of spirit possession, Rouget insisted that the possessed individual must identify with the respective form of divine being pertinent to his or her culture and attract the spirit through characteristic movements (pp. 35, 103, 105–108). Observed electroencephalogram (EEG) and experience alterations do not follow an acoustic driving model positing that EEG frequency follows mechanically the number of drumbeats (Maxfield, 1990).

In discussing the Ammassalik Eskimos of eastern Greenland, Kalweit (1988) observed the following:

> [Their] continuous rubbing of stones against each other may be seen as a simple way of inducing a trance. . . . The monotony, loneliness, and repetitive rhythmic movement join with the desire to encounter a helping spirit. This combination is so powerful that it erases all mundane thoughts and distracting associations. (p. 100)

Belo (1960) observed similarities between the behavior of Balinese mediums and hypnotized participants. Although there was no trained observer of hypnosis on Belo's field trips, a hypnotic practitioner observed several of her films and claimed to notice similarities between "hypnotic trance" and "mediumistic trance." Likewise, Bowers (1961) proposed similarities between *vodou* practices and hypnosis. There is evidence that physical movement, characteristic of *vodou* and other religious rituals, does not prevent Western hypnotic virtuosos from experiencing substantial alterations of consciousness similar, but not identical, to those produced by a motionless procedure (Cardeña, 2005). Some ingredients that share similarities between Western hypnosis and most, if not all, of the non-Western induction procedures described include a disregard of extraneous, everyday concerns (i.e., for instance by a hypnotic induction or by entering a sacred space); some means to focus the individual's experiences; and what the individual expects will happen and what his or her role will be in that situation (Shor, 1962).

Kirsch's (1990) discussion of the role of expectancies in hypnosis and psychotherapy is also relevant to each of these cases. Hypnosis, like many culturally based rituals, serves to shape and bolster relevant expectancies that reorganize consciousness and produce behavioral changes related to the goals of hypnotic participants and shamanic clients. For example, the ideomotor behavior that often characterizes hypnosis (e.g., arms becoming heavier or lighter, fingers moving to denote positive or negative responses) partly resembles the postures, gestures, collapsing motions, and rhythmic movements that occur during many native rituals. In both instances, the participants claim that the movements occur involuntarily. Also, drumming and many other ritual aspects may help maintain a continuous focus of attention, as compared with the usual shifting of attentional foci (Cardeña & Spiegel, 1991).

Navajo Healing Procedures

Despite attempts at acculturation, many Navajo men and women still follow their traditional cultural myths and participate in the corresponding rituals (Adair, Deuschle, & Barnett, 1988). In the Navajo concept of illness, the universe is an interrelated whole in which powers of both good and evil exist in a balanced and orderly relationship. When this relationship is disturbed, disharmony occurs, producing illness. Its cause, therefore, is basically metaphysical; illness takes place when the individual or group is out of harmony with the natural and supernatural worlds (Topper, 1987). When someone knowingly or accidentally breaches taboos or offends dangerous powers, the natural order of the universe is ruptured and causes "contamination" or "infection" that must be redressed (Sandner, 1979). When the family has determined that treatment is necessary, a *hataalii*, or "singing shaman," is called in, frequently accompanied by an herbalist and/or a diagnostician (both of whom are of lower status). The herbalists gather plants and make medicines, some of which are used directly and some of which are used ceremonially by the *hataalii*. The diagnosticians are usually women and "listen" to the spirits for a statement of the problem. This procedure resembles self-hypnosis in that it regulates attention and is goal-oriented in nature. Other diagnostic procedures that resemble self-hypnosis include hand trembling, star gazing, candle gazing, and crystal gazing, all of which involve the focusing of attention, with the purpose of facilitating insight into the nature of the problem.

Navajo *hataalii* use a number of therapeutic procedures, most notably one or more of the 10 basic *chantways*, complex patterns of activities centered around cultural myths in which heroes or heroines once journeyed to spiritual realms to acquire special knowledge. One can observe the resemblance of the storytelling aspect of the chant to the use of narrative "teaching stories" in Ericksonian hypnotic procedures (e.g., Erickson, Rossi, & Rossi, 1976). These stories are highly scripted and reflect the society's perspective on human nature (Lynn & Rhue, 1991). Like Milton Erickson's "teaching stories," no formal induction procedures are used in chants. However, there is an emphasis on the correctness of the procedures; as a result, the *hataalii* is in an extremely vigilant frame of mind. The ability to master the elements of a chantway has been compared with memorizing a Wagnerian opera (Kluckholn & Leighton, 1962, p. 309). An ability to remember the cultural myths used in the chantway is mandatory if a *hataalii* is to serve as an educator who can pass traditions and tribal wisdom on to the younger generation (Dixon, 1908).

The absence of a formal induction does not prevent the client from becoming receptive and motivated to follow the implicit and explicit suggestion of the ritual, just as most, if not all, hypnotic phenomena can be evoked without hypnotic induction (Kirsch, 1990). Contributing to this procedure is the multimodal approach that characterizes chants, as well as their repetitive nature and the mythic content of the words, which are easily deciphered by those clients well versed in tribal mythology. A *hataalii* usually displays a highly developed dramatic sense in carrying out the chant but generally avoids the clever sleight-of-hand effects used by many other cultural healing practitioners to demonstrate their abilities to the community. The chant is considered by Sandner (1979) to facilitate suggestibility and shifts in attention through repetitive singing and the use of culture-specific mythic themes. These activities prepare participants for a healing session that may involve symbols and metaphors acted out by performers, enacted in purification rites, or executed in "sand paintings" composed of sand, corn meal, charcoal, and flowers but destroyed once the healing session is over.

There are various steps in the typical chantway ceremony: preparation (in which the client is "purified"); presentation of the client to the healing spirits; summoning of these spirits to the place of the ceremony; identification of the clients with a positive mythic theme; transformation of the clients into a condition in which ordinary and mythic time and space merge; and release from the mythic world and return to the everyday world, where past transgressions are confessed, new learning is assimilated, and life changes are brought to fruition. These steps resemble Kirsch's (1990, p. 163) three phases of the use of hypnosis in psychotherapy: preparation, induction, and application. The client's purification and presentation are analogous to preparation, the evocation of the spirits resembles induction, and the identification and transformation represent clinical application. Throughout all of these procedures there is the assumption that the participant enters a special, sacred space, similar to attending a Western therapist's office.

Hypnotic-like procedures may affect the mentation of both the *hataalii* and the client during the chant. Sandner (1979) pointed out that the *hataalii*'s performance empowers the client by creating a "mythic reality" through the use of chants, dances, and songs (often accompanied by drums and rattles); masked dancers; purifications (e.g., sweats, emetics, herbal infusions, ritual bathings, sexual abstinence); and sand paintings. This resembles the focusing of attention characteristic of many hypnotic procedures, and the presence of culturally significant symbols may maximize clients' imagination and motivation, empowering their self-healing capacities through identification with symbols held to have therapeutic consequences. It provides the "credible rationale" that Kirsch (1990) found to enhance treatment effectiveness (see also Torrey, 1986).

Topper's (1987) study of Navajo *hataalii* indicated that they also raise their clients' expectations through the example they set of stability and competence. Politically, they are authoritative and powerful; this embellishes their symbolic value as "transference figures" in the psychoanalytic sense, representing "a nearly omniscient and omnipotent nurturative grandparental object" (p. 221; for a similar analysis to the hypnotic situation, see Shor, 1962). Frank and Frank (1991) put it more directly: "The personal qualities that predispose patients to a favorable therapeutic response are similar to those that heighten susceptibility to methods of healing in nonindustrialized societies, religious revivals, experimental manipulations of attitudes, and administration of a placebo" (p. 184). Also, in his modern classic, Ellenberger (1970, p. 12) suggested three *sine qua non* essentials of healing: the healer's faith in his or her own abilities, the patient's faith in the healer, and communal acknowledgement of the disease, the healing method, and the healer. Suggestion and expectancy are bolstered through reinforcement of the client's belief in the power of the chant and its symbols, a tight structuring of the ceremonial performance, repetition (i.e., especially in chants, songs, and prayers), physical exhaustion, the dramatization of a significant event in Navajo mythology, and, on rare occasions, the use of psychotropic herbal substances (e.g., Datura) to evoke a physical effect that convinces the client of the power of the ritual. "The chant work is a restrained and dignified procedure, and for the most part, the medicine man represents for the patient a stable, dependable leader who is a helper and guide until the work is ended" (Sanders, 1979, p. 258). In other words, two crucial factors in the client's treatment appear to be the personal qualities of the *hataalii* and the expectancies of the client.

Even though Navajo shamans use hypnotic-like procedures, they do not believe the chantway or the healing prayers induce an alteration in ordinary consciousness. To deliberately enter an altered state, or to claim that they were in such a condition, would be considered undignified by the Navajo healers. Nevertheless, the lengthy chants, songs, and prayers are so repetitive and monotonous that an outside observer might justifiably claim that they serve as consciousness-altering procedures. Furthermore, this example suggests how each culture constructs the notion of altered states differently; the spectrum of altered states is constricted and narrow among the Navajo, in contrast with the complexities of construction found in many Eastern traditions. Tibetan Buddhism, for example, contains five classes of meditation, each of which includes four levels that may incorporate dozens of specific potential alterations with a variety of outcomes (Brown, 1977).

Afro-Brazilian and Afro-Caribbean Healing Procedures

Various early West African cultures considered that an individual was closely connected with nature, the community, and his or her communal group. Each person was expected to play his or her part in a web of kinship relations and community networks. Strained or broken social relations were held to be the major cause of sickness; a harmonious relationship with one's community, as well as with one's ancestors, was important for health. At the same time, an ordered relationship with the forces of nature, as personified by the *lwas*, *orixas*, or deities, was essential for maintaining the well-being of the individual, the family, and the community. West Africans knew that disease often had natural causes, but they believed that these factors were exacerbated by discordant relationships between people and their social and natural milieu. Long before Western medicine recognized the fact, Africa's traditional healers took the position that ecology and interpersonal relations affected people's health (Raboteau, 1986).

West African healing practitioners felt that they gained access to supernatural power in three ways: by making offerings to the spirits; by foretelling the future with the help of a spirit; and by incorporating a spirit or an ancestor, who then diagnosed illnesses, prescribed cures, and provided the community with warnings or blessings. The medium, or person through whom the spirits spoke and moved, performed this task voluntarily, claiming that such procedures as dancing, singing, or drumming were needed to surrender their minds and bodies to the discarnate entities (Desmangles & Cardeña, 1996; Krippner, 1989), although it is a simplification to assume that spirit possession involves only one type of consciousness alteration (Cardeña, 1989). The slaves brought these practices to Brazil and the Caribbean with them; despite colonial and ecclesiastical repression, the customs survived over the centuries and eventually formed the basis for a number of Afro-Brazilian and Caribbean religions.

Contemporary shamans in Brazil, Haiti, and other countries still teach apprentices how to sing, drum, and dance in order to incorporate the various deities, ancestors, and spirit guides. They also teach their followers about the special herbs, teas, and lotions needed to restore health, and about the charms and rituals needed to prevent illness (McGregor, 1962). The ceremonies of the various Afro-Brazilian groups (e.g., Candomblé, Umbanda, Batuque, Caboclo, Quimbanda, Xangó) differ, but all share three beliefs: (a) Humans have a spiritual body (that generally reincarnates after physical death), (b) discarnate spirits are in constant contact with the physical world, and (c) humans can learn how to incorporate spirits for the purpose of healing.

After interviewing 40 spiritistic healing practitioners in Brazil, Krippner (1989) identified five methods of receiving the "call" to become a medium: (a) coming from a family having a history of mediumship, (b) being "called" by spirits in one's visions and dreams, (c) succumbing to a malady or "spiritual crisis" from which one recovers to serve others, (d) having a revelation while reading Afro-Brazilian spiritistic literature or attending spiritistic worship services, or (e) working as a volunteer in a spiritistic healing center and becoming inspired by the daily examples of compassion. If the call is rejected, severe illness or misfortune may result; as one Candomblé medium told Krippner, "Once the *orixa* calls, there is no other path to take" (p. 193). In a similar fashion, a *vodou oungan* (i.e., priest) told Cardeña that he had rejected his call until he had an episode of amnesia after which he found a machete wound in his leg, at which point he no longer resisted.

Once the apprentices begin to receive instruction in mediumship, such experiences as spirit incorporation, automatic writing, "out-of-body" travel, and recall of "past lives" lose their bizarre quality and seem to occur quite naturally (Cardeña, 1991). Socialization processes provide role models and the support of peers. A number of cues (e.g., songs, chants, music) facilitate spirit incorporation, and a process of social construction teaches control and appropriate role-taking and provides communal support. Richeport (1992) observed many similarities between these mediumistic behaviors and those of some hypnotized participants (e.g., dissociation and frequent amnesia for the experience).

The traits most admired in mediums resemble those that facilitate ordinary social interactions. If a spirit seems to be taking control of the medium too quickly, the other mediums may sing a song that will slow down the process of incorporation (Rouget, 1985). Leacock and Leacock (1972) observed that the Brazilian mediums usually behaved in ways that were "basically rational," communicated effectively with other people, and demonstrated few symptoms of hysteria or psychosis. They engaged in intensive training and, as mediums, pursued hard work that often put them at risk with seriously ill individuals. These are not likely to be the favorite pastimes of fragile personalities or malingerers. In fact, contrary to earlier proposals, usually without any actual data to support them, that practitioners of classical shamanism or spirit possession are psychotic or at least "hysterical," recent empirical studies have found that their psychological health is as good if not better than that of their referent groups (Cardeña, Van Duijl, Weiner, & Terhune, 2009; Moreira-Almedia, Lotufo, & Cardeña, 2008; Van Ommeren et al., 2004).

A common feature of spirit possession is the supposed inability to recall the events that transpired during the possession. Spanos and Chaves (1989) pointed out that this amnesic quality could be explained as an "achievement"; each failure to remember "adds legitimacy to a person's self-presentation as 'truly unable to remember,' hence as deeply in 'trance'" (p. 101). And there is evidence that indigenous practitioners acknowledge different levels of possession depth, some of which do not involve amnesia (Frigerio, 1989), in a similar way to the different kinds of mediumship in the West (Cardeña et al., 2009). Thus, the interpretation of hypnotic phenomena as goal-directed action is helpful in understanding mediumship as an activity that meets role demands because mediums guide and report their behavior and experience according to these demands. An alternative point of view maintains that mediums actually do lose control over their behavior, entering a "trance" or "dissociative state" that allow "hidden parts" of their minds to manifest as secondary personalities or spirits (see Krippner, 1989).

Another important consideration is that spiritistic ceremonies enable clients and mediums to arrive at a shared worldview in which an ailment can be discussed and treated (Torrey, 1986). In some spiritistic traditions, there are mediums who specialize in diagnosis, mediums who specialize in healing by a laying-on of hands, mediums who specialize in distant healing, and mediums who specialize in intercessory prayer, among others. All of these procedures contain the possibility of enhancing clients' sense of mastery, increasing their self-healing capacities, and replacing their demoralization with empowerment (Frank & Frank, 1991; Torrey, 1986).

Mediums are not the only ones who appear to manifest hypnotic-like effects. Their clients also demonstrate apparent shifts in consciousness, especially while undergoing crude surgeries without the benefit of anesthetics. Greenfield (1992) observed that Brazilian mediums make no direct effort to alter their clients' awareness, yet he attributed the benefits of these sessions to the clients' alterations of consciousness. He observed that "no one is consciously aware of hypnotizing . . . patients . . . , and unlike the mediums, patients participate in no ritual during which they may be seen to enter a trance state" (p. 23). However, there are a number of cultural procedures that Greenfield found to be hypnotic-like in nature. One of them is the relationship of client to healer, characterized by trust and resembling "that between hypnotist and client" (p. 23). Another variable is a context that allows the clients to become totally absorbed in the intervention, a healing ritual that galvanizes the clients' attention and distracts them from feeling pain. Greenfield added that the spiritistic aspects of Brazilian culture foster "fantasy proneness" because large numbers of people believe that supernatural entities help (or hinder) them in their daily lives (p. 24). In support of Greenfield's speculations, Biswas, See, Kogon, and Spiegel (2000) found that individuals consulting a faith healer in Nepal were significantly more hypnotizable than those being treated by Western medicine or ayurvedic practitioners and that their level of hypnotizability was positively correlated with their assessment of the faith healer's efficacy.

CLINICAL AND FORENSIC MATERIAL

We present in this section vignettes from diverse cultures and contexts. The first two illustrate how the construct of hypnotizability cannot always be translated directly into different cultures or socioeconomic classes. The case in Puerto Rico suggests that the effectiveness of a hypnotic procedure depends on a background knowledge of the safety of the procedure and on how to behave accordingly; the vignette from Haiti shows that participants with a talent to alter their consciousness according to their cultural practice may nonetheless not respond to Western hypnosis. Finally, the vignette of a Native American healer exemplifies how healers may integrate their traditions with Western techniques. One aspect that is common to both hypnosis and shamanic practices is the use of procedures that may start as an artifice but later become experientially and physiologically real (Cardeña & Cousins, in press; Krippner, 2005).

A Murder Case in Puerto Rico and a Haitian Oungan

Some years ago, the first author of this chapter (Cardeña) was hired by the Puerto Rican post office police to help solve a murder/robbery, with the help of hypnotic interviews. After explaining that there was no guarantee that any of the information obtained would be valid, Cardeña followed the ASCH forensic interview guidelines (Hammond et al., 1995) with two of the witnesses. The first one, a university student, had no problem with the hypnotic procedure. The second one, though an illiterate peasant with no formal education, responded in exactly the opposite way to his suggestions. So, for instance, when Cardeña mentioned that she could allow her eyes to start closing, she would open them even more. Although, this was done in the presence of a police officer, she obviously did not trust a strange man to help lead her experience, and understandably so, because there was nothing in her background to have "trained" her to just sit down and follow his instructions, and it is likely that if she had ever heard about hypnosis, it had been in the context of sensationalistic TV shows.

The second example concerns an interview with an intellectually sophisticated Haitian *oungan* who did not respond at all to a previous attempt made by a Western clinician to hypnotize him. He explained that suggestions of relaxation were trivial compared with his frequent experience of interaction with the *lwas* (i.e., spirits; Cardeña, 1991). Both examples illustrate that sociocultural context and explanation, in addition to cognitive and biological predispositions, mediate hypnotic experience.

Graywolf

A former resident of a Native American community, Graywolf was a shamanic healer whom the second author visited several times in Oregon. Graywolf held a master's degree in counseling and integrated shamanic procedures into his practice and his lifestyle after a number of transformative dreams and visions. Taking the position that dysfunctional behavior is underscored by dysfunctional images of oneself and one's world, Graywolf attempted to assist his clients in identifying and transforming them. Janis, a client of Graywolf's, exhibited behavior that manifested an excessive need for approval yet had been punctuated of late by unexpected and uncontrollable bursts of rage. One of Graywolf's procedures was hypnotic-like in that it used guided imagery to reach the "upper" or "lower" world, or to "journey" back into a recalled dream. In an "upper world" session, Janis discovered herself as a "deserted child" and gained insight into an important source of her need for approval. In a "lower world" session, Janis began swaying like a snake. Convinced that she had discovered her "power animal," Janis repeated these movements daily, noticing that her angry outbursts began to diminish. Finding ways to restore self-esteem to her "child," and express her "power animal" in her daily behavior, Janis was delighted to observe an end to her outbursts.

On one occasion, Graywolf guided Janis back into a dream in which she shot her husband because he had not given her an expensive present. By imagining herself moving into the rage, she discovered a dark tunnel at the end of which was a red-faced baby crying desperately. In her fantasy, Janis picked up the baby, held it, and dried its tears. Later, she realized that the baby was herself at a younger age, experiencing a lack of attention that still upset her. The dream was an exaggerated account of her claims on her husband's care and affection; no matter how much he gave her, it was never enough to assuage the needs of the red-faced baby and the deserted child.

Janis understood that her dysfunctional image of being "nice" had begun to break down and that the uncontrolled bursts of rage had signified its demise. By reveling in the image and movements of the snake rather than in her angry outbursts, she was able to enjoy a part of her that was not necessarily "nice" or "approved" but that was needed for her very survival. Graywolf worked with Janis, exploring the feelings accompanying the snakelike body movements to determine what new self-images they anticipated. Accepting her repressed sensuality, self-protection, and authenticity was possible because of her almost instant attraction to her "power animal." Janis associated her newly discovered self-acceptance and self-esteem with a newly discovered enjoyment of life. Graywolf's procedures mirrored the findings of Frank and Frank (1991) that effective treatment procedures involve an emotionally charged, trusting relationship with a helping person in a healing setting; a conceptual scheme or myth that provides a plausible explanation for the client's symptoms; and a ritual that requires the active participation of both client and helper and that is believed by both to be the means of combating the patient's demoralization.

RESEARCH AND APPRAISAL

Torrey (1986) surveyed indigenous psychotherapists and concluded on the basis of anecdotal reports that "many of them are effective psychotherapists and produce therapeutic change in their clients" (p. 205). The sources of that effectiveness are the four basic components of psychotherapy: a shared worldview, personal qualities of the healer, client expectations, and a process that enhances the client's learning and mastery (p. 207). Frank and Frank (1991) drew a similar conclusion after their classical study of the universal components of healing, and Jilek (1982) found support for the effectiveness of traditional healers in the Northwest. Strupp (1972) added, "The modern psychotherapist . . . relies to a large extent on the same psychological mechanisms used by the faith healer, shaman, physician, priest, and others, and the results, as reflected by the evidence of therapeutic outcomes, appear to be substantially similar" (p. 277).

A review of anomalous healing events and experiences (Achterberg & Krippner, 2000) is beyond the scope of this chapter, but it is worth mentioning that some reports support indigenous healing practices. For example, JAMA published a study of an apparently successful treatment of systemic lupus erythematosus (SLE) by a native healer (Kirkpatrick, 1981). In early 1977, a 28-year-old Philippine American woman was diagnosed as having this disease, which is notoriously resistant to treatment. After a year of unsuccessful medical attention, the patient returned to the remote Filipino village of her birth, contacting a local healer who claimed to remove a curse that had supposedly been placed on her by a previous suitor. Within 3 weeks, she returned to face her skeptical physicians. She declined further medication, appeared to be in good health, and 23 months later gave birth to a healthy girl. The physician who authored the report concluded the following:

> It is unlikely that this patient's SLE "burned out". . . . But by what mechanism did the machinations of an Asian medicine man cure active lupus nephritis, change myxedema into euthyroidism, and allow precipitous withdrawal from corticosteroid treatment without symptoms of adrenal insufficiency? (Kirkpatrick, 1981, p. 137)

Kleinman (1980) conducted a follow-up study of 19 clients treated by Taiwanese tang-kis, or shamans, at a healing shrine. All clients were visited at their homes 2 months after their initial visit to the tang-ki. Interviews could not be held with 7 of the clients, but of the 12 interviewed, 10 (83%) reported at least partially effective treatment. Six (50%) regarded themselves as completely cured, and two (17%) were "treatment failures." The evaluations of family members were also considered, and the mother of one of the "failures" felt that the treatment would have been successful had her daughter continued for a longer period of time. The father of the other failure implied that his daughter's condition had worsened after treatment. Even though the sample was small, Kleinman noted "there are virtually no other follow-up studies of indigenous practice." Even so, "these findings are in line with our findings from studies of other indigenous healers and our impressions from observation of large numbers of patients treated by [the] tang-ki" (p. 320).

Kim (1973), a psychiatrist, conducted a follow-up study of individuals treated by a shaman in South Korea. He noted that temporary symptom relief was obtained in the four cases he diagnosed with psychoneuroses. However, of the eight cases he diagnosed as schizophrenic, six deteriorated following the shamanic ceremonies.

Finkler (1985) examined spiritualist healers in a rural community in Mexico and found that their treatments were most effective for nonpathogenic diarrheas, simple gynecological disorders, psychosomatic problems, and mild psychiatric disorders. The former two ailments were treated with teas, enemas, and douches; the latter two by symbolic manipulations and ministrations. However, Finkler found that in most cases, by the patients' own accounts, spiritual practitioners had not cured them. Little change was noted in the case of serious physiological symptoms caused by physical or mental illness. The underlying factors instrumental in producing the disease expressed in physiological or somaticized symptoms continued, including the unceasing flow of untreated sewage waters in the irrigation canals and the unremitting presence of disease vectors in the open garbage pits. Of course, deaths related to alcoholism and violence continued, given the extant sociostructural conditions within this population. Of the 108 clients in the study, he judged 30% to have had successful treatments, 35% unsuccessful treatments, and the others inconclusive or unclassifiable results. Campos Navarro (1997) conducted an in-depth field study with Mexican indigenous healers and supported their efficacy for some types of malaise along the same lines described by Finkler.

Katz (1982, 1984) carried out a 22-month field study among Fijian healers, recording data on 500 clients in one community who sought help during the course of a year. He noted that in 5% of the interactions, more than one type of healer was consulted. Overall, nearly 79% of the client–healer contacts were with the local nurse, and 13% were with the traditional healer. However, the latter saw each of his clients more times, so the actual time spent in the respective healing efforts was about equal. The most frequent complaints were various aches and pains (35%). The nurse saw most of the cases of cuts and wounds, whereas the traditional healer handled all of the requests for help against misfortune. However, Katz noted considerable overlap because of the ways in which clients conceptualized the problems and their etiology.

Additional research projects are needed to follow up the leads provided by these studies, improving on their methodological shortcomings, for instance, by conducting long-term follow-ups to determine the stability of any improvement. Expectation and excitement can produce dramatic short-term effects but may not demonstrate staying power. The hypnotic-like aspects of native healing are possibilities for fruitful investigation. Scales are now available to measure absorption, imagination, suggestibility, and other human capacities that might be related to long-term improvement. Most of these scales are amenable to modification and adaptation to non-Western populations. Various instruments to evaluate variations of consciousness (Pekala & Cardeña, 2000) are promising candidates for cross-cultural studies, as are the imagery scales developed by Achterberg and Lawlis (1984), which were reported to give a better prognosis of a disease progress than the patient's blood chemistry. These imagery scales are especially suitable for cross-cultural research because they simply ask the afflicted to draw images representing their disease, the treatment they are receiving for the disease, and their body's self-healing capacities.

We also need more qualitative analyses of the experiences of both practitioners and their clients. Krippner (1990) used questionnaires to study perceived long-term effects following visits to Filipino and Brazilian folk healers, finding such variables as "willingness to change one's behavior" to significantly correlate with reported beneficial modifications in health. Cooperstein (1992) interviewed 10 prominent alternative healers in the United States, finding that their procedures involved the self-regulation of their "attention, physiology, and cognition, thus inducing altered awareness and reorganizing the healer's construction of cultural and personal realities" (p. 99). Cooperstein concluded that the concept that most closely represented his data was "the shamanic capacity to transcend the personal self, to enter into multiform identifications, to access and synthesize alternative perspectives and realities, and to find solutions and acquire extraordinary abilities used to aid the community" (p. 121). Indeed, the shaman's role and that of the alternative healer are both socially constructed, as are their operating procedures and their patients' predispositions to respond to the treatment. It is important not only to study the effects of the hypnotic-like procedures found in native healing but also to accurately describe them and to understand them within their own framework.

CONCLUSION

Although some critics continue to heap scorn on native healers, serious consideration is being given to the positive contributions that native healers may provide, either alone or in conjunction with Western health practitioners (e.g., Campos Navarro, 1997). Even in traditional Western settings, there is a long history of using alternative practices or practices complementary to the mainstream treatment. There are also instances of countries in which laws have been passed to integrate traditional healing into the national health system, for instance, in Nigeria, Swaziland, and Zimbabwe (Seligmann, 1981). In 1977, the United Malay National Organization, Malaysia's dominant political party, decided to promote the use of bomohs in the treatment of drug addicts. However, when a World Federation of Mental Health workshop in Malaysia suggested collaboration between the university's department of psychiatry and the traditional *bomoh* practitioners, the psychiatrists objected, claiming that such a move would only confirm the prejudice held by other departments in the medical school against psychiatry as unscientific (Carstairs, 1973). Despite similar complaints in Mexico, there have been encouraging events such as having indigenous healers give talks to physicians and university professors (Campos Navarro, 1997).

The professionalization of shamanic and other traditional healers may suggest their similarity to practitioners of Western medicine; nevertheless, the differences cannot be ignored. Rogers (1982) contrasted Western and native models of healing, noting that in Western medicine, "healing procedures are usually private, often secretive. Social reinforcement is rare. . . . The cause and treatment of illness are usually regarded as secular. . . . Treatment may extend over a period of months or years." In native healing, however, the following is the case:

> Healing procedures are often public: Many relatives and friends may attend the rite. Social reinforcement is normally an important element. The shaman speaks for the spirits or the spirits speak through him [or her]. Symbolism and symbolic manipulation are vital elements." (p. 169)

Rogers (1982, p. 112) divided native healing procedures into several categories: nullification of sorcery, removal of objects, exorcism of harmful entities, retrieval of lost souls, eliciting confession and penance, transfer of illness, suggestion and persuasion, and shock. In all of these procedures, hypnotic-like techniques using symbols, metaphors, stories, and rituals, especially those involving group participation, can play an important role. Ceremonial activities produce shifts of attention for both the healer and the client, and the culture's rules and regulations produce a structure through which the clients' motivations may operate to empower them and stimulate their self-healing abilities. Western practitioners of hypnosis employ the human capacities that have been used by native practitioners in their hypnotic-like procedures. These include the capacity for imaginative suggestibility; the ability to shift attentional style; the potential for intention and motivation; and the capability for self-healing made possible by neurotransmitters, internal repair systems, and other components of mind-body interaction.

By investigating ways in which different societies have constructed diagnostic categories and remedial procedures, therapists and physicians can explore changes to their own procedures, hypnotic or otherwise, that are ineffective. It is also the case that many underprivileged groups throughout the globe do not have the financial or geographical access to Western-trained practitioners and/or the latter may not understand their clients' worldview, one of the cornerstones of therapeutic interaction. Western medicine and psychotherapy have their roots in traditional practices and need to explore avenues of potential cooperation with native practitioners, whose healing methods may contain wise insights and practical applications. However, it is also dangerous to go to the other extreme and romanticize the potential efficacy of traditional healing methods, which may not be efficacious for a number of conditions. It is also the case that there are incompetent or unethical traditional healers, though the same can be said of practitioners of hypnosis or any other form of psychotherapy or medicine.

REFERENCES

Achterberg, J. (1985). *Imagery in healing: Shamanism and modern medicine*. Boston: Shambhala.

Achterberg, J., & Krippner, S. (2000). Anomalous healing experiences. In E. Cardeña, S. J. Lynn, & S. Krippner, S. (Eds.), *Varieties of anomalous experience: Examining the scientific evidence* (pp. 353–395). Washington, DC: American Psychological Association.

Achterberg, J., & Lawlis, G. F. (1984). *Imagery and disease*. Champaign, IL: Institute for Personality and Ability Testing.

Adair, J., Deuschle, K. W., & Barnett, C. R. (1988). *The people's health: Anthropology and medicine in a Navajo community* (Rev. ed.). Albuquerque: University of New Mexico Press.

Agogino, G. A. (1965). The use of hypnotism as an ethnologic research technique. *Plains Anthropologist, 10,* 31–36.

Angoff, A., & Barth, D. (Eds.). (1973). *Parapsychology and anthropology*. London: Parapsychology Foundation.

Balthazard, C. G., & Woody, E. Z. (1992). The spectral analysis of hypnotic performance with respect to "Absorption." *International Journal of Clinical and Experimental Hypnosis, 40,* 21–43.

Barber, T. X. (1969). *Hypnosis: A scientific approach*. New York: Van Nostrand Reinhold.

Barber, T. X. (1984). Changing "unchangeable" bodily processes by (hypnotic) suggestions. In A. A. Sheikh (Ed.), *Imagination and healing* (pp. 69–127). Farmingdale, NY: Baywood Publishing.

Barrett, D. (1990). Deep trance subjects: A schema of two distinct subgroups. In R. G. Kunzendorf (Ed.), *Mental imagery* (pp. 101–112). New York: Plenum Press.

Belo, J. (1960). *Trance in Bali*. New York: Columbia University Press.

Besmer, F. E. (1983). *Horses, musicians, & gods: The Hausa cult of possession-trance*. Zaria, Nigeria: Ahmadu Bello University Press.

Biswas, A., See, D., Kogon, M. M., & Spiegel, D. (2000). Hypnotizability and the use of traditional Dhami-Jhankri healing in Nepal. *International Journal of Clinical and Experimental Hypnosis, 48,* 6–21.

Bourguignon, E., & Evascu, T. (1977). Altered states of consciousness within a general evolutionary perspective: A holocultural analysis. *Behavior Science Research, 12,* 199–216.

Bowers, M. K. (1961). Hypnotic aspects of Haitian voodoo. *International Journal of Clinical and Experimental Hypnosis, 9,* 269–282.

Brown, D. P. (1977). A model for the levels of concentrative meditation. *International Journal of Clinical and Experimental Hypnosis, 25,* 236–273.

Brown, D. P., & Fromm, E. (1986). *Hypnotherapy and hypnoanalysis,* Hillsdale, NJ: Erlbaum.

Campos Navarro, R. (1997). *Nosotros los curanderos* [We the healers]. Mexico City, Mexico: Nueva Imagen.

Cardeña, E. (1989). The varieties of possession experience. *Association for the Anthropological Study of Consciousness Quarterly, 5*(2–3), 1–17.

Cardeña, E. (1990, Spring). *The concept(s) of trance.* Paper presented at the Annual Conference of the Society for the Anthropology of Consciousness, Pacific Palisades, CA.

Cardeña, E. (1991). Max Beauvoir: An island in an ocean of spirits. In R. I. Heinze (Ed.), *Shamans of the XXth Century* (pp. 27–32). New York: Irvington.

Cardeña, E. (1995). Review of "Shamans, priests, and witches: A cross-cultural study of magico–religious practitioners" by Michael Winkelman. *Transcultural Psychiatric Research Review, 32,* 69–73.

Cardeña, E. (1996). "Just floating on the sky." A comparison of shamanic and hypnotic phenomenology. In R. Quekelbherge & D. Eigner (Eds.), *6th jahrbuch für transkulturelle medizin und psychotherapie* (pp. 367–380). Berlin, Germany: Verlag für Wissenschaft und Bildung.

Cardeña, E. (1999). Culture, and psychopathology: The hidden dimensions in T. X. Barber's theory. *Contemporary Hypnosis, 16,* 132–138.

Cardeña, E. (2005). The phenomenology of deep hypnosis: Quiescent and physically active. *International Journal of Clinical and Experimental Hypnosis, 53,* 37–59.

Cardeña, E., & Beard, J. (1996). Truthful trickery: Shamanism, acting and reality. *Performance Research, 1,* 31–39.

Cardeña, E., & Cousins, W. E. (in press). From artifice to actuality: Ritual, shamanism, hypnosis and healing. In J. Weinhold & G. Samuel (Eds.), *Varieties of ritual experience. Ritual dynamics and the science of ritual, Volume II: Body, performance, agency and experience.* Weisbaden, Germany: Harrassowitz.

Cardeña, E., Kallio, S., Terhune, D., Buratti, S., & Lööf, A. (2007). The effect of translation and sex on hypnotizability testing. *Contemporary Hypnosis, 24,* 154–160.

Cardeña, E., & Spiegel, D. (1991). Suggestibility, absorption, and dissociation: An integrative model of hypnosis. In J. F. Schumaker (Ed.), *Human suggestibility: Advances in theory, research, and application* (pp. 93–107). New York: Routledge.

Cardeña, E., Van Duijl, Weiner, L., & Terhune, D. B. (2009). Possession/trance phenomena. In P. F. Dell & J. A. O'Neil (Eds.), *Dissociation and the dissociative disorders: DSM–V and beyond* (pp. 171–181). New York: Routledge.

Carstairs, G. M. (1973). Psychiatric problems in developing countries. *British Journal of Psychiatry, 123,* 271–277.

Cooperstein, M. A. (1992). The myths of healing: A summary of research into transpersonal healing experiences. *Journal of the American Society for Psychical Research, 86,* 99–133.

De Certeau, M. (2000). *The possession at Loudun* (M. B. Smith, Trans.) Chicago: University of Chicago Press.

Desmangles, L., & Cardeña, E. (1996). Trance possession and Vodou ritual in Haiti. In R. Quekelbherge & D. Eigner (Eds.), 6th jahrbuch für transkulturelle medizin und psychotherapie (pp. 297–309). Berlin, Germany: Verlag für Wissenschaft und Bildung.

Dixon, R. B. (1908). Some aspects of the American shaman. *Journal of American Folklore, 21,* 1–12.

Eliade, M. (1964). *Shamanism: Archaic techniques of ecstasy.* New York: Pantheon Books.

Ellenberger, H. F. (1970). *The discovery of the unconscious.* New York: Basic Books.

Erickson, M. H., Rossi, E. L., & Rossi, S. H. (1976). *Hypnotic realities: The induction of clinical hypnosis and the indirect forms of suggestion.* New York: Irvington.

Finkler, K. (1985). *Spiritualist healers in Mexico: Successes and failures of alternative therapeutics.* New York: Praeger.

Frank, J. D., & Frank, J. B. (1991). *Persuasion and healing* (3rd ed.). Baltimore, MD: Johns Hopkins University Press.

Frigerio, A. (1989). Levels of possession awareness in Afro-Brazilian religions. *Association for the Anthropological Study of Consciousness Quarterly, 5,* 5–11.

Furst, P. T. (1977). "High states" in culture–historical perspective. In N. E. Zinberg (Ed.), *Alternate states of consciousness* (pp. 53–88). New York: Free Press.

Gauld, A. (1992). *A history of hypnotism.* Cambridge, England: Cambridge University Press.

Gergen, K. J. (1985). The social constructionist movement in modem psychology. *American Psychologist, 40,* 266–275.

Gergen, K. J. (1990). Therapeutic professions and the diffusion of deficit. *Journal of Mind and Behavior, 11,* 353–368.

Gowan, J. C. (1975). *Trance, art and creativity.* Buffalo, NY: Creative Education Foundation, State University College.

Greenfield, S. M. (1992). Hypnosis and trance induction in the surgeries of Brazilian spiritist healer–mediums. *Anthropology of Consciousness, 2,* 20–25.

Gussow, Z. (1985). Pibloktoq (hysteria) among the polar Eskimo: An ethnopsychiatric study. In R. C. Simons & C. C. Hughes (Eds.), *The culture bound syndromes* (pp. 271–288). Boston: Reidel.

Halifax, J. (1980). *Shamanic voices*. Middlesex, England: Penguin.

Hammond, D. C., Garver, R. B., Mutter, C. B., Crasilneck, H. B., Frischholz, E., Gravitz, M. A., et al. (1995). *Clinical hypnosis and memory: Guidelines for clinicians and for forensic hypnosis*. Des Plaines, IL: American Society of Clinical Hypnosis Press.

Henney, J. H. (1974). Spirit-possession belief and trance behavior in two fundamentalist groups in St. Vincent. In F. D. Goodman, J. H. Henney, & E. Pressel (Eds.), *Trance, healing, and hallucinations: Three field studies in religious experience* (pp. 1–111). New York: Wiley-Interscience.

Hilgard, E. R. (1973). The domain of hypnosis: With some comments on alternative paradigms. *American Psychologist, 28*, 972–982.

Hilgard, J. (1979). *Personality and hypnosis: A study of imaginative involvement*. Chicago: University of Chicago Press.

Hughes, C. (1985). Glossary of "culture bound" or folk psychiatric syndromes. In R. C. Simons & C. C. Hughes (Eds.), *The culture bound syndromes* (pp. 469–505). Boston: Reidel.

Jilek, W. G. (1982). *Indian healing: Shamanic ceremonialism in the Pacific Northwest*. Blaine, WA: Hancock House.

Jung, C. G. (1966). *Two essays on analytical psychology* (2nd ed.). Princeton, NJ: Princeton University Press.

Kalweit, H. (1988). *Dreamtime and inner space: The world of the shaman*. Boston: Shambhala.

Katz, R. (1982). The utilization of traditional healing systems. *American Psychologist, 27*, 715–716.

Katz, R. (1984). Toward a paradigm of healing. *Personnel and Guidance Journal, 61*, 494–497.

Keel, P. K., & Klump, K. L. (2003). Are eating disorders culture-bound syndromes? Implications for conceptualizing their etiology. *Psychological Bulletin, 129*, 747–769

Kim, H. (1973). Review of shamanist healing ceremonies in Korea. *Transcultural Psychiatric Research Review, 10*, 124–125.

Kirkpatrick, R. A. (1981). Witchcraft and lupus erythematosus. *JAMA, 245*, 137.

Kirsch, I. (1990). *Changing expectations: A key to effective psychotherapy*. Pacific Grove, CA: Brooks/Cole.

Kleinman, A. (1980). *Patients and healers in the context of culture*. Berkeley: University of California Press.

Kleinman, A. (1988). *Rethinking psychiatry: From cultural category to personal experience*. New York: Free Press.

Kluckholn, C., & Leighton, D. (1962). *The Navaho*. Garden City, NY: Anchor Books.

Kok, L. P. (1989). Hypnotic susceptibility in kavadi carriers in Singapore. *Annals of the Academy of Medicine, Singapore, 18*, 655–657.

Krippner, S. (1987). Dreams and shamanism. In S. Nicholson (Ed.), *Shamanism: An expanded view of reality* (pp. 125–132). Wheaton, IL: Theosophical.

Krippner, S. (1989). A call to heal: Patterns of entry in Brazilian mediumship. In C. Ward (Ed.), *Altered states of consciousness and mental health: A cross-cultural perspective* (pp. 186–206). Newbury Park, CA: Sage.

Krippner, S. (1990). A questionnaire study of experiential reactions to a Brazilian healer. *Journal of the Society for Psychical Research, 56*, 208–215.

Krippner, S. (2005). Trance and the trickster: Hypnosis as a liminal phenomena. *International Journal of Clinical and Experimental Hypnosis, 53*, 97–118.

Krippner, S., & Bindler, P. (1974). Hypnosis and attention: A review. *American Journal of Clinical Hypnosis, 16*, 166–177.

Kroger, W. S. (1977). *Clinical and experimental hypnosis* (2nd ed.). Philadelphia: Lippincott Williams & Wilkins.

Laurence, J. R., & Perry, C. (1988). *Hypnosis, will, and memory: A psycho–legal history*. New York: Guilford Press.

Leacock, S., & Leacock, R. (1972). *Spirits of the deep: Drums, mediums and trance in a Brazilian city*. Garden City, NY: Doubleday.

Lewis-Williams, D., & Pearce, D. (2005). *Inside the Neolithic mind: Consciousness, cosmos, and the realm of the Gods*. London: Thames & Hudson.

Lichtenberg, P., Bachner-Melman, R., Ebstein, R. P., & Crawford, H. J. (2004). Hypnotic susceptibility: Multidimensional relationships with Cloninger's tridimensional personality questionnaire, COMT polymorphisms, absorption, and attentional characteristics. *International Journal of Experimental and Clinical Hypnosis, 52*, 47–72.

Locke, R. G., & Kelly, E. F. (1985). A preliminary model for the cross-cultural analysis of altered states of consciousness. *Ethos, 13*, 3–55.

Ludwig, A. M. (1966). Altered states of consciousness. *Archives of General Psychiatry, 15*, 225–234.

Lynn, S. J., & Rhue, J. (1988). Fantasy proneness: Hypnosis, developmental antecedents, and psychopathology. *American Psychologist, 43*, 35–44.

Lynn, S. J., & Rhue, J. (1991). An integrative model of hypnosis. In S. J. Lynn & J. Rhue (Eds.), *Theories of hypnosis: Current models and perspectives* (pp. 397–438). New York: Guilford Press.

Maxfield, M. (1990). *The effect of rhythmic drumming on EEG and subjective experience*. Unpublished doctoral dissertation, Institute of Transpersonal Psychology, Menlo Park, CA.

McGregor, P. (1962). *The moon and the two mountains*. London: Souvenir Press.

Miranda, J. (1997). *Curanderos y chamanes de la sierra mazatec* [Healers and shamans of the mazateca sierra]. Mexico City, Mexico: Gatuperio.

Moreira-Almeida, A., Lotufo Neto, F., & Cardeña, E. (2008). Comparison between Brazilian Spiritist mediumship and dissociative identity disorder. *The Journal of Nervous and Mental Disease, 196*, 420–424.

Morgan, A. H. (1973). The heritability of hypnotic susceptibility in twins. *Journal of Abnormal Psychology, 82*, 55–61.

Murphy, G. (1947). *Personality: A biosocial approach to origins and structure*. New York: Harper & Brothers.

Noll, R. (1985). Mental imagery cultivation as a cultural phenomenon. *Current Anthropology, 26*, 443–461.

O'Shaughnessy, B. (1972). Mental structure and self-consciousness. *Inquiry, 15*, 30–63.

Overton, J. A. (1998). Shamanism and clinical hypnosis: A brief comparative analysis. *Shaman, 6*, 151–170.

Oxford University Press. (1928). *Oxford English Dictionary* (1st ed.). Oxford, England: Author.

Pekala, R., & Cardeña, E. (2000). Methodological issues in the study of altered states of consciousness and anomalous experiences. In E. Cardeña, S. J. Lynn, & S. Krippner (Eds.), *Varieties of anomalous experience* (pp. 47–81). Washington, DC: American Psychological Association.

Perry, C., Nadon, R., & Button, J. (1992). The measurement of hypnotic ability. In E. Fromm & M. R. Nash (Eds.), *Contemporary hypnosis research* (pp. 459–490). New York: Guilford Press.

Price-Williams, D. (1975). *Explorations in cross-cultural psychology*. San Francisco: Chandler & Sharp.

Raboteau, A. J. (1986). The Afro-Brazilian traditions. In R. L. Numbers & D. W. Amundsen (Eds.), *Caring and curing: Health and medicine in Western religious traditions* (pp. 539–562). New York: Macmillan.

Richeport, M. M. (1992). The interface between multiple personality, spirit mediumship, and hypnosis. *American Journal of Clinical Hypnosis, 34*, 168–1 77.

Rogers, S. L. (1982). *The shaman: His symbols and his healing power*. Springfield, IL: Charles C Thomas.

Rosen, G. (1969). *Madness in society. Chapters in the historical sociology of mental illness*. New York: Harper.

Rouget, G. (1985). *Music and trance: A theory of the relations between music and possession*. Chicago: University of Chicago Press.

Sandner, D. (1979). *Navaho symbols of healing*. New York: Harcourt Brace Jovanovich.

Seligmann, J. (1981, September 21). The new witch doctors. *Newsweek*, 106.

Shor, R. E. (1959). Hypnosis and the concept of generalized reality-orientation. *American Journal of Psychotherapy, 13*, 582–602.

Shor, R. E. (1962). Three dimensions of hypnotic depth. *International Journal of Clinical and Experimental Hypnosis, 10,* 23–38.

Shweder, R. (1972). Aspects of cognition in Zinacanteco shamans: Experimental results. In W. Lessa & E. Vogt (Eds.), *Reader in comparative religion: An anthropological approach* (3rd ed., pp. 407–412). New York: Harper & Row.

Sluhovsky, M. (2007). *Believe not every spirit: Possession, mysticism, and discernment in early modern catholicism.* Chicago: University of Chicago Press.

Spanos, N. P., & Chaves, J. F. (1989). *Hypnosis: The cognitive–behavioral perspective.* Buffalo, NY: Prometheus Books.

Spanos, N. P., & Chaves, J. F. (1991). History and historiography of hypnosis. In S. J. Lynn & J. W. Rhue (Eds.), *Theories of hypnosis: Current models and perspectives* (pp. 43–78). New York: Guilford Press.

Stanford, R. G. (1992). Experimental hypnosis–ESP literature: A review from the hypothesis-testing perspective. *Journal of Parapsychology, 56,* 39–56.

Strupp, H. H. (1972). On the technology of psychotherapy. *Archives of General Psychiatry, 26,* 270–278.

Tellegen, A., & Atkinson, G. (1974). Openness to absorbing and self-altering experiences ("absorption"), a trait related to hypnotic susceptibility. *Journal of Abnormal Psychology, 83,* 268–277.

Topper, M. D. (1987). The traditional Navajo medicine man: Therapist, counselor, and community leader. *Journal of Psychoanalytic Anthropology, 10,* 17–249.

Torrey, E. F. (1986). *Witchdoctors and psychiatrists: The common roots of psychotherapy and its future.* New York: Harper & Row.

Tseng, W. S. (1997). Overview: Culture and psychopathology. In W. S. Tseng & J. Streltzer (Eds.), *Culture and psychopathology* (pp. 1–27). New York: Brunner.

van Duijl, M., Cardeña, E., & de Jong, J. (2005). The validity of *DSM–IV* dissociative disorders categories in SW Uganda. *Transcultural Psychiatry, 42,* 219–241.

Van Ommeren, M., Komproe, I., Cardeña, E., Thapa, S. B., Prasain, D., de Jong, J., & Sharma, B. (2004). Mental illness among Bhutanese shamans in Nepal. *The Journal of Nervous and Mental Disease, 192,* 313–317.

Vogel, V. J. (1990). *American Indian medicine.* Norman: University of Oklahoma Press. (Original work published 1970)

Ward, C. (1989). Introduction. In C. Ward (Ed.), *Altered states of consciousness and mental health: A cross-cultural perspective* (pp. 8–10). Newbury Park, CA: Sage.

Winkelman, M. J. (1992). *Shamans, priests, and witches: A cross-cultural study of magico–religious practitioners.* Tempe, AZ: Arizona State University.

Woody, E. Z., Bowers, K. S., & Oakman, J. M. (1992). A conceptual analysis of hypnotic responsiveness: Experience, individual differences, and context. In E. Fromm & M. R. Nash (Eds.), *Contemporary hypnosis research* (pp. 3–33). New York: Guilford Press.

INDEX

ASCH. *See* American Society of
   Clinical Hypnosis
Asclepius, 745
Ashworth, A., 709
Assimilator learning style, 695
Association (cognitive strategy), 652
Asthma, 473
Athwal, B. S., 86
Attention, focused, 268
Attentional focusing, 91–92
Attention-deficit/hyperactivity disorder
   (ADHD), 476
Attitudes, 188, 303, 343–344
Attitudes Toward Hypnosis scale, 69
Audiotapes, of hypnosis sessions
   in depression treatment, 405
   in mindfulness-based treatments,
      331–333
   for pain control, 537
   for relaxation, 578–579
Authoritarian therapy, 214–215
Authoritative suggestions, 287
Autogenic training, 646
Autohypnosis, 646
Automatic thoughts, 362, 373, 397
Automatic word processing, 478
Automatic writing, 34, 132
Automation, 31
Autonomic nervous system (ANS)
   control of, 554
   sympathetic arousal of, 552
Aversion therapy, 255
Aversive images, 249
Aviv, A., 478
Avoidance
   in anxiety disorders, 375
   dissociation as, 433–435
   in health settings, 553
Avoidant couples, 512
Azam, Eugene, 31

Baddeley, M., 513
Baker, E. L., 39, 131, 143, 561–562
Baker, S. L., 194
Baker–Nash approach, to treatment
   of anorexia nervosa, 458–462

Balsamo, Giuseppe, 683
Balzac, Honoré de, 673
Bandler, R., 225, 287
Bandura, A., 181
Banerjee, S., 477
Banich, M. T., 730
Bank, W. O., 228
Bányai, E. I., 82, 309, 312
Barabasz, A. F., 384, 476
Barabasz, M., 47, 62, 100, 288, 457–458,
   476
Barber, T. X., 40, 59, 170, 184–188,
   656, 657, 722, 745
Barber Suggestibility Scale (BSS), 56
Barlow, D. H., 258–259
Barnier, A. J., 47, 54, 156
Barrett, D., 59, 722
Barry, H., 50
Barton, R. D., 438
BASIC I.D.
   applicability of, 255
   elements of, 240–246
   second-order assessments in, 251
Bateson, Gregory, 215
Baudelaire, Charles, 673
BDI–II. *See* Beck Depression
   Inventory—II
Bean, W., 227
Beard, Dorothea, 681
Beauchamp, Sally, 61
Beck, Aaron, 180, 394–397
Beck Depression Inventory—II
   (BDI–II), 627, 630
Behar, E., 385
Behavior
   and BASIC I.D., 241–243, 245
   maladaptive, 249
Behavioral analysis, 363
Behavioral generation, 191–192
Behavioral practice, 191–192
Behavioral problems, 476–478, 556–559
Behavioral rehearsal, 558, 559
Behavioral rigidity, 401–403
Behavioral skills, 595
Behavioral state, hypnosis as, 80
Behavioral task assignments, 403

Hilgard, E. R., 38, 50, 52–56, 62–63, 82, 125, 151–155, 162, 172, 434, 618, 634, 722–724, 729

Hilgard, J. R., 54, 62–63, 417, 468, 469, 483

Hiltunen, J., 103

HIP. *See* Hypnotic Induction Profile

Histoire Critique de Magnétisme Animal (Joseph Deleuze), 27–28

The History of Pendennis (William Makepeace Thackeray), 675

Hocus Pokus (film), 684

Hofbauer, R. K., 104, 106

Hoffman, Lynn, 232

Holding environment, 131–132, 455

Hollon, S. D., 483, 565, 608

Homeostasis, 126–127

Homework assignments, 294

Hoogduin, C. A., 165

Hopwood, S., 202

Horevitz, R., 47, 164

Horne, R. L., 62

Hornyak, L. M., 457

Hornyak, Lynne, 279

Horror genre (fiction), 678–679

Hostile/detached couples, 512

Hostile/engaged couples, 512

Host personality, 433

The House of Seven Gables (Nathaniel Hawthorne), 672

Huckleberry Finn (Mark Twain), 675

Huesmann, L. R., 726

Hull, C. L., 37, 656, 657

Human performance, 643

Hummel, K. E., 473

Hunt, T., 61

Husband, R. W., 50

Hyperempiria, 275–276, 309

Hyperideation, 31

Hypermnesia, 712, 713, 717

Hypnosis, 19–42. *See also specific headings*
in 20th century, 36–41
alert, 276
atheoretical formulation of, 745
client attitudes toward, 252–253
controversy surrounding, 41–42

definitions of, 5–8
as distinct mode of treatment, 4
in Ericksonian therapy, 212–217
and exorcism, 20–22
fluidist vs. animist approach to, 26–29
and magnetism, 29–32
and mesmerism, 20–26
Nancy school of, 33–35
potential misuse of, 41
and psychotherapy, 34–35, 394–395
at Salpêtrière Clinic, 32–34
solution-focused, 232

Hypnosis: A Scientific Approach (Theodore X. Barber), 186

Hypnosis in the Relief of Pain (E. R. Hilgard, J. R. Hilgard), 63

Hypnosis studies, 90–99

Hypnotherapy
cautions when using, 13–14
indications/contraindications for, 9–13

Hypnotically augmented mindfulness, 379

Hypnotically susceptible clients, 252–253

Hypnotic amnesia, 160

Hypnotic analgesia
altering awareness with, 163
EEG-related studies on, 100–101
Ericksonian approach to, 531
interest in, 521
method for, 580–582
in neodissociation theory, 154
with open surgery, 577
and pain perception, 187–188

Hypnotic anesthesia, 531

Hypnotic "dance," 513–514

Hypnotic depth, 49

Hypnotic dissociation, 532

Hypnotic distortion of memory, 160

Hypnotic dreams, 136

Hypnotic induction(s), 182, 267–291
alert, 275–276
alter hypnotic, 191
brief, 535
with children, 276–277

ABOUT THE EDITORS

Steven Jay Lynn is a professor of psychology and director of the Psychological Clinic at the State University of New York at Binghamton. He is a licensed psychologist and a diplomate (ABPP) in both clinical and forensic psychology, and he has served as a past president of the American Psychological Association's Division of Psychological Hypnosis. Dr. Lynn has received the Chancellor's Award of the State University of New York for Scholarship and Creative Activities, and he serves on 11 editorial boards, including the *Journal of Abnormal Psychology*. Dr. Lynn has published more than 260 articles and book chapters, as well as 18 books on the topics of psychotherapy, psychopathology, memory, and hypnosis. His research has been featured in numerous media venues, including popular magazines, television programs, and film documentaries. His research program has been funded by the National Institute of Mental Health.

Judith W. Rhue is a professor in the Department of Family Medicine at the Ohio University College of Osteopathic Medicine. She has coedited four books, as well as numerous book chapters, papers, workshops, and presentations. She maintains a clinical practice in addition to her teaching.

Irving Kirsch is a professor of psychology at the University of Hull. He has published 10 books and more than 200 scientific journal articles and book chapters on placebo effects, antidepressant medication, hypnosis, and suggestion. His meta-analyses on the efficacy of antidepressants have been covered extensively in the international media and have influenced the official guidelines for the treatment of depression in the United Kingdom. His most recent book, *The Emperor's New Drugs*, was published in the United Kingdom and Canada in 2009 and will be published in the United States in February 2010.